MICROSURGICAL ENDODONTICS

Arnaldo Castellucci

MICROSURGICAL ENDODONTICS

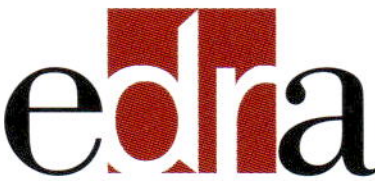

Publishing Manager
Costanza Smeraldi

Editor
Paola Sammaritano

Paper, Printing and Binding Manager
Michele Ribatti

Cover Design
Barbara Vallini

Drawings
Elisa Botton

Photographs of the instruments
Luca Ciapetti

■

ISBN: 978-88-214-4818-8
eISBN: 978-88-214-4819-5

■

Edra S.p.A.
Via G. Spadolini 7, 20141 Milano
Tel. 02 881841

www.edizioniedra.it

Printed in Italy in July 2019 by "Printer Trento" S.r.l., Trento

(*) Edra S.p.A. is part of LSWR GROUP

The Author

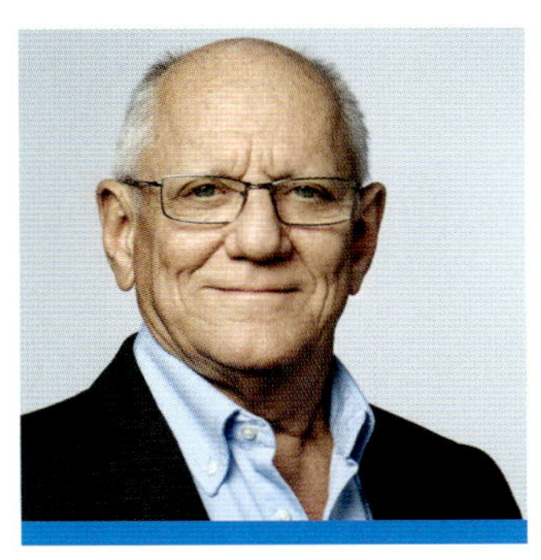

Arnaldo Castellucci

Dr. Castellucci graduated in Medicine at the University of Florence in 1973 and he specialized in Dentistry at the same University in 1977. From 1978 to 1980 he attended the Continuing Education Courses on Endodontics at Boston University and in 1980 he spent four months in the Endodontic Department of Prof. Herbert Schilder. Since then, he has a limited practice on Endodontics.
He is Past President of the Italian Endodontic Society S.I.E. and Active Member of the European Society of Endodontology E.S.E., where he was the Secretary in 1981-83. He is Active Member of the American Association of Endodontists A.A.E. since 1985.
He has been the President of the International Federation of Endodontic Associations I.F.E.A. in 1990-92.
He is Assistant Professor of Endodontics at the University of Cagliari Dental School and Professor of Microsurgical Endodontics at the Specialty of Oral Surgery of the University Federico II of Naples.
He has been the Editor of *The Italian Endodontic Journal* and of *The Endodontic Informer*. He is also the Founder and President of the "Warm Gutta-Percha Study Club". Today is Editor in Chief of *Endo Tribune* and is Editorial Advisor of the journals *Endodontic Practice* and *Endodontic Practice US*.
He is Founder and President of the Micro-Endodontic Training Center in Florence, where he teaches and gives hands-on courses on nonsurgical and surgical endodontics.
He published more then 60 articles on endodontics in the most prestigious endodontic journals.
In 1993 he published the text *EndodonziA*", edited by Martina, which in 2004 has been updated and translated in the English language with the title *EndodonticS*.
He wrote the chapter on Obturation of the Radicular Space for the 7th edition of textbook *Ingle's Endodontics*, and the chapter "Internal Tooth Anatomy and Root Canal Obturation" for the text *The Root Canal Anatomy in Permanent Dentition* edited by Springer.
International lecturer, he gave presentations at national and international congresses in more than 50 different countries in the world.
He can be reached at castelluccіarnaldo@gmail.com or through his website www.endocastellucci.com.

Co-Authors

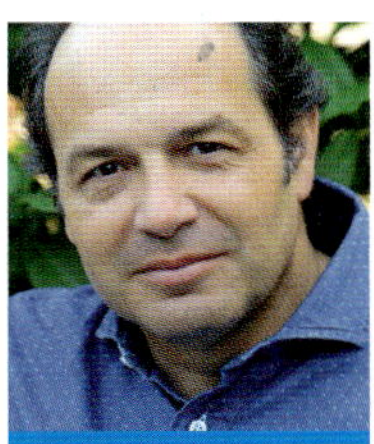

Massimo Gagliani MD, DDS

Active on Restorative Dentistry and Endodontics since 1990, he became Researcher at the University of Milan in 1992; in the same University was upgraded to Associate Professor in 2000. Member of the major international and national Society on Restorative & Endodontics, he is one of the five founders of the Digital Dental Academy (DDA).
He published in all the major international journals several papers on restorative & endodontics topics. Since 2014 is the Scientific Coordinator for Editorial Group EDRA.

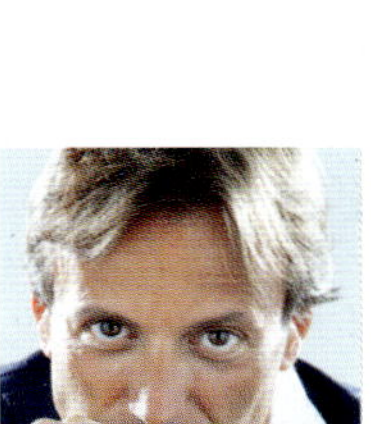

Fabio Gorni MD, DDS

Was Consulting Professor in Endodontics at the University of Milan, H. San Paolo. He is active member of the Italian Society of Endodontics, of the Italian Academy of Microdentistry, specialist member of the European Society of Endodontology and member of the American Association of Endodontists. He is speaker in several courses and congresses in Italy and in the entire world and published numerous scientific articles on national and international papers. He produced a series of scientific videos in collaboration with Dr. C.J. Ruddle, named "The Endodontic Game" distrubuted in Europe, USA, Canada, Australia and Asia. Co-founder of StyleItaliano Endodontics.

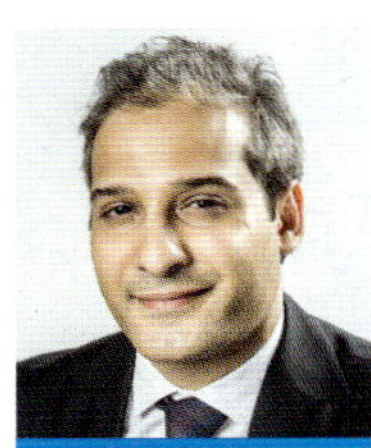

Naheed Mohamed DMD, MSD, Dip Perio, DABP, FRCD©

Is a Board-certified periodontist and Diplomate of the American Academy of Periodontology. He is a partner in a group periodontal practice in Mississauga and maintains his own private practice in Oakville. He can be reached at naheedm@gmail.com.

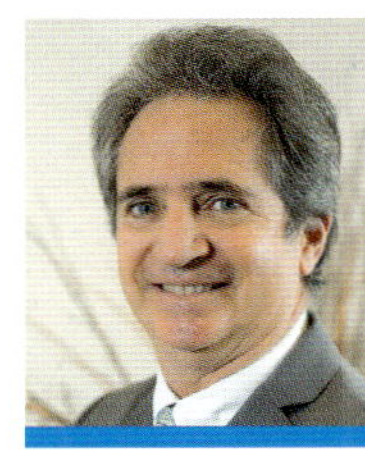

Yosef Nahmias DDS, MSc

Was born and raised in Mexico City. After he graduated from the Universidad Tecnologica de Mexico, School of Dentistry, in 1980, he decided to advance his education and chose Endodontics as his specialty. Dr. Nahmias earned his Master's of Science degree in Endodontics in 1983 at Marquette University in Milwaukee, Wisconsin. He has authored many articles and continues to lecture in Canada and internationally. Dr. Nahmias has been a practicing Endodontist in Oakville, Ontario since 1983. He can be reached at yosi@allianceds.com.

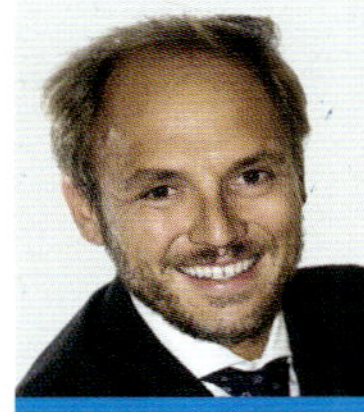

Matteo Papaleoni DDS

Graduated from the University of Florence School of Dentistry in 2004. Dr. Papaleoni earned his II Level Master in Endodontics and Restaurative Dentistry in 2006 at the University of Siena. Active Member of the Italian Society of Endodontics, he published several scientific articles and chapters of endodontic textbooks. He can be reached at matteo.papaleoni@gmail.com

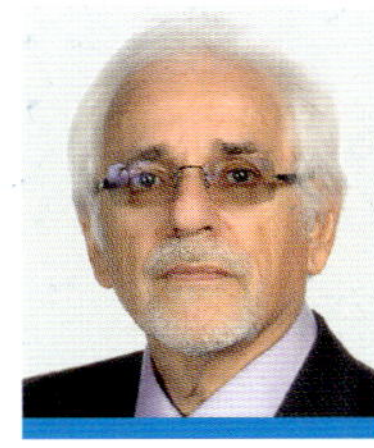

Ken Serota DDS MMSc

Graduated from the University of Toronto Faculty of Dentistry in 1973 and received his Certificate in Endodontics and Master of Medical Sciences degree from the Harvard-Forsyth Dental Center in Boston, Massachusetts. Active in online education since 1998, he is the founder of the online forums ROOTS and NEXUS. Dr. Serota is a clinical instructor in the University of Toronto Postdoctoral Endodontics Department.

Table of Contents

FROM A LECTURE OF PROF. HERBERT SCHILDER IN FLORENCE
AT THE LOCAL SECTION OF THE ITALIAN DENTAL ASSOCIATION IN NOVEMBER 1987

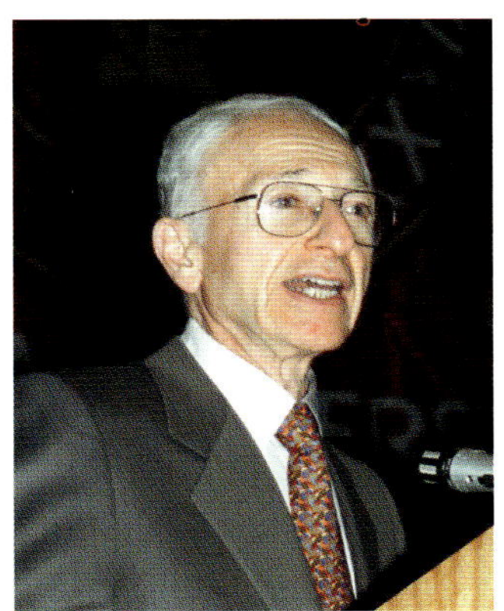

I am happy to tell you that I have seen a greater change in Endodontics in Italy, being from a very, very medically oriented base, but a bigger change than I have ever seen in any other country in the world.

However, now I am concerned that a retrogression in a way might be taking place, because I understand that again people are concerned about the tissue at the end of the root, and people are concerned about excess material, and people are concerned about things that I thought we had learned not to be concerned about anymore.

What I tried to teach through the years is a discipline to a technique, and if there is a discipline, then the work succeeds. If one cannot apply the discipline, then he doesn't get the results, and in order to stay sane, one invents a lot of reasons for not getting those results, many of which are fabrications and dreams.

Twenty-five years ago everyone knew that there was epithelium at the end of lesions of endodontic origin and everyone knew for a fact that epithelium doesn't heal. Now it heals! Now, there is only one biology. There are not two different biologies. There isn't a biology for 1962 and another for 1987. There isn't a biology for Boston and a different biology for Firenze.

There is only one biology and one cannot fight clinical reality.

Herbert S Schilder

Foreword

"Endodontic Surgery" or "Surgical Endodontics"; that is the question!
This could be the opening words of a drama, but it's the right goal this milestone book wants to achieve.
In this field of endodontics, over the past decades several transformations have been added in both technological aspects and materials.
In periapical surgery magnification, operating microscope, ultrasonic retrotips, biocompatible and bioactive materials have had a synergistic effect on the outcome of the surgical procedure formerly accomplished with means and materials of the lowest quality.
Arnaldo Castellucci's great effort has been to gather a huge amount of studies, clinical experiences and cases, squeeze them into a readable content and summarize them in a book that could guide both the expert endodontist and the young colleague to face all the critical points of the surgical procedure. This surgical procedure has to be done by the specialist in the field of dental pulp and periapical diseases: this is the fundamental message that comes out of the text. The philosophy that drove Arnaldo in his valuable career, devoted, with keen precision, to solve the problems related to root canal treatment failures that lead one to a retrograde approach for treatment of the periapical lesion of endodontic origin.
This keen precision means attention to all the details, accuracy in the use of magnification from loops up to the dental microscope, attention in the surgical operation during apical resection and, last but not least, deep "cleaning and shaping" of the retrograde root canal system to prepare an adequate endodontic space to be sealed by the best available root-end filling material.
All these steps are fully described in the textbook that perfectly represents Arnaldo Castellucci's philosophy presenting, with a didactical approach, his extended knowledge in all the fields of endodontics.
Finally, the definitive answer to the long standing dilemma: Surgical Endodontics should be considered as endodontic treatment done using a surgical approach and not surgery done for endodontic reasons and therefore we should all thank Arnaldo for his fundamental contribution on this topic.

Massimo Gagliani, MD, DDS

Preface and Acknowledgements

The idea that motivated me to write this text was the absolute belief that this branch of the dental profession should always and only be the pertinence of the Specialist in Endodontics. Only the Endodontist in fact has the knowledge of the endodontic anatomy, knows what the causes were that necessitated a surgical approach for the tooth, as well as the instrumentation and materials needed to transform, with a percentage well above 90%, an endodontic failure into a new long term success.
It is no longer acceptable to see patients that have been scheduled, maybe under general anaesthesia, for an apicectomy to remove a cystic wall which does not need any removal. We were taught this by Prof. Herbert Schilder right from the first time he came to Italy (we are talking about long ago in 1962!) when he started teaching the principles of Endodontics to the whole world. He taught us that we should not consider any difference between a granuloma and a cyst in that they are both simply "lesions of endodontic origin" and that will heal with a correct endodontic therapy, with or without a surgical approach, that can be used only in cases where an orthograde treatment to obtain an apical seal is mechanically impossible.
It is no longer acceptable to see cases treated surgically where a retrograde filling of the root canal system has not been done. This means that the cause of the apical lesion had not been understood, that is, the bacteria left inside the root canal system.
Therefore, if they want to, then the maxillofacial and oral surgeons who want to do this surgery as well, should do it with the knowledge and instrumentation that the Endodontist has. It is years now that we know that this kind of surgery is not done with the naked eye but with the use of the operatory microscope (introduced and widely used since the '90s). No longer are burs used but dedicated ultrasonic tips (introduced at the end of the '80s) and neither is amalgam used but new biocompatible materials (introduced at the beginning of the '90s)

The first person I feel the need to thank is my friend and colleague Dr. Massimo Gagliani, who was the person who gave me the impetus to start writing a text on this fascinating topic.
I obviously and equally want to thank my wife Sandra, who for years has patiently stood by my side without ever complaining about the time I dedicated to finish my various projects rather than to her.
A sincere thank you to my precious dental assistants, Isabella Talone and Denise De Santis, for the care they have taken for years in archiving my radiographs, clinical photographs and video clips.
A special thanks to the graphic designer, Elisa Botton, who produced the images that I feel can only be described as truly "unique".

Thank you to the graphic photographer, Luca Ciapetti, who produced the splendid highly detailed photographs.
A heartfelt thank you to my friend and colleague, John Theunissen, who did the translation into English of the entire text.
A sincere thank you to my colleagues who helped me with the drawing up of some chapters namely Dr. Matteo Papaleoni, my valulable and valid associate in the dental office, who helped me with the preparation of chapter 3, my good friend Dr. Domenico Riccucci who gave me precious histologic images for chapter 2, Dr. Yosi Nahmias, Ken Serota and Naheed Mohamed who wrote chapter 9 on the new technique of the cortical window, Dr. Fabio Gorni and Dr. Massimo Gagliani, who contributed to the preparation of chapter 13 and 15 and who enriched other chapters with their beautiful cases.
Finally but not of lesser importance, a heartfelt thanks to the publisher EDRA, namely Mr. Giorgio Albonetti and Ms. Paola Sammaritano, for the confidence they showed in me by deciding to publish this text.

Good reading and good Microsurgical Endodontics to all.

This book is dedicated to Sandra,
my loyal companion of my life, with eternal gratitude
and recognition for her love, understanding,
remarkable patience and incredible moral support
that daily for a long time she has shown me
and without which I could not have started and
completed this exhilarating work.

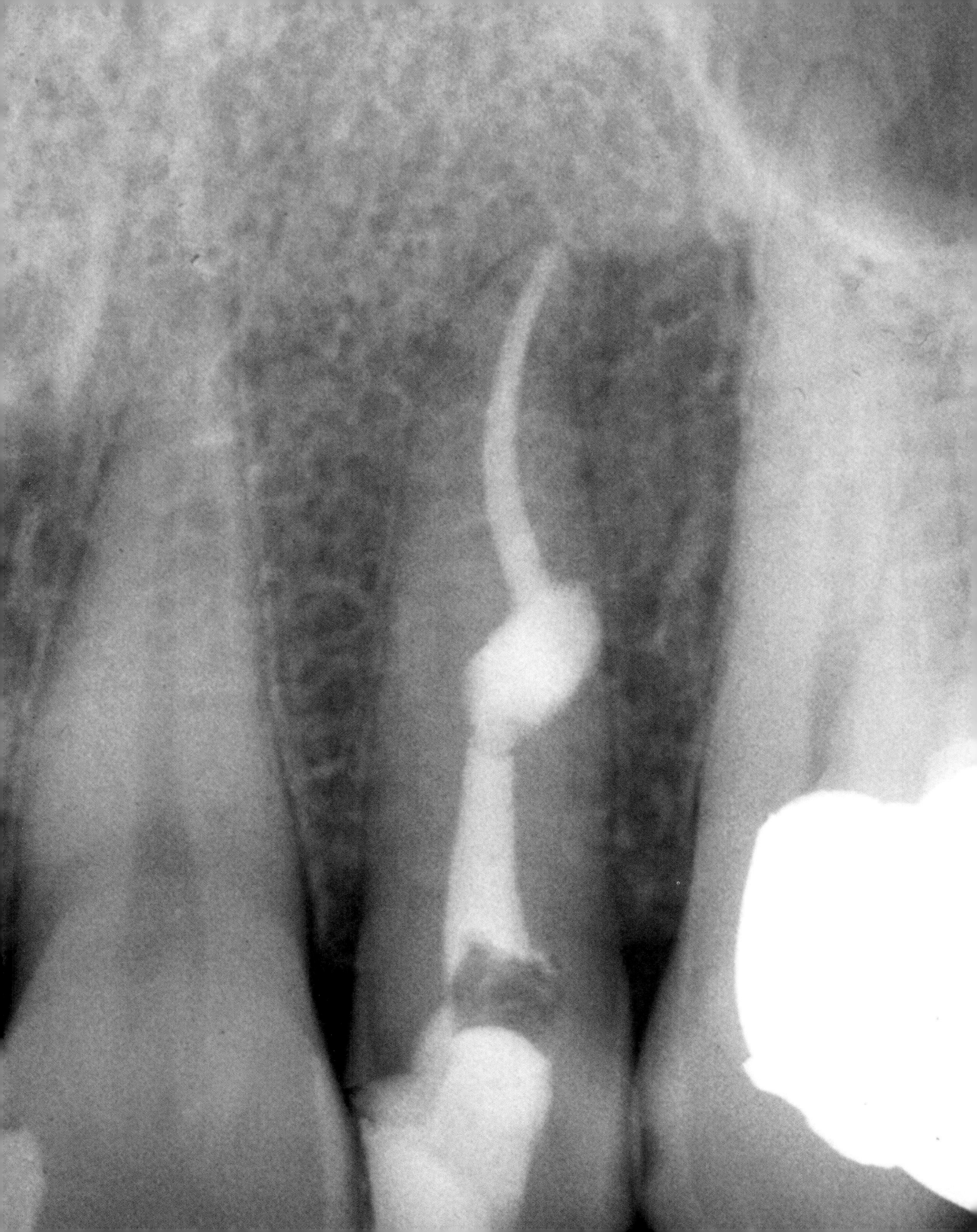

Why Microsurgical Endodontics?

By surgical endodontics one refers to the branch of Dentistry that is concerned with the diagnosis and treatment of lesions of endodontic origin that do not respond to conventional endodontic therapy or that cannot be treated by conventional endodontic therapy.[1] The scope of surgical endodontics is to achieve the three-dimensional cleaning, shaping and obturation of the apical portion of the root canal system that is not treatable via an access cavity, but only accessible via a surgical flap (📷 1.1). For this reason, it is preferable to use the term "Surgical Endodontics" instead of "Endodontic Surgery", in as much as the procedure should be planned and carried out as an *endodontic* procedure via *surgical* access and not a *surgical* procedure done for *endodontic* reasons: the tooth has a granuloma or a cyst at the apex and therefore a surgical operation is needed for the removal of the inflammatory tissue.

Until the end of the 80s, endodontic surgery was considered as a last resort; this was based on past experience when unsuitable instruments and inadequate vision were used, postoperative complications were quite frequent, and many cases ended in failure with the resultant extraction of the tooth. For these reasons, endodontic surgery was not considered to be important within the endodontic domain, was taught with very little enthusiasm at dental schools and was practiced by very few dentists in their private practice.

At the beginning of the 90s, the new era of endodontic microsurgery began. Several important developments were introduced in microsurgical endodontics: the surgical operating microscope, microinstruments, the ultrasonic root-end preparation and the use of more biologically acceptable, biocompatible, root-end filling materials. The concurrent development of better techniques has resulted in greater understanding of the apical anatomy, greater treatment success and a more favorable patient response.[2]

The incorporation of the new technology has evolved the classical apicoectomy into modern microsurgical endodontics. All steps of microsurgical endodontics are carried out under varying degrees of magnifications, including anesthesia, flap preparation, osteotomy, identification of root apices, root-end resection, inflammatory tissue removal, observation of the resected root surface, root-end preparation, root-end filling, and suturing.

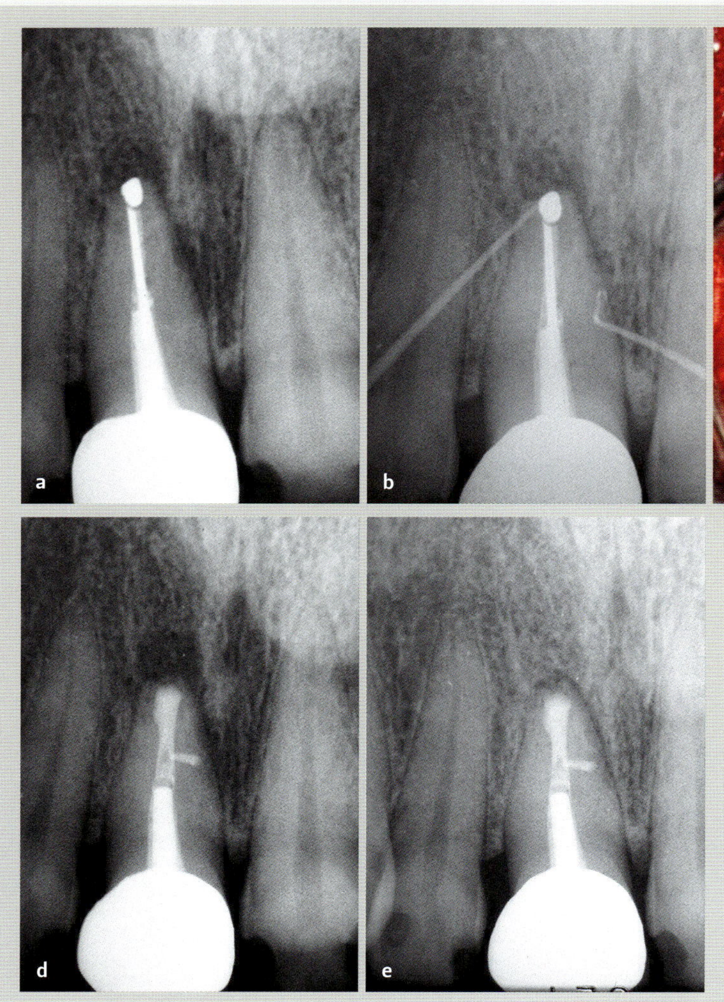

1.1 Typical example of microsurgical endodontic treatment. **a)** Preoperative radiograph. **b)** The central incisor has two lesions and two sinus tracts, one apical and one lateral. **c)** SuperEBA material is filling both the main canal and the lateral canal. **d)** Postoperative radiograph. **e)** Two-year follow-up.

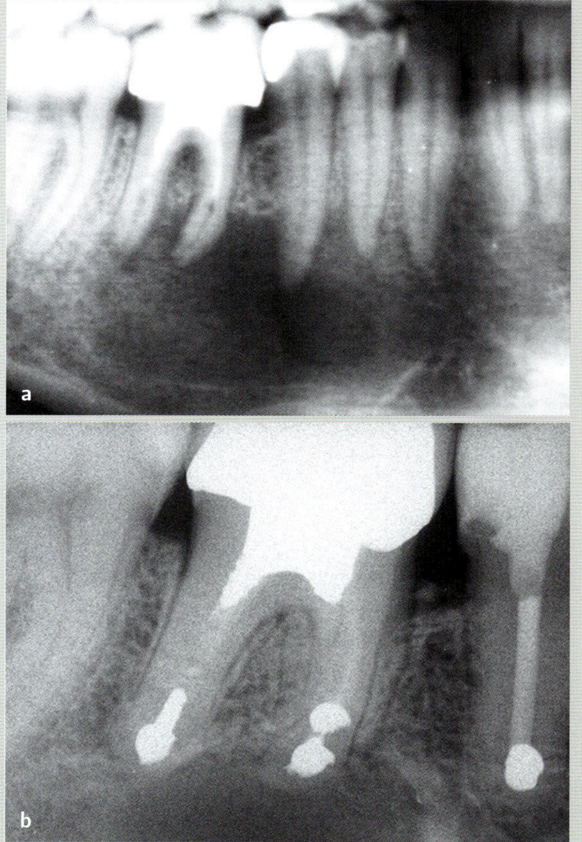

1.2 Typical example of endodontic surgery performed using traditional surgical techniques. **a)** Panoramic radiograph showing a large lesion involving the first mandibular molar and the second lower premolar. **b)** Patient was treated three years earlier by an oral surgeon using traditional technique, bur and amalgam. The patient had been scheduled for extraction, accurate curettage of the cyst and implant. The patient had also been informed of possible damage to the inferior alveolar nerve as a consequence of curettage of the lesion.

In a recent article, Setzer et al.[3,4] conducted a met-analysis and a systematic review of the literature. The authors compared the outcomes of contemporary root-end surgery techniques with microinstruments and only loupes or no visualization aids with the outcomes of endodontic microsurgery using the same instruments and materials but with high power magnification as provided by the surgical operating microscope. The conclusion of the study was that the probability for success was significantly greater if the surgical procedure was performed using the high power magnification rendered by the dental operating microscope. This conclusion is in agreement with the most recent literature,[5-10] and depending on different studies, a success rate of 98% has been described!

In 1992, Frank et al.[11] reported that success rates in apical surgeries sealed with amalgam, which had been considered successful, dropped to 57.7% after 10 years. Their study concluded that the responsibility for the failure was the root-end filling material, amalgam, which at that time was the material of choice. They speculated that probably amalgam could expand and lead to root fracture. They also noticed failing cases with apical root resorption, but they admitted that they couldn't tell if the resorption was the cause or the consequence of the failure. They finally concluded that an alternative filling material should have been considered to replace the amalgam, which in their opinion was the only reason for so many failures. In 1991, Friedman et al.[12] reported successful treatment results as 44.1% in teeth that were observed over a period of 6 months to 8 years after surgery and amalgam as a root-end filling material. In a randomized study, Kvist and Reit[13] compared results of surgically and nonsurgically treated cases. They could find no systematic difference in the outcome of treatment, which ranged in success from 56% to 60%. They noticed that surgical retreatments seemed to result in a more rapid periapical bone fill; however, the surgically treated cases showed a higher risk of "late failures", suggesting the necessity of a long follow-up period.

All of the above-mentioned studies used a conventional surgical protocol, without the benefit of the operating microscope, microsurgical instruments and biocompatible materials. Kvist and Reit[13] concluded and anticipated that the advent of the microscope, ultrasonic retrotips, and new retrofilling materials would have completely changed their surgical protocol in the near future.

The dental operating microscope has become an integral part of endodontic practice, both for nonsurgical and surgical therapy, and today it is considered indispensable to achieve excellence. Besides the obvious benefits for clinical practice, evidence has become available that demonstrates better outcomes compared to treatment without vision enhancement. Treatment rendered using the dental operating microscope results in superior care for patients, and modern endodontic therapy is more effective because of it.[14]

If we agree that the success of endodontic therapy depends on the complete removal of all necrotic and infected tissue and on the complete sealing of the entire root canal system, then the reasons why the traditional surgical approach sometimes fails are obvious: the surgeon cannot predictably locate, clean and fill all the complex apical ramifications using the traditional surgical techniques (1.2). These limitations can only be overcome with the use of the microscope with magnification and illumination, microsurgical instruments, ultrasonic retrotips and the new biocompatible materials.

Using microsurgical endodontics will make it easier to identify root apices and anatomical details such as isthmuses, canal fins, microfractures and lateral canals. Furthermore, the osteotomies will be smaller and the resection angles will be shallower, allowing the saving of cortical bone, tooth structure and root length.[2]

For this reason, it is correct to speak in terms of "Micro" (because the use of the microscope is today mandatory to perform the entire procedure) and then "surgical endodontics" because, as stated before, it is an endodontic procedure performed through a surgical flap, and not a surgical procedure performed just to remove periapical inflammatory tissue. Therefore, it is something that is pertinent to the endodontist and must be carried out with the knowledge, the skill and the hand of the endodontist. He or she will take care of cleaning, shaping and three-dimensionally obturating the root canal system with a surgical approach, only because (this is what happens most of the time) the root canal system was not negotiable without surgery (1.3).

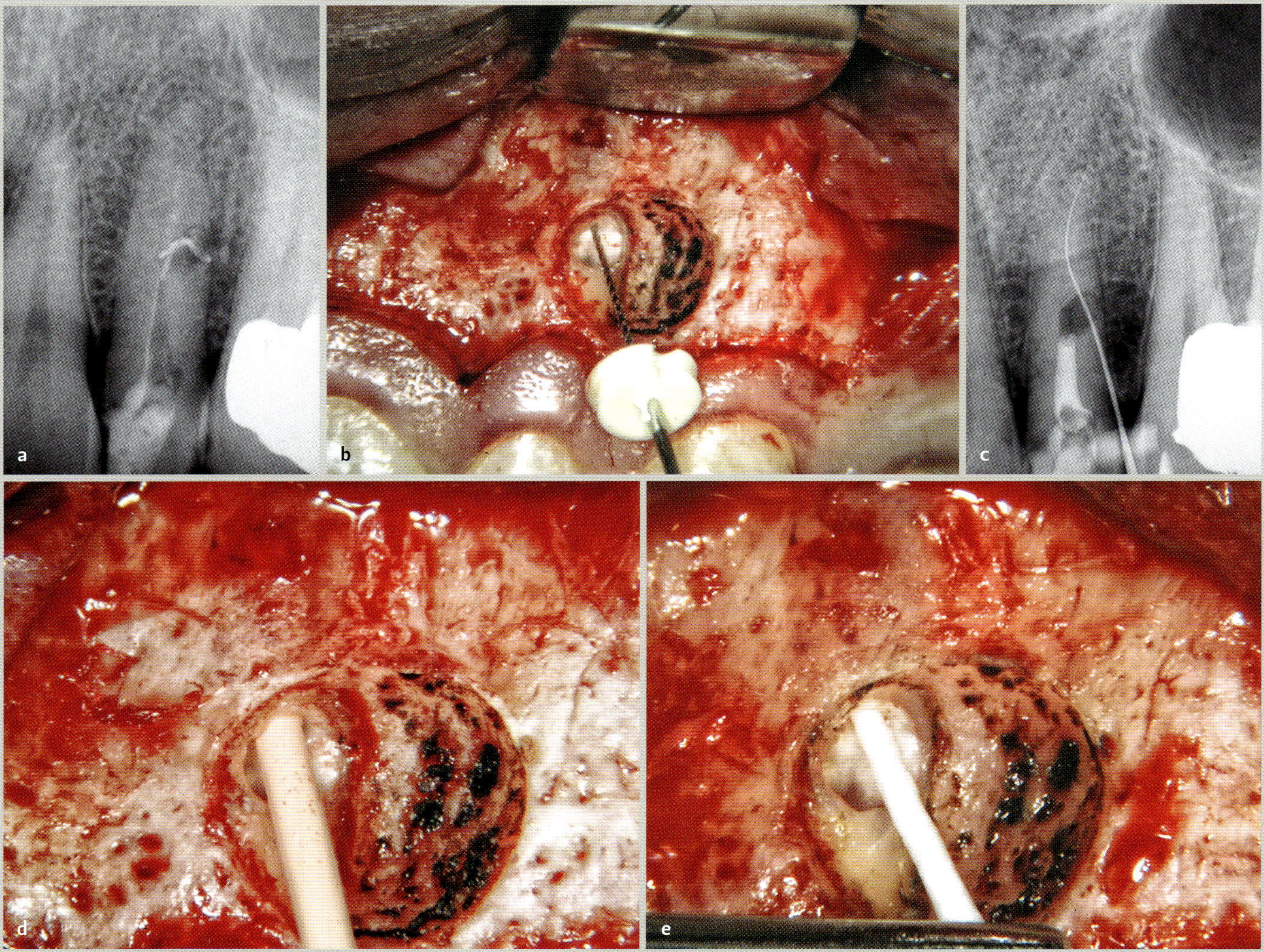

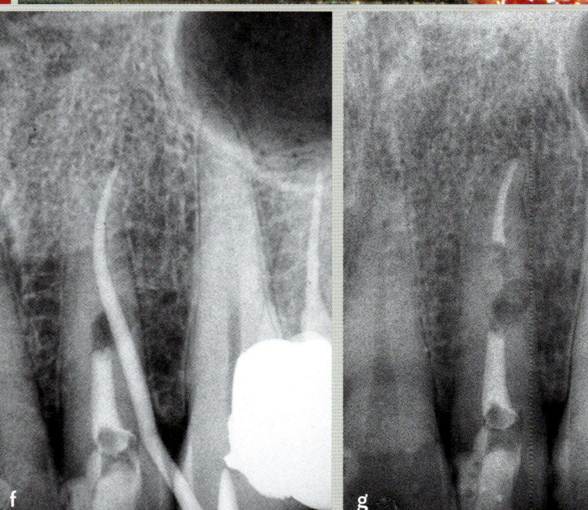

1.3 Endodontic treatment done via a surgical flap. **a)** Preoperative radiograph of the upper left lateral incisor. During the nonsurgical retreatment, it was impossible to remove the piece of gutta-percha and to negotiate the canal apical to the defect. It was then decided on surgical approach. **b)** Surgical negotiation of the root canal. **c)** Intraoperative radiograph to check the working length. The coronal portion of the root canal was filled with thermoplastic gutta-percha before surgery. **d)** The canal has been shaped with hand instruments first and then with rotary NiTi instruments. Cone fit. **e)** After irrigation with sodium hypochlorite and EDTA 17%, the canal is now dried with paper points. **f)** Intraoperative radiograph of the cone fit. **g)** Downpack with the Schilder technique. **h)** Backfill with thermoplastic gutta-percha up to the resorption defect. **i)** The defect has been filled with white MTA. **j, k)** 6-0 suture. **l)** Postoperative radiograph. **m)** The sutures are removed 24 hours after surgery. **n)** Perfect healing with no scar. **o)** Nineteen-year follow-up.

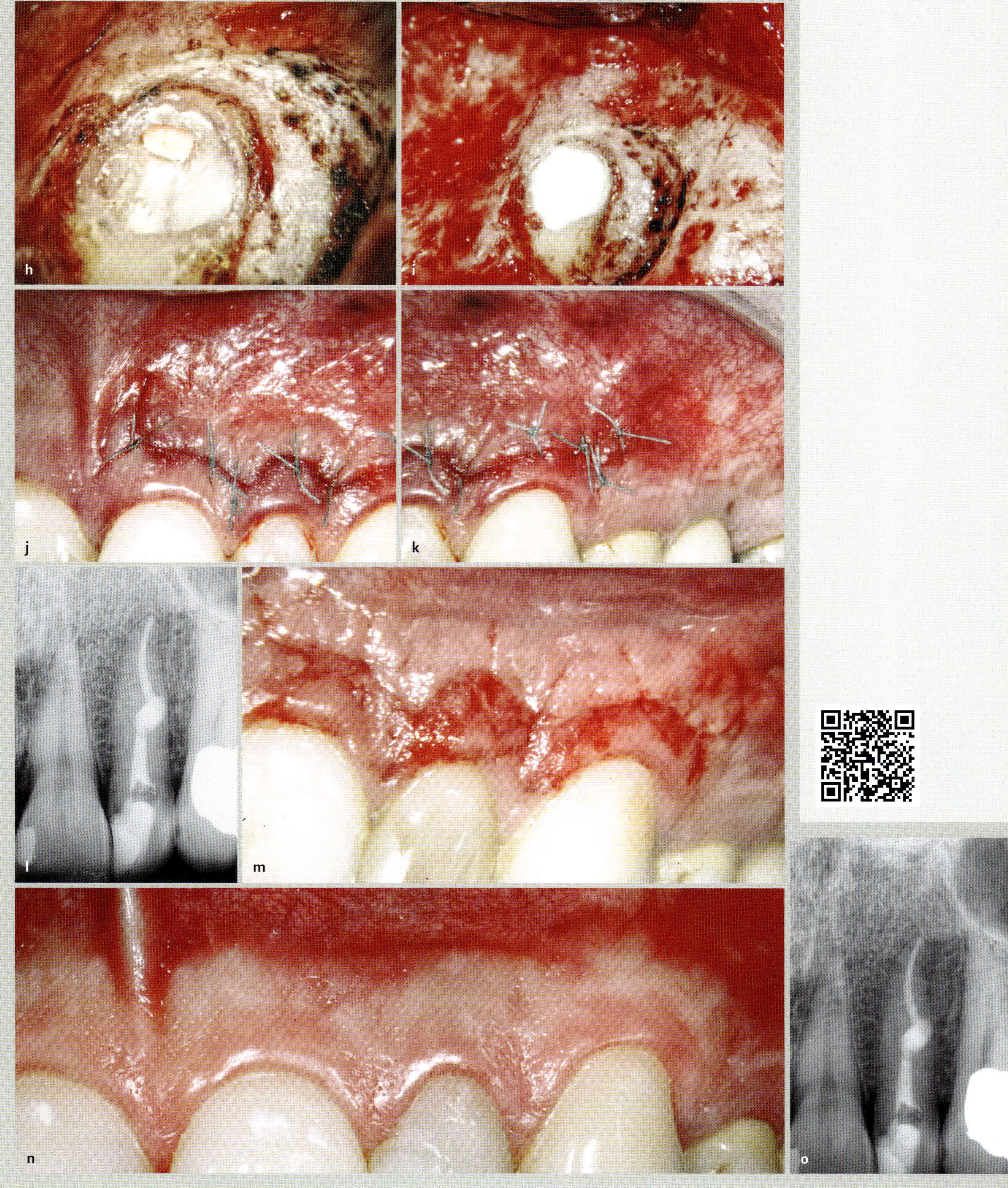
h
i
j
k
l
m
n
o

Quality assurance of endodontic therapy is an important issue[15] and microsurgical techniques have been applied in surgical endodontics for several years.[16] They have even become a standard in postgraduate education in endodontics.[17] Many endodontic surgical failures have been attributed to poor visibility and ability to diagnose and treat the minute causes of apical pathology.[18] The microsurgical approach has been purported to improve the prognosis of surgical treatment outcomes.[19]

With the aid of contemporary techniques such as magnification under a microscope, suitable materials and the use of microinstruments, endodontic surgery has evolved into microsurgical endodontics and will result in a predictably successful outcome in treated teeth (1.1).[18–21] Studies looking at the success of traditional apical surgery indicate that it is almost 50% less successful than that reported in current microsurgical success data.[7,19,20,22–26]

Surgical Advances in the Last Decades and Their Positive Effects on Outcome

These are some of the specific changes in the microsurgical approach, that are proven to increase the success of the procedure:[27]

- a smaller osteotomy, approximately 3-4 mm in diameter (1.4)

1.1 Comparison between microsurgery and traditional surgery

Author/Year	Follow-up Years	Magnification	Root-end Preparation	Root-end Filling	Success
Microsurgery					
Christiansen[22]	1	Microscope	Ultrasonic	MTA	96%
Kim[23]	2	Microscope	Ultrasonic	IRM/EBA/MTA	95.2%
Rubinstein, Kim[20]	1	Microscope	Ultrasonic	EBA	96.8%
Traditional Surgery					
Tsesis[7]	1 to 4	None	Bur	IRM	44.2%
Arad[24]	11.2	None	Bur	Amalgam/IRM	44.3%
Wessen[25]	5	None	Bur	Amalgam	57%
Haise[26]	1	None	Bur	Amalgam	68.7%

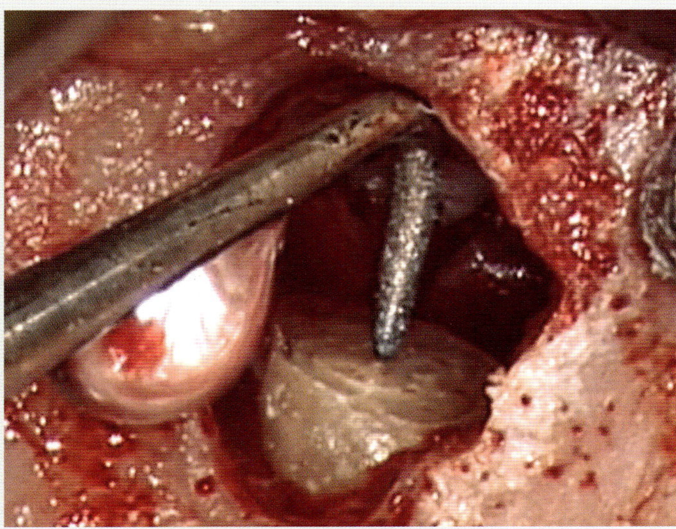

1.4 The osteotomy is just a little bit larger than the ultrasonic tip, which is 3 mm long.

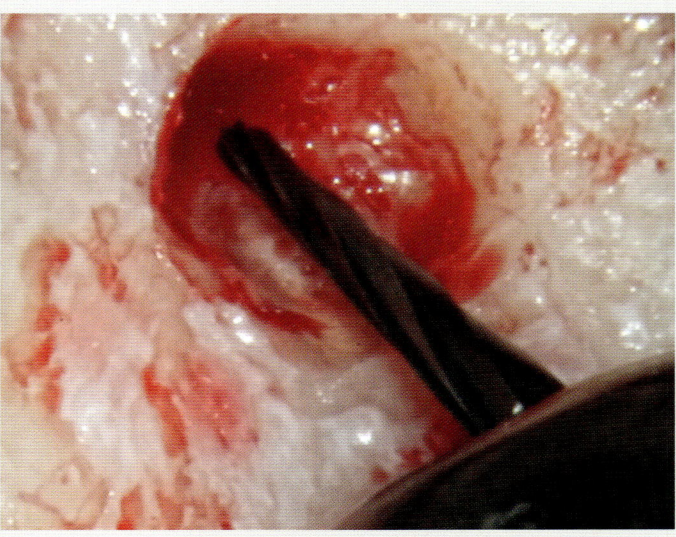

1.5 The Lindemann bur is resecting the apical 3 mm of the root-tip.

- root-tip resection of 3 mm to eliminate lateral canals and apical ramifications (1.5)
- a decreased or no root resection bevel angle (1.6)
- clear inspection of the resected root surface to visualize fractures, isthmuses or other anatomical complexities (1.7)
- 3 mm-depth preparation of the long axis of the canal (1.8)
- root-end filling with biocompatible materials (1.9).

In conclusion, microsurgical endodontics should not be viewed as the last resort. It should be an integral part of endodontic retreatment regimens.[2] It should be used where indicated to save natural teeth, since it is a predictable method to effectively eradicate the causes of

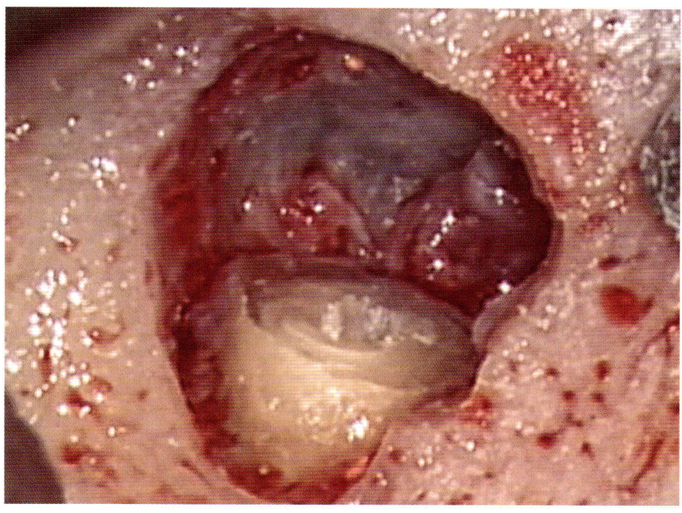

1.6 The resection is made with a 90° angle to the long axis of the root.

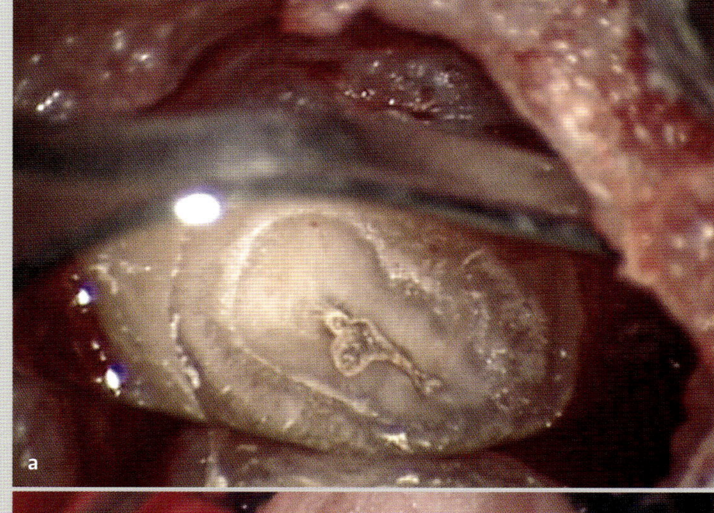

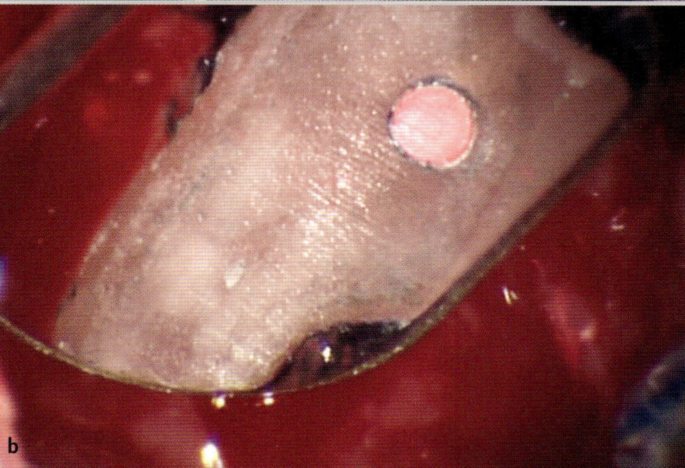

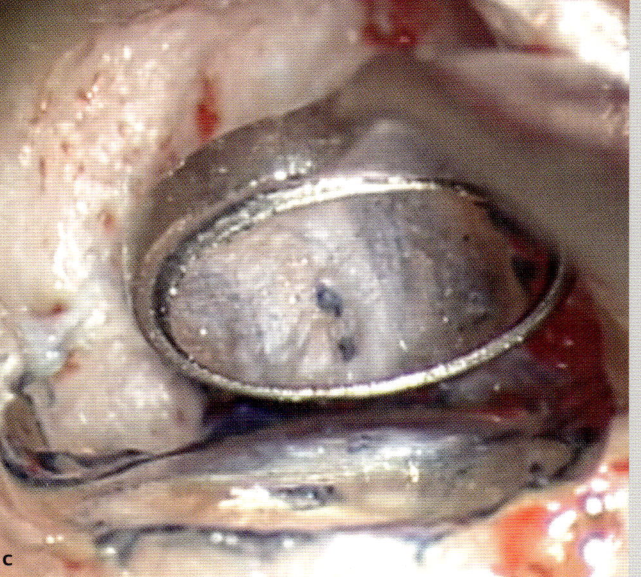

1.7 a–c) The use of a micro-mirror allows an accurate inspection of the resected root surface.

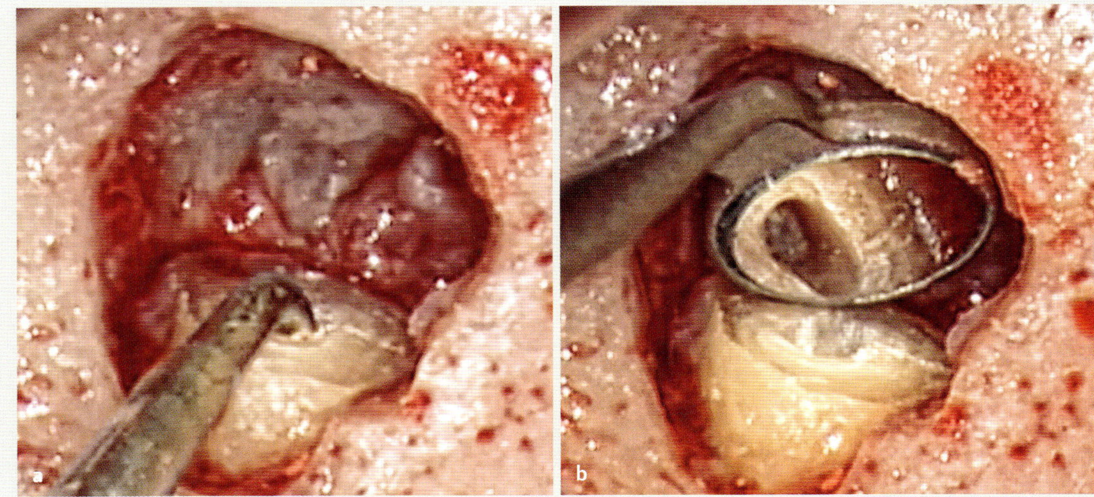

1.8 **a)** The ultrasonic tip prepares a cavity 3 mm deep. **b)** The micro-mirror allows an accurate inspection of the root-end cavity.

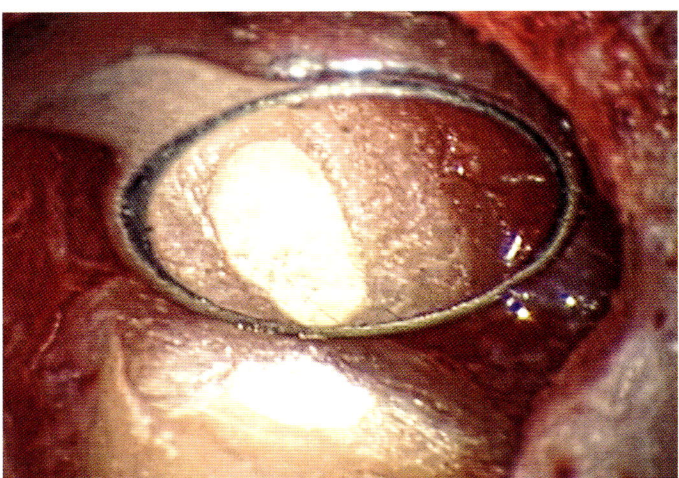

1.9 The root-end cavity has been filled with a biocompatible material.

persistent periapical pathosis with very little or no postoperative discomfort.[28,29] When a tooth has been endodontically treated but still has persisting symptoms and the patient wants to save the tooth, retreatment of the root canal system should be considered.[27] There are two options: nonsurgical retreatment through the access cavity or a surgical approach, directly accessing the root apices and periapical pathosis. Both procedures are very effective and supporting research shows that these procedures will result in the healing of apical periodontitis on an average of 80%.[30] The decision to retreat a case surgically or nonsurgically can be a challenge and should be based on individual circumstances. Current research has shown that when the previous root canal treatment appears to be adequately performed, the success of a nonsurgical retreatment is significantly decreased, meaning that apical surgery may be the preferred option.[31] However, the clinician must advise patients that the microsurgical approach is a treatment option that is preferred to nonsurgical retreatment, extraction or implant placement. Implants are a marvel of modern-day dentistry where indicated, but abuse of this technique can be catastrophic for patients.[27]

REFERENCES

1. **Friedman S, Stabholz A.** *Endodontic retreatment – case selection and technique. Part 1: criteria for case selection.* J Endod. 1986;12:28-33.
2. **Kim S, Kratchman S.** *Modern endodontic surgery concepts and practice: a review.* J Endod. 2006;32(7):601-623.
3. **Setzer FC, Shah SB, Kohli MR, Karabucak B, Kim S.** *Outcome of endodontic surgery: a meta-analysis of the literature-Part 1: Comparison of traditional root-end surgery and endodontic microsurgery.* J Endod. 2010;36:1757-65.
4. **Setzer FC, Kohli MR, Shah SB, Karabucak B, Kim S.** *Outcome of endodontic surgery: a meta-analysis of the literature-Part 2: Comparison of endodontic microsurgical techniques with and without the use of higher magnification.* J Endod. 2012;38(1):1-10.
5. **Song M, Shin S-J, Kim E.** *Outcomes of endodontic micro-resurgery: a prospective clinical study.* J Endod. 2011;37:316-20.
6. **Song M, Jung I, Lee SJ, Lee CY, Kim E.** *Prognostic factors for clinical outcomes in endodontic microsurgery: a retrospective study.* J Endod. 2011;37(7):927-33.
7. **Tsesis I, Rosen E, Schwartz-Arad D, et al.** *Retrospective evaluation of surgical endodontic treatment: traditional versus modern technique.* J Endod. 2006;32:412-6.
8. **Tsesis I, Faivishevsky V, Kfir A, Rosen E.** *Outcome of surgical endodontic treatment performed by a modern technique: a meta-analysis of literature.* J Endod. 2009;35:1505-11.
9. **Tsesis I, Rosen E, Taschieri S, Strauss YT, Ceresoli V, Del Fabbro M.** *Outcomes of surgical endodontic treatment performed by a modern technique: an updated meta-analysis of the literature.* J Endod. 2013;39(3):332-39.
10. **Gutmann J, Harrison J.** *Success, failure, and prognosis in periradicular surgery.* In: Gutmann J, Harrison J, eds. *Surgical endodontics.* Oxford: Blackwell Scientific Publications. 1991:338-84.
11. **Frank AL, Glick DH, Patterson SS, Weine FS.** *Long term evaluation of surgically placed amalgam fillings.* J Endod. 1992;18(8):391-398.
12. **Friedman S, Lustmann J, Shaharabany V.** *Treatment results of apical surghery in premolar and molar teeth.* J Endod. 1991;17(1):30-33.
13. **Kvist T, Reit C.** *Results of endodontic retreatments: a randomized clinical study comparing surgical and nonsurgical procedures.* J Endod. 1999;25(12):814-817.
14. **Setzer FC.** *The dental operating microscope in endodontics.* AAE Colleagues for Excellence. 2016;2:1-8.
15. **Maggio JD, Bray KE, Hartwell GR, Lindemann MB, Pisani JV, E.M.R.** *Appropriateness of care and quality assurance guidelines,* 3rd. Chicago: American Association of Endodontists. 1998:24-32.
16. **Velvart P, Peters C.** *Soft tissue management in endodontic surgery.* J Endod. 2005;31(1):4-16.
17. **Commission on Dental Accreditation of the American Dental Association.** *Standards for Advanced Specialty Education Programs in Endodontics 1998 (revised 2004).* http://www.ada.org/prof/ed/accred/standard/endo.pdf.Accessed Nov. 16;2004.
18. **Kim S.** *Principles of endodontic microsurgery.* Dent Clin North Am. 1997;41:481-497.
19. **Rubinstein RA, Kim S.** *Long-term follow-up of cases considered healed one year after apical microsurgery.* J Endod. 2002;28:378-383.
20. **Rubinstein RA, Kim S.** *Short-term observation of the results of endodontic surgery with use of a surgical operation microscope and Super-EBA as root-end filling material.* J Endod. 1999;25:43-48.
21. **Zuolo ML, Ferreira MO, Gutmann JL.** *Prognosis in periradicular surgery: a clinical prospective study.* Int Endod J. 2000;33:91-98.
22. **Christiansen R, Kirkevang LL, Horsted-Bindslev P, Wenzel A.** *Randomized clinical trial of root-end resection followed by root-end filling with mineral trioxide aggregate or smoothing of the orthograde gutta-percha root filling - 1-year follow-up.* Int Endod J. 2009;423:105-114.
23. **Kim E, Song JS, Jung IY, Lee SJ, Kim S.** *Prospective clinical study evaluating endodontic microscurgery outcomes for cases with lesions of endodontic origin compared with cases with lesions of combined periodontal-endodontic origin.* J Endod. 2008;34:546-551.
24. **Schwartz-Arad D, Yarom N, Lustig JP, Kaffe I.** *A retrospective radiographic study of root-end surgery with amalgam and intermediate restorative material.* Oral Surg Oral Med Oral Pathol Oral Radiol Endod. 2003;96:472-477.
25. **Wesson CM, Gale TM.** *Molar apicoectomy with amalgam root-end filling: results of a prospective study in two district general hospitals.* Br Dent J. 2003;195:707-714.
26. **Halse A, Molven O, Grung B.** *Follow-up after periapical surgery: the value of the one-year control.* Endod Dent Traumatol. 1991;7:246-250.
27. **AAE Endodontics. Colleagues for Excellence.** *Contemporary endodontic microsurgery: procedural advancements and treatment planning considerations.* Fall 2010. https://www.aae.org/specialty/wp-content/uploads/sites/2/2017/07/ecfefall2010final.pdf
28. **Iqbal M, Kratchman S, Guess G, Karabucakl K, Kim S.** *Microscopic periradicular surgery: perioperative predictors for postoperative clinical outcomes and quality of life assessment.* J Endod. 2007;33:239-244.
29. **Penarrocha M, Barcia B, Mart E, Balaguer J.** *Pain and inflammation after periapical surgery in 60 patients.* J Oral Maxillofac Surg. 2006;64:429-433.
30. *Toraninejad M*, **Corr R, Handysides R, Shabahang S.** *Outcomes of nonsurgical retreatments and endodontic surgery. A systematic review.* J Endod. 2009;35:930-937.
31. **De Chevigny C, Dao T, Basrani B, Marquis V, Farzaneh M, Abitbol S, Friedman S.** *Treatment outcome in endodontics: the Toronto study - Phases 3 and 4: orthograde retreatment.* J Endod. 2008;34:131-137.

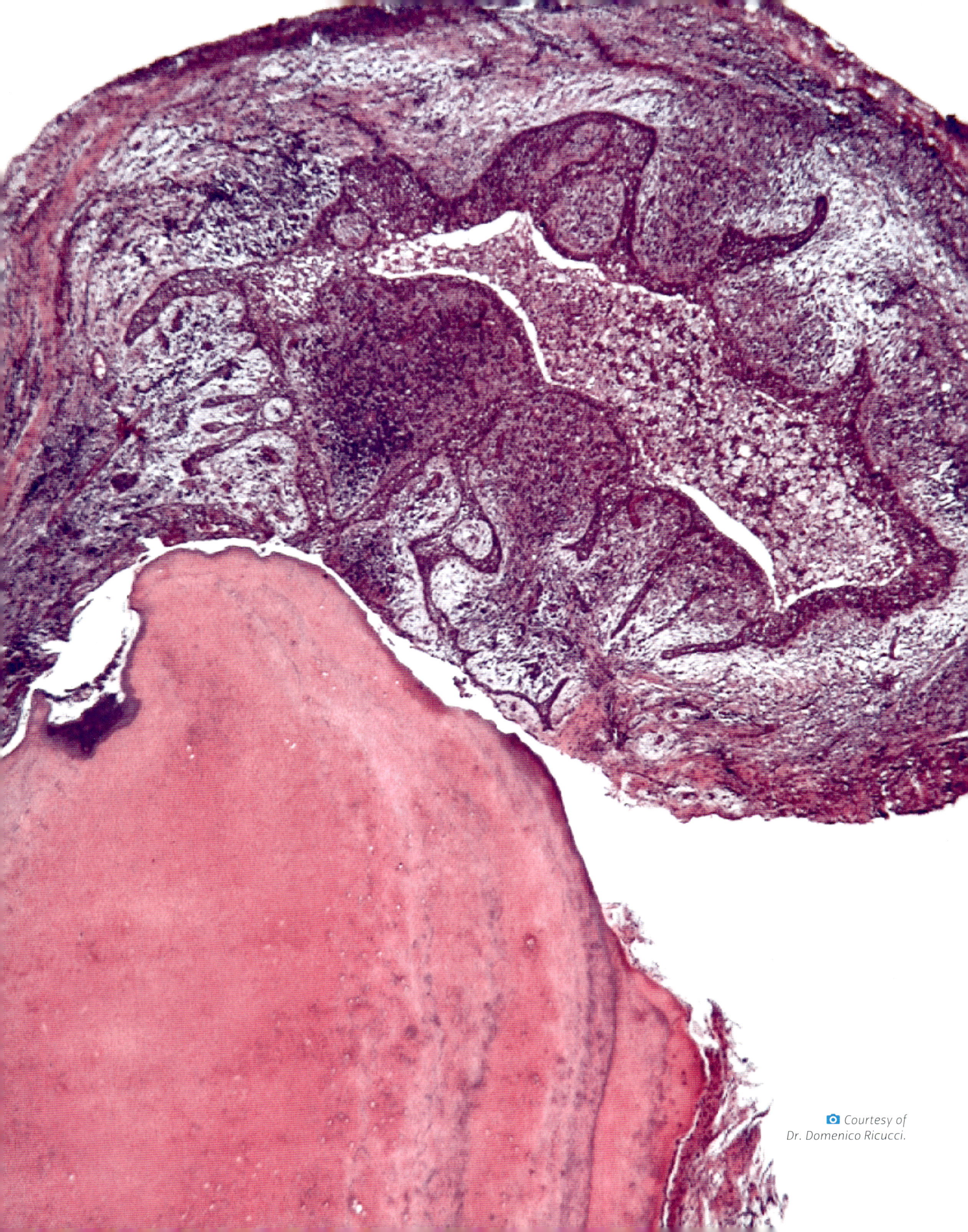

Courtesy of
Dr. Domenico Ricucci.

Diagnosis and Treatment Plan

Informed Patient Consent

Before starting any nonsurgical or surgical procedure, it is important and necessary to inform the patient about the treatment and its alternatives, which should be explained in a clear, complete and understandable way. The results of clinical and radiographic examinations, the diagnosis and the treatment options should be discussed with the patient and he/she should confirm that they understood the proposed treatment plan to solve their clinical problem.

The patient must be thoroughly advised of the benefits, risks, and other treatment options and must be given any opportunity to ask questions.[1] Regarding the risks, the patients must be informed that the surgical procedure might involve important neurovascular bundles that may be traumatized, and the maxillary sinus that might be exposed. Paresthesia after mandibular posterior surgery is uncommon, but should be discussed with the patient because this potential complication is a risk that some patient may be unwilling to assume. 1 Other possible complications that are self-limiting and easily manageable are swelling, bleeding and infections. However, these complications, like pain, swelling, bleeding, ecchymosis, are more frequent if the surgical procedure is performed without using the modern technology, instruments and materials that will be discussed in all the chapters of this textbook. Especially in cases where the patient already had a bad experience due to a previous surgical treatment not performed the way it should be, the doctor should convince the patient to literally forget the old experience and understand the "new" surgery that they will receive is a completely "new" experience, where they will not feel any pain during the procedure and no pain or very little pain during the first hours after the surgery. They also should be informed that some little swelling will be present the second and the third day following the surgical procedure, and this is not due to any infection, but it is rather the consequence of the "moderate" trauma given to the tissue during the surgery.

The patient should sign the consent form to document that he/she understood and accepted or rejected the treatment options. This written and signed document will not only protect the patient and the doctor from a medical-legal standpoint, but also will confirm the existence of a mutual trust, which is the "condition sine qua non" to start any kind of treatment.

Informed Consent for Microsurgical Procedures

Last Name	First Name	Date
Date of Birth	City of Birth	State

I declare that I was thoroughly informed by Doctor ______________________________
who explained clearly my clinical situation, the treatment options and the suggested treatment to solve my problem.

The doctor also informed about the discomfort, the side effects and the consequences of the surgical procedure that he will perform to treat the disease which is affecting my tooth/teeth.

I was also informed about the consequences and possible complications that I will have in case I refuse the surgical treatment.

I have been advised that this surgery is performed through external incisions in the mucosa, which could leave permanent scars to the extent and location of which I have been described and demonstrated to me.

The doctor has fully explained, in terms clear to me, the effect and nature of the procedure to be performed. The doctor answered to all my questions and I completely understood.

I know that the practice of dentistry is not an exact science and therefore the results cannot be guaranteed. I acknowledge that no guarantee or assurance has been made by anyone regarding the operation I have herein authorized.

I give permission to doctor who will perform the procedure to take photographs or video for diagnostic and teaching purposes and I agree that this material will remain his/her property.

I authorize the doctor to use such material to illustrate scientific papers, books or lectures.

I also give permission to the doctor to take a Cone Beam Computed Tomography of the involved area for diagnostic purposes, in case the doctor needs the three-dimensional information provided by the CBCT examination.

I assume all financial responsibilities for the proposed treatment.

Date: ______________________

Patient's signature ______________________________

Diagnosis and treatment plan

Once a diagnosis of endodontic failure has been made, it is necessary to understand what the cause of the failure was so that, successively, the possibility of correcting the failure by orthograde retreatment or by surgical retreatment can be evaluated. The decision-making process should consider the many different variables, as clearly illustrated by Reit and Dahlen.[2] Some authors have reported better clinical results with surgical procedures compared with orthograde retreatment,[3] although others have reported similar clinical outcomes using both techniques with slight differences related only to the time element.[4] According to Gorni and Gagliani,[5] during the diagnostic phase, only clinical signs and symptoms are available for dentists. Further information should be collected using radiographic analysis of the tooth to be retreated. In their article, the two authors have classified the different clinical situations encountered in retreatment cases and related them to the outcome after an observation period of 24 months. After radiographic analysis, which was occasionally performed with two different projections, the root canal systems were classified into two large groups as follows: teeth with root canal morphology that has been respected by previous endodontic treatment, root-canal-morphology-respected (RCMR), and teeth with root canal morphology altered by previous endodontic treatment, root-canal-morphology-altered (RCMA). In their study, the success percentage differs greatly in the two groups considered: the group having dental elements with canal and apical morphology alterations (RCMA), and groups with dental elements in which previous treatment had not determined this kind of problem (RCMR). The conclusion of the study was that the alterations performed on the natural course of root canal systems by previous endodontic treatments seem to have a key role. The apical morphology alteration is what should guide the treatment plan and decision making; when there is evidence of anatomic alteration, the best option is the surgical approach.

Only in those cases where nonsurgical therapy is not possible or following failure of the nonsurgical therapy conducted to resolve the problem, is surgical intervention indicated. Apical surgery in other words is not a substitute for incomplete debridement and poor endodontics (📷 2.1). In agreement with what Nygaard-Ostby and Schilder[6] confirmed, surgical endodontics must be reserved for those cases in which the preparation and obturation of the root canal appear impossible right from the beginning or when the nonsurgical retreat-

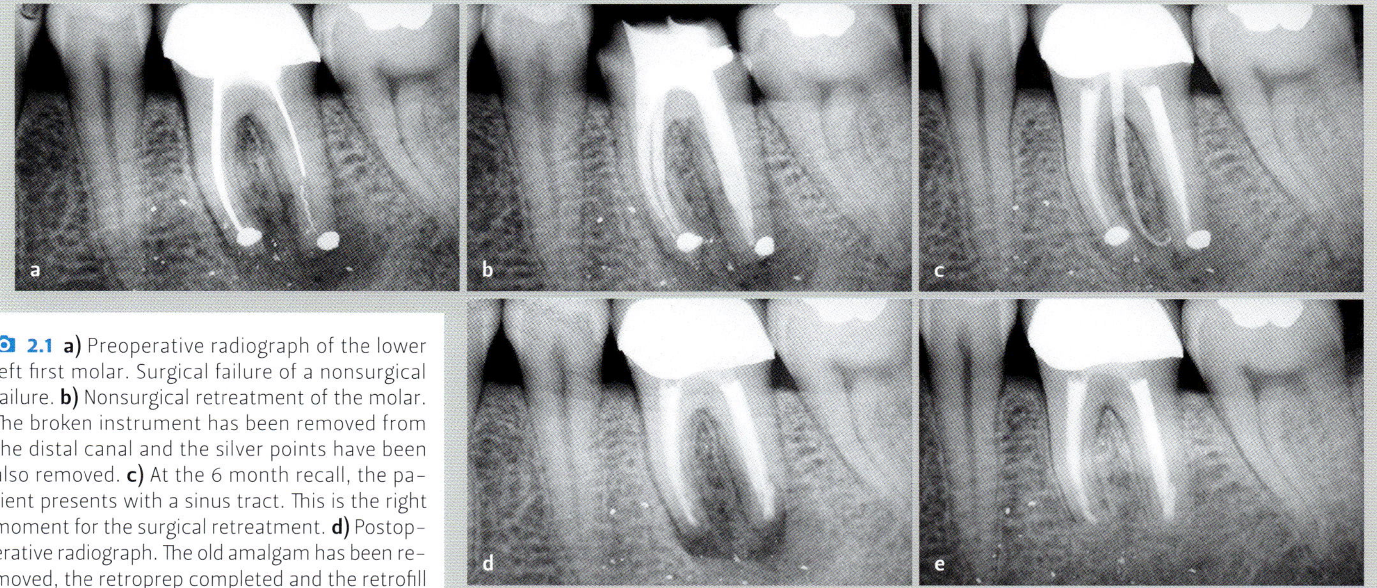

📷 **2.1 a)** Preoperative radiograph of the lower left first molar. Surgical failure of a nonsurgical failure. **b)** Nonsurgical retreatment of the molar. The broken instrument has been removed from the distal canal and the silver points have been also removed. **c)** At the 6 month recall, the patient presents with a sinus tract. This is the right moment for the surgical retreatment. **d)** Postoperative radiograph. The old amalgam has been removed, the retroprep completed and the retrofill positioned under the operating microscope. **e)** The two-year recall radiograph shows perfect healing.

ment attempts have failed. Nevertheless, even in such cases, the authors recommend filling as much of the root canal by conventional method as possible.

Ultimately, even after the indication for surgery has been established, in agreement with Weine and Gerstein,[7] it is recommended to remove as much as possible of the inadequate previous canal obturation material and replace it with well-compacted gutta-percha: in this way lateral canals and forgotten additional canals can be filled, often removing the need for surgery (2.2). For those cases in which surgery is still indicated, there is now a notably increased percentage of success with surgical treatment compared to that which could be achieved up until a few years ago, and this is thanks to recent technological progress that has happened in the field of surgical endodontics: the sur-

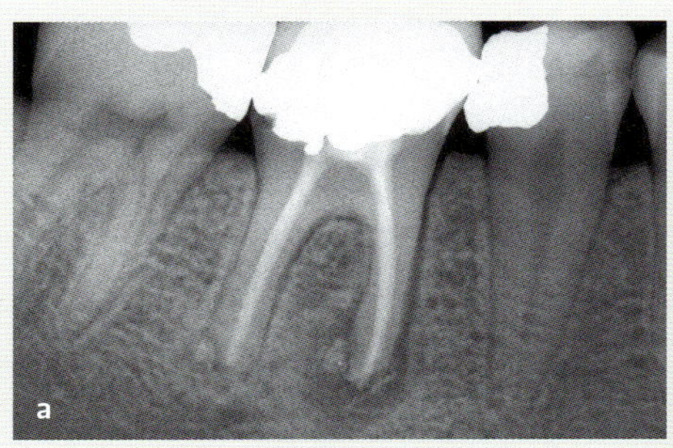

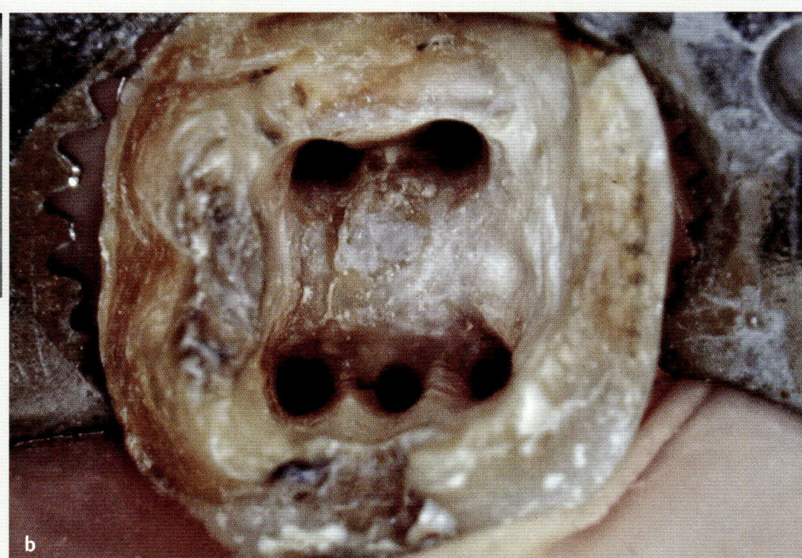

2.2 **a)** Preoperative radiograph of the lower right first molar. Even though there is some extruded material, the nonsurgical retreatment was scheduled. **b)** The tooth had two missed canals: the disto-lingual and the mesio-medial canal. **c)** Postoperative radiograph. **d)** The seven-year recall radiograph shows the healing of the lesion and the complete resorption of the extruded material.

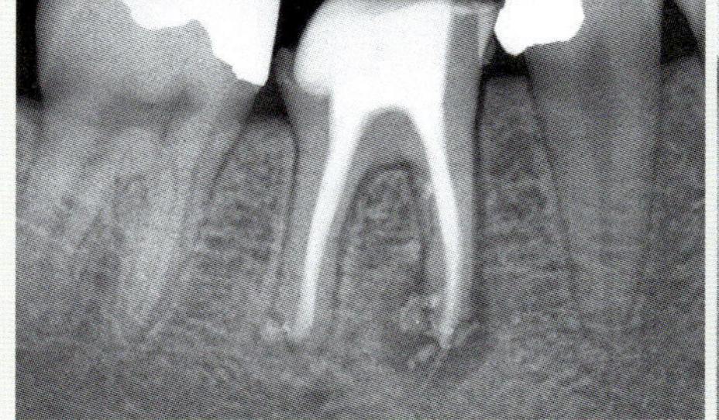

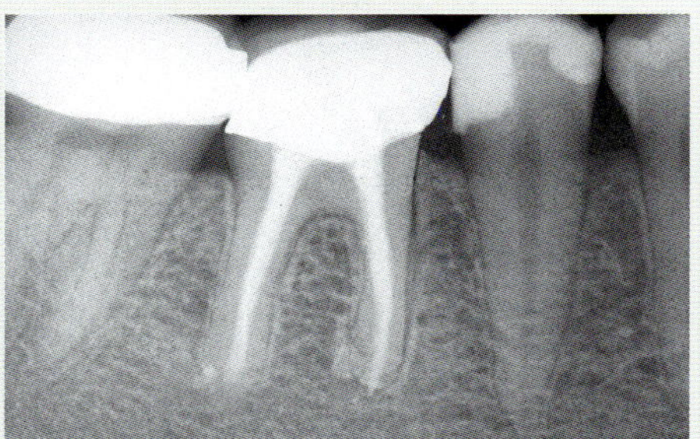

2.3 **a)** Preoperative radiograph of the lower left first molar. The tooth presents small lesions at the apex of both roots and it is sensitive to percussion. Due to the presence of a crown and a cast post, in agreement with the patient a surgical approach was elected. **b)** Postoperative radiograph. **c)** Two-year recall radiograph.

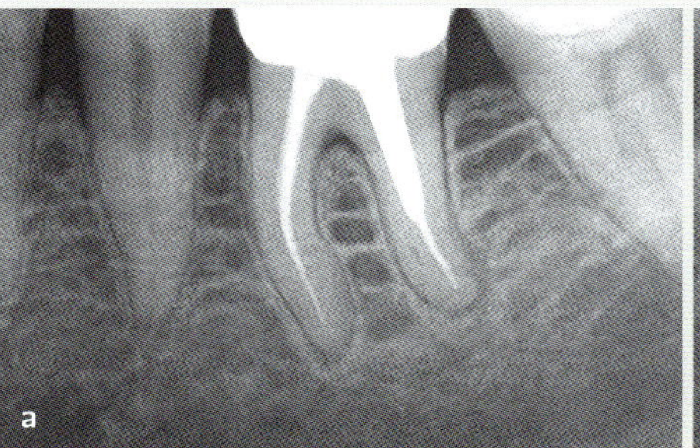

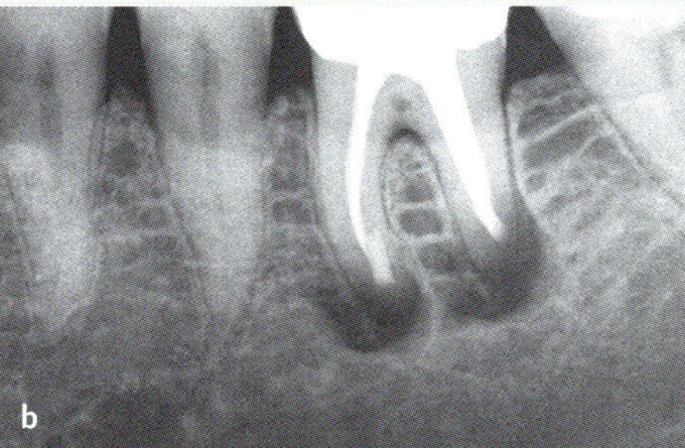

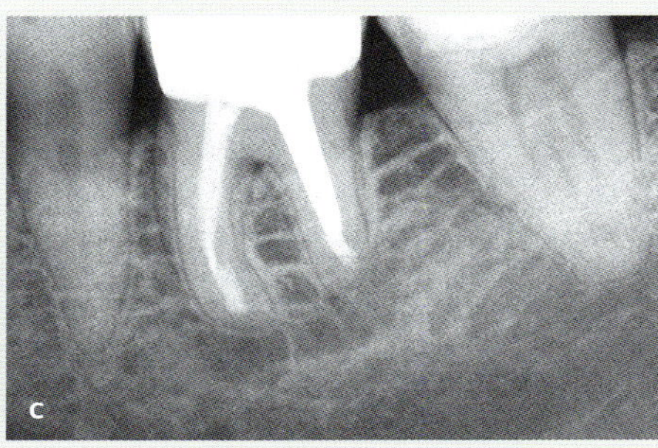

gical operating microscope, the ultrasonic retro-tips and the new biocompatible materials.

In conclusion, when we examine the different treatment options, the surgical approach is more conservative treatment than nonsurgical treatment for certain cases. A typical example is a tooth with acceptable endodontics and a new post and crown restoration, but a persistent or enlarging periapical lesion (2.3). Breaking or disassembling the crown, removing the post and retreating the root canals would be more dramatic, more time-consuming, costlier and less predictable than root-end microsurgical retreatment.[8] This surgical retreatment approach has been shown to have a higher success rate than nonsurgical retreatment, provided that periodontal conditions are not compromised.[9] Of course the patient must be informed of the prognosis for a successful outcome and the risks involved in the surgical procedure in addition to the benefits. It is also important to inform the patient about the possible short-term effects of the surgery, such as pain, swelling and bruising discoloration.[10]

Indications and Contraindications

All teeth can be treated successfully endodontically, which means that in theory there are no contraindications to such therapy, as long as the tooth is periodontally sound or can be made so, if its foramen or foramina can be sealed, independent of the approach that is chosen, that is, either the conservative, traditional, or nonsurgical one (isolating the tooth with a rubber dam and approaching it by means of the access cavity), or the retrograde, surgical one (raising a flap and performing an apicoectomy with retrofilling)[11] (2.4).

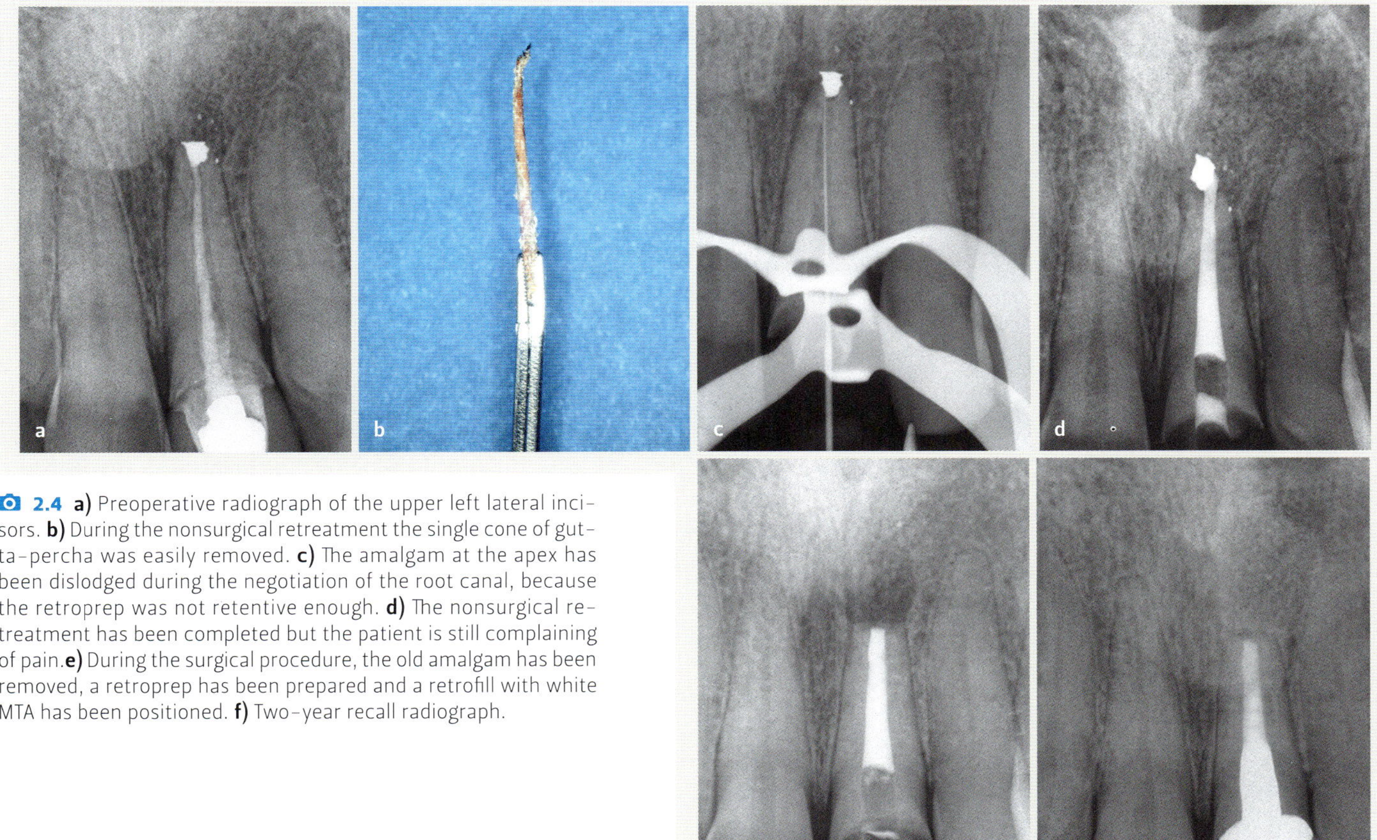

2.4 **a)** Preoperative radiograph of the upper left lateral incisors. **b)** During the nonsurgical retreatment the single cone of gutta-percha was easily removed. **c)** The amalgam at the apex has been dislodged during the negotiation of the root canal, because the retroprep was not retentive enough. **d)** The nonsurgical retreatment has been completed but the patient is still complaining of pain. **e)** During the surgical procedure, the old amalgam has been removed, a retroprep has been prepared and a retrofill with white MTA has been positioned. **f)** Two-year recall radiograph.

False Indications

Some previous indications for apical surgery are no longer valid due to advancements in techniques, equipment and materials. The following sections offer some examples.

LARGE LESIONS (2.5)

In the 10th edition of his textbook, Louis Grossman[12] mentions as the first indication for periapical surgery the extensive destruction of the periapical tissue, bone or periodontal ligament, involving one-third or more of the root apex. On the other hand, we know today that the size of the lesion (big or small), the geography of the lesion (periapical or lateral) and the histology of the lesion (granuloma or cyst) play no role in the healing process. It doesn't matter what the size, location or the histology is, they all are lesions of endodontic origin and they can heal with the correct endodontic therapy, with or without the surgical approach.

PRESENCE OF A CYST (2.6)

The second indication mentioned in the same edition of Grossman's textbook was the apex being involved in a

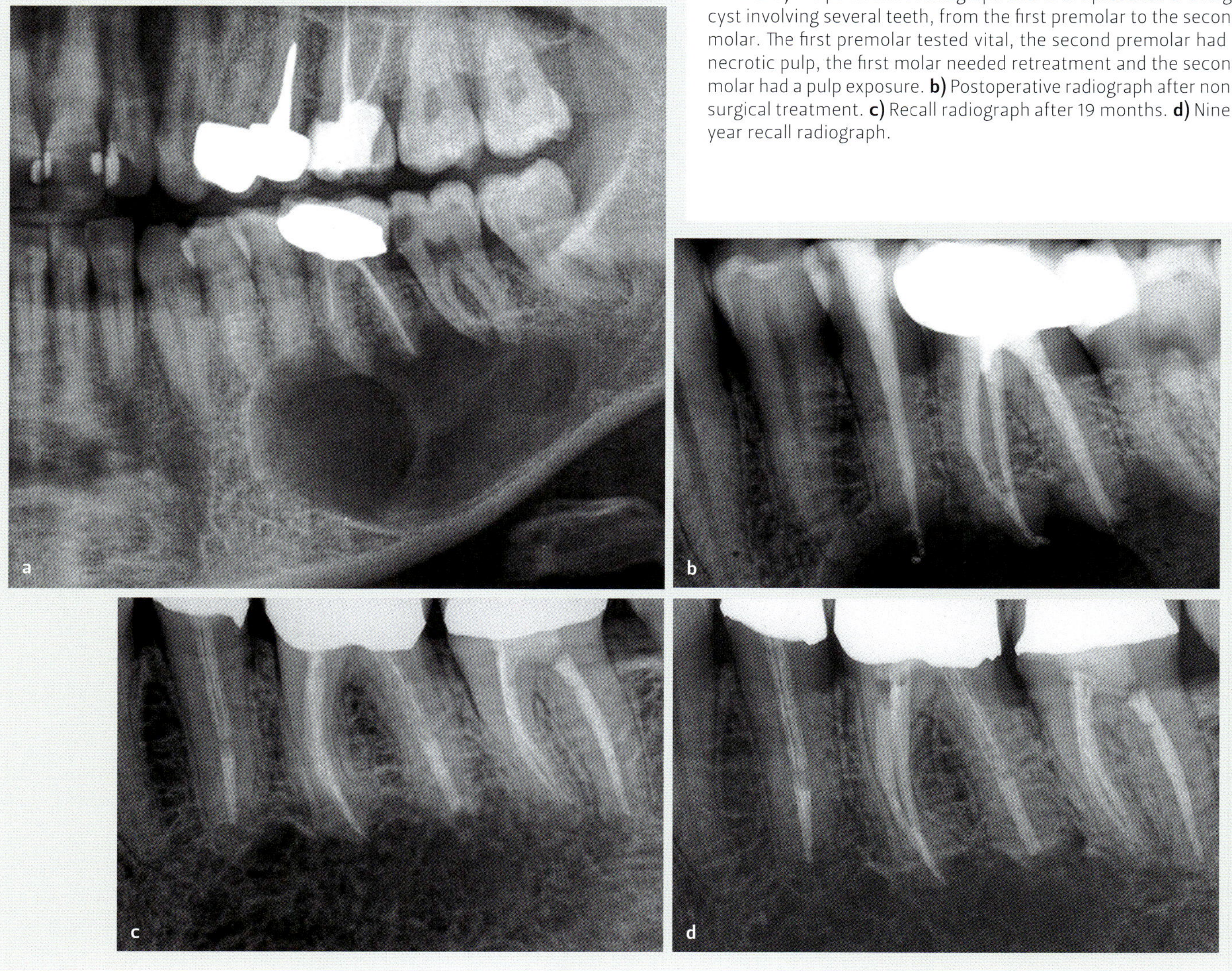

2.5 **a)** The panoramic radiograph shows the presence of a large cyst involving several teeth, from the first premolar to the second molar. The first premolar tested vital, the second premolar had a necrotic pulp, the first molar needed retreatment and the second molar had a pulp exposure. **b)** Postoperative radiograph after non-surgical treatment. **c)** Recall radiograph after 19 months. **d)** Nine-year recall radiograph.

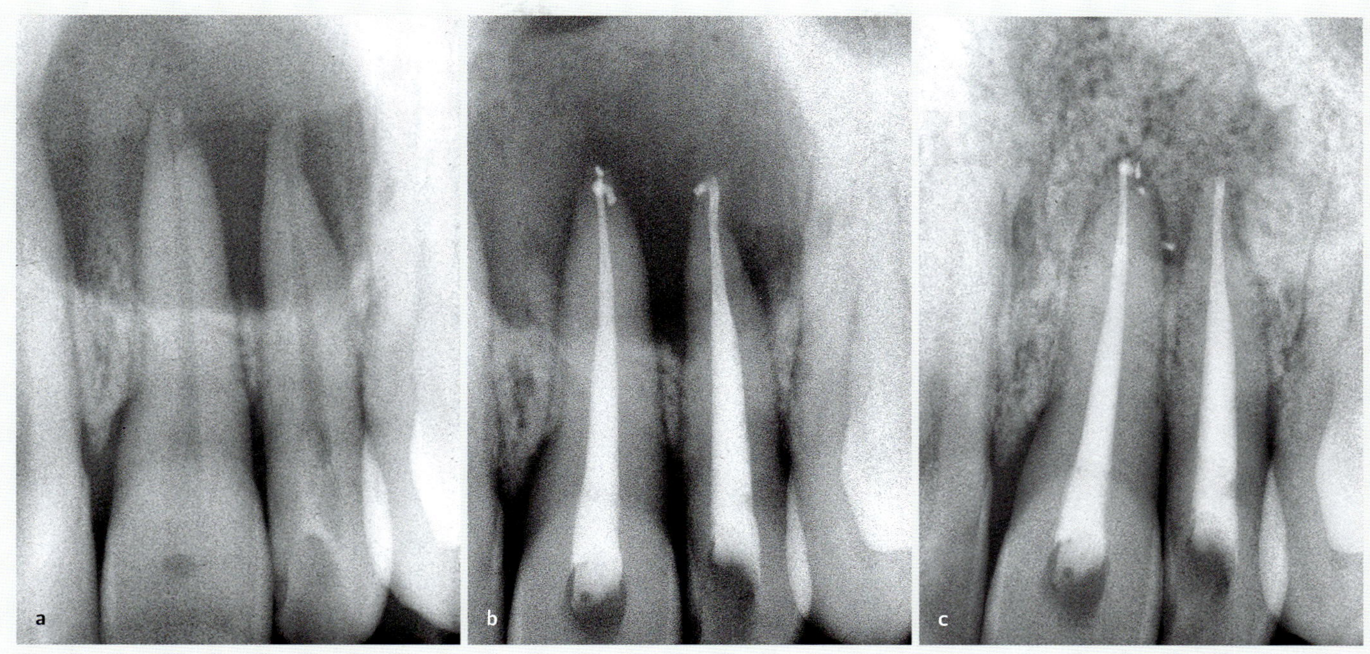

2.6 **a)** Preoperative radiograph of the upper left central and lateral incisors. The two teeth do not respond to the pulp vitality tests. The radiographic appearance of the large lesion which surrounds the two apices suggests a cyst. **b)** Postoperative radiograph. **c)** Two-year recall radiograph.

cystic condition.[12] This is an old theory, still followed by many oral surgeons and maxillo-facial surgeons. Many are still convinced that the epithelial cystic wall needs to be completely surgically removed, in order for the lesion to heal.

Regarding the pathogenesis of cysts, we know that epithelial cell rests of Malassez, the remnants of Hertwig's epithelial root sheath, which disintegrates after tooth development, are natural components of the attachment apparatus of the tooth and are found in the periodontal ligament near the root surface in all teeth after root formation.[13] Normally, they are of no clinical significance since they are quiescent in the normal periodontal ligament, but they may be stimulated to proliferate in apical periodontitis.[14]

When a lesion of endodontic origin develops at the level of the periodontal ligament, the inflammatory process inevitably also involves these cellular nests. Due to this irritating stimulus, they may proliferate and constitute the nucleus of a cystic formation.[15–17] There are several pathogenic theories of cyst formation. One of the most credited is the "breakdown theory".[17,18] This theory suggests that the continued growth of epithelium removes central cells from their nutrition and therefore the distance between the central cells and their nutritive source increases; consequently, the innermost cells of this actively proliferating cellular nest die, and their degenerative products attract fluid by simple osmosis, with a consequent increase in size of the lesion. However, it is important to realize that it is an inflammatory process. Therefore, once the stimulus is removed, there is no reason why it should not heal, like any other lesion of endodontic origin.[18] The diagnosis of the cyst is based on radiographic findings. Several authors maintain that the radiographic image of a round, sharply-demarcated radiolucency 1 cm or greater in diameter suggests a cyst, while a smaller, less well-defined radiolucency indicates a granuloma.[19] As already stated, there is no practical need to distinguish the two entities; in fact, it is not possible to do so by radiographic criteria alone (2.7).[20–27] Numerous studies[25–30] have confirmed the lack of correlation between the size and shape of the radiolucencies and their histology. Furthermore, even histologically, there is no clear division between granulomas and cysts: small lesions may contain cystic vacuoles, and large lesions may consist entirely of granulation tissue (2.8). The only way to make a correct

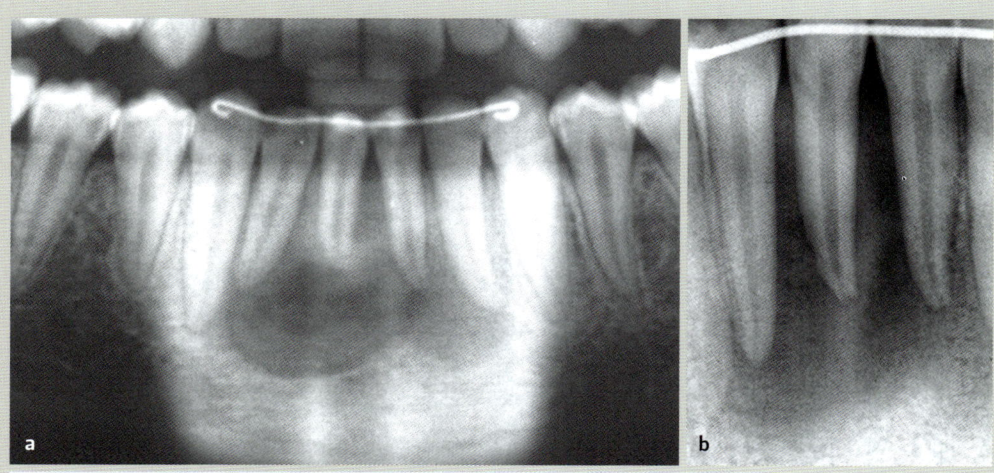

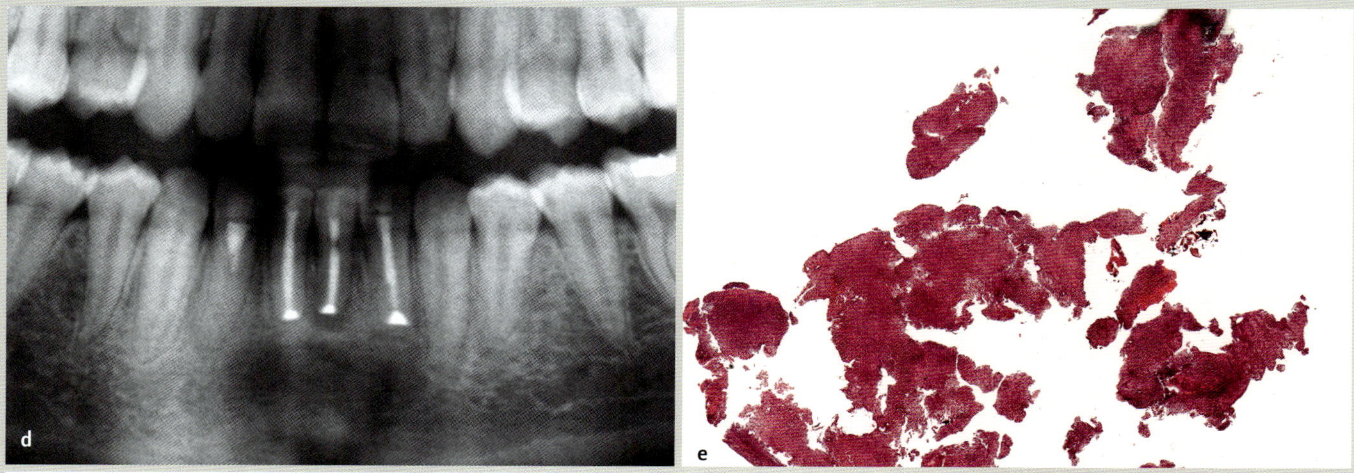

c

In data 17/1/2006 la paziente è stata sottoposta ad intervento chirurgico in anestesia generale consistito in:

- Enucleazione di neoformazione cistica in regione 42-41-31-32;
- Accurato curettage osseo:
- Apicectomia con otturazione retrograda in amalgama dei 41,31,32;
- Lavaggi della cavità residua;
- Sutura in seta.

E' in corso esame istologico.

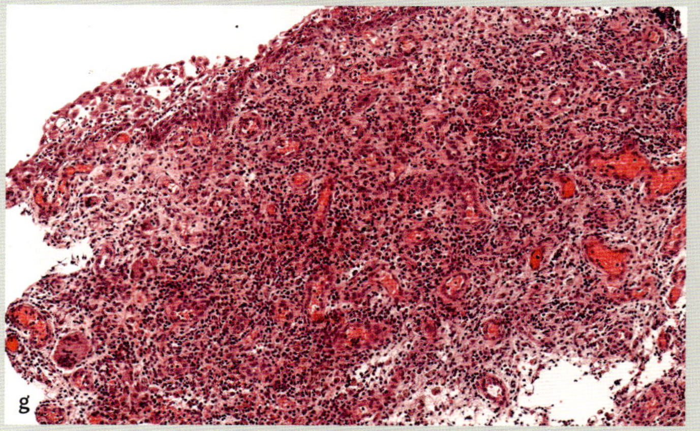

d

e

f

Azienda U.S.L. di

ANATOMIA ISTOLOGIA PATOLOGICA E CITODIAGNOSTICA

Esame Istologico n.

01/02/06

MARIANNA
nata il 21/05/89
Esame richiesto il 19/01/06 da:
CASA DI CURA HOSPITAL

BIOPSIA - MANDIBOLA

Inclusioni:

A x1

Diagnosi
Cheratocisti odontogena, flogosata.

T-11180 M-92700

Il Direttore

g

2.7 **a)** The panoramic radiograph shows the presence of a large lesion in a 15-year-old girl. The maxillo-facial surgeon made the diagnosis of a cyst. **b)** Intraoral radiograph of the same lesion involving four lower incisors. **c)** The young patient has been treated in the hospital by a maxillo-facial surgeon under general anesthesia for the removal of the "cystic lesion" and an accurate bone curettage. **d)** Two years after surgery. **e)** During surgery, a biopsy was taken for histologic examination. **f)** The histo-pathologist made the diagnosis of inflamed "odontogenic keratocyst". **g)** The histologic section at higher magnifications shows just a simple granuloma.

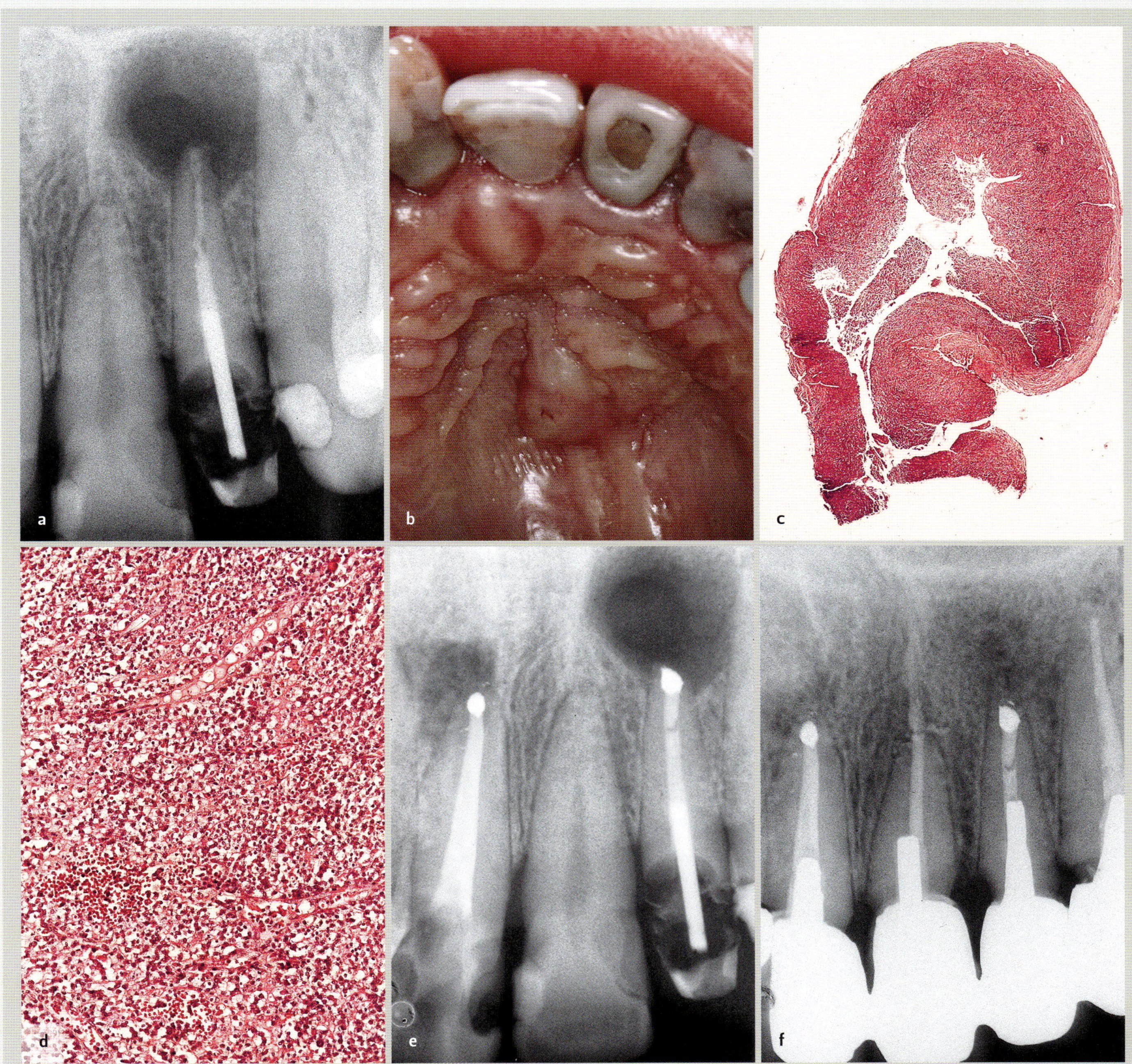

2.8 a) Preoperative radiograph of the upper left lateral incisor. The shape, degree of radiolucency, sharp borders, and size suggest a cystic lesion. **b)** A palatal swelling is present. **c)** Histologic appearance of the lesion (×2,5). **d)** At high magnification, the lesion has all the characteristics of a granuloma (×250). **e)** Postoperative radiograph. Retrofilling has also been performed on the right central incisor. **f)** One year later. Note the "apical scar" several millimeters above the root of the lateral incisor.

diagnosis is by histopathological examination, but there are numerous histological transitional forms.[20] However, the differential diagnosis must be made with other radiolucencies that cannot be attributed to pulp necrosis and that radiographically may resemble odontogenic cysts. These are lateral periodontal cysts, cysts of the incisor canal, cysts of the naso-palatine duct (📷 2.9), traumatic cysts,[31] also called hemorrhagic[32] or solitary[33] cysts (📷 2.10) which are bony cavities lacking an epithelial lining,[34] and keratocysts[35,36] (📷 2.11).

Cysts should be treated by endodontic therapy, by which even unsuspected or undiagnosed cysts are treated with resolution. Bhaskar[22] claims that cysts represent about 42% of bony rarefactions at the apices of teeth with a necrotic pulp. The high success rate of endodontic therapy, which according to Ingle[37] ranges from 80% to 90%, is indirect confirmation that odontogenic cysts resolve with proper endodontic therapy (admittedly, though, many oral surgeons would not concur) (📷 2.12).

The treatment of choice for cysts is therefore not surgical enucleation, but endodontic therapy of the diseased necrotic tooth, followed, as per usual, by periodic check-ups and radiographs[38] (📷 2.5). Surgical treatment is indicated only *after* traditional nonsurgical therapy has failed or if new symptoms develop[39]

Cont'd on page 23

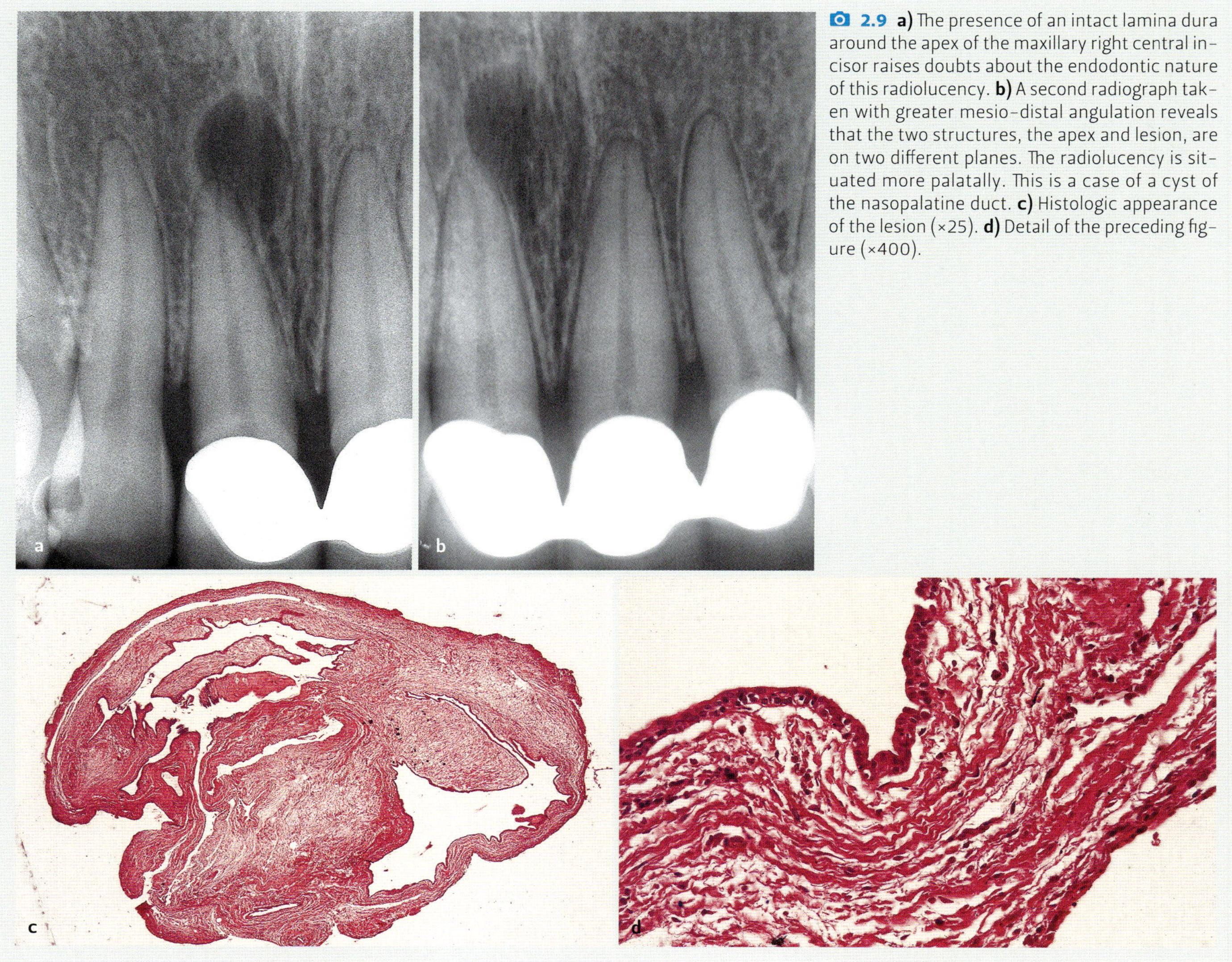

📷 **2.9 a)** The presence of an intact lamina dura around the apex of the maxillary right central incisor raises doubts about the endodontic nature of this radiolucency. **b)** A second radiograph taken with greater mesio-distal angulation reveals that the two structures, the apex and lesion, are on two different planes. The radiolucency is situated more palatally. This is a case of a cyst of the nasopalatine duct. **c)** Histologic appearance of the lesion (×25). **d)** Detail of the preceding figure (×400).

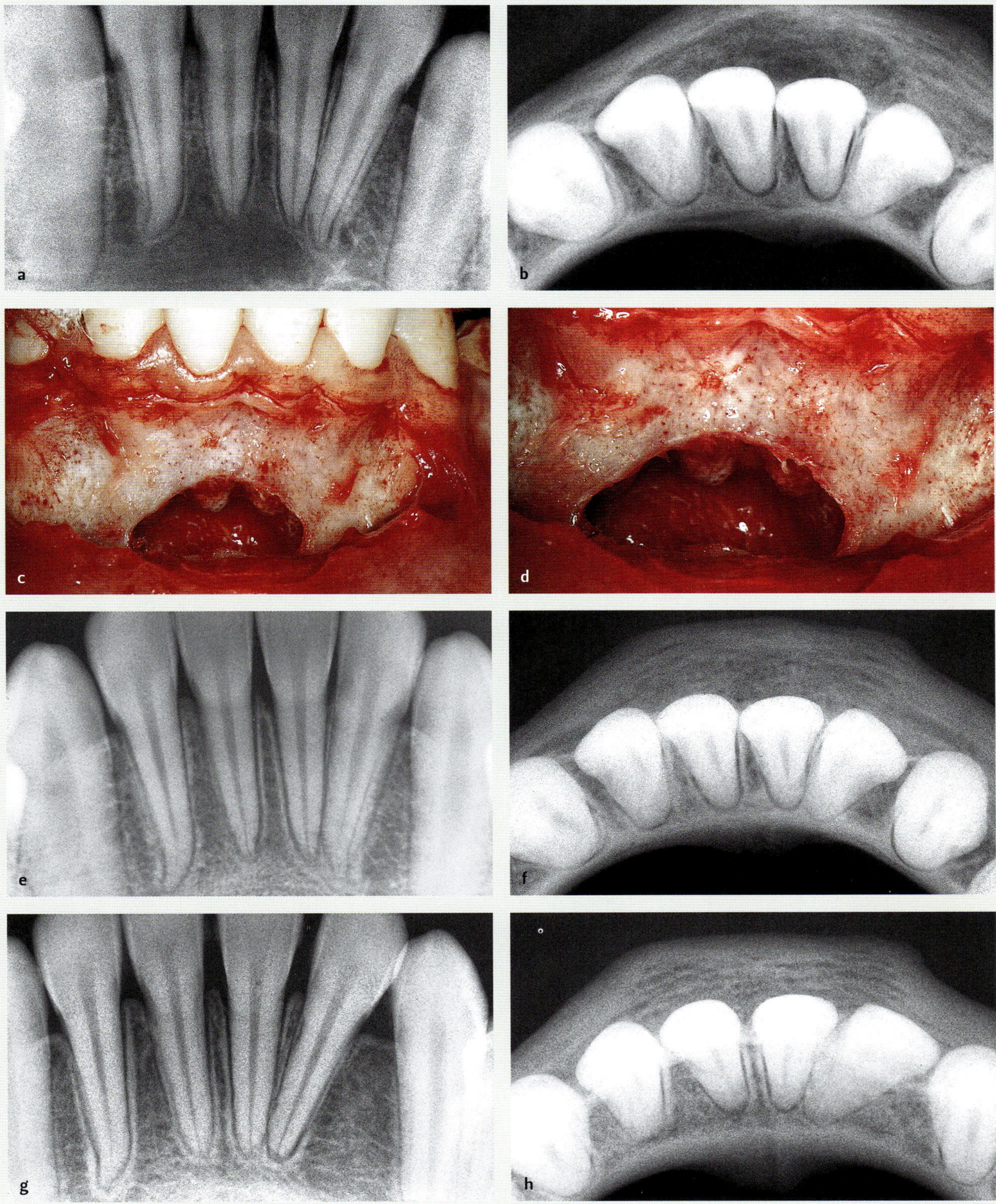

2.10 **a)** Preoperative radiograph of the lower incisors. A large radiolucency with sharp borders is present. It seems to involve the apices of the four incisors and that of the right canine. All the teeth respond positively to the vitality tests. The young patient recounted a history of trauma in this area about two years before. The diagnosis of traumatic cyst was made. **b)** The same lesion seen in an occlusal radiograph. **c)** The flap has been raised and the thin layer of vestibular bone has been removed. The cavity appears empty, lacking any hemorrhagic or cystic content, and it is not lined by epithelium. Note that the apices of the two incisors seem to dip into the cyst. **d)** The bony cavity at higher magnification. The two apical foramina of the right central incisor are visible. **e)** Eight months later. **f)** The same area seen in an occlusal radiograph. **g)** Four years later. The teeth have preserved their pulp vitality. **h)** The same area radiographed in an occlusal projection.

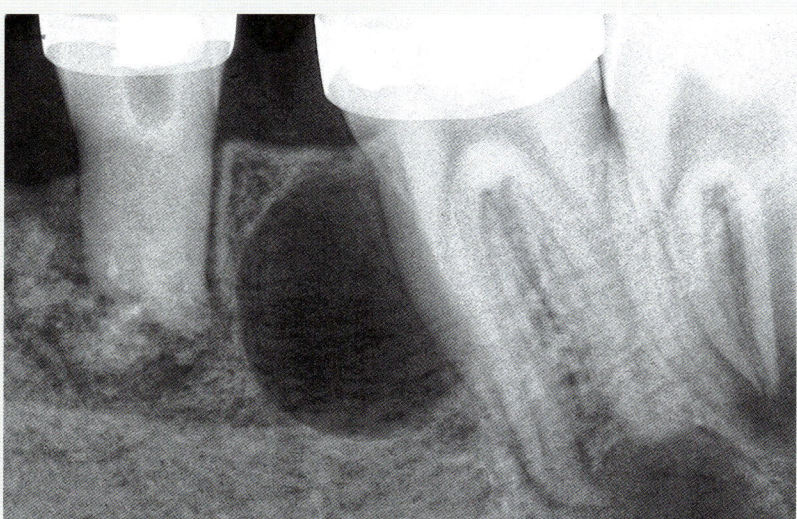

2.11. Keratocysts in a patient with Gorlin-Golz Syndrome, or basocellular nevomatosis. (*Case published by Gazzotti et al.*[32])

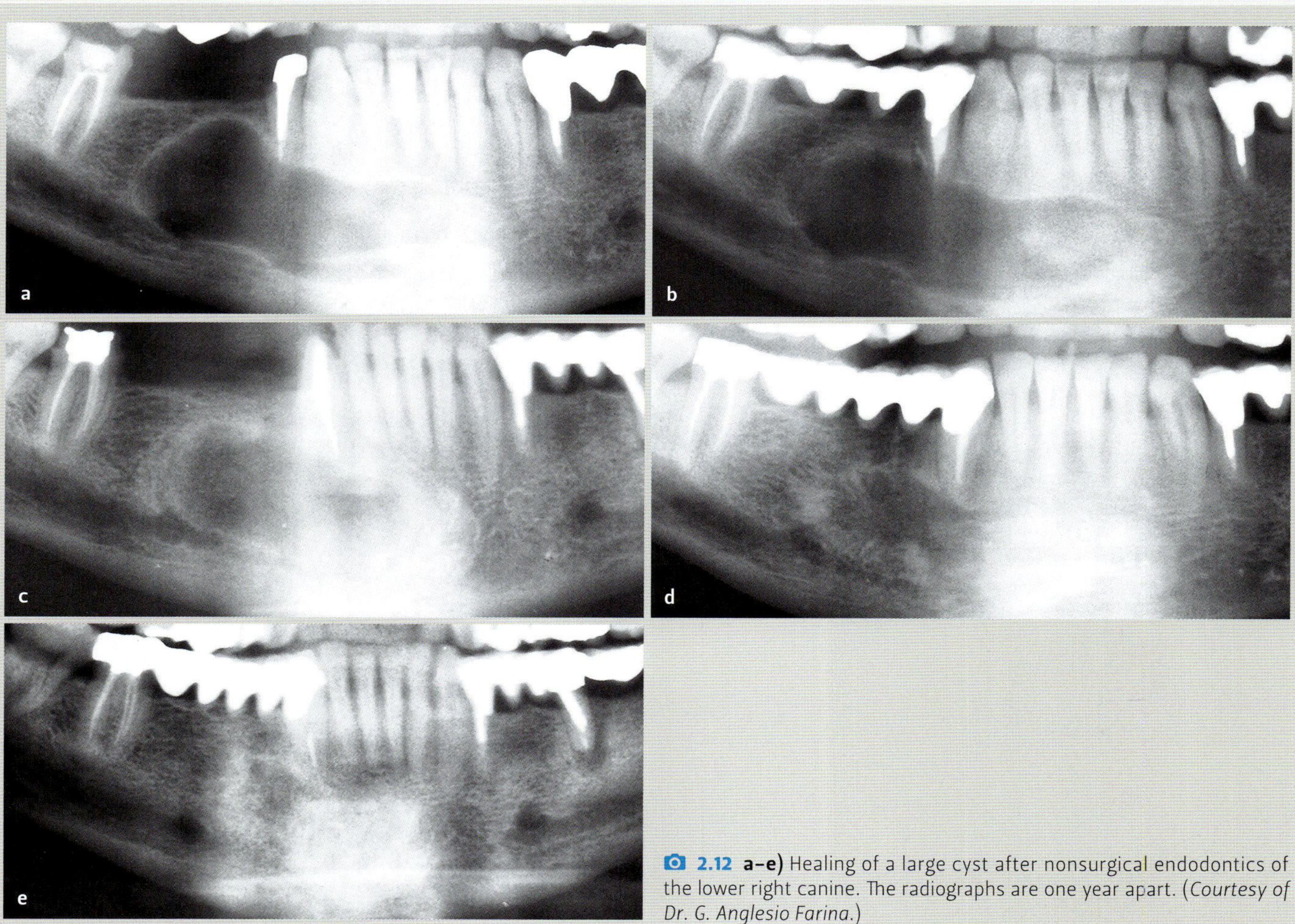

2.12 a–e) Healing of a large cyst after nonsurgical endodontics of the lower right canine. The radiographs are one year apart. (*Courtesy of Dr. G. Anglesio Farina.*)

(2.13, 2.14). Furthermore, when intervening surgically, enucleation of the cyst may be indicated only if it is absolutely certain that it will not compromise the vascular peduncles of nearby apices or important adjacent anatomical structures, such as the floor of the maxillary sinus, nasal fossae, mental nerve, or inferior alveolar nerve. If there is even the slightest doubt, it is preferable to excise a small flap of the cystic wall, which will suffice to assure adequate surgical access to the apex of the involved tooth. The remains of the lesion may be left in place (2.13, 2.15) without concern.[40]

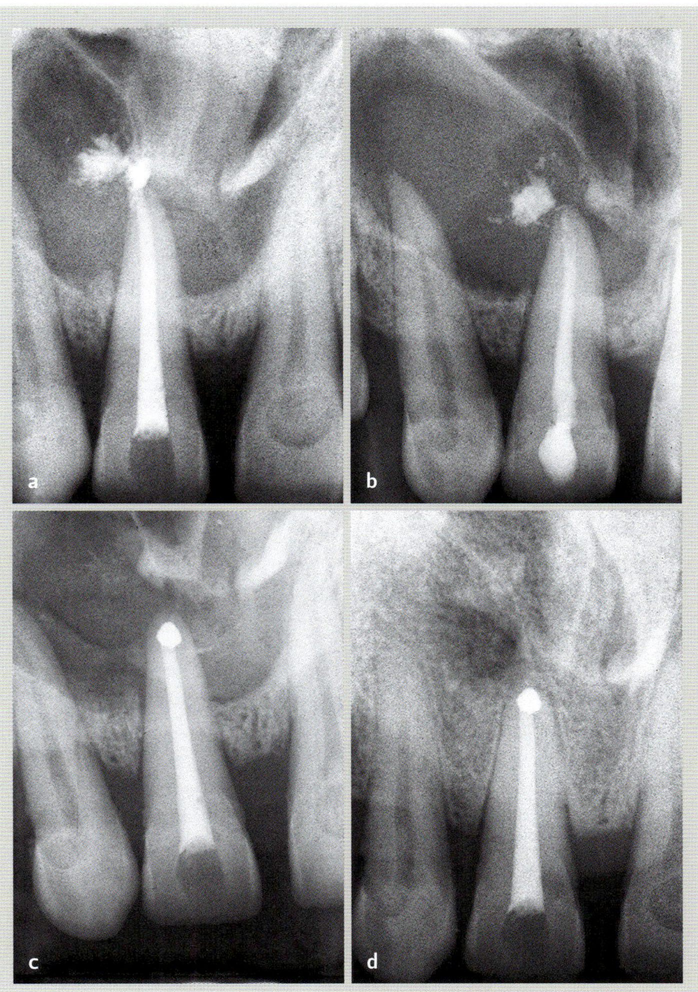

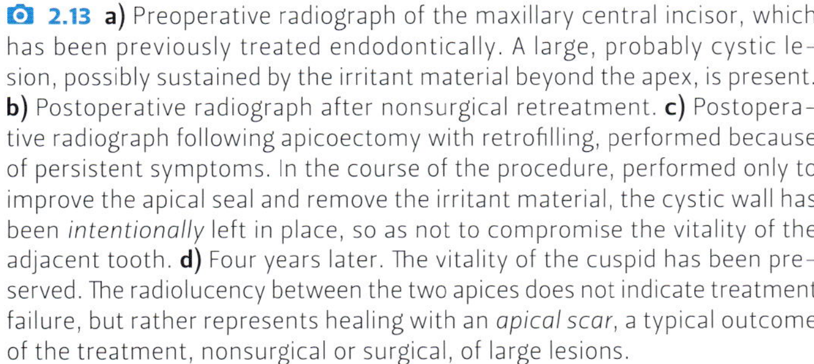

2.13 a) Preoperative radiograph of the maxillary central incisor, which has been previously treated endodontically. A large, probably cystic lesion, possibly sustained by the irritant material beyond the apex, is present. **b)** Postoperative radiograph after nonsurgical retreatment. **c)** Postoperative radiograph following apicoectomy with retrofilling, performed because of persistent symptoms. In the course of the procedure, performed only to improve the apical seal and remove the irritant material, the cystic wall has been *intentionally* left in place, so as not to compromise the vitality of the adjacent tooth. **d)** Four years later. The vitality of the cuspid has been preserved. The radiolucency between the two apices does not indicate treatment failure, but rather represents healing with an *apical scar*, a typical outcome of the treatment, nonsurgical or surgical, of large lesions.

2.14 a) Preoperative radiograph of the upper right lateral incisor. A large, abscess-like cystic lesion is present. The canine and the first premolar respond positively to the vitality tests, while the central incisor gives a negative response. **b)** An acute alveolar abscess has developed from a chronic lesion and is visible on the palate. **c)** Postoperative radiograph. **d)** Eight years following apicoectomy. Following the recurrence of acute symptoms (presumably related to inadequacy of the apical seal consequent to the difficulty of achieving a dry canal), apicoectomy with amalgam retrofilling was performed on both the lateral and central incisors.

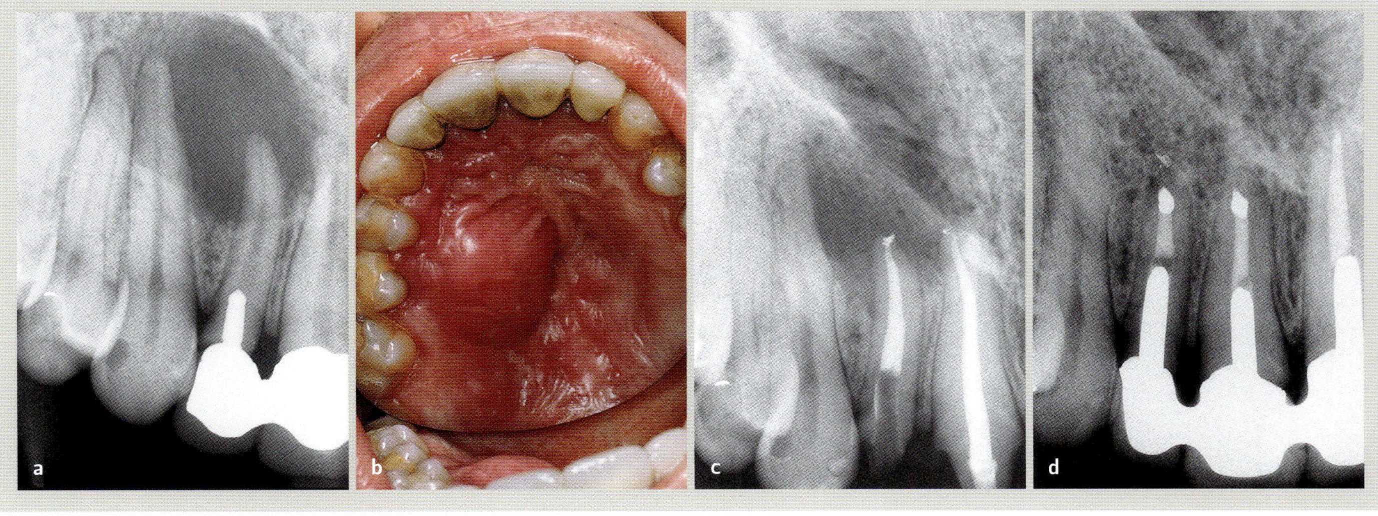

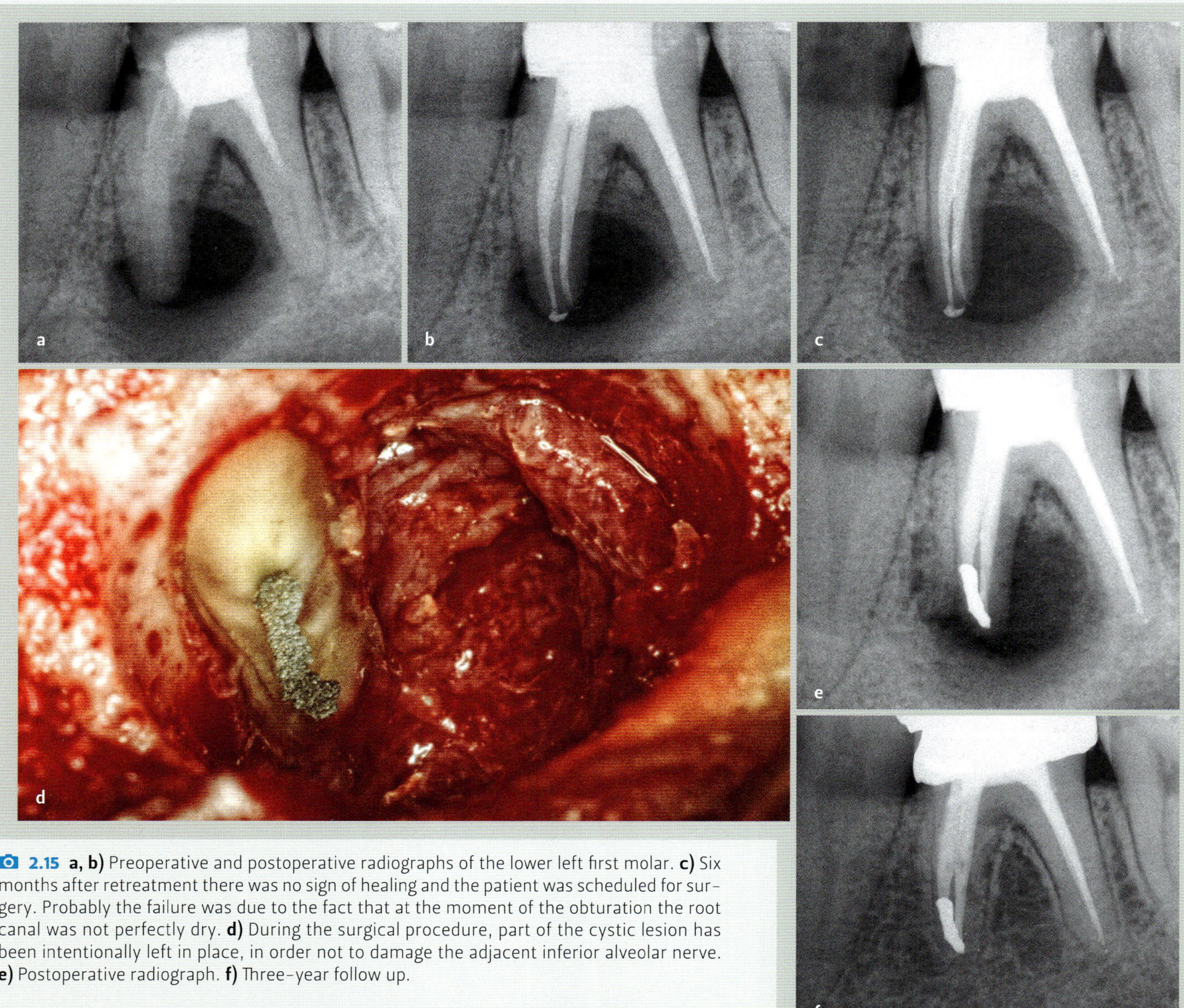

2.15 **a, b)** Preoperative and postoperative radiographs of the lower left first molar. **c)** Six months after retreatment there was no sign of healing and the patient was scheduled for surgery. Probably the failure was due to the fact that at the moment of the obturation the root canal was not perfectly dry. **d)** During the surgical procedure, part of the cystic lesion has been intentionally left in place, in order not to damage the adjacent inferior alveolar nerve. **e)** Postoperative radiograph. **f)** Three-year follow up.

2.16 Disto-buccal root of a maxillary first molar extracted with a periapical lesion attached. **a)** Section encompassing one apical foramen. A central cavity filled with necrotic debris and completely lined by epithelium is present. No communication between the cyst cavity and the foramen can be observed (hematoxylin and eosin, original magnification ×16). **b)** Section cut 100 sections away from that in **(a)**. One foramen is present at the geometrical top of the root and another on the right profile. The cyst cavity is still independent from the root canal space. No communication was found in any of the serial sections, and the histologic diagnosis was "true cyst". Note that the lumen of the large ramification is completely filled with a bacterial biofilm (Taylor's modified Brown & Brenn, original magnification ×16). (*Courtesy of Dr. Domenico Ricucci.*)

"True cyst" and "Pocket cyst"

Two types of cysts have been described in chronic apical periodontitis lesions: the true cyst (2.16) and the pocket cyst (2.17). The true cyst is completely enclosed by a lining epithelium, and its lumen has no communication with the root canal of the involved tooth[41,42] while the pocket cyst is a sack-shaped apical inflammatory lesion, with the epithelium-lined cystic lumen open to and continuous with the root canal.[41]

True cysts are characterized by the presence of one or more cavities completely enclosed in an epithelial lining, which in none of the serial sections show connection with the canal lumen.

The lesions classified as pocket cysts show a cystic space surrounded by an epithelial wall that joins the external root surface forming a "sac", insulating the foramen from the rest of the lesion. The cystic cavity has direct communication with the canal lumen.

According to Ricucci and Siqueira,[41] it can be extremely difficult to clearly differentiate between pocket cysts and true cysts, especially in cases of complex root canal anatomy in the apical third, with multiple ramifications that end at a certain distance from one another on the root surface. In fact, this differential diagnosis can only be delivered easily in the presence of a single large root canal that ends near the geometric tip (anatomic apex) of the root. The studies by Nair and his group[43–45] have repeatedly shown only sections of roots with simple root canal anatomy, not even mentioning the possible frequent variations. In other words, in cases of complex apical root canal anatomy, depending on the histological sections of the same sample, both diagnosis can be made, depending on whether the cyst is in communication with the root canal or not.

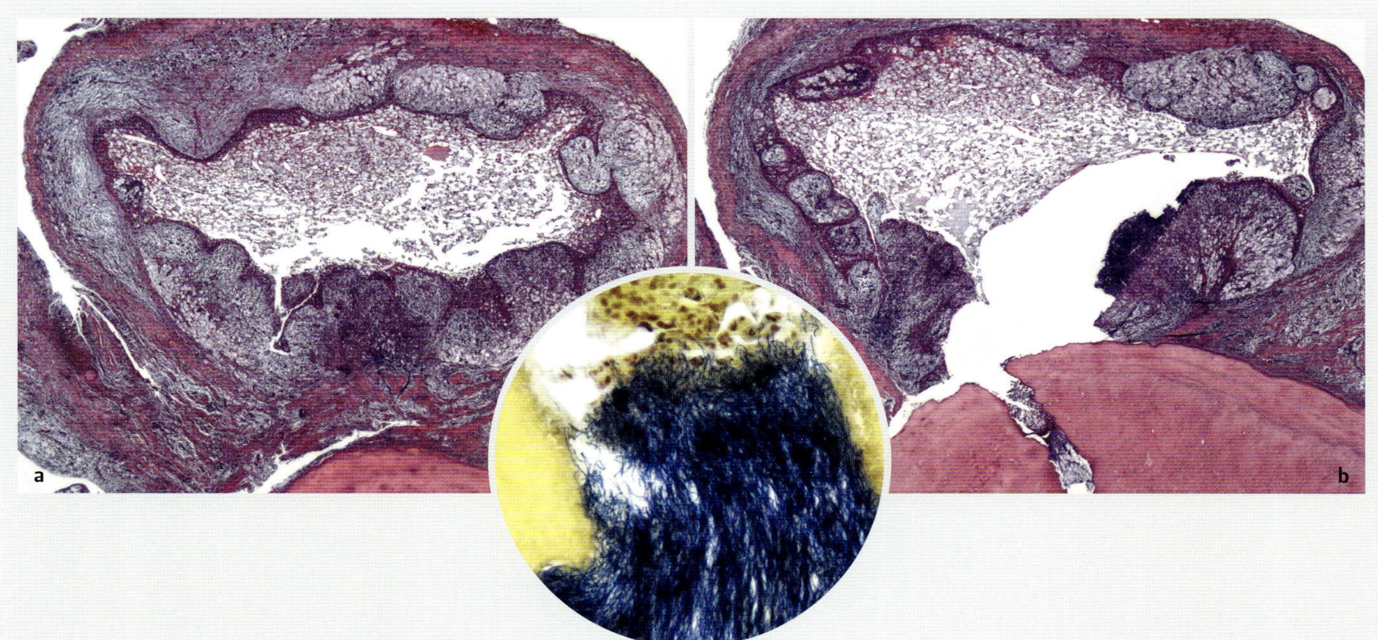

2.17 Maxillary third molar extracted with a large periapical lesion. **a)** Section cut approximately at the center of the mass, not encompassing the apical foramen. The center of the lesion is occupied by a space filled with debris and cholesterol crystals, completely lined by epithelium. Based on this section only, the histologic diagnosis of this lesion would be "true cyst" (hematoxylin and eosin, original magnification ×16). **b)** Section taken approximately 120 sections away from that in **(a)** showing a completely different morphology of the lesion. The cyst lumen is contiguous with the root canal space, the reason for which the correct diagnosis is "pocket cyst" (original magnification ×16). **Inset.** Section proximal to that in **(b)**. High power view from the foramen shows the presence of a thick bacterial biofilm faced with a concentration of PMNs (Taylor's modified Brown & Brenn, original magnification ×400).

Considerations. 1) The histologic diagnosis of "true" or "pocket" cyst can be made exclusively when a serial sectioning procedure is adopted. 2) Irrespective of the morphologic type of cyst, the etiology is infection of the apical canal space. There is no reason why the "true" cyst should not heal if infection is controlled by treatment procedures. (*Courtesy of Dr. Domenico Ricucci.*)

At the same time, it is important to discuss whether or not apical cysts cause a treatment problem. Based on morphological observation, Nair speculated that the so-called true cyst are refractory to conventional endodontic treatment due to the lack of direct communication between the cystic lumen and the canal space. The pathologic process would be self-sustaining and, therefore, able to continue to expand independently of the influence of the root canal infection.[46,47] On the other hand, according to Ricucci and Siqueira, there is still no confirmation of this hypothesis, which is recognizably difficult to obtain based on clinical and radiographic data.[41] It is also important to point out that based on current knowledge, there is no apparent reason to believe that the two morphological varieties of cysts respond differently to root canal treatment, since they have the same pathogenic origin (infection of the endodontic space); therefore they should *not* be regarded as two distinct pathological entities.[41] As already stated, cysts should be treated by endodontic therapy alone, and surgical treatment is indicated only *after* traditional nonsurgical therapy has failed or if new symptoms develop.[39]

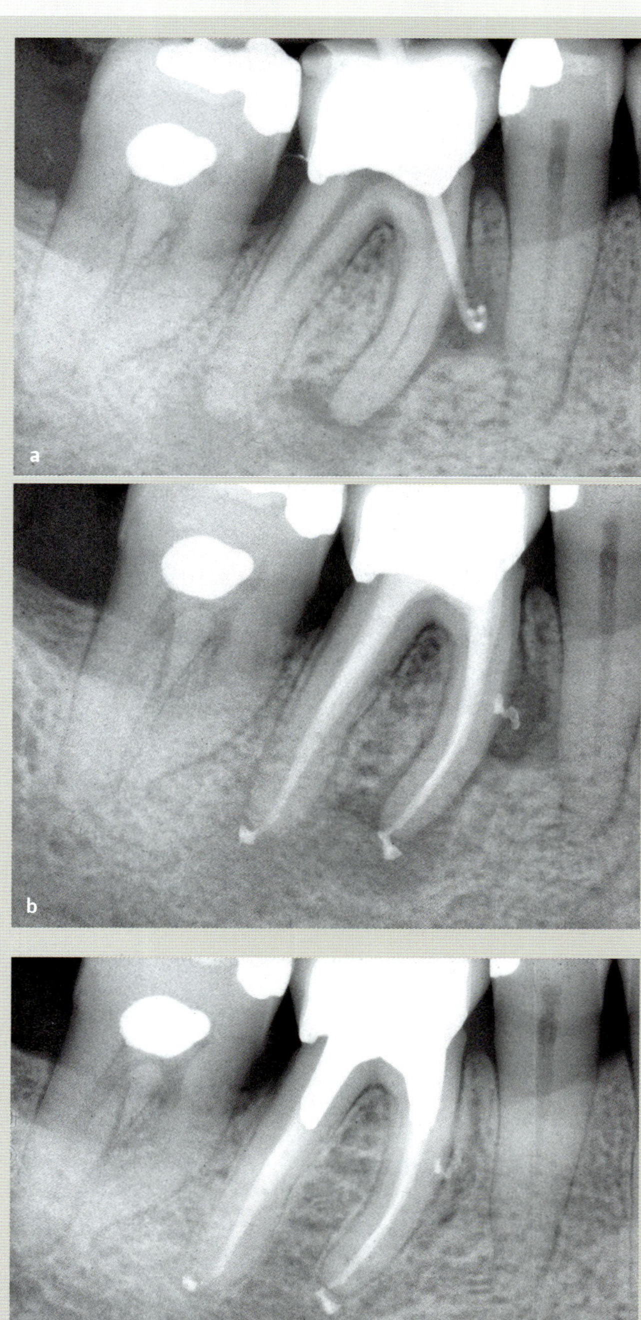

2.18 **a)** Preoperative radiograph of a lower right first molar: the tooth has a sinus tract arising from a lateral canal. **b)** Postoperative radiograph: note the filling of the lateral canal. **c)** The recall radiograph twentyfour months later shows the complete healing of both the apical and the lateral lesions.

PRESENCE OF A SINUS TRACT (2.18)

On occasion, a chronic endodontic infection will drain through an intraoral communication to the gingival surface and is known as a sinus tract.[48] This pathway, which is sometimes lined with epithelium, extends directly from the source of the infection to a surface opening, or *stoma*, on the attached gingival surface.[49] As will be described later, it can also extend extraorally. The term *fistula* is often inappropriately used to describe this type of drainage. The fistula, by definition, is actually an abnormal communication between two internal organs or a pathway between two epithelium-lined surfaces.[50]

Some authors[51–55] are still convinced that the presence of a sinus tract indicates a more serious lesion that requires special intervention, such as surgical incision and excision of the entire sinus tract, in addition to extraction of the diseased tooth (2.19), and this because of the presence of an epithelium lining of the sinus tract itself. Histologic studies have found that most sinus tracts are not lined with epithelium throughout their entire length. Harrison and Larson[56] found only 1 of the 10 sinus

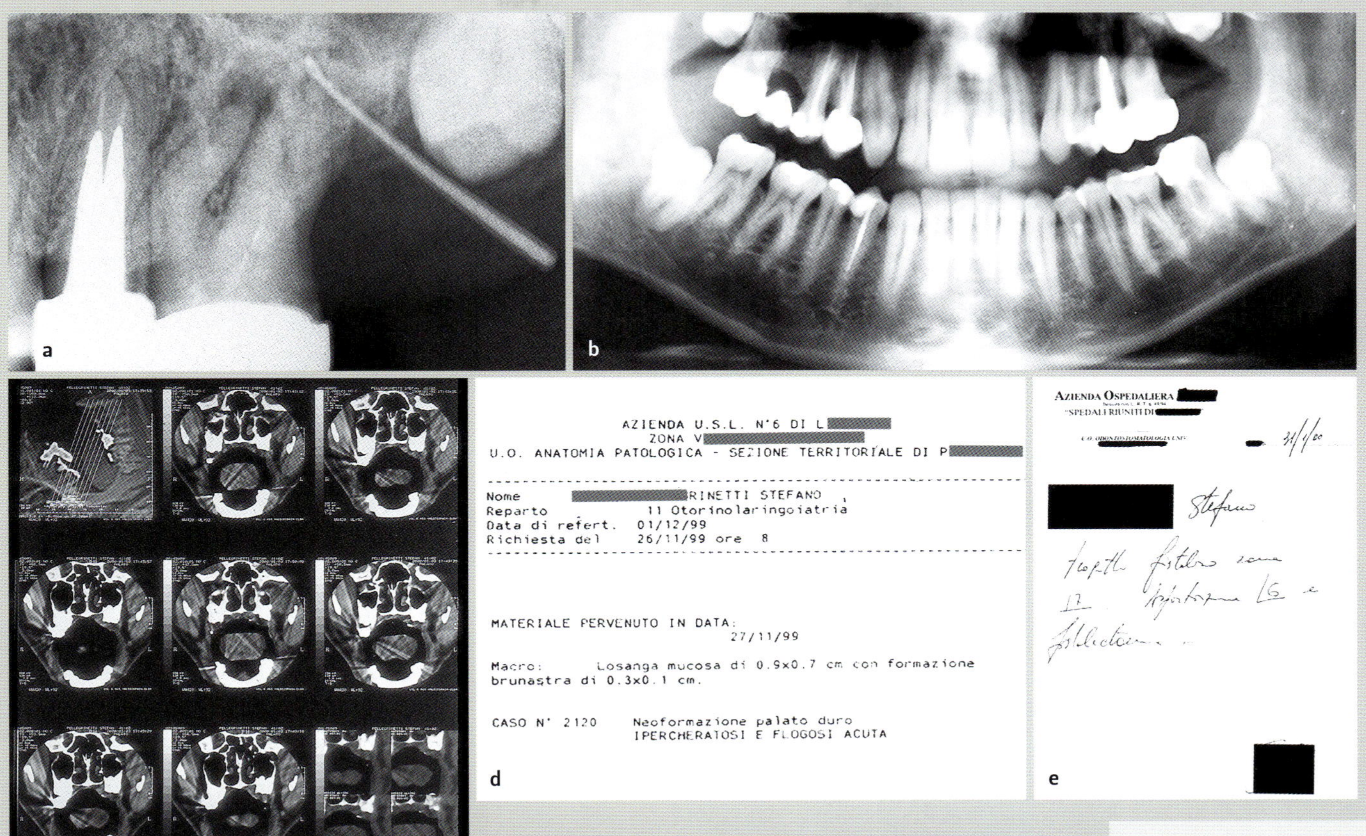

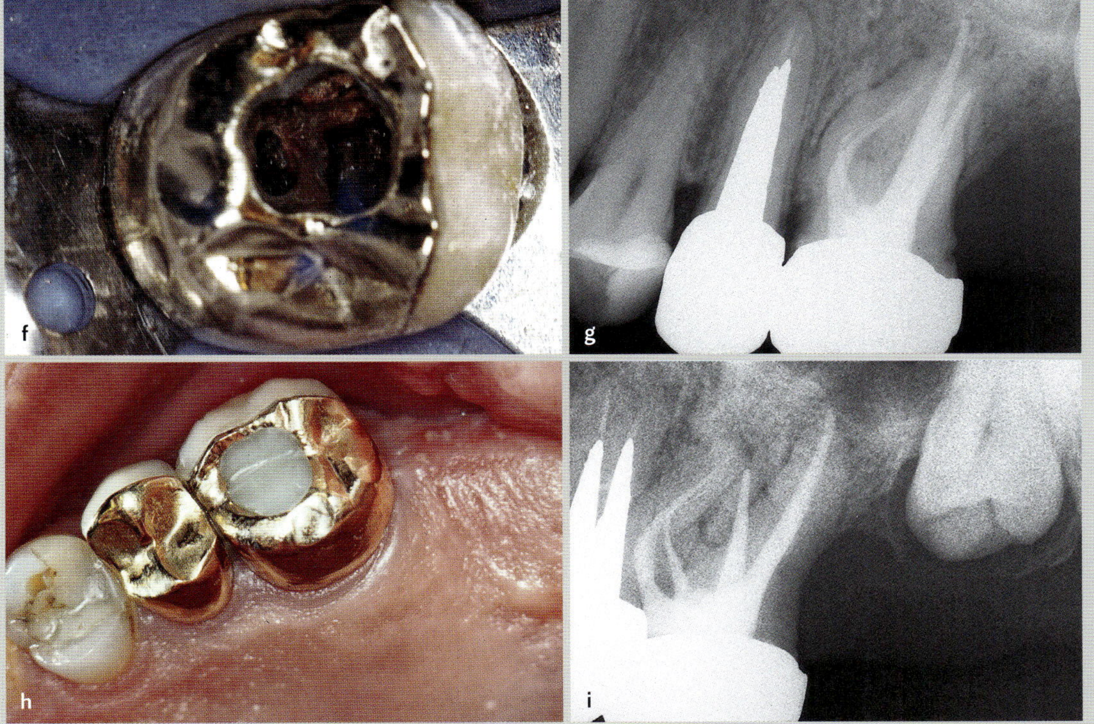

2.19 a) The endodontic treatment of the upper left first molar is completely inadequate. A gutta-percha cone is tracing a sinus tract, originating on the palate, in the area of the missing second molar. The patient was firstly examined in a hospital by an oral surgeon and was already subjected to a panoramic radiograph (**b**), a computerized tomography (**c**), a biopsy (hyperkeratosis and acute inflammation!) (**d**) and scheduled for tooth extraction and a *fistulectomy*(!) (**e**). **f)** After the removal of the old restoration, it is evident the way the access cavity was previously made: the pulp horns have been misdiagnosed for canal orifices and the clinician forgot to remove a big portion of the roof of the pulp chamber. **g)** Postoperative radiograph. **h)** The sinus tract is healed. **i)** Two-year recall radiograph.

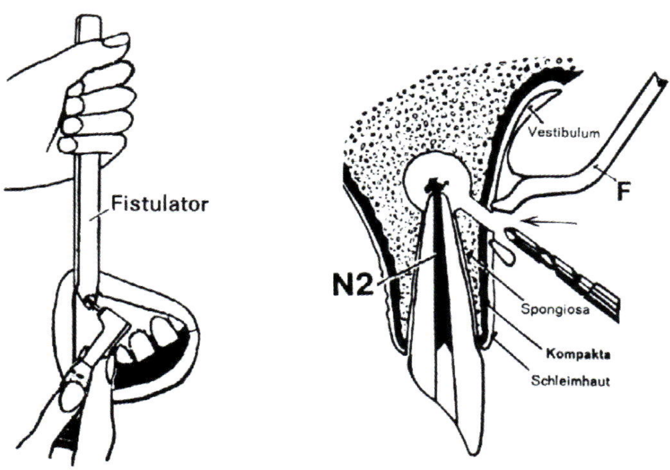

2.20 The Fistulator invented by Dr. Sargenti to create a fistula when it was not present, in order to avoid flare up![61]

tracts they studied were lined with epithelium. The other nine specimens were lined with granulation tissue. The presence or absence of an epithelial lining does not seem to prevent closure of the tract as long as the source of the problem is properly diagnosed and adequately treated and the endodontic lesion has healed. Failure of a sinus tract to heal will necessitate further diagnostic procedures to determine whether other etiologic factors are present or whether a misdiagnosis occurred.[48] In fact, the presence of a sinus tract should be seen as a favorable sign, since it is associated with a number of advantages, so much so that some authors[57–64] suggest that if there is none, one should be created (2.20).

It may be extremely helpful in diagnosis. Tracing of the sinus tract by the insertion of a gutta-percha cone

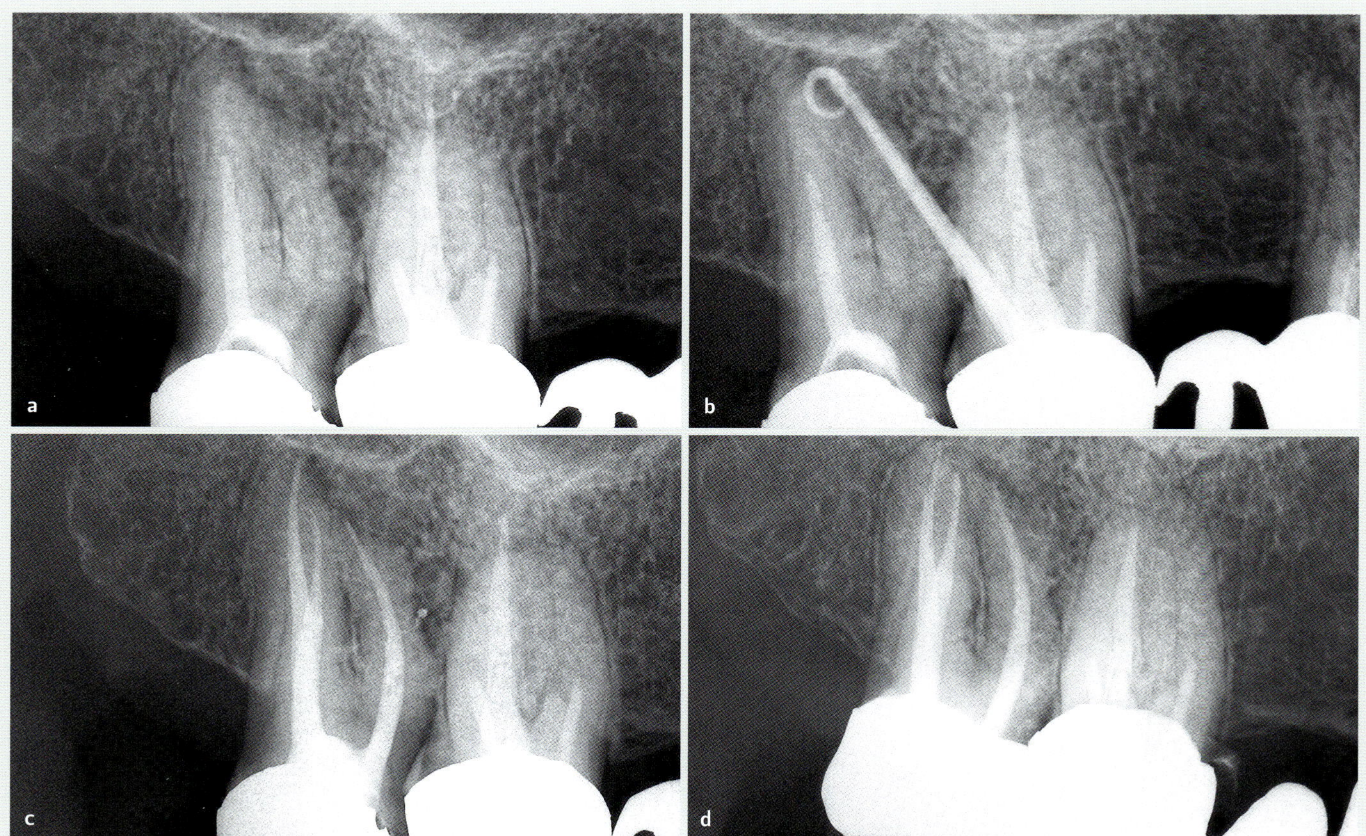

2.21 **a)** Preoperative radiograph of the upper right first and second molars. Note the round radiolucency between the mesio-buccal root of the second molar and the distobuccal root of the first. The patient had presented with a vestibular fistula at the level of the first molar, and for financial reasons only wanted to retreat the diseased tooth. **b)** A gutta-percha cone placed in the fistula indicates that the fistulous tract arises from the second molar. **c)** Postoperative radiograph of the second molar. Note that a small lateral canal in the mesio-buccal root, which was apparently responsible for the lesion seen in the preoperative film, is filled up. **d)** Five-year recall.

will provide objectivity in diagnosing the location of the problematic tooth[63] (2.21). Once the causative factors related to the development of the sinus tract are removed, the stoma and the sinus tract will close within just a few days.[48] In other situations, the sinus tract may run in the space of the periodontal ligament of the same tooth (2.22). It may even traverse the periodontal ligament of the adjacent healthy tooth,[65] thus simulating a lesion of periodontal origin (2.23, 2.24). Furthermore, healing of the lesion about one week after cleaning and shaping of the infected root canals without the use of any medications within the canal (2.25) confirms that the diagnosis was correct and testifies to the efficacy of the treatment. This also suggests a favorable prognosis for the lesion.

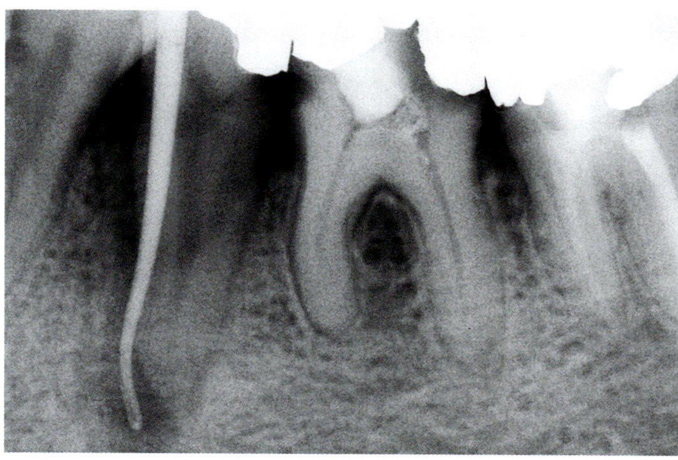

2.22 Preoperative radiograph of a necrotic lower left second premolar with a fistula opening into the space of the periodontal ligament. A gutta-percha cone has been inserted into the fistula.

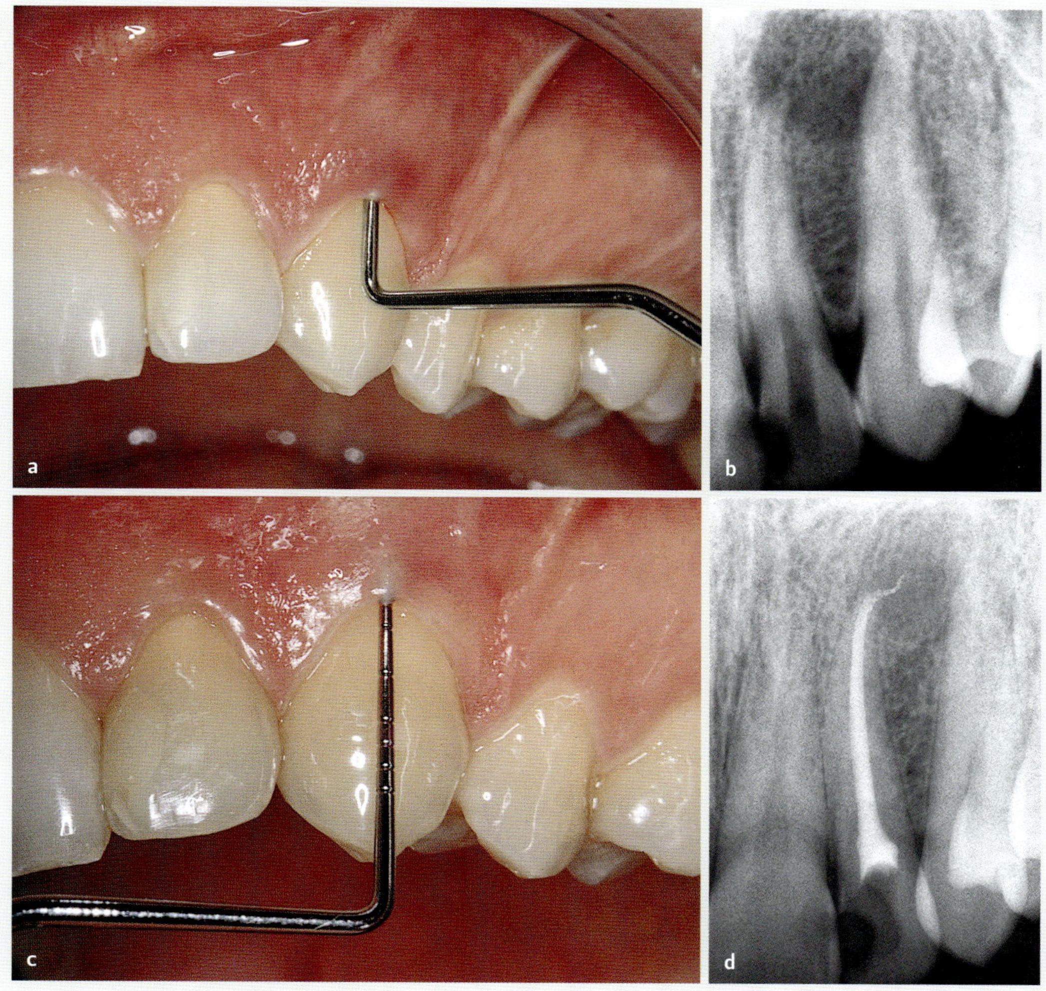

2.23 **a)** The periodontal probe disappears in the sulcus of the canine in a patient with good oral hygiene and healthy periodontium in the other quadrants. The canine responds positively to the tests of vitality, while the lateral incisor is necrotic. **b)** Preoperative radiograph of the lateral incisor. Note that the lesion "rests" on the mesial side of the root of the adjacent canine. **c)** Clinical appearance of the canine gingiva one week after cleaning and shaping of the lateral incisor. **d)** Postoperative radiograph.

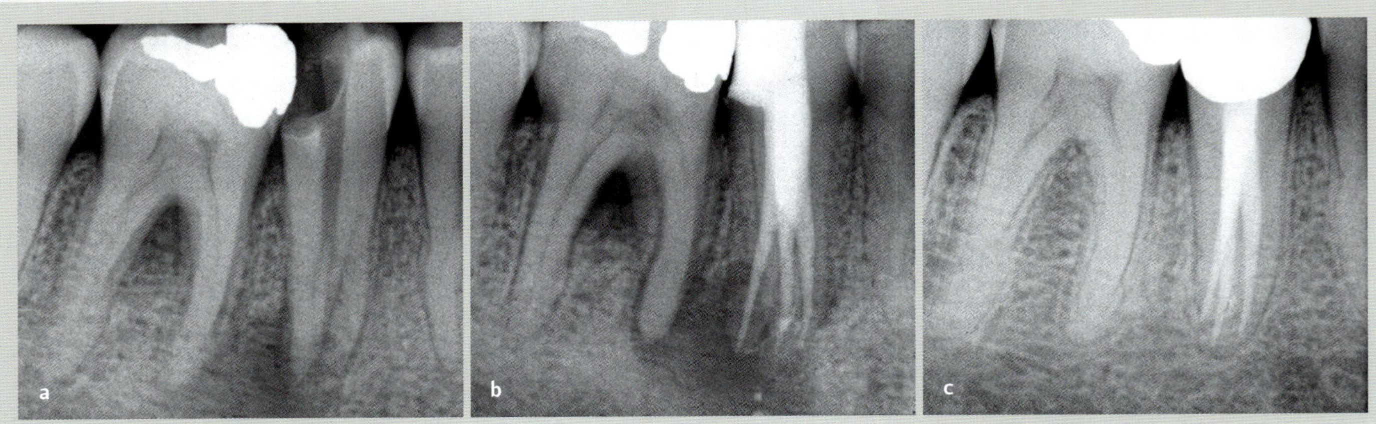

2.24 The first mandibular molar has a furcation involvement. The tooth has a vital pulp and the patient has no periodontal disease in the other quadrants of his mouth. The radiolucency is not of periodontal origin but rather is a primary endodontic lesion caused by the necrotic pulp of the second premolar. Its lesion is draining through the periodontal ligament of the molar, in the area of the furcation. **a)** Preoperative radiograph. **b)** Postoperative radiograph. **c)** Four-year recall.

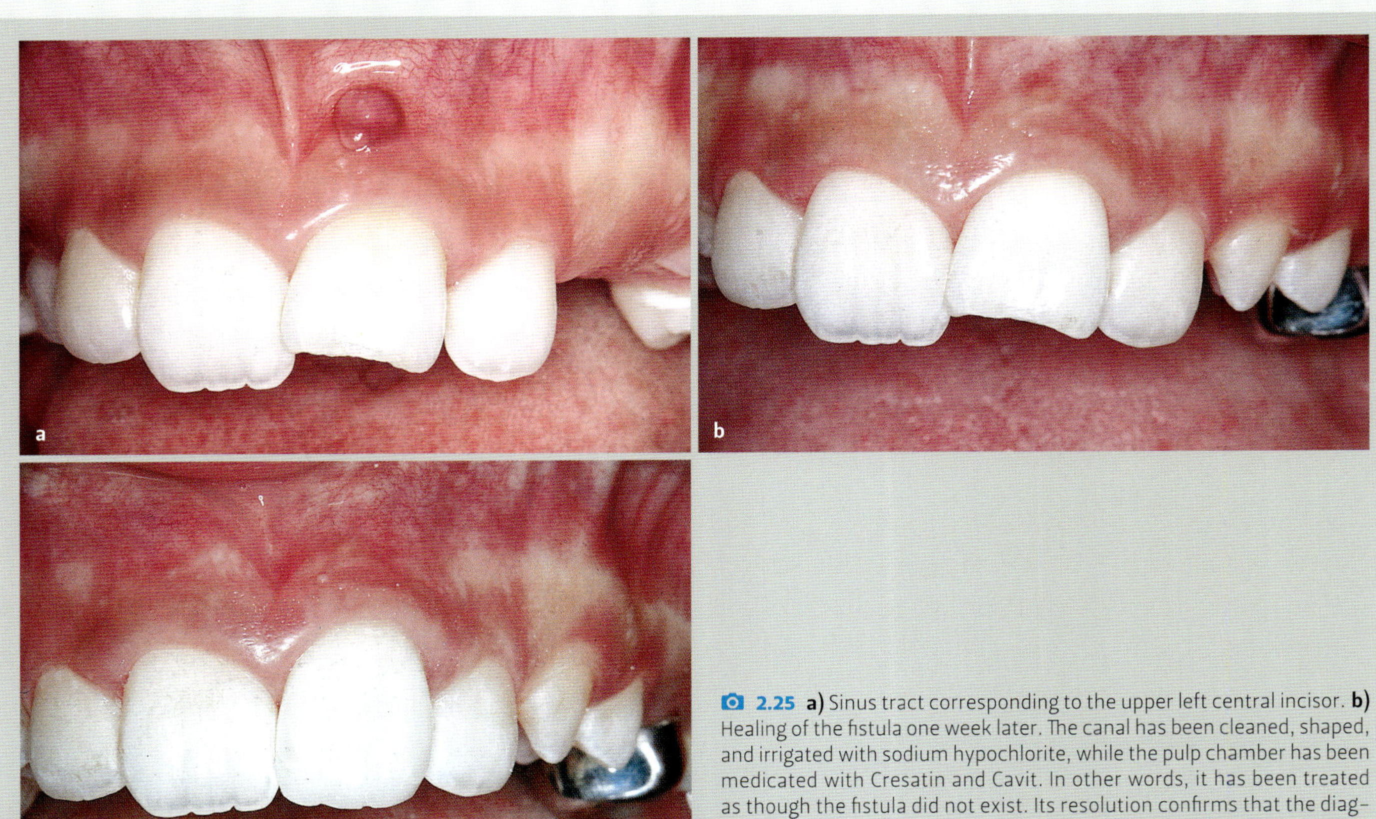

2.25 **a)** Sinus tract corresponding to the upper left central incisor. **b)** Healing of the fistula one week later. The canal has been cleaned, shaped, and irrigated with sodium hypochlorite, while the pulp chamber has been medicated with Cresatin and Cavit. In other words, it has been treated as though the fistula did not exist. Its resolution confirms that the diagnosis and therapy were correct and justifies proceeding with three-dimensional filling of this root canal system. **c)** Another view one year later.

The pus creates a tract in the surrounding tissues, following the *loci minoris resistentiae*. It may exit at any point of the oral mucosa or even the skin.[66] It is not uncommon, particularly in young patients, to find extraoral stoma at the level of the mental symphysis, if lower incisors are involved (2.26), or in the submandibular region, if a lower first molar is involved (2.27), or in the floor of the nasal fossa, if a central incisor is involved.[67,68]

Extraoral sinus tracts, which unfortunately are sometimes treated as though they were independent dermatologic lesions, have the same pathogenic and prognostic significance as mucosal sinus tracts and require the same therapy.[69,70] A review of the literature[71–74] reveals that patients with extraoral sinus tracts are sometimes subjected to repeated surgical excisions and biopsies (2.19d) before it is clear that the sinus tract is none other than an extension of pulp disease in the periradicular tissues. Many patients with extraoral sinus tracts will give a history of being treated by general physicians and dermatologists with systemic or topical antibiotics and/or surgical procedures in attempts to heal the extraoral stoma. In these particular cases, only after multiple treatment failures are the patients finally referred to a dental clinician to determine whether there is a dental etiology.[75]

Trying to treat such lesions with a circular incision of the orifice of the extraoral sinus tract and excision of its entire tract, with all the ramifications – particularly esthetic – of such an intervention, is not consistent with the present standard of care and can be considered pure folly.

The diseased tooth associated with the sinus tract must be identified and the root canal system cleaned, shaped and obturated to have complete healing after about one week.

If the tooth presents any obstacles to nonsurgical treatment or retreatment, or if the patient specifically requests surgery, one may proceed surgically, but one's attention must be directed solely to achieving a retro-

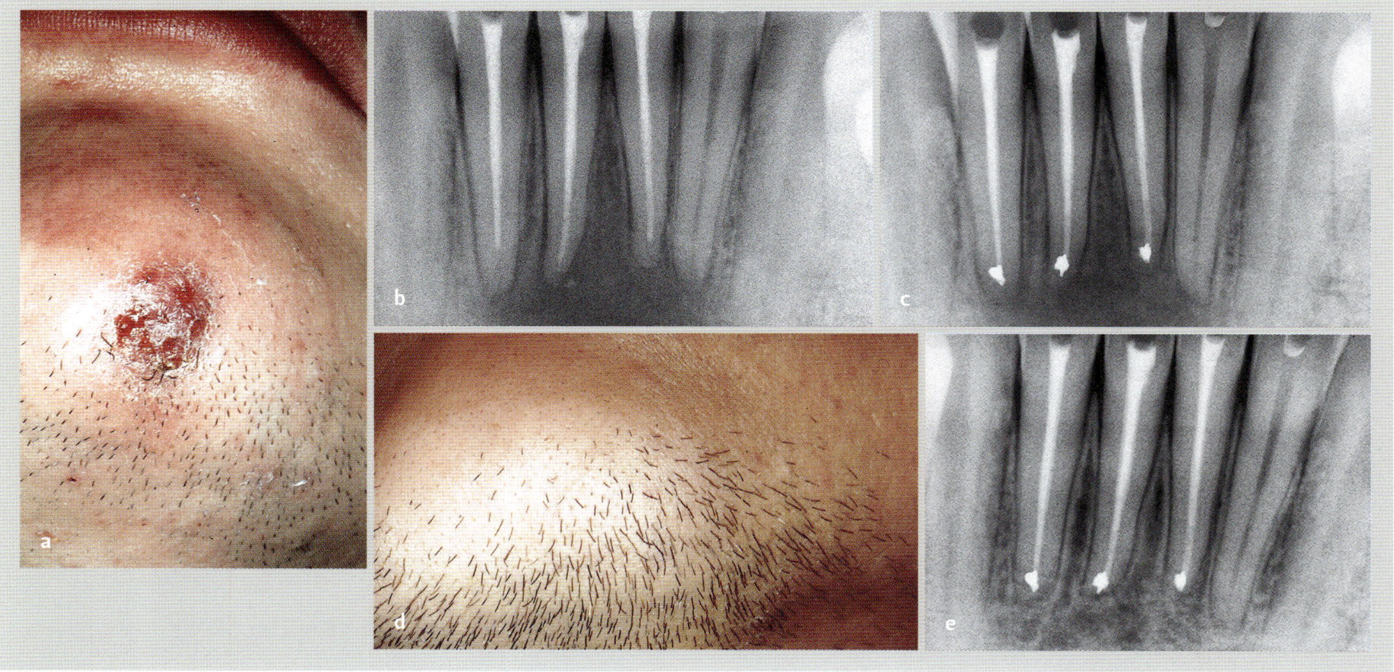

2.26 **a)** Cutaneous sinus tract in the mental region. **b)** Preoperative radiograph of the lower incisors. The patient elected surgical therapy for economical reasons. The left lateral incisor had already been subjected to a cavity test. **c)** Postoperative radiograph. Three apicoectomies with amalgam retrofilling have been performed. **Not** the least attention has been paid to removal of all the granulation tissue **or** to curettage of the surrounding bone or apices, **or** to removal of the sinus tract, **or** even to circular incision of the cutaneous orifice of the sinus tract. **d)** Complete healing of the cutaneous sinus tract without any residual scarring after two years. **e)** Radiograph two years later confirms total resolution of the previous radiolucency. The patient was treated several years before ultrasonic tips and MTA became available.

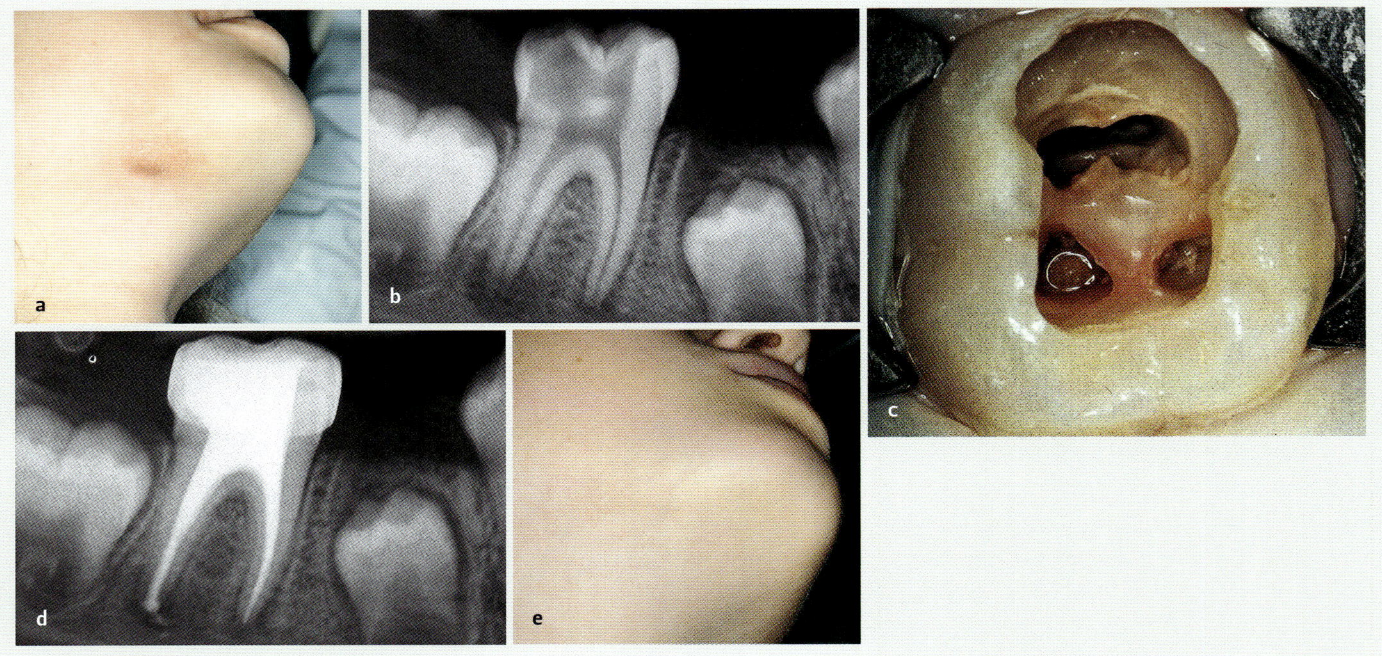

2.27 **a)** Cutaneous fistula in the right submandibular region. **b)** Preoperative radiograph of the ipsilateral lower first molar. The tooth had been "opened" one month before and left open "to drain". Note the small radiopacity at the center of the access cavity, due to remnants of the chamber's roof left in place. **c)** Clinical appearance of the access cavity: three openings have been made in the roof of the pulp chamber! One, corresponding to the distal canal, is shaped like an "8"; the two round ones correspond to the mesial canals: the pulp horns have been misdiagnosed for canal orifices. **d)** Postoperative radiograph. The tooth has been pretreated with a copper band. **e)** Healing of the fistulous tract two years later. Note the complete absence of any scarring.

grade apical seal, and not eliminating the sinus tract or its cutaneous orifice (2.26). As already stated, the reason why some authors believe in the need for surgical removal of the sinus tract lies in the mistaken conviction that it is lined by an epithelium.[76] Grossman[39] states, however, that such tracts are lined by granulation tissue. In his study, he was unable to identify any epithelium at all.

Bender and Seltzer[77] have also made histologic studies of numerous sinus tracts without finding an epithelial lining.

Other authors[49,63,78] agree that the sinus tract may be lined by flat, multilayered epithelial cells, but that more often it is lined by granulation tissue, with acute and chronic inflammatory cells.

Given the current state of knowledge, there is no reason to recommend surgical removal of such tracts. There is no reason that even epithelium-lined fistulous tracts should not heal after appropriate endodontic therapy.

When it is present, the epithelium may arise from the oral mucosa or proliferating epithelial cells from the periapical lesion. However, there is no correlation between the presence or absence of an epithelium and the clinical appearance of the fistula or its chronicity. In animal experiments, Ordman and Gillman[79] have demonstrated that cutaneous sutures may become completely epithelialized if the sutures are left in place for several weeks. Once they are removed, on the other hand, the epithelium-lined tract always heals completely.

There is no reason that the same should not happen to the possibly present epithelium of the sinus tract of a necrotic tooth once the inflammatory stimulus is removed.

Obviously, these sinus tracts must be distinguished from congenital fistulae of the neck, both lateral (arising from the second branchial cleft) and medial (arising from rests of the thyroglossal duct), which are lined by an epithelium. Such fistulae, however, have a different pathogenesis and obviously do not resolve spontaneously, but only after careful surgical excision of the entire tract.[79] The differential diagnosis includes the following:[67,69]

- localized skin infections, such as pyoderma, pimples, ingrown hairs, and obstructed sweat glands
- traumatic or iatrogenic lesions
- osteomyelitis
- neoplasia
- tuberculosis
- actinomycosis.

EXCESS FILLING MATERIAL (2.28)

First of all, it is necessary to make a distinction between over – and underfilling and between over – and underextension.

Over- and underextension refer only to the vertical component of the obturation; either beyond or short of the apical foramen.

Underfilling refers to an obturation that has been performed inadequately in all dimensions (e.g., a short and narrow silver cone in a longer and wider root canal, or a short obturation only in cement full of voids).

Overfilling refers to an obturation that has been performed in three dimensions in which a small portion of material extrudes beyond the foramen.

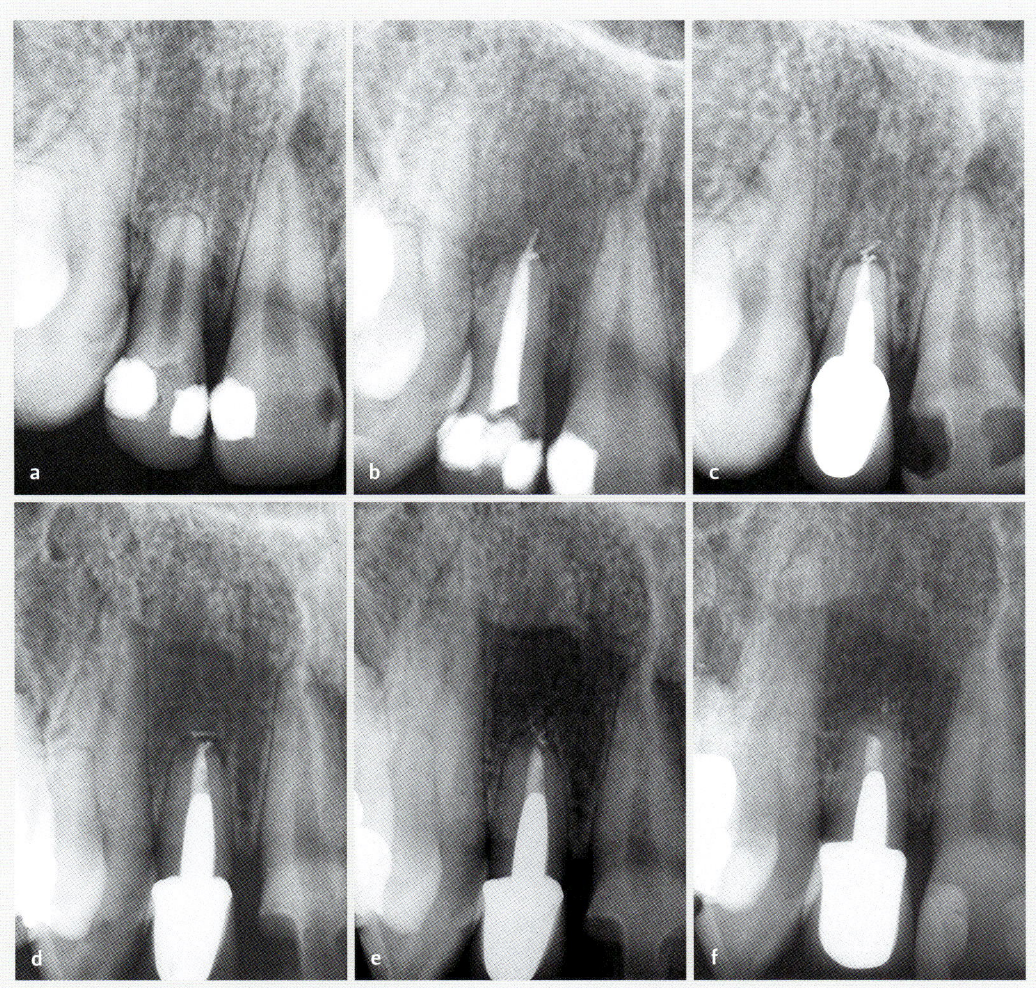

2.28 **a)** Preoperative radiograph of an upper right lateral incisor. **b)** Postoperative radiograph: the tip of the cone has slid 2-3 mm beyond the apex, probably because the "tug-back" of the cone was half-way along its length rather than at the tip. **c)** Six months later: the excess material appears to be sectioned at the apical foramen. **d)** Twelve months postoperative: the tip of the cone lies horizontally over the root apex. **e)** Five years postoperative: of the excess material nothing has remained except for a minimum trace. **f)** The 34-year recall confirms that an overfilling in a three-dimensionally obturated root canal is **not** an indication for surgery **neither** is it a cause of endodontic failure.

The situation of a canal with a slight overfilling is quite different from that of a canal with a vertical overextension and underfilling. In the former, the obturation fills the entire endodontium in its three dimensions and an excess of material extrudes from the apical foramen. In the latter case, the obturation material protrudes beyond the apex without sealing the apical foramen and thus without three-dimensionally obturating the root canal system.

The cause of failure in these cases is not the tip of the silver cone or of the gutta-percha that "pricks" the periodontium, but the fact that it does not seal the apical foramen. Surgery may be indicated, just to improve the apical seal of the root canal system (📷 2.29).

Ingle[81] stated that in Endodontics one achieves a high success rate in spite of overfillings.

Weine[82] stated that fortunately, since gutta-percha is so well tolerated by periapical tissue, only rarely is a post-treatment failure noted in conjunction with an overfilling. Most instances show no abnormal radiographic evidence (📷 2.30), and in some cases there is an actual amputation of the overfilling with phagocytosis of the extra mass (📷 2.28).

Schilder[83] claims that he has never found a case of failure as a result of overfilling.

Those cases that are labeled failures because of the presence of material beyond the apex are actually cases of underfilling with vertical overextension of the obturation and the failure depends on the presence of bacteria left inside the root canal system which has not been three-dimensionally obturated.[84] In the literature it has been widely demonstrated that the major factors associated with endodontic failures are inadequate root canal debridement or incomplete root canal seal,[85-87] while the apical extent of root canal fillings is not a determining factor.[88-90]

The excess material beyond the cemento-dentinal junction plays no role in healing[91,92] and may be considered irrelevant. It should, however, be avoided as it is unnecessary and because it may bother the patient at the time of obturation.[83]

Exclusive clinical research on the influence of the excess material on the treatment failure cannot be taken into consideration, since they exclude too many variables regarding the cleaning and shaping of these root canals and the true three-dimensionality of their obturation.

Histologic studies on experimental animals by Deemer and Tsaknis,[93] and by Tavares et al.[94] have demonstrated that gutta-percha is perfectly tolerated by the surrounding tissues. Their results agree with those of Schilder[92] on human specimens.

Bergenholtz et al.[95] stated that in the case of overfillings the filling material *per sé* is not necessarily the immediate cause of failure. Gutta-percha, both *in vitro* in cell cultures,[96] and in *in vivo* implants in experimental animals,[97,98] has been shown to be compatible with living tissues. Recent radiographic studies have shown that, over time, the extruded canal filling materials would not cause chronic inflammation and could eventually be removed from the periradicular tissues.[89,99] Consequently, the factors that impede healing in cases of overfilling are to be investigated elsewhere.

Regarding the greatly feared foreign body reaction around the excess material, Yusuf[100] has demonstrated inflammation around the small pieces of dentin and cement found beyond the apex in granulation tissue, where they act like a foreign body. In contrast, small pieces of dental amalgam or other canal obturating materials were usually associated with a fibrous reaction and encapsulation, without active inflammation.

This is further confirmation of the tissue tolerance of canal filling material. Thus, accidental minor overfilling of a properly cleaned, shaped, and three-dimensionally filled canal is *not* desired but is *not* an indication for surgical removal of the excess (📷 2.31), unless there are clear signs of treatment failure.

If this is true for the excess of gutta-percha, it is even more so the case when the excess is made with sealer which, in the case of Pulp Canal Sealer, has been demonstrated to have good biocompatibility. Pertot et al.[101] in experimental animals have demonstrated that 12 weeks after the root canal sealer was implanted into the

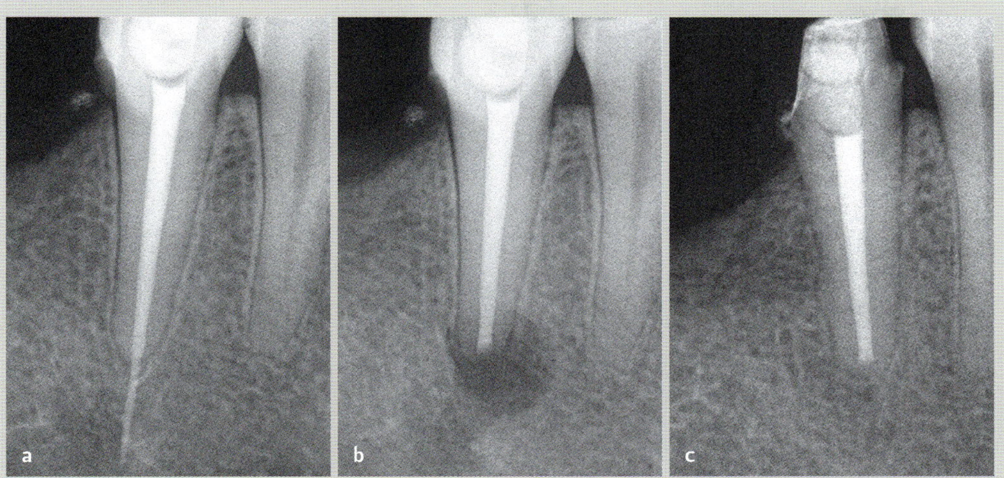

2.29 **a)** Preoperative radiograph of a lower right second premolar. Several millimeters of gutta-percha have been pushed over the mental nerve and the patient is complaining of paraesthesia and pain. **b)** Postoperative radiograph. During the surgical procedure, the gutta-percha piece has been removed, the root apex has been beveled with an ultrasonic tip instead of using the Lindeman bur, because of the extreme proximity of the mental nerve, a retro cavity has been prepared and then obturated with white MTA. With the same ultrasonic tip used for the bevel, small pieces of the endodontic sealer have also been removed from the surface of the nerve. **c)** Six-year recall.

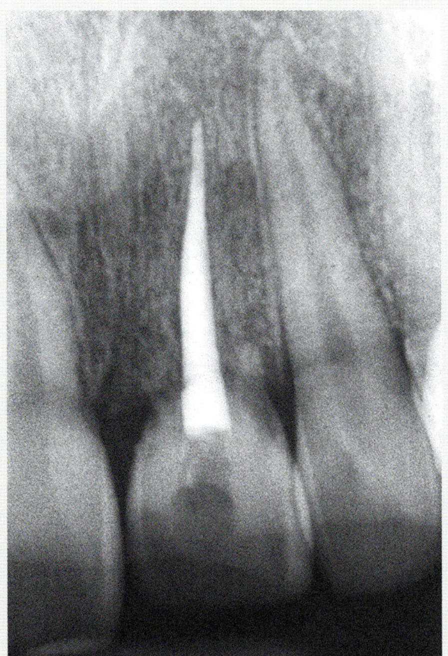

2.30. Radiograph of the upper left central incisor, reimplanted three years before after a traumatic avulsion. The root had a replacement resorption. The gutta-percha radiographically appears to be in direct contact with bone and there is no radiographic evidence of inflammation.

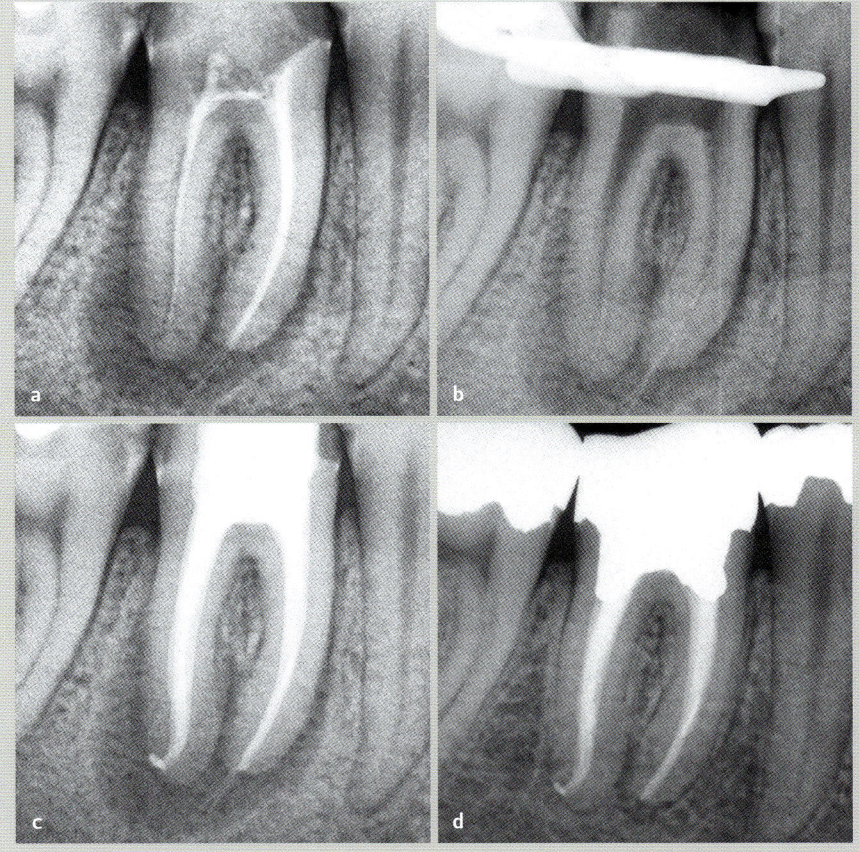

2.31 **a)** Preoperative radiograph of the lower right first molar improperly treated endodontically: the distal canal is underfilled and each one of the mesial canals has a gutta-percha cone overextending into the periapical tissues. **b)** Intraoperative radiograph: the attempt to remove the gutta-percha from beyond the foramen failed. **c)** Postoperative radiograph: the two cones are still present in the lesion. **d)** Three-year recall: the lesion is completely healed and the two gutta-percha cones have completely disappeared. The radiolucency was obviously a lesion of endodontic origin maintained by bacteria left in the root canal system and **not** a foreign body reaction, maintained by two pieces of gutta-percha!

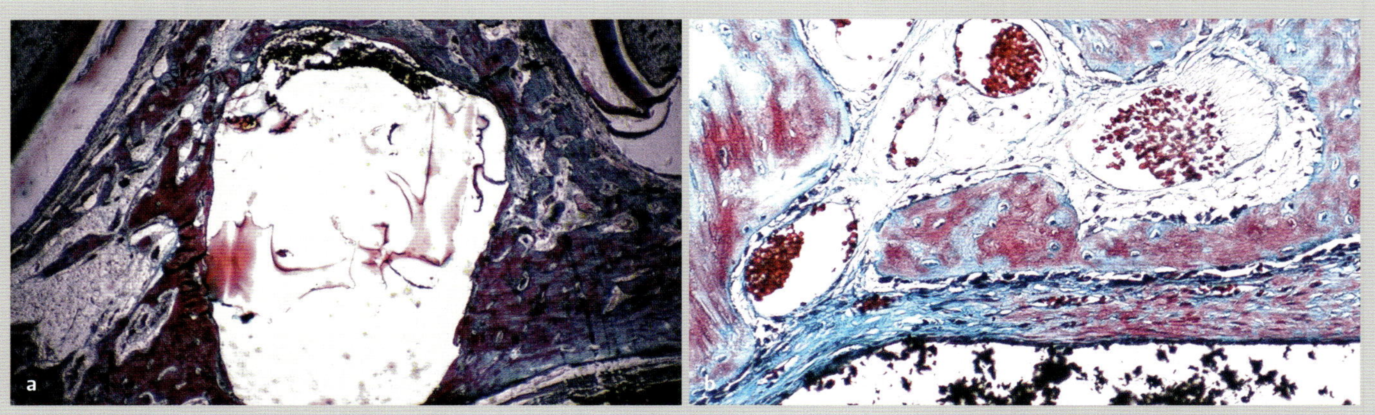

2.32 Osseous reaction to implanted pulp canal sealer at four weeks. **a)** Normal bone marrow spaces (original magnification: ×5. Masson's Trichrome). **b)** Layer of fibrous connective tissue between pulp canal sealer and bone, without evidence of inflammatory cells. Normal appearance of the bone with living osteocytes and surrounded by a layer of osteoblasts (original magnification ×25. Masson's Trichrome). (*Courtesy of Dr. Wilhelm-Joseph Pertot.*)

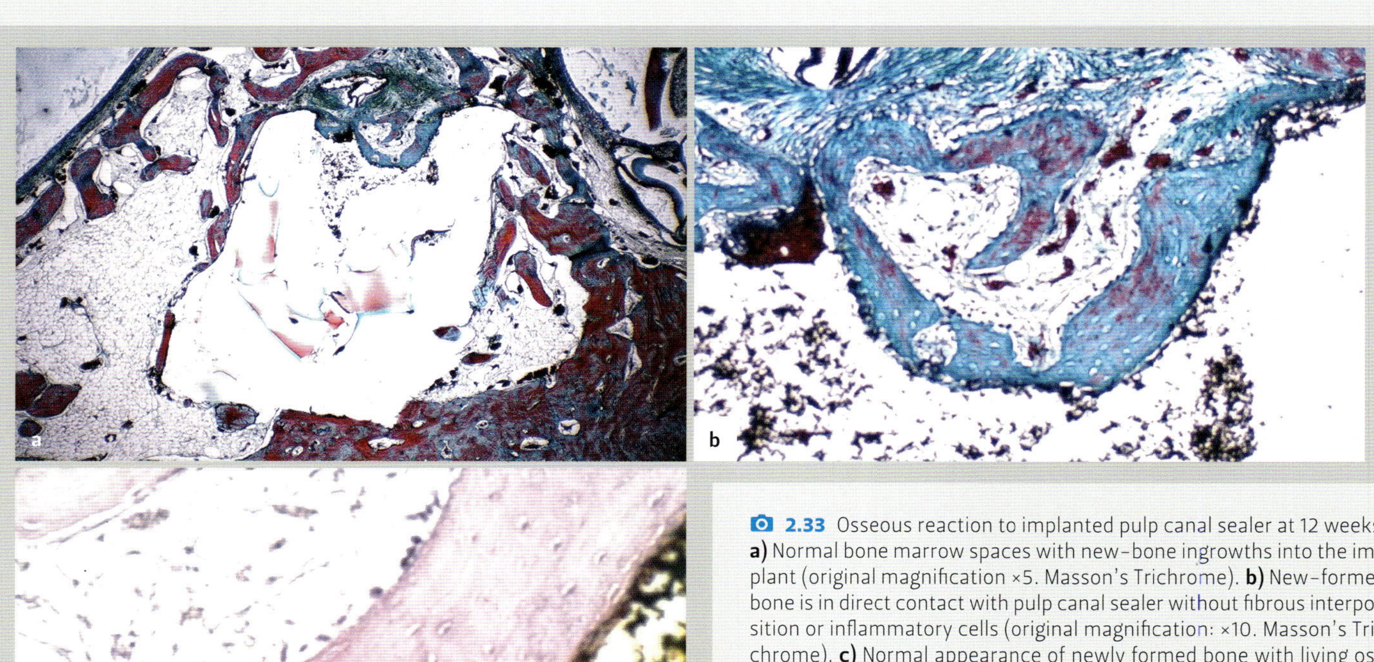

2.33 Osseous reaction to implanted pulp canal sealer at 12 weeks. **a)** Normal bone marrow spaces with new-bone ingrowths into the implant (original magnification ×5. Masson's Trichrome). **b)** New-formed bone is in direct contact with pulp canal sealer without fibrous interposition or inflammatory cells (original magnification: ×10. Masson's Trichrome). **c)** Normal appearance of newly formed bone with living osteocytes and normal bone marrow (original magnification ×50. Hematoxylin-eosin). (*Courtesy of Dr. Wilhelm-Joseph Pertot*).

mandibular bone, macrophages, lymphocytes and plasma cells were no longer present (2.32). In most cases, new bone was observed in direct contact with the sealer. The absence of an even moderate inflammatory reaction at 12 weeks seemed to indicate that the reported *in vitro* toxicity of the freshly mixed sealers[102–104] decreases and disappears with time (2.33).

If we can accept the material that protrudes by many millimeters beyond the apical foramen in cases of endodontic implants, even more so can the fraction of a millimeter of gutta-percha that may accidentally protrude beyond the apex in a three-dimensionally filled canal be accepted (2.34, 2.35).

In conclusion, the presence of protruded gutta-percha in a failing case must be interpreted not as responsible for the failure but as the consequence of a transportation of the apical foramen and, therefore, as a consequence of a lack of apical seal (2.36, 2.37).

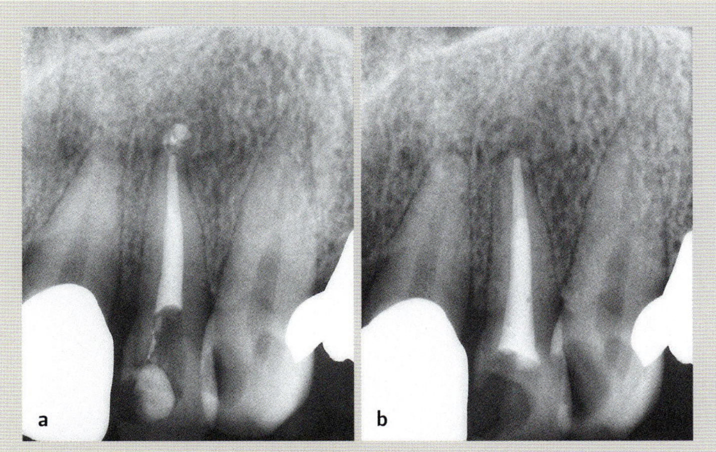

2.34 **a)** Postoperative radiograph of an upper left lateral incisor. **b)** Seven months later: the excess sealer has disappeared.

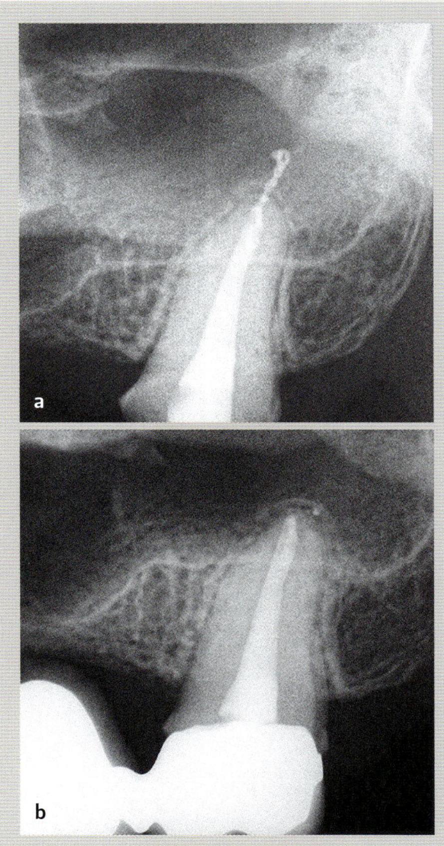

2.35 **a)** Postoperative radiograph of an upper left second molar. **b)** Eight months later: the excess material is no longer present.

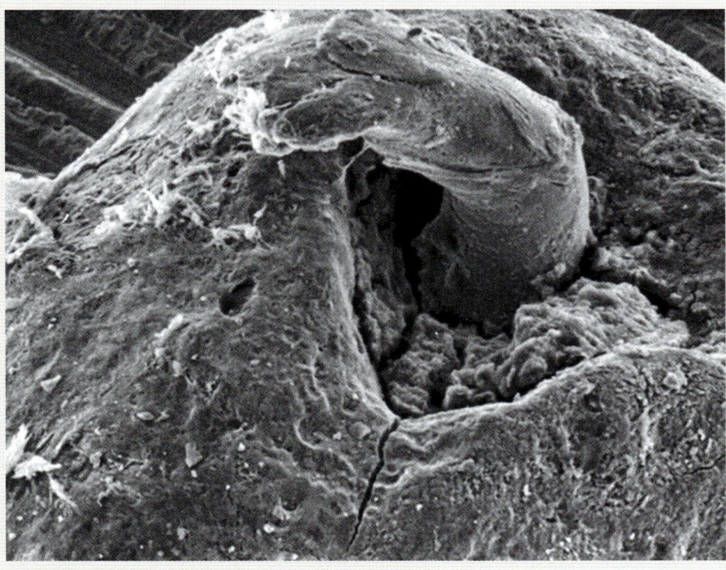

2.36 S.E.M. photograph of a tear drop foramen with extrusion of obturating material (x65).

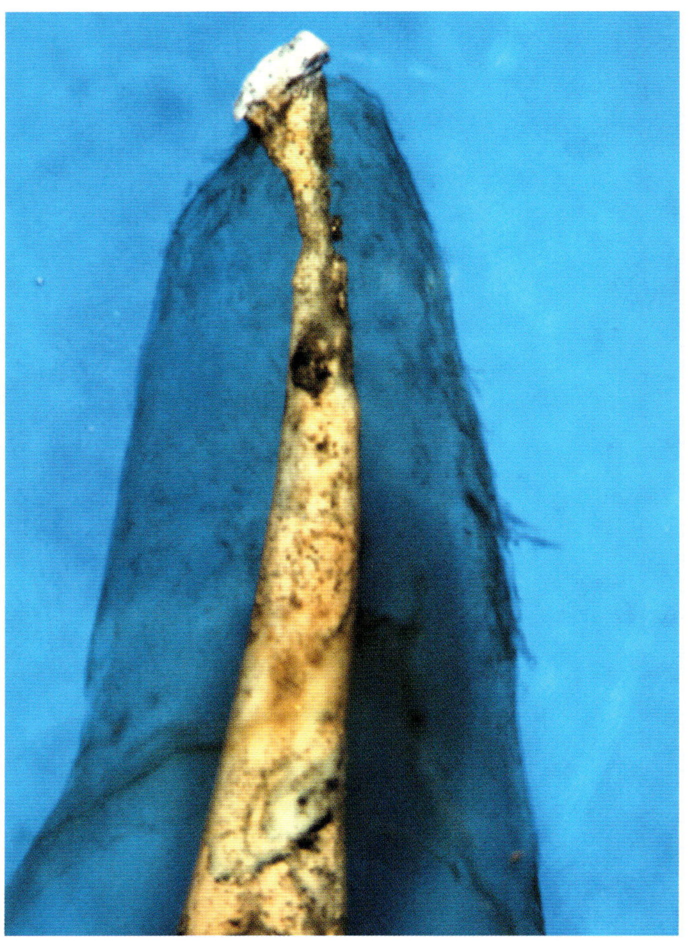

2.37 The transparent tooth is showing the hourglass shape of the apical one third, due to the tear drop foramen.

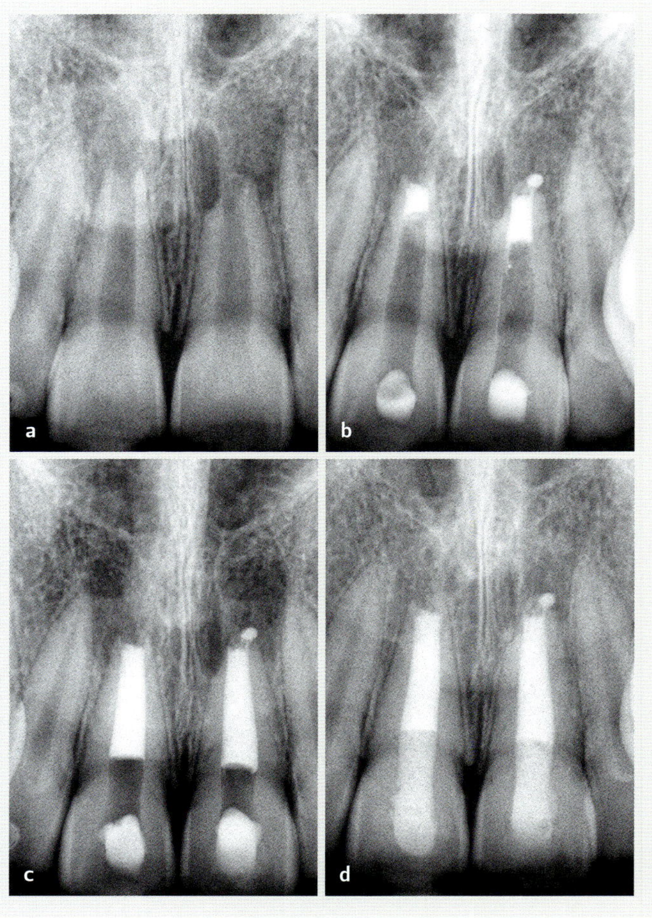

2.38 **a)** Preoperative radiograph of the upper central incisors. The teeth have open apices and necrotic pulps. **b)** After one week of calcium hydroxide, 3 mm of MTA has been positioned at the foramina. **c)** Postoperative radiograph. **d)** Two-year recall.

OPEN APEX (2.38)

For many years, teeth with immature apices and necrotic pulp have been treated with a form of therapy called "apexification", the aim of which was to induce the formation of a calcific barrier at the open apex against which the conventional obturating materials could be condensed without overfilling. This was obtained using medications with calcium hydroxyde for several months, until the calcific barrier was formed and became visible on the radiograph. More recently, these teeth started to be treated with the "apical barrier technique",[105] where 3 or 4 mm of MTA is positioned at the open apex to act as a barrier against which the obturating material can be condensed. Another re-

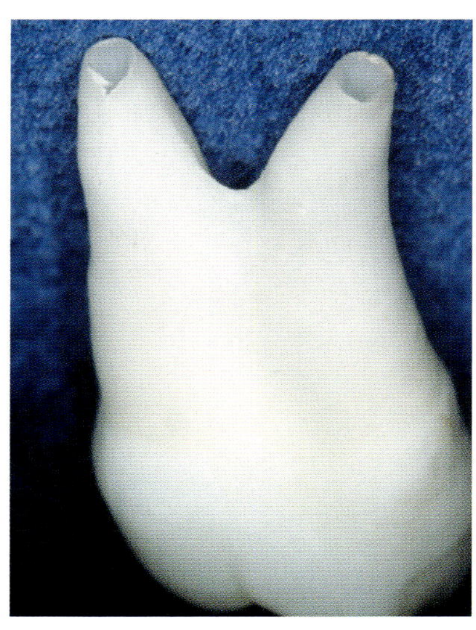

2.39 An upper first premolar with immature apices. Note the thinness and fragility of the roots.

cent technique suggested in the case of a necrotic pulp in an immature tooth is the revascularization, to obtain both the healing of the periapical lesion and the complete maturation of the root development, thanks to the presence of living tissue inside the root canal. However, according to the recent literature, the predictability of this technique does not seem to be consistently established.[106]

Prior to the advent of these techniques, the therapy of these teeth was surgical, with the anatomical and psychological implications of such a procedure.[107,108] The tooth with an immature apex has extremely thin, fragile walls surrounding a very wide canal (2.39). Consequently, an enormous amount of amalgam was introduced into a cavity with extremely weak walls, with a high risk of fracture.[109] The surgically-treated cases often failed because the fragile canal walls permitted neither the preparation of an undercut - and thus of a retentive cavity - nor the application of the pressure necessary for the condensation of the amalgam, so that it was often impossible to obtain a good apical seal.[110] Instead of retrofilling, some authors at that time suggested overfilling of the root canal, followed by periapical curettage. In all cases, however, an unfavorable crown-root ratio resulted.

Furthermore, teeth with immature apices were very often found in very young patients, who were apprehensive and fearful of the dentist. Because of their poor cooperation, they were not ideal candidates for a surgical procedure. Even though there are some authors[111] who even today consider the tooth with necrotic pulp and an immature apex to be an indication for retrograde endodontic treatment, the vast majority agree that apexification or the apical barrier technique is the treatment of choice in these cases. In certain cases, when the patient is an adult and a root canal therapy has already been performed unsuccessfully on a toot that was immature at the time of treatment, then subsequent surgical therapy could be the correct treatment option (2.40).

CALCIFIED ROOT CANALS (2.41)

It is well known that calcifications progress in a coronal to apical direction, which means that even though the pulp chamber, the coronal one third and may be the middle one third are completely calcified, today using the surgical operating microscope and the CBCT it is always possible to find the root canal and to complete the therapy with a nonsurgical approach. Therefore, the

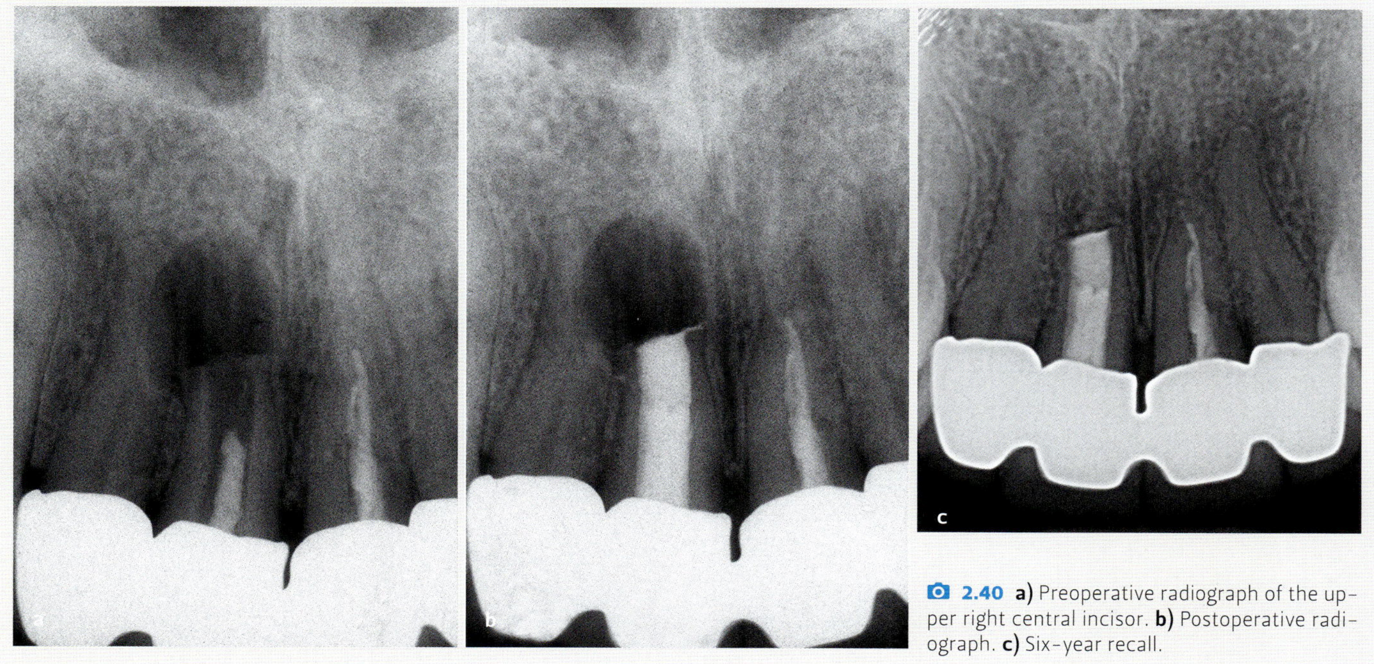

2.40 **a)** Preoperative radiograph of the upper right central incisor. **b)** Postoperative radiograph. **c)** Six-year recall.

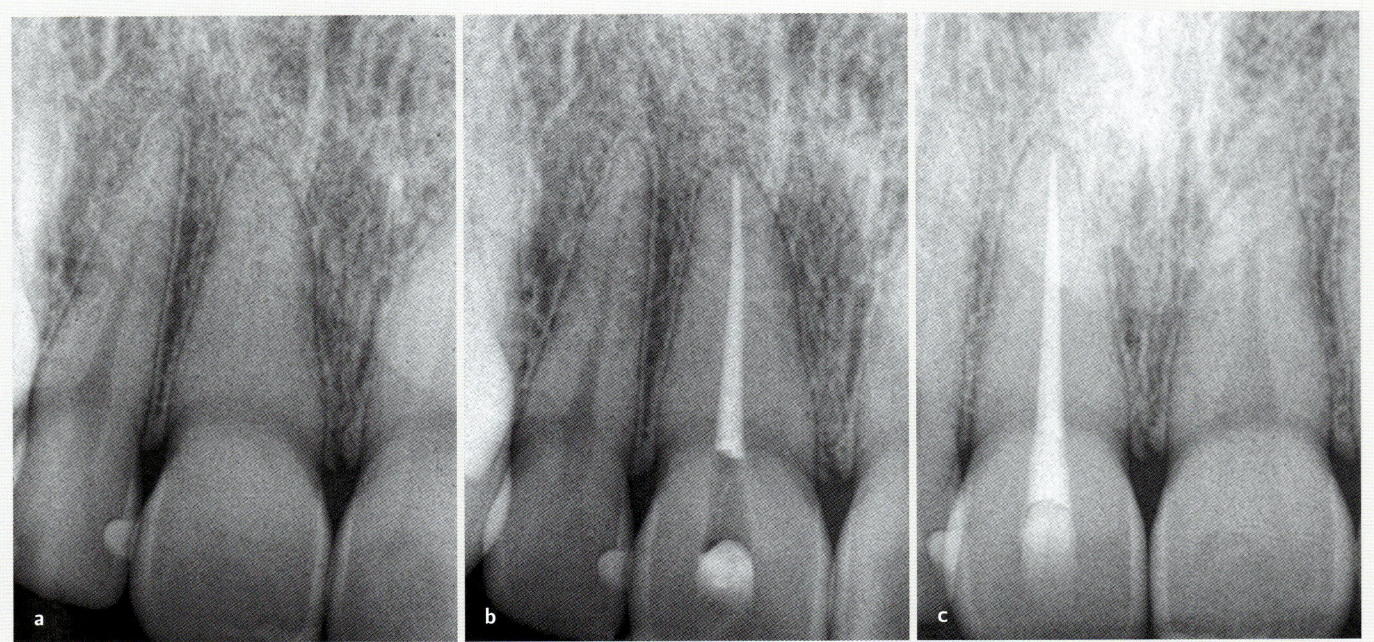

2.41 **a)** Preoperative radiograph of the upper right central incisor. Because of a previous trauma the pulp space seems to be completely calcified and now the tooth is symptomatic and requires a root canal treatment. **b)** Postoperative radiograph. Using the operating microscope and ultrasonic tips the patent canal has been found and treated. **c)** Two-year recall.

calcified root canal should not be considered an indication for a surgical procedure.

The aforementioned "false indications for surgery" can actually be successfully treated with a nonsurgical treatment or retreatment. If the root canal system can be negotiated, cleaned, shaped and three-dimensionally filled, it will respond favorably to the conventional procedure.

True Indications

The true indications for apical surgery are the following.

PRESENCE OF OBSTACLES (2.42)

If the root canal system can be successfully negotiated and eventually obturated, as already stated, it will respond favorably to conventional treatment. On the other hand, if any obstacle prevents the instruments, the irrigating solutions and the obturating materials from reaching the working length, then in such a situation the only way to get healing of the existing lesion is the use of the surgical approach.

The obstacles may be represented by a ledge, a calcification, a broken instrument, a perforation or post (2.43). However, many procedures previously considered impossible to accomplish, are now becoming a matter of routine. The removal of a broken instrument can be accomplished safely with the new technology available today, the CBCT can be used to locate missed canals, thanks to the new biocompatible materials perforations can be repaired nonsurgically in many circumstances, posts can be safely removed, so that the clinician can expect predictable results also from a nonsurgical endodontic procedure.

In conclusion, the only time surgical endodontics should be considered is when it is impossible to get a good apical seal in a "virgin" case, or to improve the apical seal by "retreating" a case with a nonsurgical approach. As already stated at the beginning of this chapter, in agreement with what Nygaard-Ostby and Schilder[5] said, surgical endodontics must be reserved for those cases in which the nonsurgical therapy appears impossible right from the beginning or when the nonsurgical retreatment attempts have failed. Nevertheless,

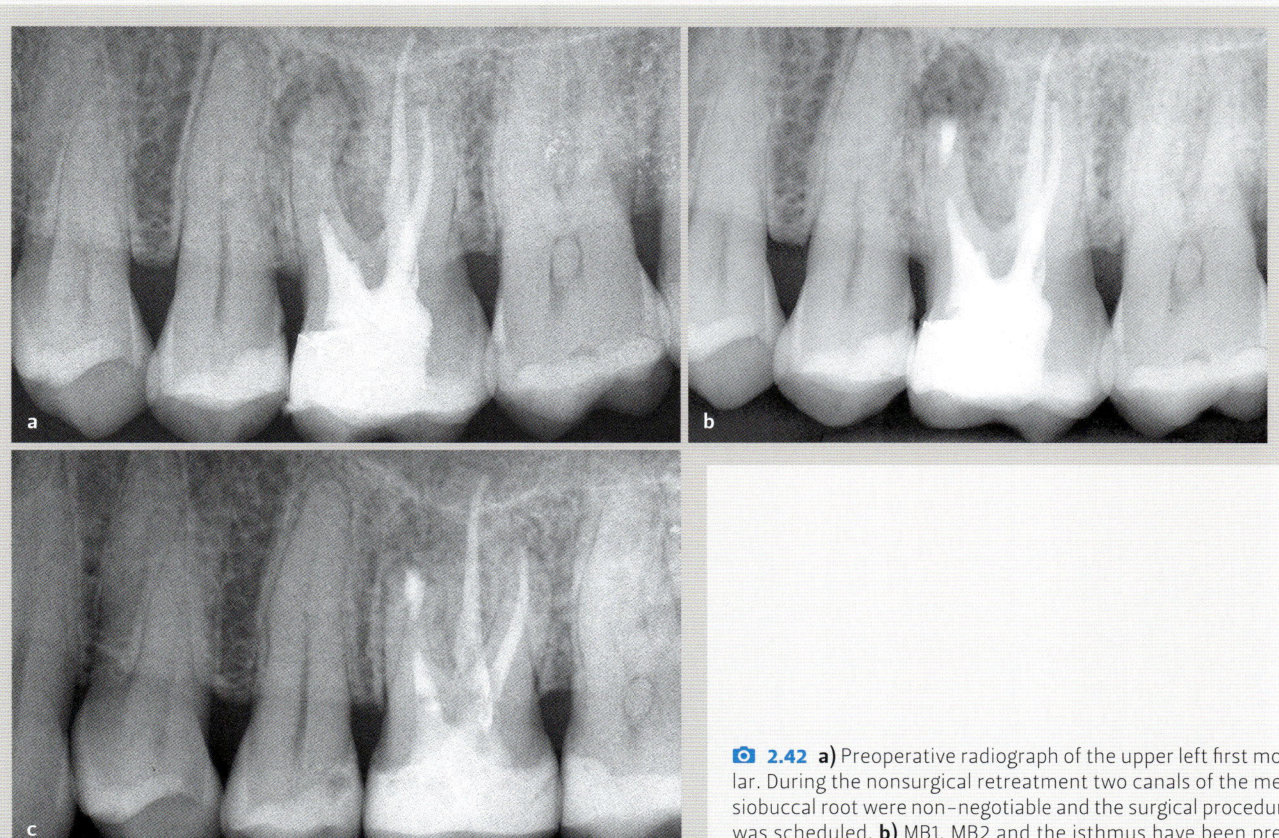

2.42 **a)** Preoperative radiograph of the upper left first molar. During the nonsurgical retreatment two canals of the mesiobuccal root were non-negotiable and the surgical procedure was scheduled. **b)** MB1, MB2 and the isthmus have been prepared and sealed with white MTA. **c)** Two-year recall.

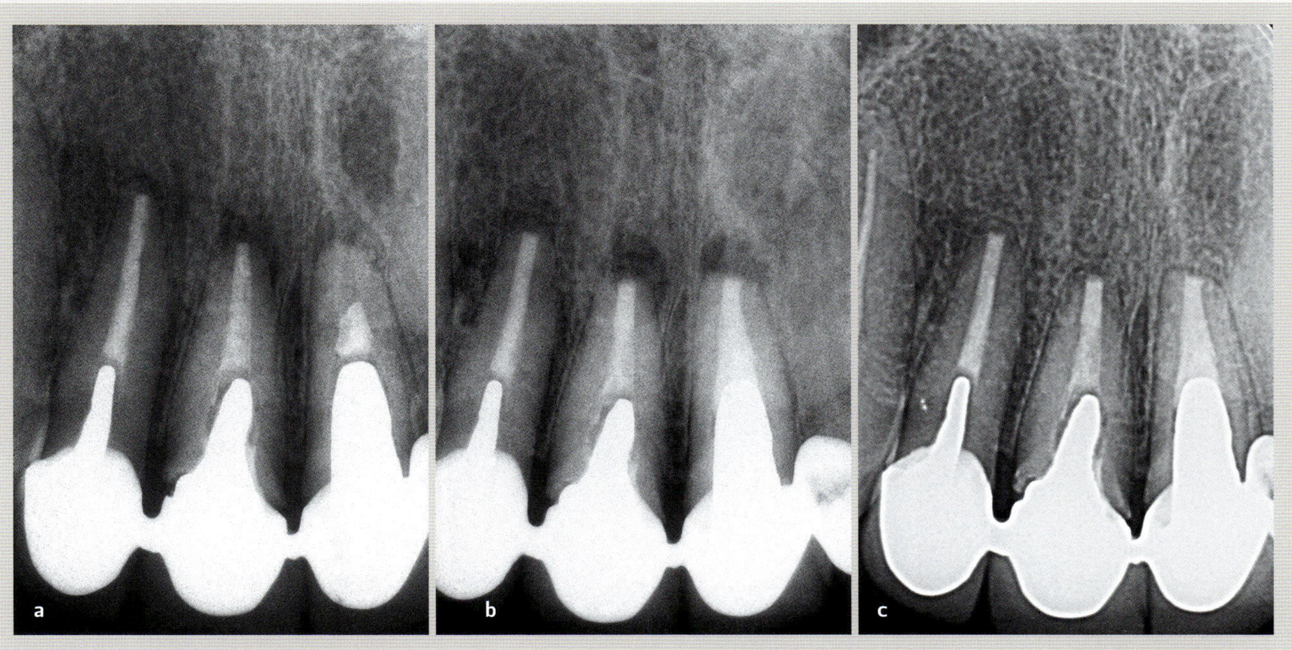

2.43 **a)** Preoperative radiograph of the upper left incisors. **b)** Postoperative radiograph. **c)** One-year recall.

even in such cases, the authors recommend filling as much of the root canal by conventional method as possible (2.1). If the proper protocol is followed, the current apical microsurgical technique should have a healing rate of between 91-96%.[112–115]

PERFORATIONS (2.44)

Perforations are pathologic or iatrogenic communications between the root canal system and the attachment apparatus. The perforation creates an "additional" portal of exit in the root canal system and, once identified, it must be sealed as quickly as possible, since periodontal involvement arising from the perforation can become irreversible with time. Treating a perforation may often require a multidisciplinary approach in order to establish the appropriate treatment plan. The decision must be made to either extract the tooth or direct efforts towards nonsurgical retreatment or surgical correction. If the nonsurgical approach seems to be impossible or if the previous attempts have failed, only then the surgical endodontic retreatment should be considered.

DENS IN DENTE AND DENS INVAGINATUS (2.45)

The root canal anatomy of such teeth can be sometimes so bizarre as to become extremely difficult to be treated only with a nonsurgical approach. However, the surgical procedure should be considered only "a posteriori", when the previous therapy has failed. In such a case, the

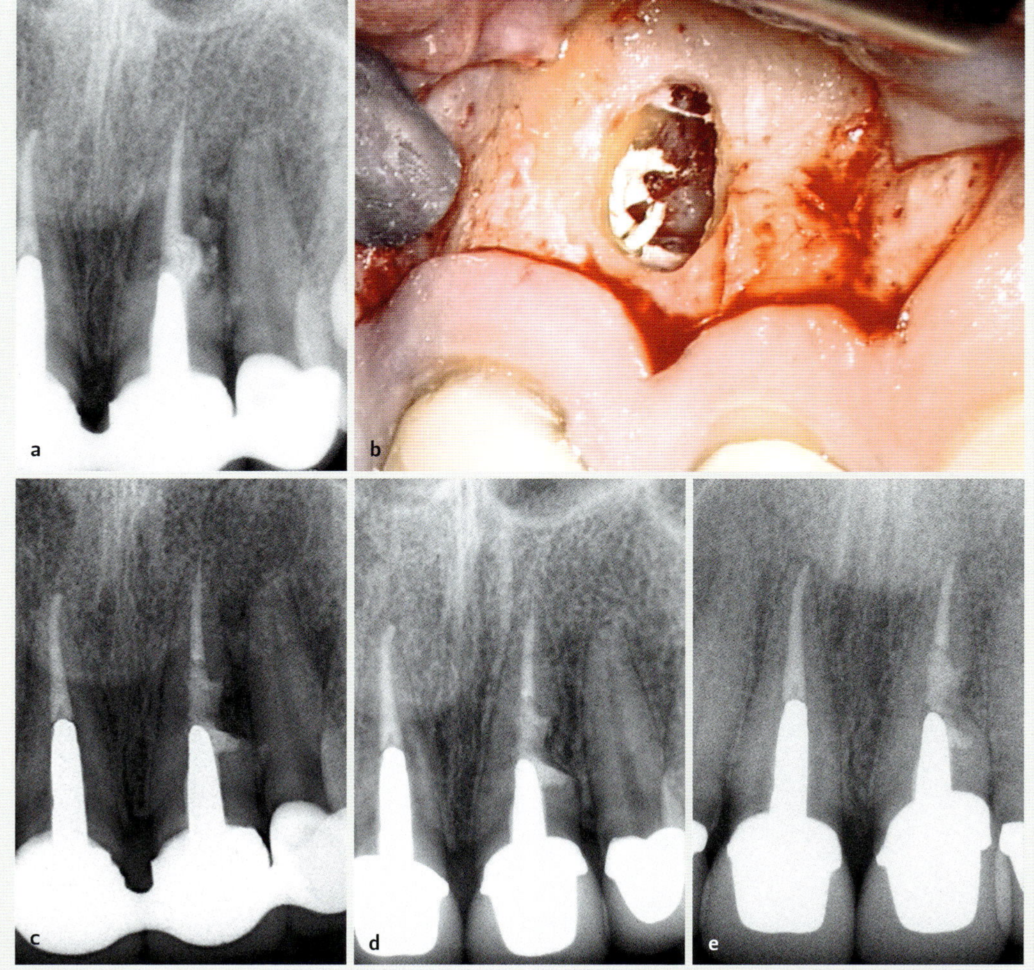

2.44 a) Preoperative radiograph of the upper left central incisor. The external resorption has been obturated with cold lateral condensation. **b)** The defect filled with many gutta-percha cones. **c)** The defect has been filled with grey MTA. **d)** Nineteen months recall radiograph. **e)** Nineteen-year recall radiograph.

surgery can be considered to be successful and can be performed just to increase the apical seal.

EXPEDIENCY AND CONVENIENCE[116] (2.46, 2.47)

In some particular situation, the surgical procedure can be used as an expedient to treat a challenging case, keeping in mind that it is not the best choice.

SYMPTOMATIC CASES (2.48)

When symptoms persist after the nonsurgical retreatment, in such cases surgical endodontics should be considered to relieve pain and discomfort to the patient.

According to Weine and Bustamante,[117] when pain persists after canal filling, surgery may be needed. The complaint of pain after canal filling is not unusual. In most cases, the tenderness dissipates after a few days and rarely lasts for more than one week. When post-treatment pain fails to subside, surgery is usually suggested so that an accurate examination of the periapical tissues where the pain resides can be made and any discrepancy corrected. Often the flapping of the tissue reveals an unexpected picture, and the cause of the pain becomes apparent. Examples of teeth that appear satisfactory on radiographs but have an obvious problem when exposed surgically are those with apical fenestrations (2.49, 2.50) and root fractures (10.13).

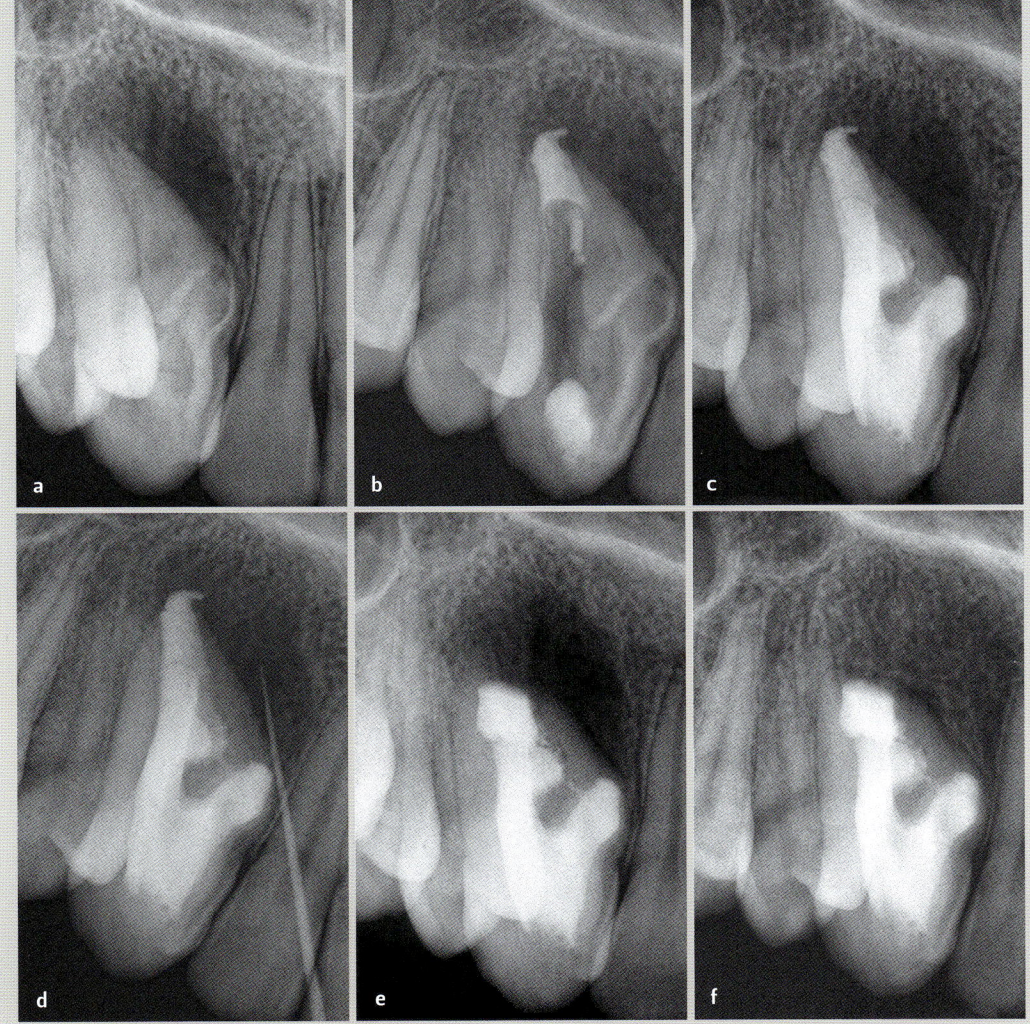

2.45 a) Preoperative radiograph of the upper right cuspid. The tooth presents as a "dens invaginatus" in a 13-year-old girl. The patient was scheduled by an oral surgeon for extraction and implant. **b)** The open apex has been sealed with MTA, according to the Apical Barrier Technique. **c)** Postoperative radiograph. **d)** Six months later the young patient presented with a sinus tract and she was scheduled for surgery. **e)** Postoperative radiograph. The seal of the only apical foramen has been improved during the surgical procedure. **f)** The one-year recall radiograph shows healing of the lesion.

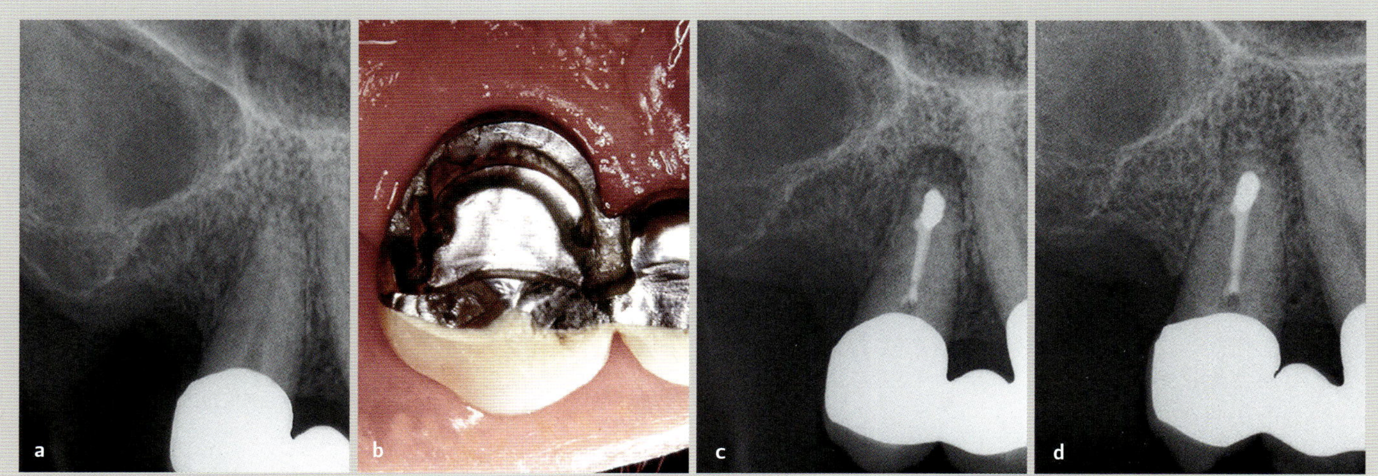

2.46 a) Preoperative radiograph of an upper right cuspid with pulpitis. The onset of acute symptoms started one week after definitive cementation of the prosthesis. **b)** Palatal view of the prosthetic crown on the cuspid, which has a removable prosthesis attached. It was not possible to perform an adequate access cavity, since this would have entailed destruction of the intracoronal attachment and thus the need to remake the prosthesis, therefore a surgical approach was chosen. **c)** Postoperative radiograph. **d)** Recall radiograph ten years later.

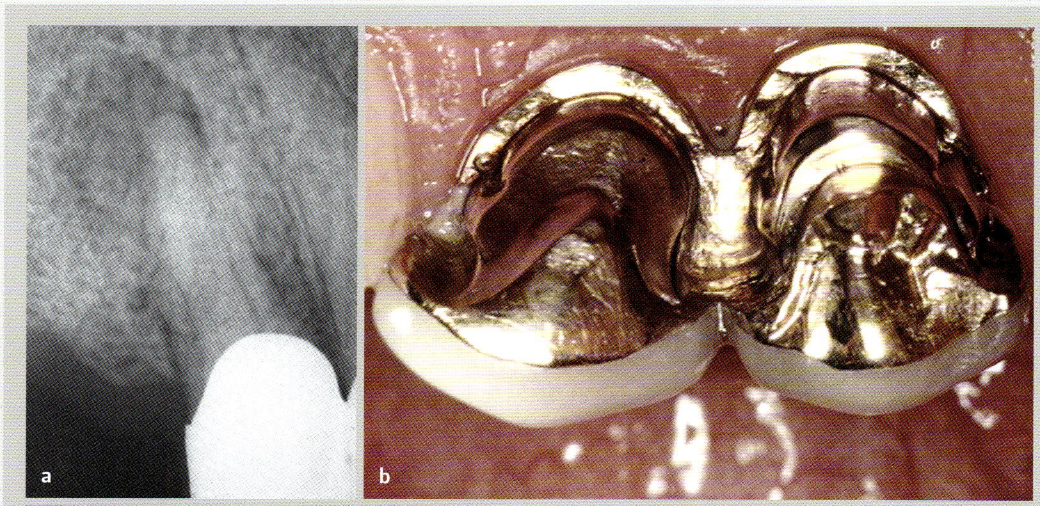

2.47 a) Preoperative radiograph of an upper left first premolar with a necrotic pulp and a periapical lesion. **b)** Occlusal view of the prosthetic crown of the first premolar, on which the removable prosthesis is attached. The prosthodontist specifically requested a surgical approach not to damage the intracoronal attachment with a regular access cavity. **c)** Both canals are instrumented with hand files. **d)** Both canals have been obturated with gutta-percha and sealer. **e)** Postoperative radiograph. **f)** Recall radiograph three years later.

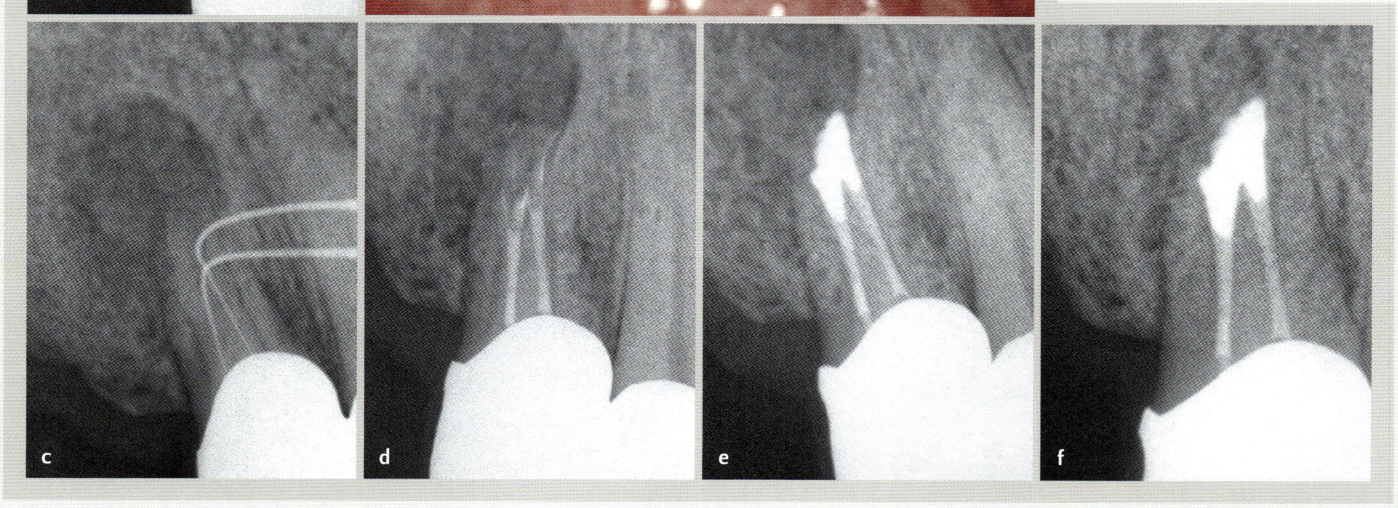

Apical fenestrations are localized defects of the cortical bone covering the teeth, a "window" in the bone through the apex protrudes. These defects occur almost exclusively on the buccal surfaces of the alveolar bone and maxillary teeth appear to be more frequently affected. Although they are usually symptoms-free if left alone, these fenestrations may give rise to pain when a root canal treatment is done on a tooth that already has this type of bone defect.[118] This phenomenon was first described by Spasser and Wend,[119] and later by Patterson[120] and Weine and Bustamante.[117] Upon palpation, the vestibular area in the region of the involved tooth is sensitive. The diagnosis can be easily confirmed with a CBCT and the treatment plan consists of raising a flap, making an apical resection, reducing some of the labial portion of the root, and remodeling the root in such a way as to reposition it in the bony housing. The bone may then repair itself, and the pain will disappear.

Persistent pain can also follow the fracture of a root during canal filling due to excessive forces used in condensation of gutta-percha or insertion of a dowel.[117] Because these fractures are usually vertical, the line of the fracture is rarely discernible on the radiograph, but when the affected root is exposed by surgical means, the fracture line may be visualized. These fractures run in an apical to coronal direction. The prognosis for such a condition depends on the extension of the fracture line. If the portion of the root containing the fracture can be removed without compromising the tooth stability, the prognosis remains excellent.

The aforementioned "true indications for surgery" can successfully be addressed by a surgical approach only, since the root canal system is not negotiable or not all the portals of exit can be successfully sealed nonsurgically or all our previous nonsurgical efforts were unsuccessful.

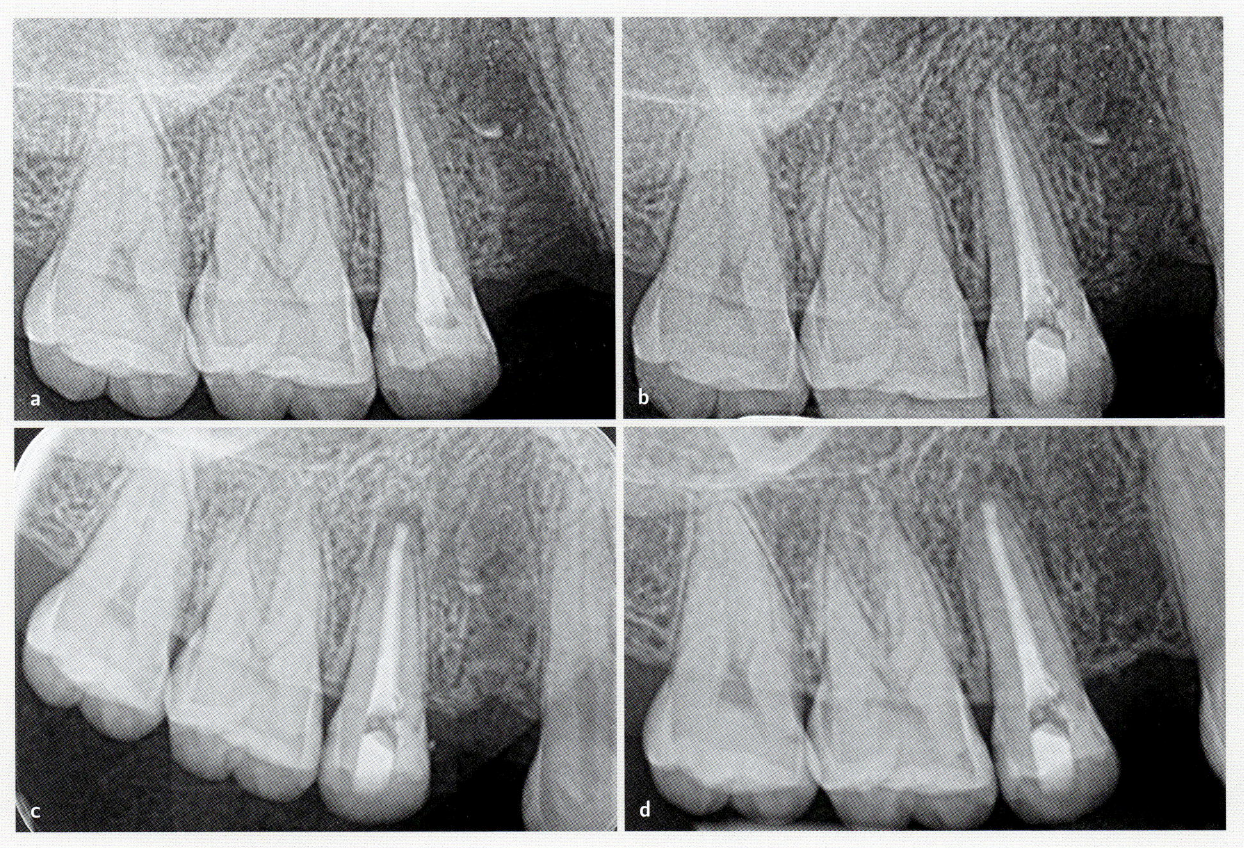

2.48 a) Preoperative radiograph of an upper right second premolar. The tooth is sensitive to percussion and needs to be retreated. **b)** Postoperative radiograph after nonsurgical retreatment. After a few months the tooth is still sensitive to percussion and a surgical retreatment is scheduled. **c)** Postoperative radiograph after surgery. **d)** Two-year recall.

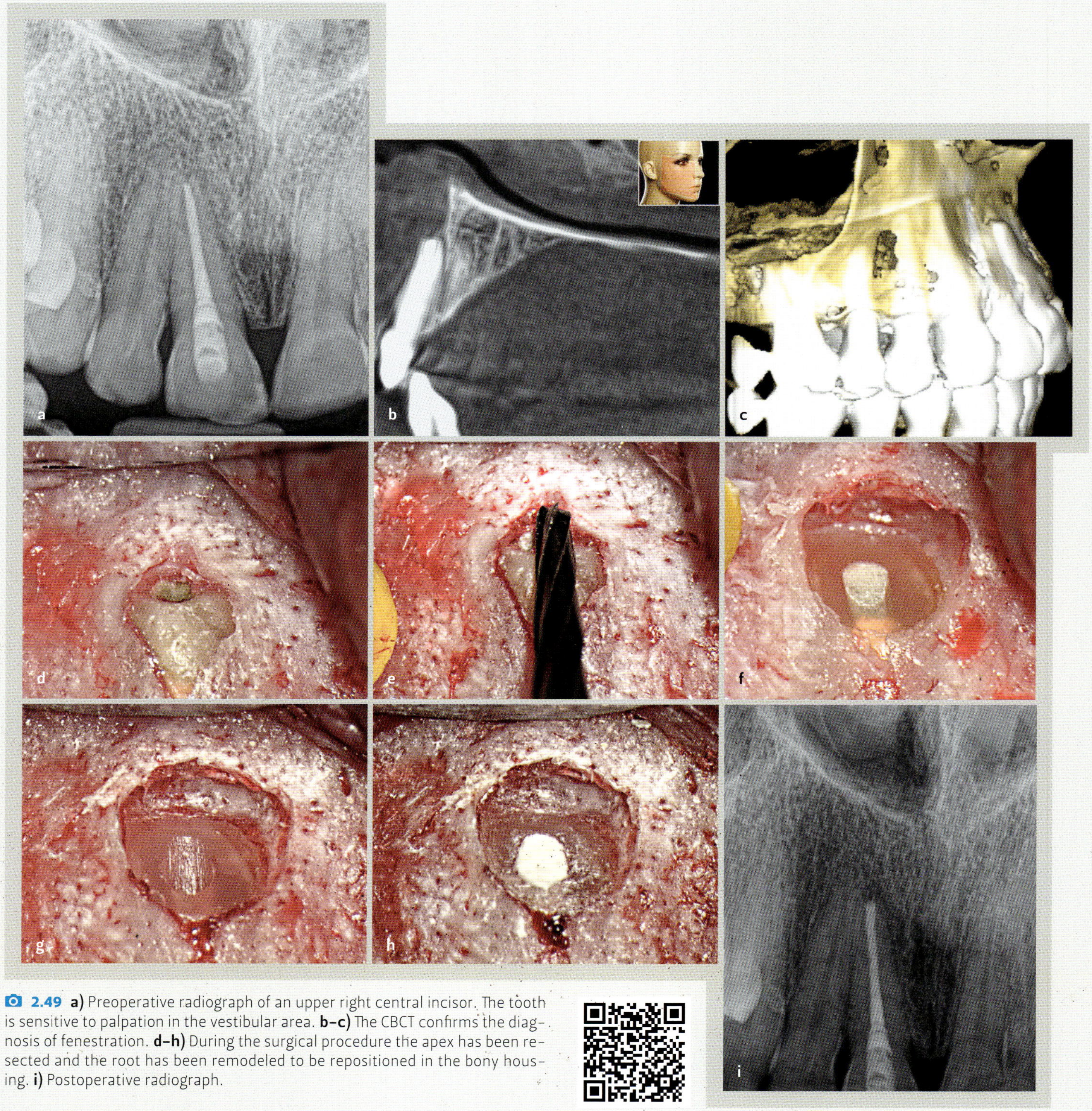

2.49 a) Preoperative radiograph of an upper right central incisor. The tooth is sensitive to palpation in the vestibular area. **b–c)** The CBCT confirms the diagnosis of fenestration. **d–h)** During the surgical procedure the apex has been resected and the root has been remodeled to be repositioned in the bony housing. **i)** Postoperative radiograph.

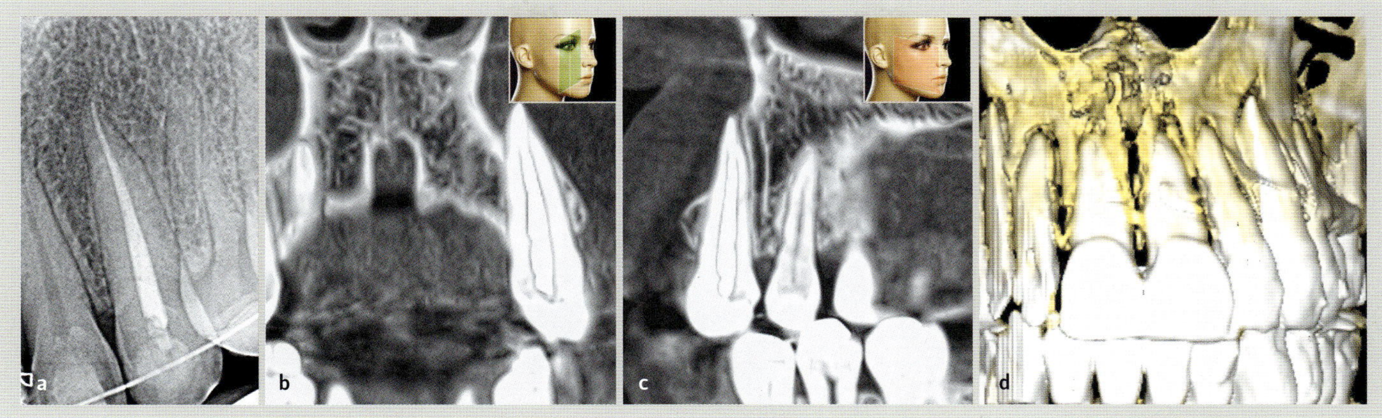

2.50 **a)** The upper left cuspid has been endodontically treated two years before and the tooth is sensitive on palpation of the buccal area. **b–d)** The CBCT confirms the diagnosis of fenestration but the patient refused the surgical treatment.

EXTRARADICULAR INFECTIONS

It is well known that the development of periradicular lesions create a barrier within the body to prevent further spread of microorganisms.[121] This barrier is formed of a concentration of mononuclear cells and PMNs. It is conceivably very difficult for viable bacteria cells to cross this defense barrier and establish an extraradicular infection.

The most common form is the acute alveolar abscess, which is a transitory event dependent on the intraradicular infection. Once the drainage of pus is established (spontaneously or after surgical incision), infection is once again confined to the canal and the balance between aggression and defense is reestablished.[121]

There are two other forms of infection that may, however, become established outside the limits of the canal, and have been regarded as being independent of the intraradicular infection. This would make them play an important role in determining failure of even adequately treated root canals. These two distinct forms of extraradicular infection include:

- bacterial colonization of the external root surface forming extraradicular biofilms
- apical actinomycosis.

Extraradicular biofilms from a pathological point of view are actually an extension of the intraradicular infection and are biologically part of the intracanal infection. As such they survive only to the extent they maintain themselves adhered to the root surface, not being able to propagate within the apical periodontitis lesion.[121] From a clinical point of view the entity assumes great importance, because the infection established on the external root surface is beyond the reach of treatment measures and calculus-like deposits formed on the external surface of the root apex may be a direct cause of persistent apical periodontitis (2.51).[122–124] The calculus-like structures are certainly a result of calcification of the extraradicular biofilm adhered on the external root surface. In several cases reported in the literature[122] a sinus tract was also present. The possibility exists that, by allowing the traffic of fluids in both directions between the lesion and the oral environment, the sinus tract may have permitted minerals from saliva to reach the extraradicular biofilm and precipitate.[121] Another source of mineral is the hydroxyapatite of bone and cementum, which may dissolve and give rise to a fluid around the tissue that is rich of calcium and phosphate. Thus, the extraradicular biofilm may have become calcified even in the absence of contact with saliva. Obviously, this biofilm cannot be destroyed by conventional root canal treatment procedures and antimicrobial agents, because it remains out of reach for instruments, irrigants and medicaments. These calcified structures maintain apical periodontitis and lead to treatment failure, and only apical surgery can successfully manage these refractory cases.[121]

The clinical relevance of *apical actinomycosis* resides is the fact that this entity has been assigned with the ability to establish itself in the inflamed periradicular tissues and is claimed to survive independently of the intraradicular microbiota, thereby preventing healing even after proper root canal treatment procedures.[125–129] This helped perpetuate the belief that apical actinomycosis can be a direct cause of apical periodontitis.[121] However Ricucci and Siqueira[130] pointed out that at the present time there is no scientific evidence to support apical actinomycosis as an autonomous entity, able to sustain apical periodontitis in the absence of a

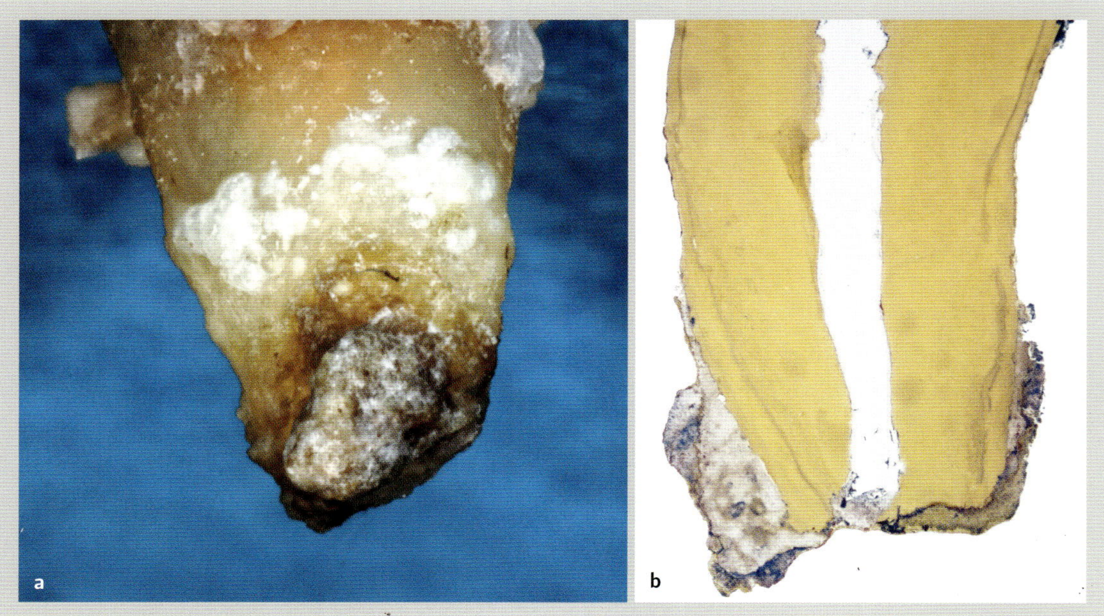

2.51 **a)** Exuberant calculus observed on the root tip of a mandibular canine after extraction. Note that this is not continuous with any periodontal calculus. **b)** The tooth was processed for histology. Calculus exhibits a sandwich-like appearance, with several layers and abundance of bacteria (original magnification ×16. Taylor modification of the Brown and Brenn technique). (*Courtesy of Dr. Domenico Ricucci.*)

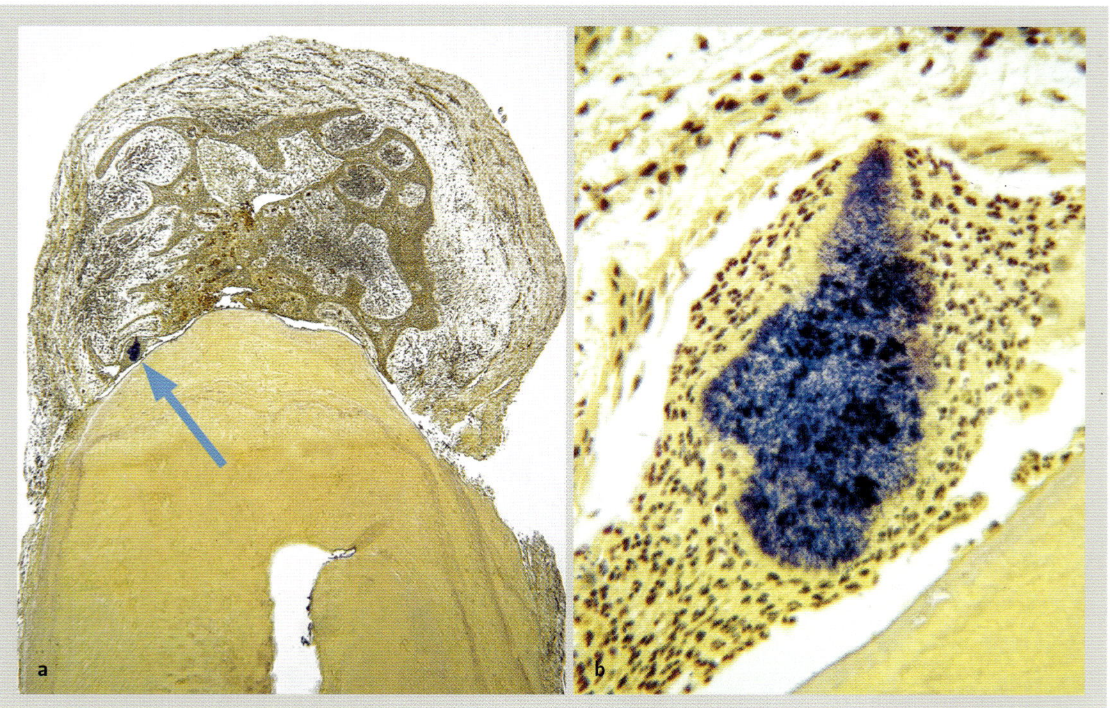

2.52 **a)** Disto-buccal root of a maxillary first molar, extracted with a periapical lesion attached. The lesion is epithelialized (original magnification ×16. Taylor modification of the Brown and Brenn technique). **b)** Middle magnification of the area indicated by the arrow in **(a)**. A large bacterial colony with branching intertwining filamentous bacteria at the periphery can be observed. The colony is surrounded by a severe concentration of polymorphonuclear leukocytes. This morphology is typical of actinomycosis (original magnification ×200). (*Courtesy of Dr. Domenico Ricucci.*)

concomitant intraradicular infection. Actinomycotic colonies observed in periradicular biopsy specimens are just an extension of a persistent intraradicular infection. In conclusion, according to Ricucci and Siqueira, the existence of apical actinomycosis as a pathologic entity independent of the root canal infection and its involvement as an exclusive cause of treatment failure are questionable and remain to be proven. Therefore, these failing cases need for a microsurgical endodontic procedure (2.52), which means not only curettage of the lesion but also resection of the root apex and retrofill of the root canal, to remove both the intraradicular and the extraradicular components of infection.[121]

FAILURE OF AN APPARENTLY SATISFACTORY ROOT CANAL TREATMENT

In order to be considered satisfactory, a root canal treatment should radiographically demonstrate a dense and homogeneous obturation, extending to the canal terminus, with the maximum respect of the original root canal anatomy. On the other hand, it is well known from the famous study by Walter Hess[131] of 1928 that the root canal anatomy it is not represented by a single and hopefully straight canal. As a matter of fact, we speak in terms of "Root Canal System", since root canals have irregular canal cross-sections, accessory and lateral canals, apical deltas, isthmuses and many areas that are mostly inaccessible to mechanical preparation.[132,133] Several studies demonstrated that with both current NiTi instrument systems and traditional stainless steel instruments a large percentage of root canal surface area remains unprepared.[134,135] Several studies of cases of endodontic failures[136] have demonstrated the presence of bacterial biofilm in all these areas not reached by conventional instrumentation. The impossibility of eliminating these biofilms are most certainly responsible for the failures of cases that radiographically can be defined as satisfactory (2.15, 2.53, 10.20).

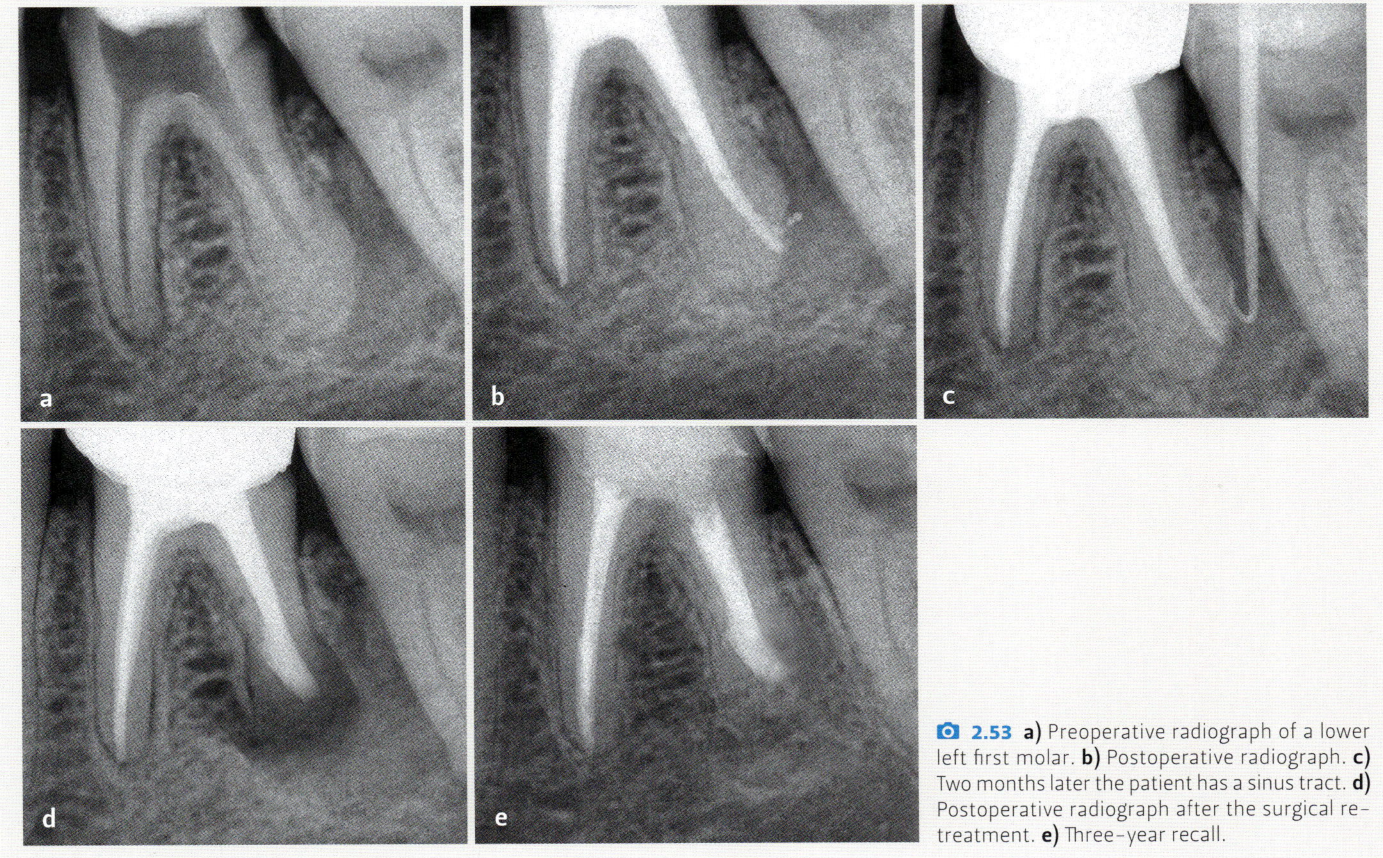

2.53 **a)** Preoperative radiograph of a lower left first molar. **b)** Postoperative radiograph. **c)** Two months later the patient has a sinus tract. **d)** Postoperative radiograph after the surgical retreatment. **e)** Three-year recall.

LEDGES

Ledges are *internal* transportations of the canal and frequently results when clinicians are preparing a curved canal and work short of length (📷 2.54). Ledges are typically on the outer wall of the canal curvature and many of them are successfully bypassed using precurved stainless steel and NiTi instruments of the latest generation, like ProTaper Gold or WaveOne Gold. In case the ledges cannot be bypassed, surgical endodontics is indicated.

SURGICAL FAILURES

Surgical failures are an obvious indication for retreatment, however it is necessary to make a distinction depending of the quality of the previous nonsurgical root canal treatment, knowing that periapical surgery it is not an excuse to position plugs of any material at the apex of infected root canals. In some case it is sufficient a nonsurgical retreatment only (📷 2.55), in some other case it is indicated a surgical retreatment only (📷 1.1, 📷 10.26), while in some more cases both the nonsurgical and the surgical retreatments are necessary (📷 2.1, 2.4).

EXPLORATORY SURGERY

The last indications for surgery are the radiolucencies that are not caused by root canal infection and which may mimic a lesion of endodontic origin (📷 2.56). Such radiolucencies require exploratory surgery including a biopsy for histologic examination.[137]

Contraindications

Apical surgery is contraindicated in the following circumstances:

1. *Lateral lesions of endodontic origin* (📷 2.57). As regards the presence of a lateral lesion due to the

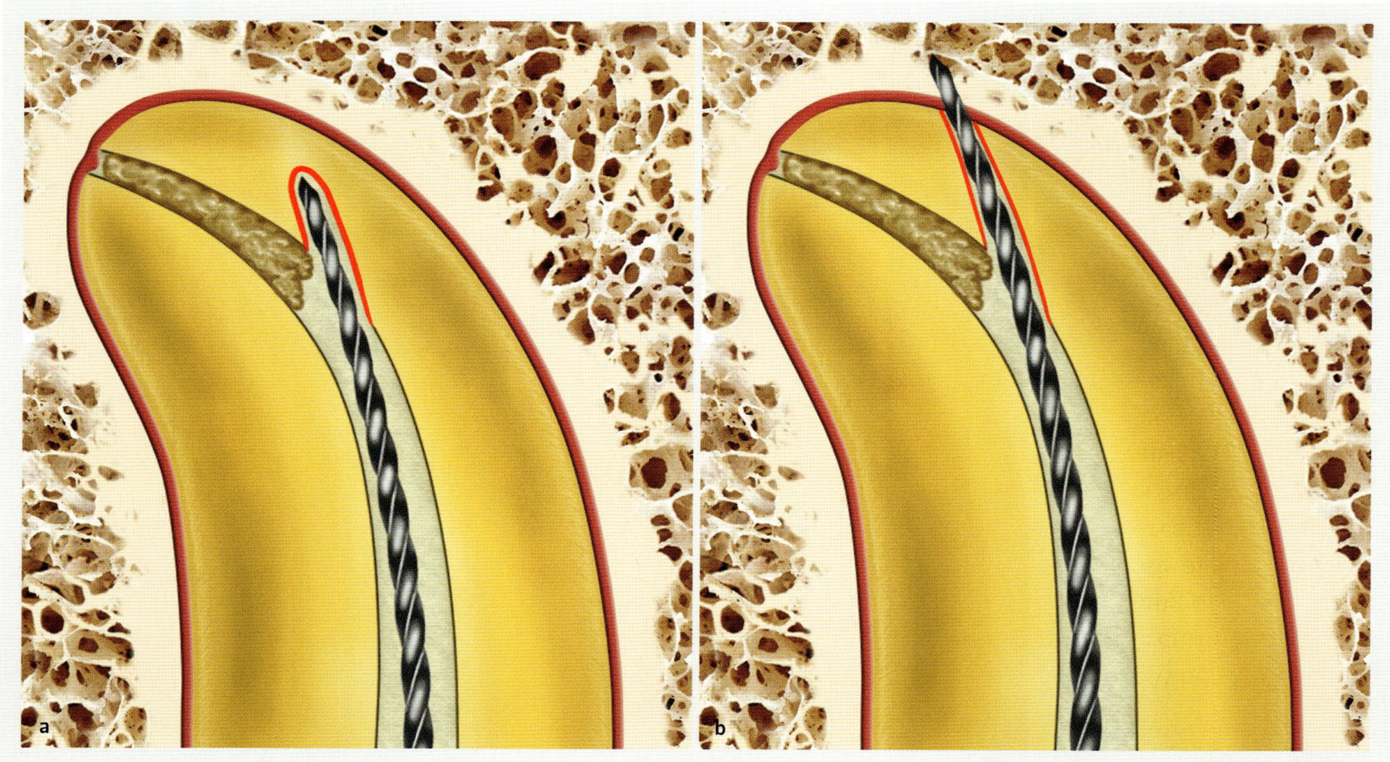

📷 **2.54 a, b)** In the attempt to bypass the ledge, a perforation could occur.

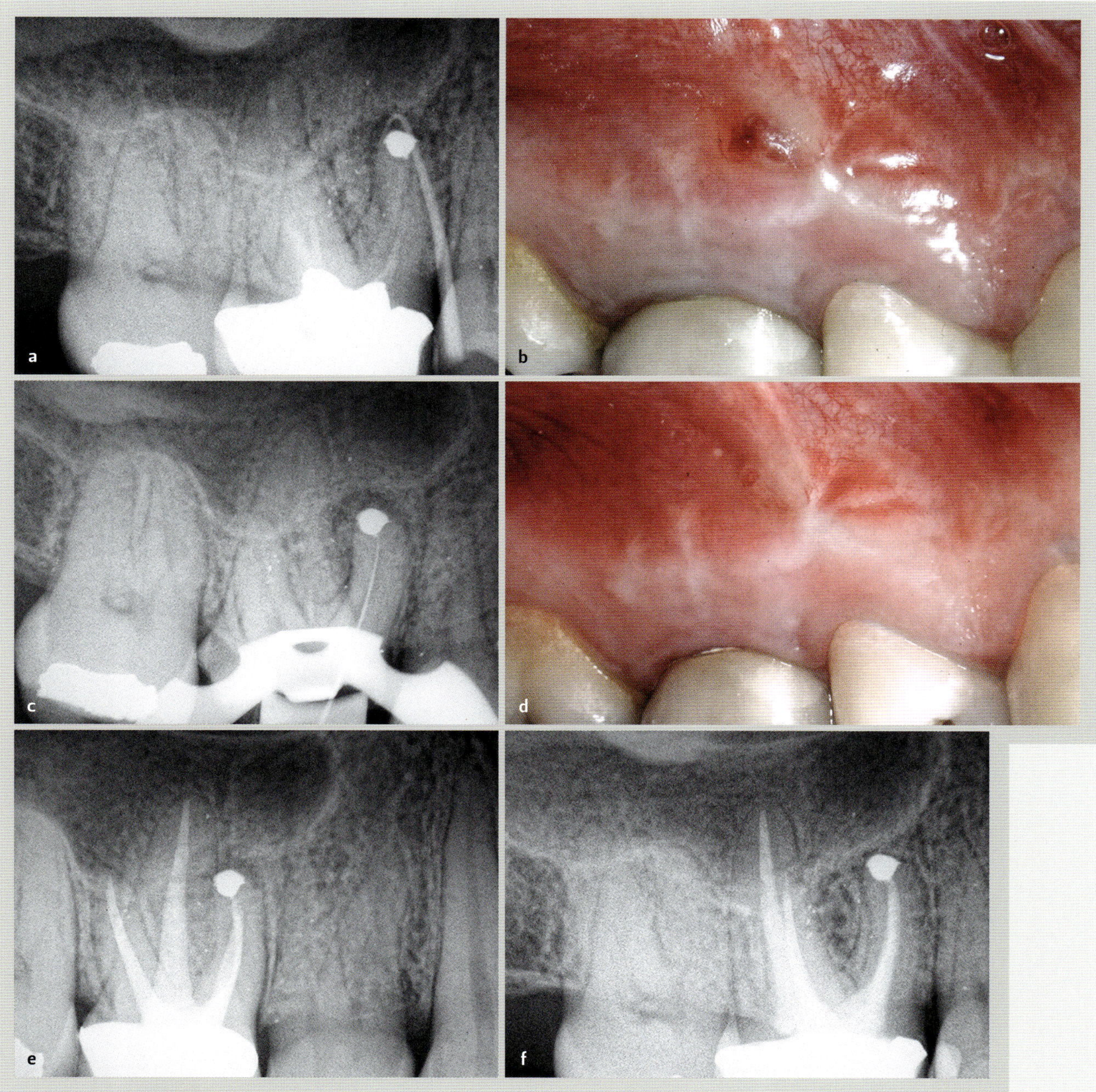

2.55 a) Preoperative radiograph of an upper right first molar showing a gutta-percha point introduced in a sinus tract. The case had been treated surgically by someone who positioned and amalgam retrofill on top of a root with a very poor endodontic treatment. It is obvious that the case could and should have been treated nonsurgically. **b)** The sinus tract is evident and also the scar of the previous surgical procedure is evident. Then scar is showing that the flap used before was a semilunar flap. **c)** The crown has been removed and the molar has been retreated nonsurgically. **d)** One week after cleaning and shaping the four canals of the molar the sinus tract is completely healed. **e)** Postoperative radiograph. **f)** Recall radiograph two years later.

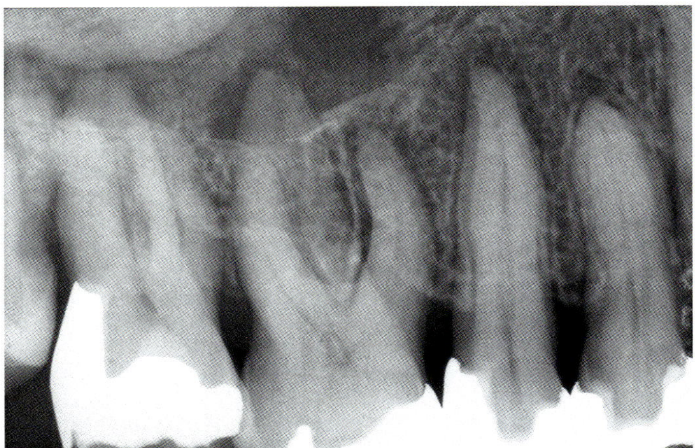

2.56 Every tooth of this radiograph test vital, therefore the apical radiolucencies are not lesions of endodontic origin. The biopsy confirmed that the patient has an adenocarcinoma of the maxillary sinus.

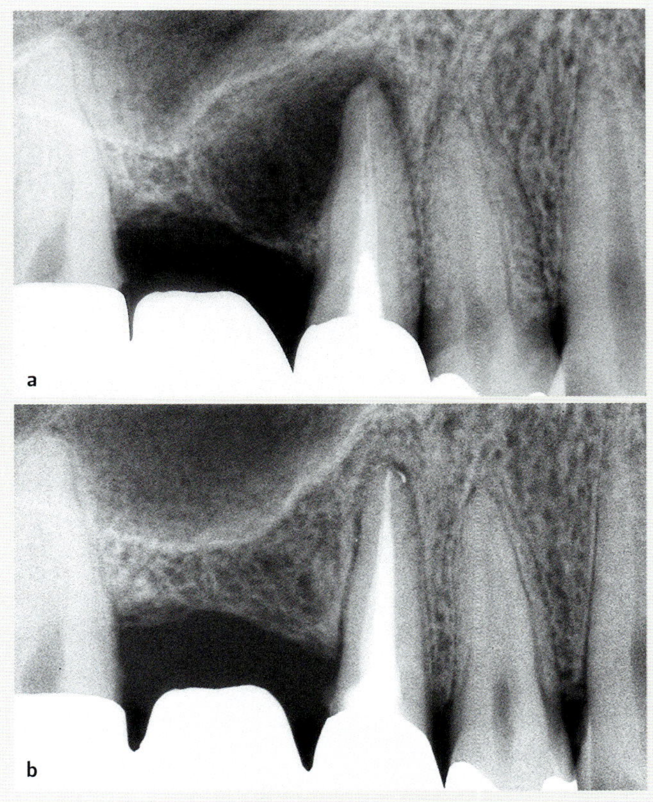

2.57 **a)** The radiograph shows a lateral lesion: this is an indication for a nonsurgical retreatment, since the lesion is maintained by bacteria in a lateral canal, which could be difficult or impossible to treat surgically. **b)** Two-year recall: a small lateral canal has been filled on the distal aspect of the root and the lesion is completely healed.

existence of a lateral canal, this is often impossible to access surgically; therefore, these cases should be treated conventionally first, in the attempt to fill the lateral canal responsible for the lesion. On the other hand, thanks to magnification, to the ultrasonic tips, and thanks to the carrier available today, many times the lateral canal can be accessed, prepared and filled through a surgical approach (2.58, 2.59).

2. *Periodontal pockets and combined endodontic-periodontic lesions* (2.60). In such cases, the prognosis of the lesions depends on the severity of the periodontal desease. If the prognosis is poor, the tooth needs to be extracted.
3. *Unfavorable crown-to-root ratio* (2.61). As will be discussed in other chapters, the surgical procedure involves the removal of few millimeters of the root length. If this compromises the stability of the tooth itself, the tooth needs to be extracted.
4. *Vertical root fractures* (2.62). When a "J" shaped radiolucency is present along the entire root length, associated with the typical probing of a small, narrow and deep defect, the diagnosis of a vertical root fracture is obvious and the only treatment is extraction. To confirm the diagnosis of vertical root fracture, a marginal flap can be raised to expose the entire fracture line. However, when possible, the diagnosis can today be confirmed examining the root canal wall under the operating microscope. In such cases, instead of raising a surgical flap, it will be less traumatic for the patient to have the access cavity opened and some obturating material removed. If a vertical line is visible on the canal wall and in correspondence with it there is probing on the external surface of the root, then the diagnosis of a vertical root fracture is obvious (2.63)
5. *Risk of osteonecrosis due to the use of bisphosphonates* (see 5.12). Bisphosphonates and other drugs

Cont'd on page 57

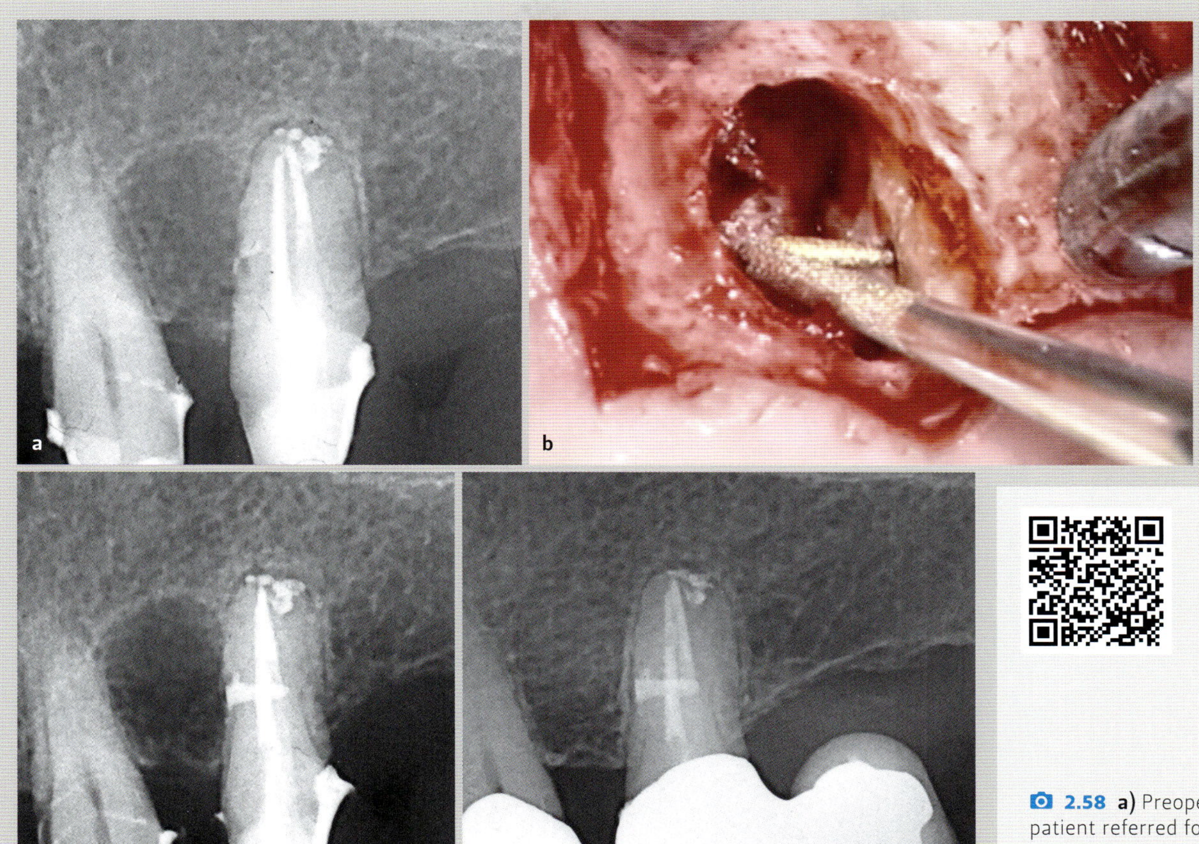

2.58 a) Preoperative radiograph of patient referred for surgical endodontics. Notice the lateral lesion. **b)** The ultrasonic tip is preparing the lateral cavity for the retrofill. **c)** Postoperative radiograph. **d)** Two-year recall.

2.59 a) Preoperative radiograph of an upper right second premolar with both a periapical and a lateral lesion. **b)** The micro-probe is showing the presence of the lateral canal. **c)** The ultrasonic tip is making the root-end preparation for the retrofill of the main canal. **d)** The ultrasonic tip is now making the root-end preparation for the retrofill of the lateral canal. **e)** The micro-probe is showing the lateral canal prepared and communicating with the main retroprep. **f)** The MAP System is carrying white MTA in the main canal. **g)** The micro-mirror is showing the MTA which is filling the lateral canal. **h)** The main canal and the lateral canal are now obturated with white MTA. **i)** The bony krypt is now bleeding and the flap can be sutured. **j)** Postoperative radiograph. **k)** Recall radiograph two years later.

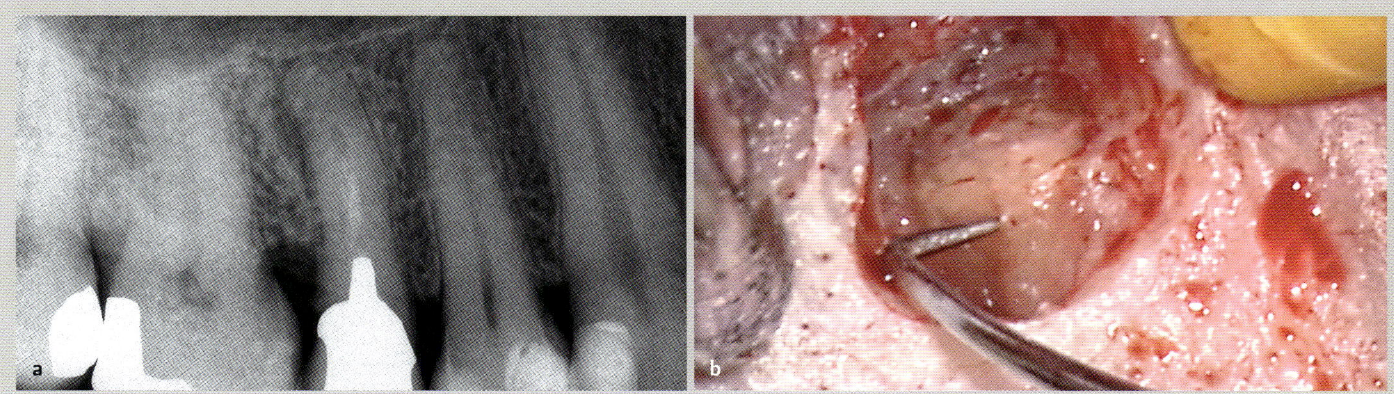

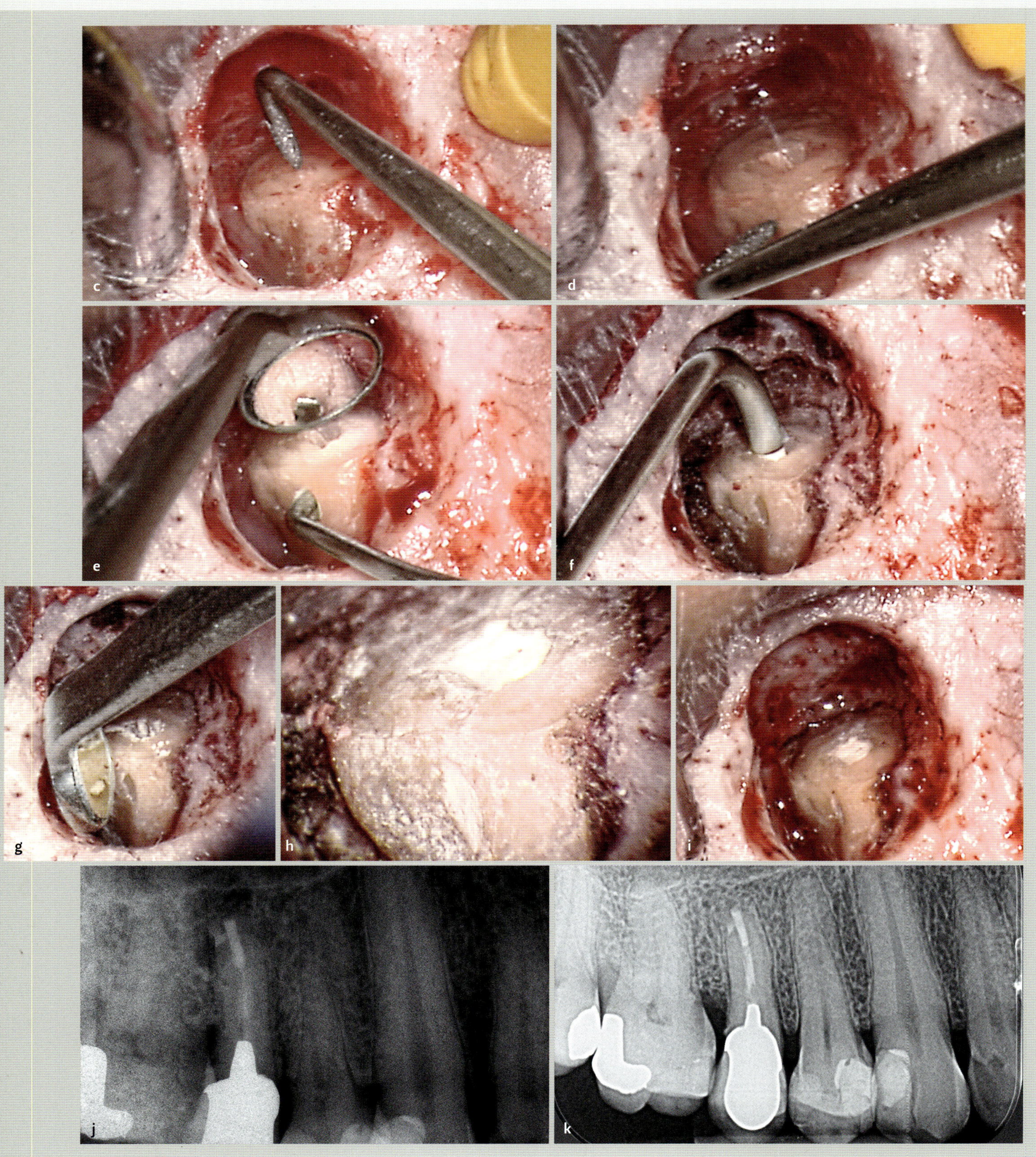
c
d
e
f
g
h
i
j
k

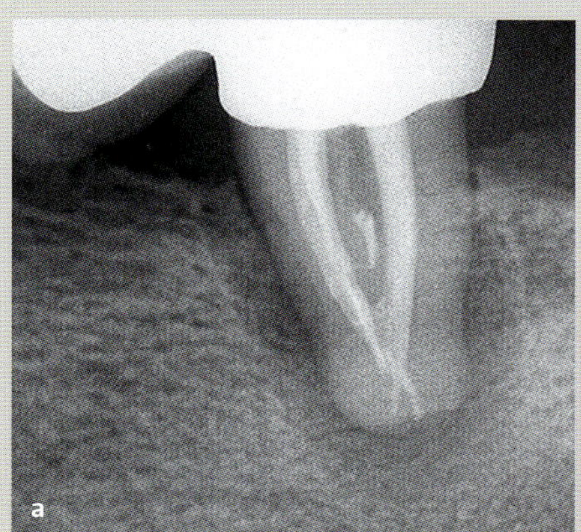

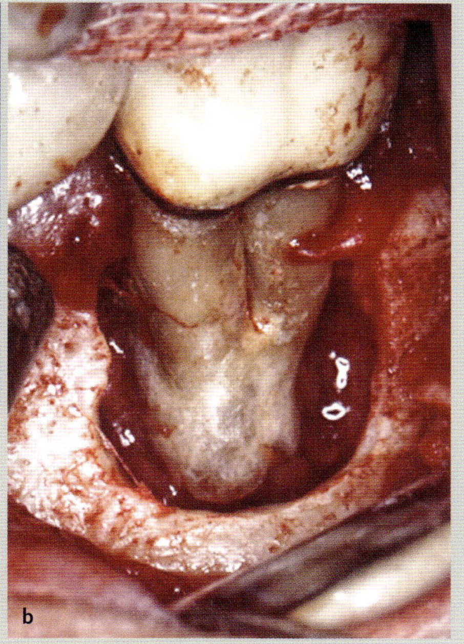

2.60 **a)** The lower left second molar has a periapical lesion and also a periodontal involvement. **b)** Due to the severity of the periodontal disease, the tooth will be extracted.

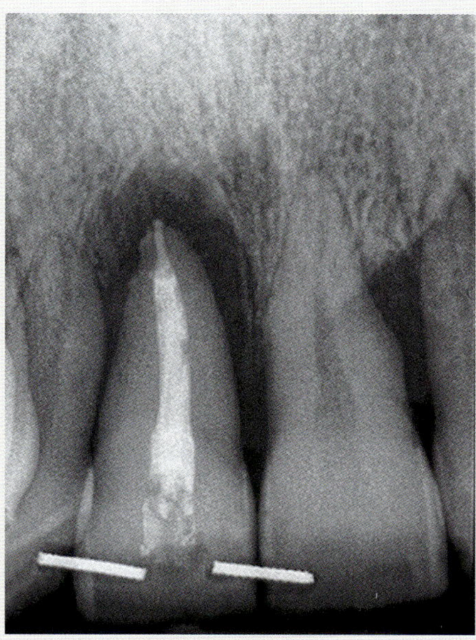

2.61 The central incisor was referred for surgical endodontics. The contraindication is obvious.

2.62 Vertical fracture of an upper left first premolar. **a)** The preoperative radiograph gives no information about the existence of the vertical fracture, except for the small radiolucency distal to the screw post. **b)** The periodontal probe indicates the existence of a tubular defect. **c)** Schematic representation of a periodontal defect that has developed at a vertical fracture. **d)** A small, exploratory full-thickness marginal flap confirms the suspicion of a vertical fracture, which could not be diagnosed radiographically. **e)** The extracted tooth.

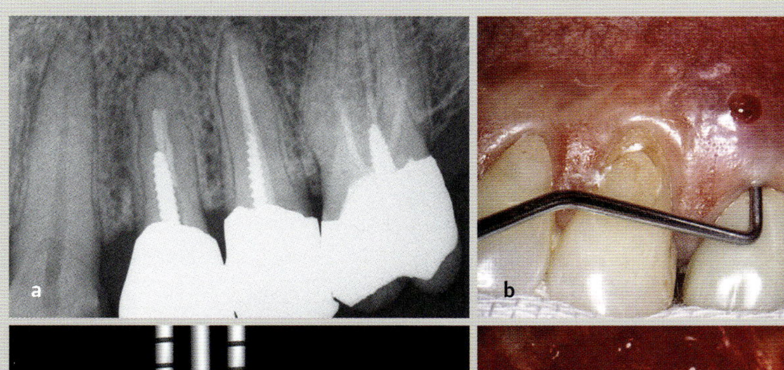

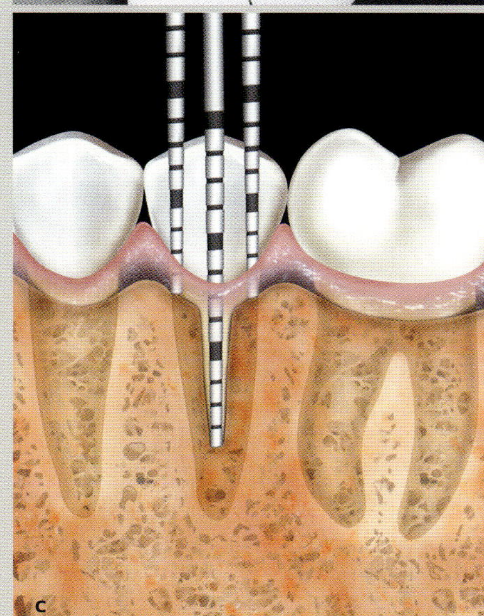

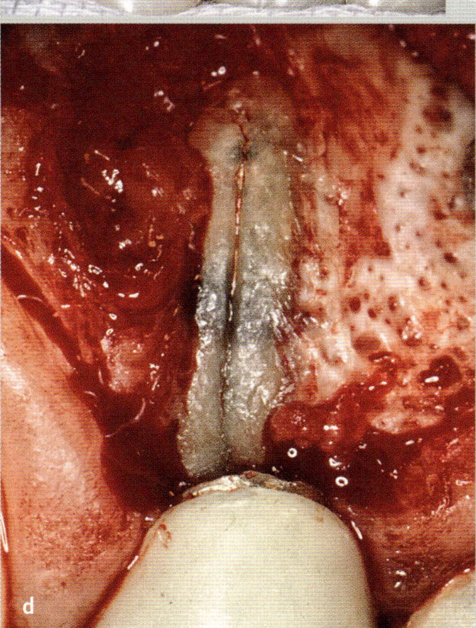

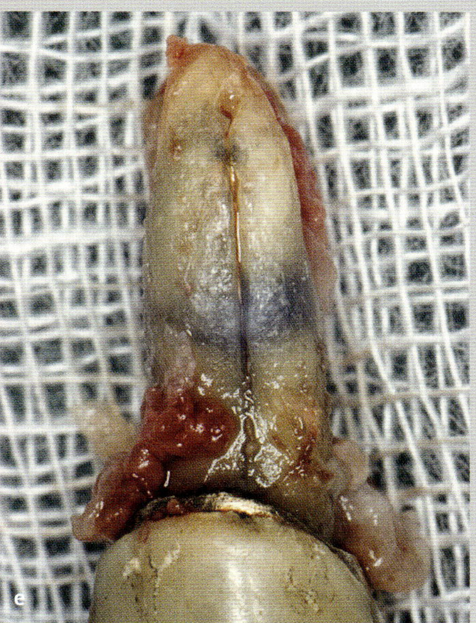

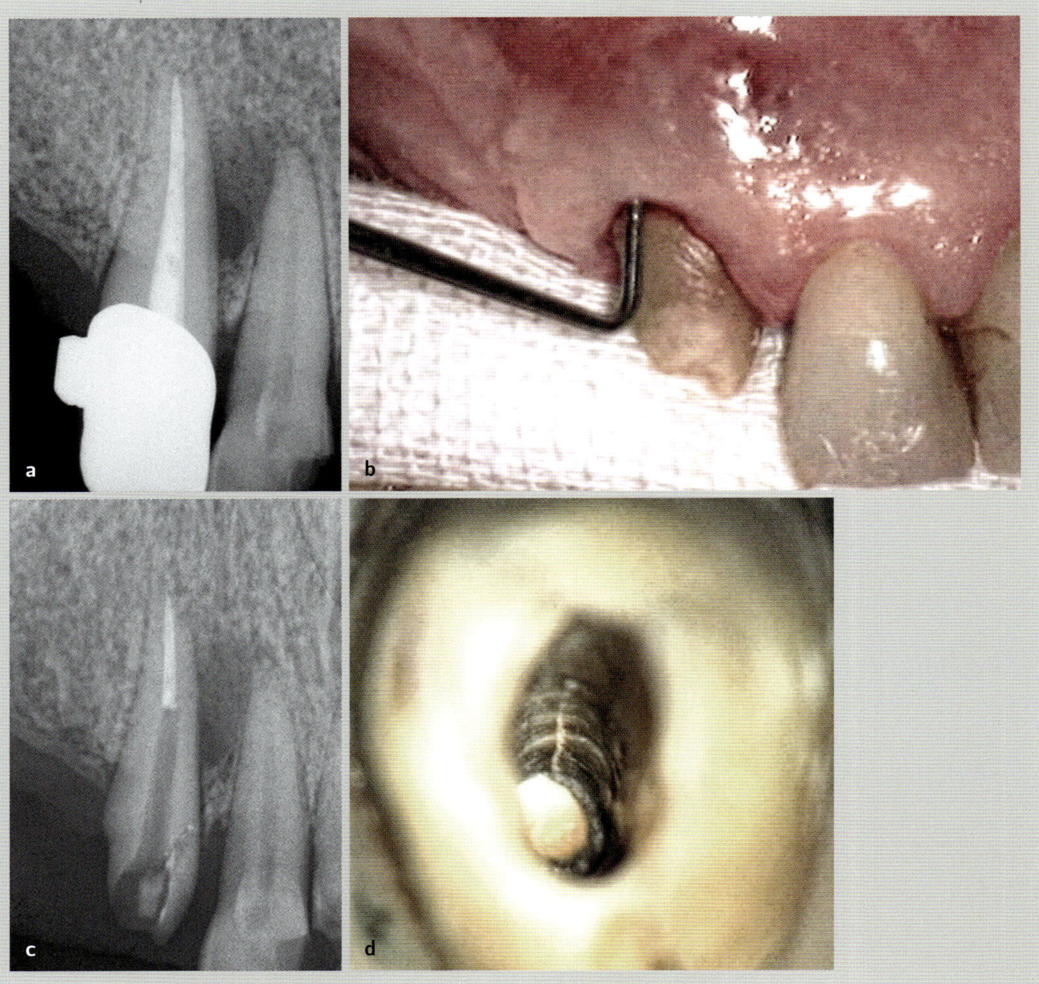

2.63 **a)** The upper right cuspid was successfully treated fifteen years before and recently became the only abutment for a posterior removable prosthesis. A lesion is present on the mesial aspect of the root. The adjacent lateral incisor tests vital. **b)** The prosthetic crown has been removed and the periodontal probe is showing a narrow and deep defect. **c)** The gutta-percha has been easily removed to explore the root canal walls under the microscope. **d)** A vertical line is evident on the buccal surface of the canal wall, exactly in correspondence with the external defect.

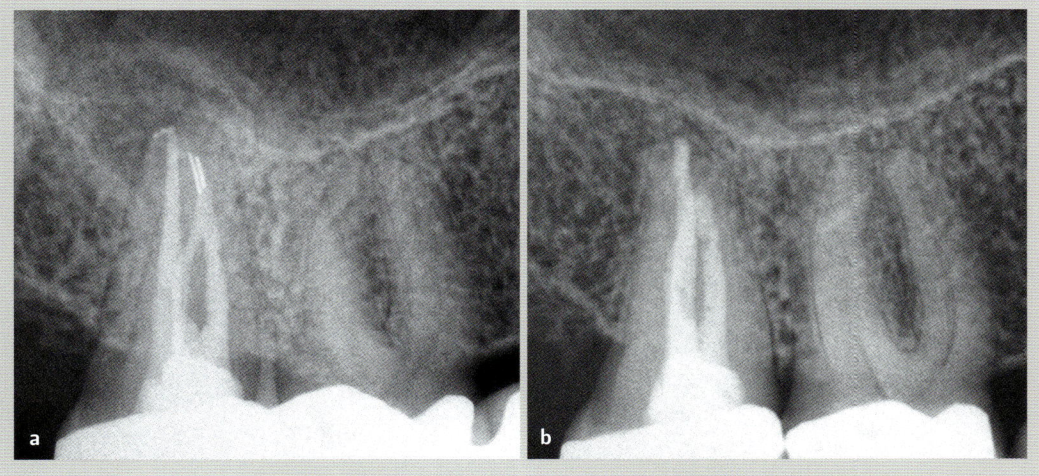

2.64 **a)** The upper right second molar has two broken instruments in the mesio-buccal canals. The cheek of the patient has enough retractability, therefore the surgical procedure can be successfully performed. **b)** Recall radiograph two years later.

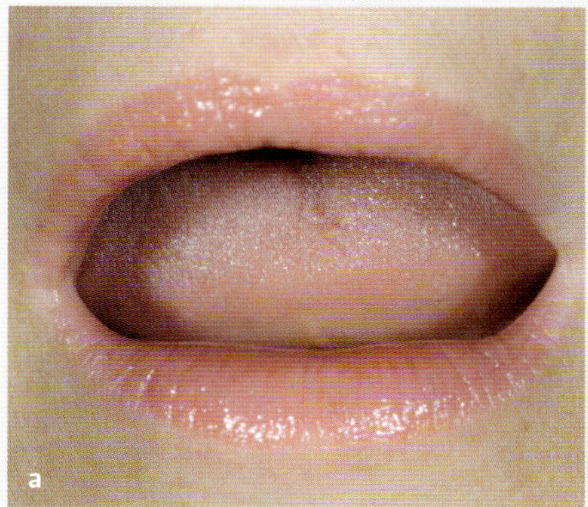

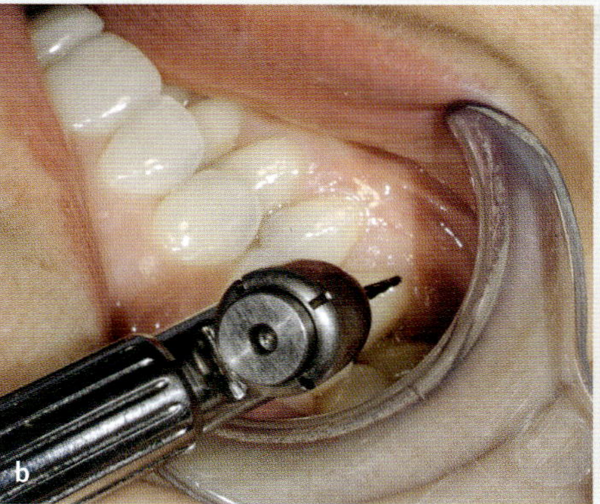

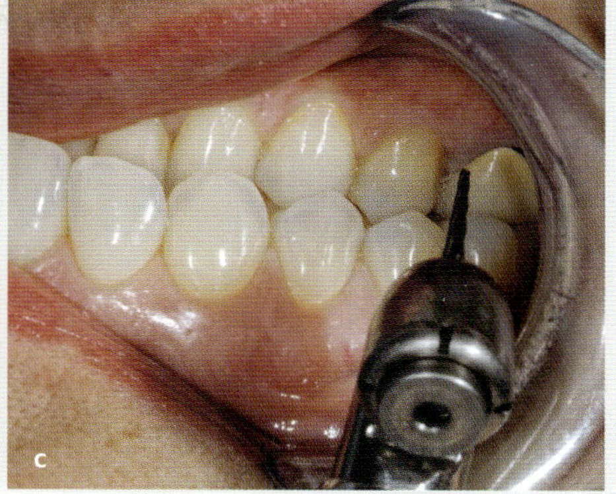

2.65 a) The labial perimeter is quite limited. **b, c)** The patient is positioned in the dental chair simulating the surgical procedure. There is a very limited access to the first molar, therefore on that tooth the surgical procedure is contraindicated.

used to treat osteoporosis and some malignancies occasionally produce a rare and dangerous reaction in the maxilla and mandible called "bisphosphonates-associated osteonecrosis of the jaw".[138] Patients on intravenous therapy for more than 2 years are at the greater risk for developing osteonecrosis.[139] Patients on oral bisphosphonates have a significantly lower risk. The exact mechanism for this osteonecrosis is still unknown but may be related to the fact that bisphosphonates inhibit angiogenesis and osteoclast function. Endodontic surgical procedures present an increased risk for developing osteonecrosis of the jaw in patients with a history of intravenous bisphosphonate use, and these procedures should be avoided.[133]

6 *Limited access to posterior teeth.* Periapical surgery is performed having patient with a closed mouth. For this reason, patients don't need to have a large mouth, but it is essential the retractability of their cheek (2.64). A small labial perimeter and an abundant thickness of the muscles can make the surgical procedure quite complicate or even make it impossible. For this reason, it is always mandatory to see the patient at a first consultation before scheduling the surgical appointment. During this occasion the patient will be positioned in the dental chair simulating the surgery, just to make sure there is an adequate access and visibility to the surgical site (2.65).

7 *Indiscriminate use of surgery* (see 2.55). Indiscriminate use of surgery for those cases that can be handled nonsurgically is unethical and should not be practiced.[116] Periapical surgery is contraindicated when nonsurgical treatment or retreatment is feasible and has a good chance of a successful outcome. In conclusion, the nonsurgical retreatment should always be the first choice before attempting a surgical procedure.

8 *Anatomic contraindications.* The unusual location of the mental foramen coronal to the apex of the premolar that needs surgery is an obvious contraindication for the surgical procedure (6.11), as well as the unusual location of the distobuccal root of the first molar of the 6.12.

REFERENCES

1. Johnson BR, Fayad M. *Periradicular surgery. In Hargreaves KM, Berman LH, eds. Pathways of the Pulp. 11th ed.* St. Louis, MO: Elsevier; 2016:402.
2. Reit C, Dahlen G. *Decision making analysis of endodontic treatment strategies in teeth with apical periodontitis.* Int Endod J. 1988;21:291-9.
3. Danin J, Stromberg T, Forsgren H, et al. *Clinical management of non-healing periradicular pathosis. Surgery versus endodontic retreatment.* Oral Surg Oral Med Oral Pathol Oral Radiol Endod. 1996;82:213-7.
4. Kvist T, Reit C. *Result of endodontic retreatment: a randomized clinical study comparing surgical and nonsurgical procedures.* J Endod. 1999;25:814-7.
5. Gorni FM, Gagliani MM. *The outcome of endodontic retreatmnent: a 2-year follow-up.* J Endod. 2004; 30(1):1-4.
6. Nygaard-Ostby B, Schilder, H. *Inflammation and infection of the pulp and periapical tissues: a synthesis.* Oral Surg Oral Med Oral Pathol Oral Radiol Endod. 1972;34:498.
7. Weine FS, Gerstein H. *Periapical Surgery.* In Weine FS: Endodontic Therapy. 3rd ed. St. Louis: The C.V. Mosby Company. 1982;408-76.
8. Kim S, Kratchman S. *Modern endodontic surgery concepts and practice: a review.* J Endod. 2006; 32(7): 601-23.
9. Rubinstein RA, Kim S. *Short-term observation of the results of endodontic surgery with use of a surgical operation microscope and Super-EBA as root-end filling material.* J Endod. 1999;25:43-48.
10. Torabinejad M, Sabeti M, Glickman G. *Surgical endodontics.* In: Rotstein I, Ingle JI (eds). Ingle's Endodontics, 7th ed. Shelton, CT: People's Medical, 2017 (in press).
11. Schilder H. *Nonsurgical endodontics. Continuing education course.* Boston University. Nov. 1978.
12. Grossman L. *Endodontic Practice.* 10th ed. Philadelphia: Lea & Febiger. 1981:348-83.
13. Ten Cate AR. *Development of the tooth and its supporting tissues.* In Oral Histology: Development, structure and function. 2nd ed. St. Louis: The CV Mosby Company. 1985:223.
14. Luukko K, Kettunen P, Fristad VI, Bergreen E. *Structure and function of the dentin-pulp complex.* In Hargreaves KM, Cohen S, eds. Pathways of the Pulp. 10th ed., St. Louis: The CV Mosby Company, 2011:457.
15. Lin LM, Huang GTJ, Rosenberg P. *Proliferation of epithelial cell rests, formation of apical cysts, and regression of apical cysts after periapical wound healing.* J Endod. 2007; 33:908.
16. Nair PNR, Sundqvist G, Sjögren U. *Experimental evidence supports the abscess theory of development of radicular cysts.* Oral Surg Oral Med Oral Pathol Oral Radiol Endod. 2008;106:294.
17. Ten Cate AR. *The epithelial cell rests of Malassez and the genesis of the dental cyst.* Oral Surg Oral Med Oral Pathol. 1972;34:56.
18. Shafer W, Hine M, Levy B. *A textbook of oral pathology.* 3rd ed. Philadelphia: WB Saunders. 1974.
19. McCall JO, Walds SS. *Clinical dental roentgenology.* 3rd ed. Philadelphia: WB Saunders. 1952:192.
20. White SC, Sapp JP, Seto BG, Mankovich NJ. *Absence of radiometric differentiation between periapical cysts and granulomas.* Oral Surg Oral Med Oral Pathol. 1994;78:650.
21. Baumann L, Rossman SR. *Clinical, roentgenologic, and histopathologic findings in teeth with apical radiolucent areas.* Oral Surg Oral Med Oral Pathol. 1956;9:1330.
22. Bhaskar SN. *Periapical lesions-types, incidence, and clinical features.* Oral Surg Oral Med Oral Pathol. 1966;21:657.
23. Lalonde ER. *A new rationale for the management of periapical granulomas and cysts: an evaluation of histopathological and radiographic findings.* J Am Dent Assoc. 1970;80:1056.
24. Linenberg WB, Westfield NJ, Waldron CA, Delaune GF. *A clinical, roentgenographic, and histopathologic evaluation of periapical lesions.* Oral Surg Oral Med Oral Pathol. 1964;17:467.
25. Morse DR, Schacterle GR, Wolfson EM. *A rapid chairside differentiation of radicular cysts and granulomas.* J Endod. 1976;2:17.
26. Priebe WA, Laxansky JP, Wuehrmann AH. *The value of the roentgenographic film in the differential diagnosis of periapical lesions.* Oral Surg Oral Med Oral Pathol. 1954;7:979.
27. Wais FT. *Significance of findings following biopsy and histologic study of 100 periapical lesions.* Oral Surg Oral Med Oral Pathol. 1958;11:650.
28. Cunningham CJ, Penick EG. *Use of roentgenographic contrast medium in the differential diagnosis of periapical lesions.* Oral Surg Oral Med Oral Pathol. 1968;26:96.
29. Forsberg A, Hagglund G. *Differential diagnosis of radicular cyst and granuloma: use of X-ray contrast medium.* Dental Radiogr Photogr. 1960;33:84.
30. Howell FV, De La Rosa VM, Abrams AM. *Cytologic evaluation of cystic lesions of the jaws: a new diagnostic technique.* J So Cal Dent Assoc. 1968;36:161.
31. Abbott PV. *Traumatic bone cyst: case report.* Endod Dent Traumatol. 1992;8:170.
32. Polastri F, Barbero P, Gallesio C, Cappella M. *Le cisti emorragiche della mandibola.* Min Stom. 1989;38:1279.
33. Rushton MA. *Solitary bone cysts in the mandible.* Br Dent J. 1946;81:37.
34. Newton CW, Zunt SL. *Endodontic intervention in the traumatic bone cyst.* J Endod. 1987;13:405.
35. Gazzotti A, Collini M, Raffaini M, Fiamminghi L, Bozzetti A. *Problemi diagnostico-terapeutici delle cisti epidermoidi dei mascellari.* Dental Cadmos. 1983;12:105.
36. Saccardi A, Ficarra G. *Cheratocisti delle ossa mascellari. Sindrome di Gorlin.* Dental Cadmos. 1993;18:76.
37. Cummings RR, Ingle JI, Frank AL, Gloick DH, Antrim, DD. *Endodontic Surgery.* In: Ingle JI. *Endodontics.* 3rd ed. Philadelphia: Lea & Febiger. 1985:618-707.

38. **Bhaskar SN.** *Non surgical resolution of radicular cysts.* Oral Surg Oral Med Oral Pathol. 1972;34:458.
39. **Grossman LI, Oliet S, Del Rio CE.** *Endodontic Practice.* 11th ed. Philadelphia: Lea & Febiger. 1988:88.
40. **Natkin E, Oswald RJ, Carnes LI.** *The relationship of lesion size to diagnosis, incidence, and treatment of periapical cysts and granulomas.* Oral Surg Oral Med Oral Pathol. 1984;57:82.
41. **Ricucci D, Siqueira JF.** *Periradicular pathology.* In *Endodontology. An integrated biological and clinical view.* Quintessence Publishing. 2013;125.
42. **Roda RS, Gettleman BH.** *Nonsurgical retreatment.* In Hargreaves KM, Berman LH, eds. Cohen's Pathways of the Pulp. 11th ed. Elsevier. 2016:326.
43. **Nair PNR, Pajarola G, Schroeder HE.** *Types and incidence of human periapical lesions obtained with extracted teeth.* Oral Surg Oral Med Oral Pathol. 1996;81:93.
44. **Nair PNR.** *Apical periodontitis: a dynamic encounter between root canal infection and hot response.* Periodontol 2000. 1997;13:121.
45. **Nair PNR.** *On the cause of persistent apical periodontitis: a review.* Int Endod J. 2006;39:249.
46. **Nair PNR.** *New perspectives on radicular cysts: do they heal?* Int Endod J. 1998;31:155.
47. **Nair PNR, Sjögren U, Schumacher E, Sundkvist G.** *Radicular cyst affecting a root-filled human tooth: a long-term post-treatment follow-up.* Int Endod J. 1993;26:225.
48. **Berman LH, Hartwell GR.** *Diagnosis.* In Hargreaves KM, Cohden S, eds. Pathways of the Pulp. 10th ed. St. Louis: The CV Mosby Company. 2011:13.
49. **Baumgartner JC, Picket AB, Muller JT.** *Microscopic examination of oral sinus tracts and their associated periapical lesions,* J Endod. 1984;10(4):146.
50. **American Association of Endodontists.** *Glossary of Endodontic Terms,* 7th ed, 2003.
51. **Bella G, Russo S, Messina G, Badalà A.** *Considerazioni sulle fistole cutanee odontogene.* Il Dentista Moderno. 1989;10:2353.
52. **Calvarano G, De Paolis F, Bernardini G.** *Fistole cutanee e salivari: soluzioni terapeutiche.* Odontostomatologia e Implantoprotesi. 1991;1:82.
53. **Galli S, Galli G.** *Considerazioni anatomiche e cliniche su un caso di fistola odontogena.* Odontostomatologia e Implantoprotesi, 1989;6:50
54. **Harnisch H.** *Apicectomia. Scienza e Tecnica Dentistica.* Milano: Edizioni Internazionali. 1981:30.
55. **Palattella G, Mangani F, Palattella P, Palattella D, Mauro R.** *Fistole cutanee da estrinsecazioni perimandibolari di parodontiti apicali croniche.* Dental Cadmos. 1987;2:57.
56. **Harrison JW, Larson WJ.** *The epithelized oral sinus tract.* Oral Surg Oral Med Oral Pathol. 1976;42:511.
57. **Bence R.** *Trephination technique.* J Endod. 1980;6:657.
58. **Elliot JA, Holcomb JB.** *Evaluation of a minimally traumatic alveolar trephination procedure to avoid pain.* J Endod. 1988;14:405.
59. **Cummings RR, Ingle JJ, Frank AL, Glick DH, Antrim DD.** *Endodontic Surgery.* In Ingle JI. Endodontics. 3rd ed. Philadelphia: Lea & Febiger. 1985:618-707.
60. **Peters DD.** *Evaluation of prophilactic alveolar trephination to avoid pain.* J Endod. 1980;6:518.
61. **Sargenti A.** *Apical aeration made easy by a new instrument.* J Br Endod Soc. 1972;6:49.
62. **Seldon HS, Parris L.** *Management of endodontic emergencies.* J Dent Child. 1970;37:260.
63. **Weine FS.** *Endodontic therapy,* 2nd ed. St. Louis: The CV Mosby Company. 1976:138.
64. **Wolch I.** *A new approach to the basic principles of endodontics.* Int Dent J. 1975;25:179.
65. **Kaufman AY.** *An enigmatic sinus tract origin.* Endod Dent Traumatol. 1989;5:159.
66. **McWalter GM, Alexander JB, Del Rio CE, Knott JW.** *Cutaneous sinus tracts of dental etiology.* Oral Surg Oral Med Oral Pathol. 1988;66:608.
67. **Heling I, Rotstein I.** *A persistent oro-nasal sinus tract of endodontic origin.* J Endod. 1989;15:132.
68. **Strader RJ, Seda HJ.** *Periapical abscess with intranasal fistula.* Oral Surg Oral Med Oral Pathol. 1971;32:881.
69. **Pagavino G, Pace R, Giachetti L.** *Le fistole cutanee odontogene: diagnosi e terapia,* R.I.S., Anno LIX, 11;1990;12:6.
70. **Zerman N, Urbani G, Menegazzi G, Cavalleri G.** *Il trattamento di fistole cutanee da lesioni endodontiche.* Il Dentista Moderno 1990;7:1381.
71. **Braun RJ, Lehman J.** *A dermatologic lesion resulting from a mandibular molar with periradicular pathosis.* Oral Surg Oral Med Oral Pathol. 1981;52:210.
72. **Cioffi GA, Terezhalmy GT, Parlette HL.** *Cutaneous draining sinus tract: an odontogenic etiology.* J Am Acad Dermatol. 1986;14:94.
73. **Lewin-Epstein J, Taicher S, Azaz B.** *Cutaneous sinus tract of dental origin.* Arch Dermatol 1978; 114:1158.
74. **Spear KL, Sheridan PJ, Perry HO.** *Sinus tracts to the chin and jaws of dental origin.* J Am Acad Dermatol. 1983;8:486.
75. **Johnson BR, Remeikis NA, Van Cura JE.** *Diagnosis and treatment of cutaneous facial sinus tracts of dental origin.* J Am Dent Assoc. 1999;130:832.
76. **Sommer RF, Ostrander FD, Crowley M.C.** *Clinical Endodontics,* 3rd ed., Philadelphia: WB Saunders Company. 1966:306.
77. **Bender IB, Seltzer S.** *The oral fistula: its diagnosis and treatment.* Oral Surg Oral Med Oral Pathol. 1961;14:1367.
78. **Ogilvie AL.** *Periapical Pathosis.* In: Ingle JI. Endodontics. Philadelphia: Lea & Febiger. 1965:361-62.
79. **Ordman LJ, Gillman T.** *Studies in the healing of cutaneous wounds. II. The healing of epidermal, appendageal and dermal injuries inflicted by suture needles in the skin of pigs.* Arch Surg. 1966;93:883.
80. **Sicher H.** *In: Orban's Oral Histology and Embriology,* 6th ed., St. Louis: The CV Mosby Company. 1966:1-17.
81. **Ingle JI.** *Root canal obturation.* J Am Dent Assoc. 1956;53:47.
82. **Weine FS, Gerstein H.** In: *Endodontic therapy.* 3rd ed. St. Louis: The CV Mosby Company. 1982;409-476.

83. SCHILDER H. *Filling root canals in three dimensions.* Dent Clin North Amer. 1967:723-44.

84. LIN LM, SKRIBNER JE, GAENGLER P. *Factors associated with endodontic treatment failures.* J Endod. 1992;18:625.

85. FUKUSHIMA H, YAMAMOTO K, HIROHATA K, SAGAWA H, LEUNG K, WALKER CB. *Localization and identification of root canal bacteria in clinically asymptomatic periapical pathosis.* J Endod. 1990;16:534.

86. LIN LM, PASCON EA, SKRIBNER J, GAENGLER P, LANGELAND K. *Clinical, radiographic, and histologic study of endodontic treatment failures.* Oral Surg Oral Med Oral Patol. 1991;71:603.

87. NAIR PNR, SJÖGREN U, KREY G, KAHNBERG KE, SUNDQVIST G. *Intraradicular bacteria and fungi in root-filled, asymptomatic human teeth with therapy-resistant periapical lesions: a long-term light and electron microscopic follow-up study.* J Endod. 1990;16:580.

88. SJÖGREN V, FIGDOR D, PERSSON S, SUNDQUIST G. *Influence of infection at the time of root filling on the outcome of endodontic treatment of teeth with apical periodontitis.* Int Endod J. 1997;30:297.

89. HALSE A, MOLVEN O. *Overextended gutta-percha and kloropercha N-O root canal filling. Radiographic findings after 10-17 years.* Acta Odontol Scand. 1987;45:171.

90. SJOGREN U, HAGGLUND B, SUNDQVIST G, WING K. *Factors affecting the long-term results of endodontic treatment.* J Endod. 1990;16:498.

91. TAVARES T, SOARES IJ, SILVEIRA NL. *Reaction of rat subcutaneous tissue to implants of gutta-percha for endodontic use.* Endod Dent Traumatol. 1994;10:174.

92. SCHILDER H. *Advanced course in Endodontics.* Boston, MA: Boston University of Graduate Dentistry. 1978.

93. DEEMER JP, TSAKNIS PJ. *The effects of overfilled polyethylene tube intraosseous implants in rats.* Oral Surg Oral Med Oral Pathol. 1979;48:358.

94. TAVARES T, SOARES IJ, SILVEIRA NL. *Reaction of rat subcutaneous tissue to implants of gutta-percha for endodontic use.* Endod Dent Traumatol. 1994;10:174.

95. BERGENHOLTZ G, LEKHOLM U, MILTHON R, ENGSTROM B. *Influence of apical overinstrumentation and overfilling on retreated root canals.* J Endod. 1979;5:310.

96. SPANGBERG L. *Biological effects of root canal filling materials. Toxic effect in vitro of root canal filling materials on HeLa cells and human skin fibroblasts.* Odontol Revy. 1969;20:427.

97. FELDMANN G, NYBORG H. *Tissue reactions to filling materials. Comparison between gutta-percha and silver amalgam implanted in rabbit.* Odontol Revy. 1962;13(1):1.

98. SPANGBERG L. *Biological effects of root canal filling materials. Reaction of bony tissue to implanted root canal filling material in Guinea pigs.* Odontol Tidskr. 1969;77:133.

99. AUGSBURGER RA, PETERS DD. *Radiographic evaluation of extruded obturation materials.* J Endod. 1990;16:492.

100. YUSUF H. *The significance of the presence of foreign material periapically as a cause of failure of root treatment.* Oral Surg Oral Med Oral Pathol. 1982;54:566.

101. PERTOT WJ, CAMPS J, REMUSAT M, PROUST JP. *In vivo comparison of the biocompatibility of two root canal sealers implanted into the mandibular bone of rabbits.* Oral Surg Oral Med Oral Pathol. 1992;73:613.

102. LINDQVIST L, OTTESKOG P. *Eugenol liberation from dental materials and effect on human diploid fibroblast cells.* Scand J Dent Res. 1981;89:552.

103. MERYON SD, JAKERMAN, KJ. *The effects in vitro of zinc released from dental restorative materials.* Int Endod J. 1985;18:191.

104. MERYON SD, JOHNSON SG, SMITH AJ. *Eugenol release and the cytotoxicity of different zinc oxide-eugenol combinations.* J Dent Res. 1988;16:66.

105. TORABINEJAD M, CHIVIAN N. *Clinical applications of mineral trioxide aggregate.* J Endod. 1999;25:197.

106. NAGATA JY, GOMES BP, ROCHA LIMA TF, MURAKAMI LS, ET AL. *Traumatized immature teeth treated with 2 protocols of pulp revascularization.* J Endod. 2014;40:606-612.

107. BARONE M. *Gli apici beanti.* Attualità Dentale 1991;32:6.

108. BARONE M, CIANCONI L. *Il trattamento endo-conservativo combinato di un incisivo superiore ad apice immaturo in presenza di estesa lesione periapicale.* Pratica odontoiatrica 1991;8:30.

109. AMATO M, RICCITIELLO F, FORTUNATO L, MARTUSCELLI R. *Nuovo cemento all'idrossido di calcio nella tecnica dell'apecificazione.* R.I.S. 1990;1-2:4.

110. BRADLEY HL. *The management of the non-vital anterior tooth with an open apex.* J Brit Endod Soc. 1977;10:77.

111. HAM JW, PATTERSON SS, MITCHELL DF. *Induced apical closure of immature pulpless teeth in monkeys.* Oral Surg Oral Med Oral Pathol. 1972;33:438.

112. CHRISTIANSEN R, KIRKEVANG L, HØRSTED-BINDSLEV P, WENZEL A. *Randomized clinical trial of root-end resection followed by root-end filling with mineral trioxide aggregate or smoothing of the orthograde gutta-percha root filling-1-year follow-up.* Int Endod J. 2009;42:105-14.

113. KIM E, SONG JS, JUNG IY, LEE SJ, KIM S. *Prospective clinical study evaluating endodontic microsurgery outcomes for cases with lesions of endodontic origin compared with cases with lesions of combined periodontal-endodontic origin.* J Endod. 2008;34:546-51.

114. TASCHIERI S, DEL FABBRO M, TESTORI T, WEINSTEIN R. *Microscope versus endoscope in root-end management: a randomized controlled study.* Int J Oral Maxillofac Surg. 2008;37:1022-6.

115. TSESIS I, ROSEN E, SCHWARTZ-ARAD D, FUSS Z. *Retrospective evaluation of surgical endodontic treatment: traditional versus modern technique.* J Endod. 2006;32:412-6.

116. ARENS D. *Practical lessons in endodontic surgery.* Quintessence Publishing Co. Inc., 1998:4.

117. WEINE FS, BUSTAMANTE MA. *Periapical surgery.* In: Weine FS, ed. Endodontic therapy, 5th ed. St. Louis: Mosby. 1995:536-39.

118. BOUCHER Y, SOBEL M, SAUVEUR G. *Persistent pain related to root canal filling and apical fenestration: a case report.* J. Endod. 2000;26(4): 242-44.

119. **Spasser HF, Wendt R.** *A cause for recalcitrant post endodontic pain.* NY State Dent J 1973;39:25-6.
120. **Patterson SA.** *Considerations and indications for endodontic surgery.* In: Arens DE, Adams WR, DeCastro RA, eds. Endodontic surgery. Philadelphia: Harper & Row. 1981:4-5.
121. **Ricucci D, Siqueira JF.** *Failure of the endodontic treatment.* In: *Endodontology. An integrated biological and clinical view.* Quintessence Publishing. 2013;354.
122. **Harn WM, Chen YH, Yuan K, Chung CH, Huang PH.** *Calculus-like deposit at apex of tooth with refractory apical periodontitis.* Endod Dent Traumatol. 1998;14:237-40.
123. **Noiri Y, Ehara A, Kawahara T, Takemura N, Ebisu S.** *Participation of bacterial biofilm in refractory and chronic periapical periodontitis.* J Endod. 2002;28:679-83.
124. **Ricucci D, Martorano M, Bate AL, Pascon EA.** *Calculus-like deposit on the apical external root surface of teeth with post-treatment apical periodontitis: report of two cases.* Int Endod J. 2005;38:262-71.
125. **Bystrom A, Happonen RP, Sjgren U, Sundquist G.** *Healing of Periapical lesions of pulpless teeth after endodontic treatment with controlled asepsis.* Endod Dent Traumatol. 1997;3:58-63.
126. **Happonen RP.** *Periapical actinomycosis: a follow up study of 16 surgically treated cases.* Endod Dent Traumatol. 1986;2:205-209.
127. **Nair PN, Sjogren U, Figdor D, Sundquist G.** *Persistent periapical radiolucencies of root-filled human teeth, failed endodontic treatments, and periapical scars.* Oral Surg Oral Med Oral Pathol Oral Radiol Endod. 1999;87:617-27.
128. **Nair PNR, Schroeder HE.** *Periapical actinomycosis.* J Endod. 1984;10:567-70.
129. **Sjögren U, Happonen RP, Kahnberg KE, Sundquist G.** *Survival of Arachnia propionica in periapical tissue.* Int Endod J. 1988;21:277-82.
130. **Ricucci D, Siqueira JF Jr.** *Apical actinomycosis as a continuum of intraradicular and extraradicular infection: case report and critical review on its involvement with treatment failure.* J Endod. 2008;34:1124-129.
131. **Hess W, Zurcher E..** *The anatomy of the root canals of the teeth of the permanent dentition. The anatomy of the root canals of the teeth of the deciduos dentition and of the first permanent molars.* London, J. Bale Sons & Danielsson, 1925.
132. **Ida RD, Gutmann JL..** *Importance of anatomic variables in endodontic treatment outcomes: case report.* Endod Dent Traumatol 1995;11:199-203.
133. **Siqueira JF, Araujo MCP..** *Histological evaluation of the effectiveness of five instrumentation techniques for cleaning the apical third of root canals.* J Endodon 1997;23:499-502.
134. **Peters OA..** *Current challenges and concepts in the preparation of root canal systems: a review.* J Endod. 2004;30:559-567.
135. **Paqué F, Balmer M, Attin T, Peters OA.** *Preparation of Oval-shaped Root Canals in Mandibular Molars Using Nickel-Titanium Rotary Instruments: A Micro-computed Tomography Study.* J Endod. 2010;36:703-707.
136. **Carr GB, Schwartz RS, Schaudinn C, Gorur A, J. William Costerton JW..** *Ultrastructural Examination of Failed Molar Retreatment with Secondary Apical Periodontitis: An Examination of Endodontic Biofilms in an Endodontic Retreatment Failure.* J Endod. 209;35:1303-1309.
137. **Torabinejad M.** *Diagnosis and treatment planning. In: Torabinejad M, Rubinstein R. The art and science of contemporary surgical endodontics.* Quintessence Publishing Co. Inc. 2017:75-96.
138. **Jursky K.** *Wound healing. In The art and science of contemporary surgical endodontics.* Quintessence Publishing. 2017;239.
139. **Goodell GG.** *Biphosphonate-associated osteonecrosis of the jaw.* Endodontics. Colleagues for excellence. 20\12;(2):1-8.

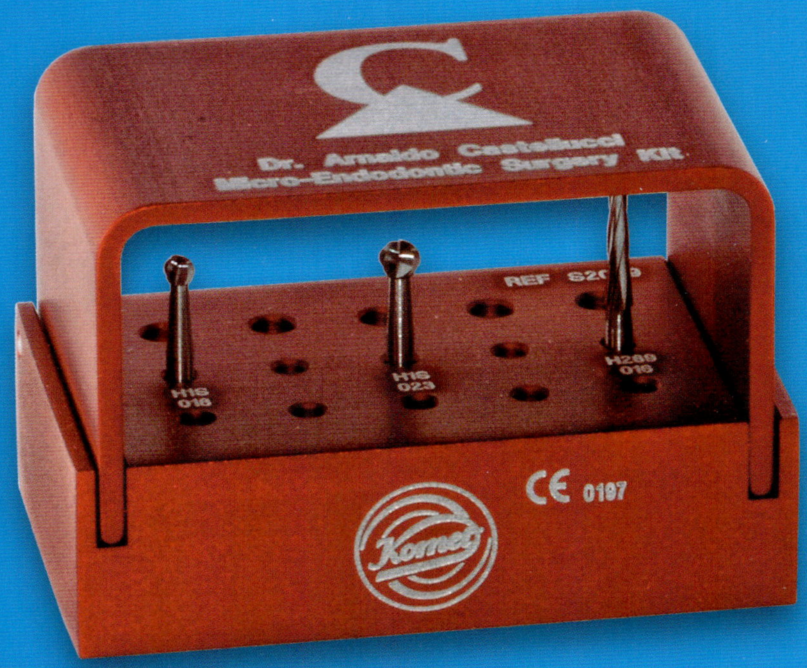

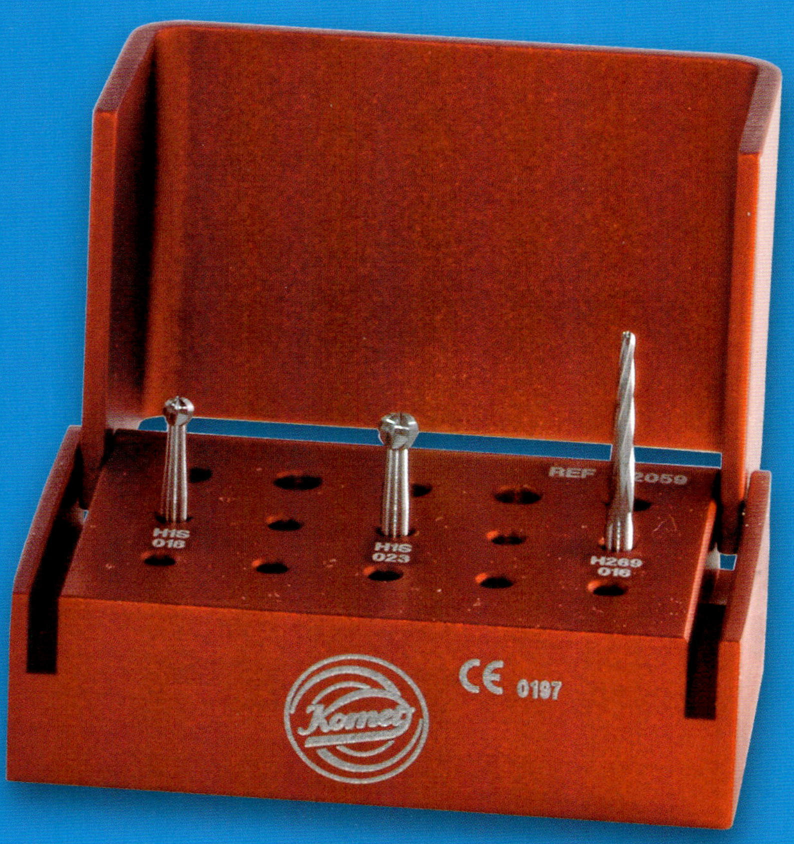

The complete kit of burs used in surgery: #6, #8 round burs to make the access opening to the root apex and the Lindemann bur for the root-end resection and bevel.

Microsurgical Instruments

Matteo Papaleoni, DDS, Arnaldo Castellucci, MD, DDS

As will be described in Chapter 4, the introduction of the operating microscope has been one of the most significant developments in the past three decades in endodontics.[1–6] In the early 1990s, operating microscopes were introduced into endodontics and endodontic residency programs in the United States. It is well recognized today that performing apical surgery without magnification is no longer adequate or defensible.[7] On the other hand, it is obvious that performing surgical endodontics under high magnification without specifically designed "micro" instruments is nearly impossible. Gary Carr has been the first designer and manufacturer of the first generation of microsurgical instruments for endodontics and surgical endodontics. Some of these instruments are just a miniaturized version of traditional instruments, while many others have been specifically designed to be used in microsurgical endodontics.

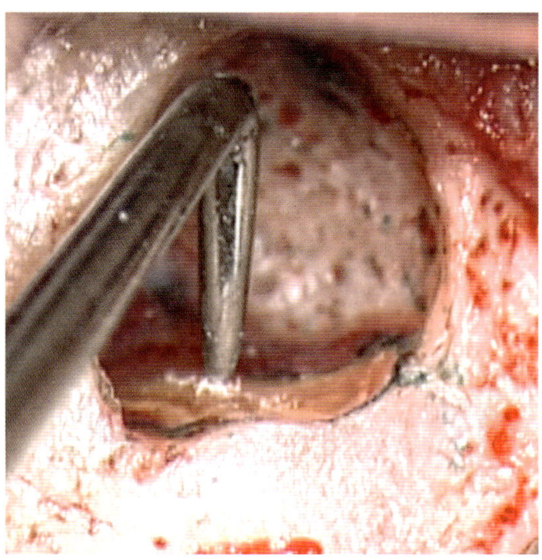

3.1 The Carr explorer is creating a tracking groove in the isthmus that later will be deepened by the ultrasonic tip.

Examination Instruments

Examination instruments are the same used in endodontic practice, like the mirror, periodontal probe and endodontic explorer. The "microexplorer" has been specifically designed for microsurgery and can be used to confirm the presence of a fenestration on the cortical bone before starting the preparation of the bony crypt, to make the initial groove to prepare the isthmus or to

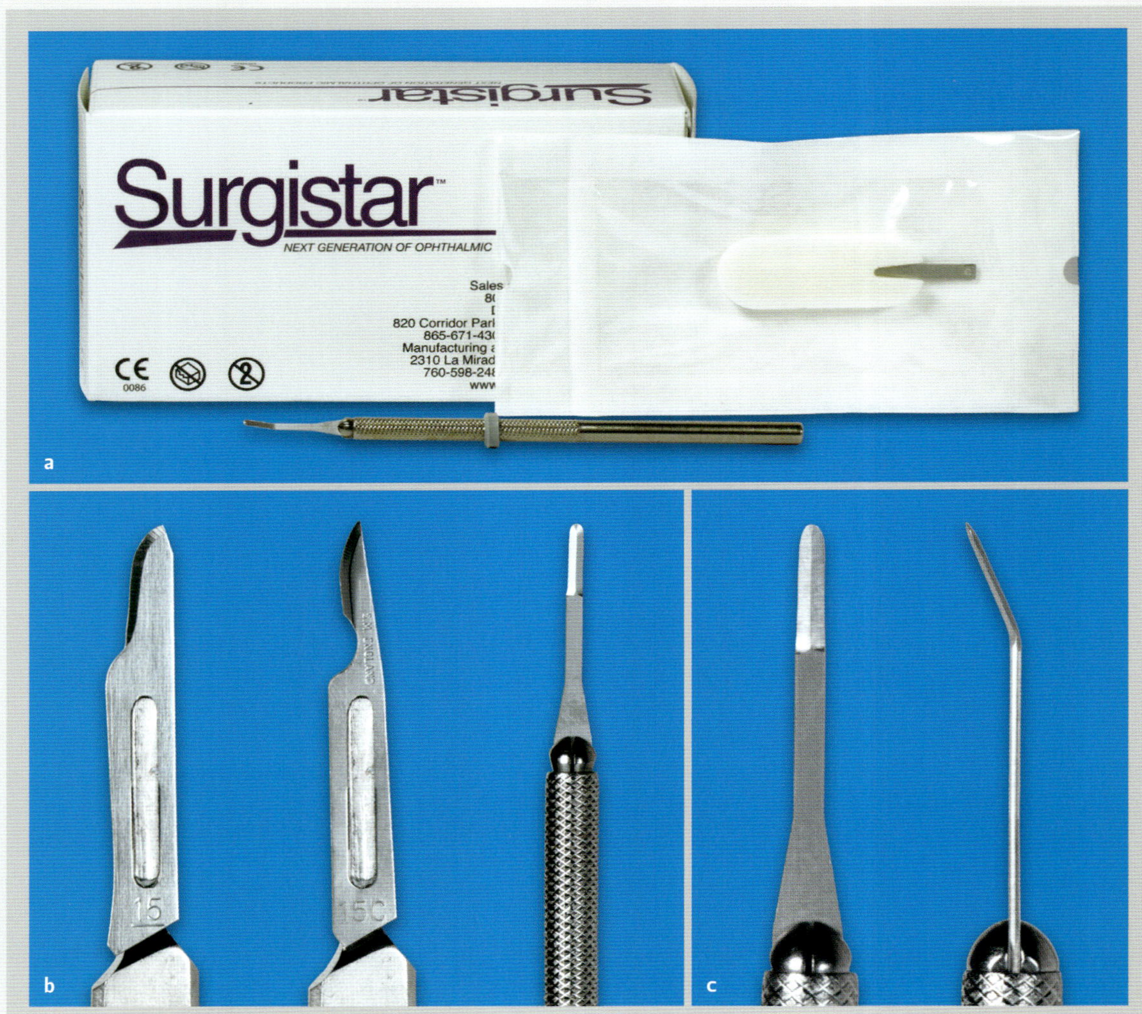

3.2 **a)** The microsurgical blade Surgistar (Micro-Mini Blade Surgistar USM6910, Vista, CA). **b)** Comparison of BP #15 blade, BP #15 C blade and the microsurgical blade. **c)** The microsurgical blade Surgistar has a rounded tip and two cutting sides, with a 10° angle.

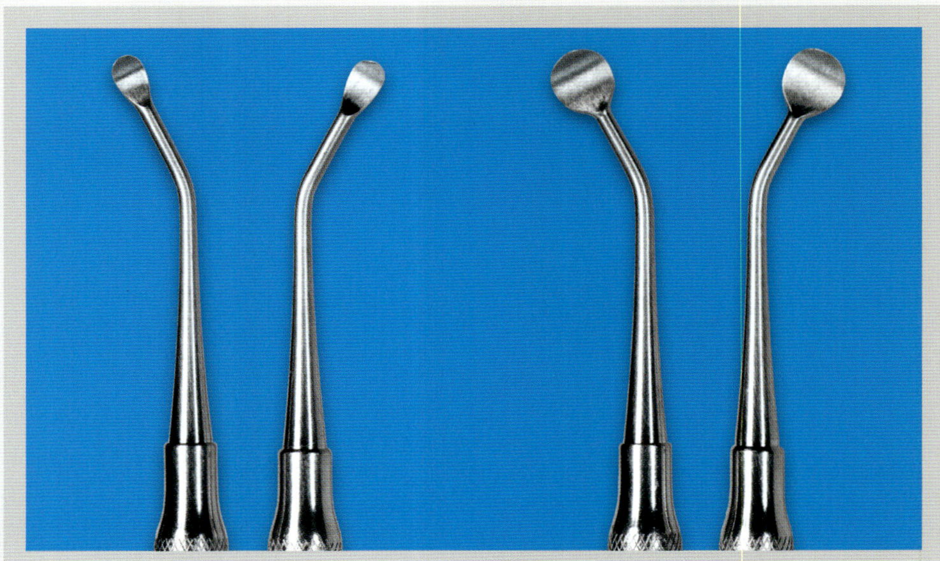

3.3 The Ruddle elevators. They are intended to dissect and lift the full thickness flap from the osseous surface.

locate a lateral canal. It was designed by Gary Carr and is the explorer CX 1 (3.1).

Incision and Elevation Instruments

The ideal blade is a microsurgical blade like the microsurgical blade Surgistar (Micro-Mini Blade Surgistar USM6910, Vista, CA) which is much smaller than the BP #15 and smaller than the BP #15C (3.2). The soft tissue elevators are used to elevate the full thickness flap from the underlying cortical bone in an atraumatic manner, in order not to cause postoperative discomfort to the patient and to guarantee fast and uneventful healing. As will be described in Chapter 7, a sharp periosteal elevator is used, like one of the Ruddle elevators (American Eagle, Missoula, MT) (3.3), so as to gently dissect the periosteum from the osseous surface, without leaving fragments of the periosteum that later will cause continuous bleeding.

Retraction Instruments

Once the elevation is completed, retraction of the tissue is necessary to provide surgical access to the apex of the involved tooth or teeth. The retractor must always rest on cortical bone with light but firm pressure, in an atraumatic manner, in order not to cause postoperative discomfort to the patient. As will be described in more detail in Chapter 7, there are many retractors available

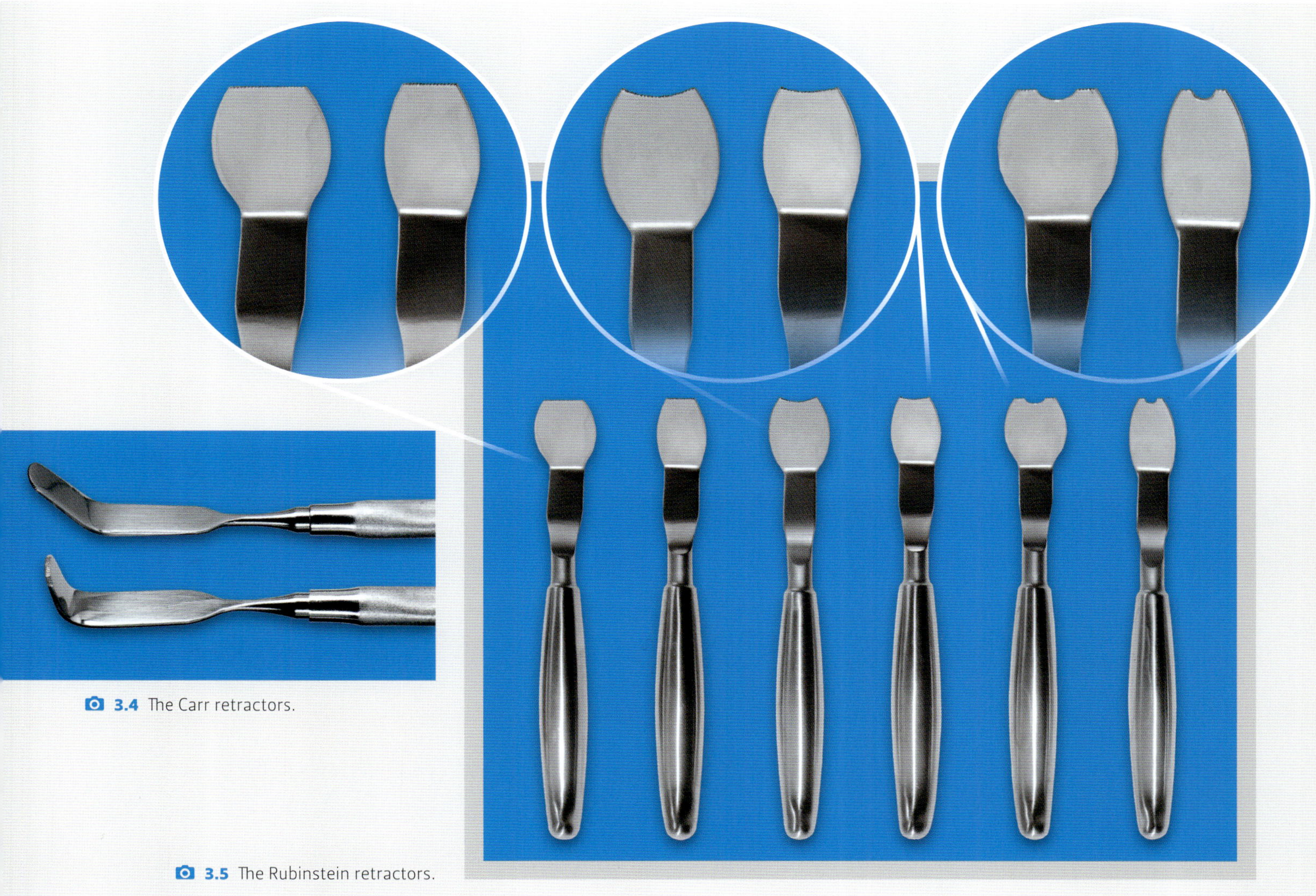

3.4 The Carr retractors.

3.5 The Rubinstein retractors.

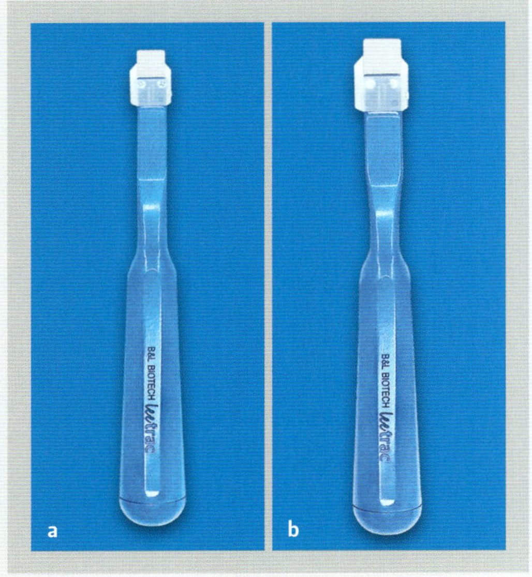

3.6 The Lee Trac Retractors, narrow **(a)** and wide **(b)** (B&L Biotech).

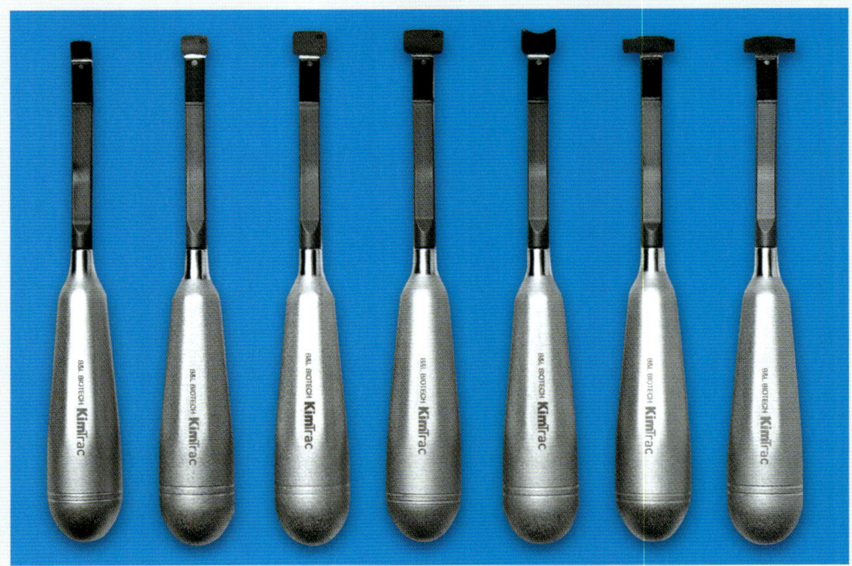

3.7 The Kim retractors (B&L Biotech).

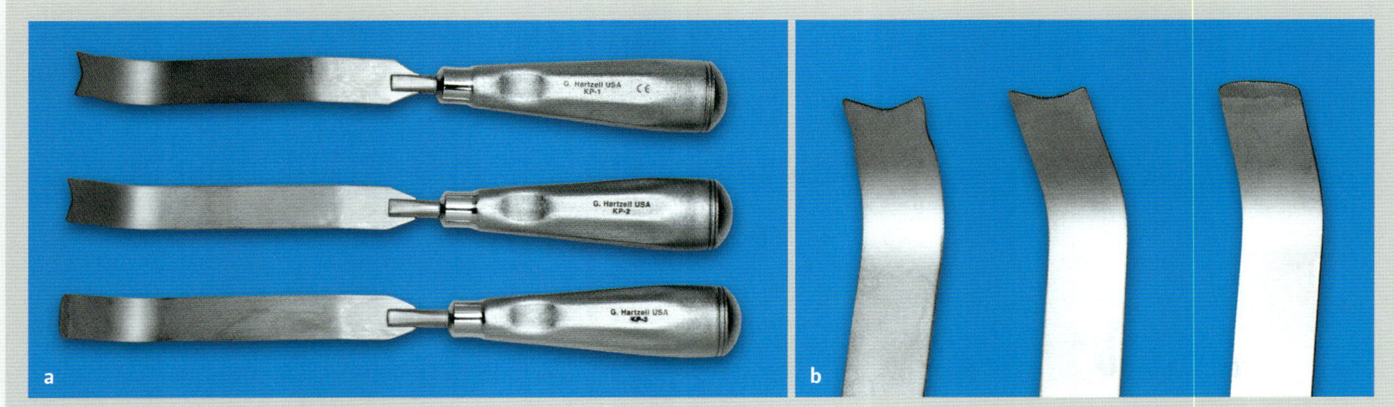

3.8 **a)** The Kim and Pecora retractors (KP Retractors by Obtura/Spartan). **b)** The retractors at higher magnification.

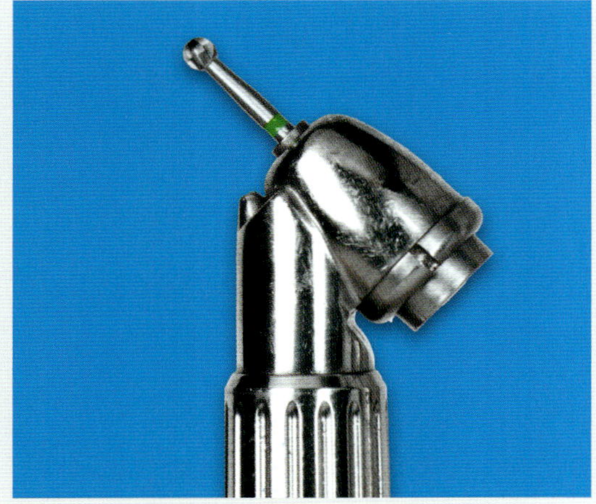

3.9 The Impact Air 45 (Palisades Dental, NJ, USA) with the #8 round bur.

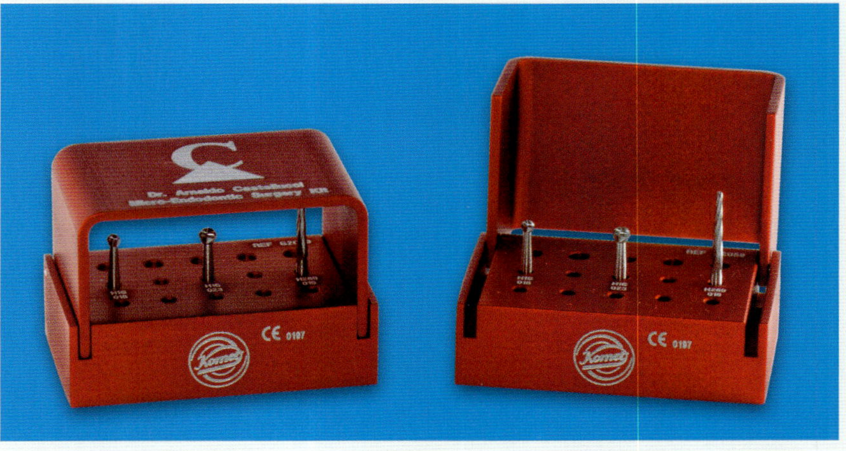

3.10 The complete kit of burs used in surgery: #6, #8 round burs to make the access opening to the root apex and the Lindemann bur for the root-end resection and bevel.

on the market. The most popular are the Carr retractors (3.4), the Rubinstein retractors (3.5), the Lee Trac retractors (3.6) and the Kim retractors (3.7). The Kim retractors (KimTrac retractors by B&L Biotech) are available in different widths (from 8 to 14 mm). They also have wings to separate the elevated soft tissue from the area of surgery and additional plastic protectors for soft tissue elevation, to provide better visibility. These retractors have serrated ends to guarantee a very precise and stable anchorage against the cortical bone plate. Similar retractors have been designed by Kim and Pecora (KP Retractors by Obtura/Spartan) (3.8). They have serrated ends and wide tips of 15 mm.

Osteotomy and Root-end Resection Instruments

The osteotomy and the root-end resection are done using a specifically designed high speed handpiece, like the Impact Air 45 (Palisades Dental, NJ, USA) (3.9). This handpiece delivers only irrigating solution and has no air exiting from the working end, in order to avoid the risk of creating air emphysema or embolism in the soft tissue around. The 45° surgical handpiece makes it easier to work in and to visualize difficult to reach areas, like posterior quadrants. The osteotomy is made using a surgical length round bur #6 or #8 (3.10). The root-end resection is made using a Lindemann bur on the same 45° surgical handpiece. This bur has fewer flutes compared to conventional burs, with the advantage of less clogging, less frictional heat and more efficiency (3.11).

Curettage Instruments

To curette the granulation tissue any periodontal curette can be used. Usually, the granulation tissue is not adherent to the surrounding bone, while is well attached to the root surface through the periodontal ligament, since it starts developing at the expenses of the periodontal ligament space. Therefore, the curette should be able to guarantee an efficient curettage of the root surface.

Inspection Instruments

It is well known that the use of the operating microscope in surgical endodontics doesn't require a steep "learning curve", for the simple reason that the operator can work in direct vision. The only time a "micro" mirror is needed is when it is necessary to examine the resected root surface, to evaluate the apical seal, to check the presence of an apical root fracture or to inspect the root-end preparation. Microsurgical mirrors are available in several different shapes, but the most popular are the round 3 mm and the oval 3 mm × 6 mm (3.12). The round mirror is particularly indicated for

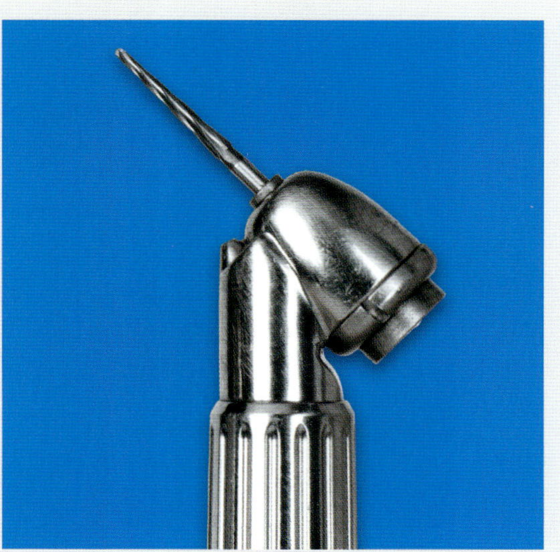

3.11 The Lindemann bur mounted on the Impact Air 45 high-speed handpiece.

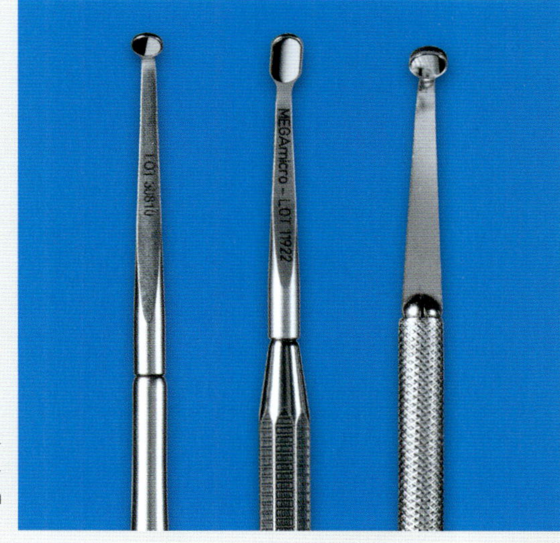

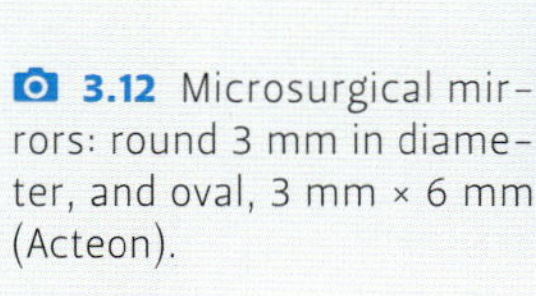

3.12 Microsurgical mirrors: round 3 mm in diameter, and oval, 3 mm × 6 mm (Acteon).

round single rooted teeth, while the oval is best indicated for roots with two canals, like the mesiobuccal root of upper molars and mesial root of lower molars. Another important characteristic that the microsurgical mirrors should have is the flexibility of their handle, to allow the reflection of the entire resected root surface using the correct angulation.

Ultrasonic Units

As it will be described in Chapter 11, at the end of the 80s, Gary Carr made a big revolution in the field of the surgical endodontics, introducing the ultrasonic retrotips specifically designed for the root-end cavity preparation during surgical endodontics. The ultrasonic units have a piezoelectric crystal made of quartz or ceramic located in the handpiece, which vibrates at 28,000 to 40,000 cycles per second. The energy is transferred to the ultrasonic tip, which then moves forward and backward in a single plane, brushing away the dentin with gentle strokes.[3] The most widely used ultrasonic units are the Spartan Wave (Spartan/Obtura) (3.13), the Piezon 250 EMS (3.14) and the Newtron Booster (Acteon) (3.15). They should always work at the minimum power and with continuous irrigation along the working portion of the cutting tip. The irrigation should also be minimized in order to maintain good visibility during the root-end preparation.

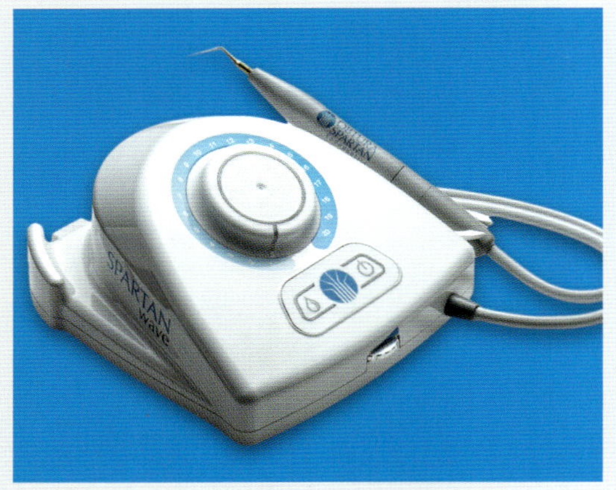

3.13 The Spartan Wave (Spartan/Obtura).

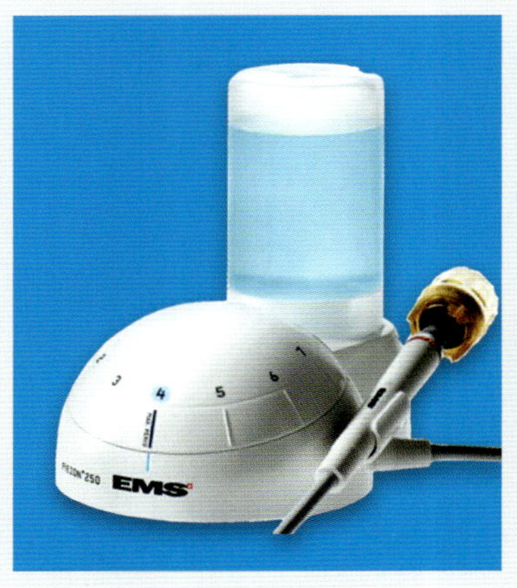

3.14 The Piezon 250 EMS.

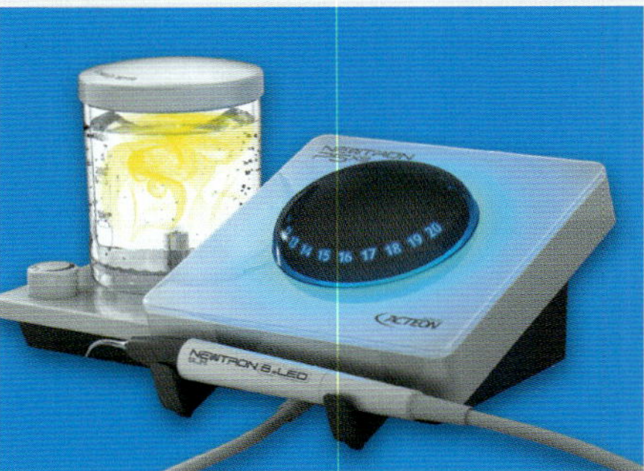

3.15 The Newtron Booster (Acteon).

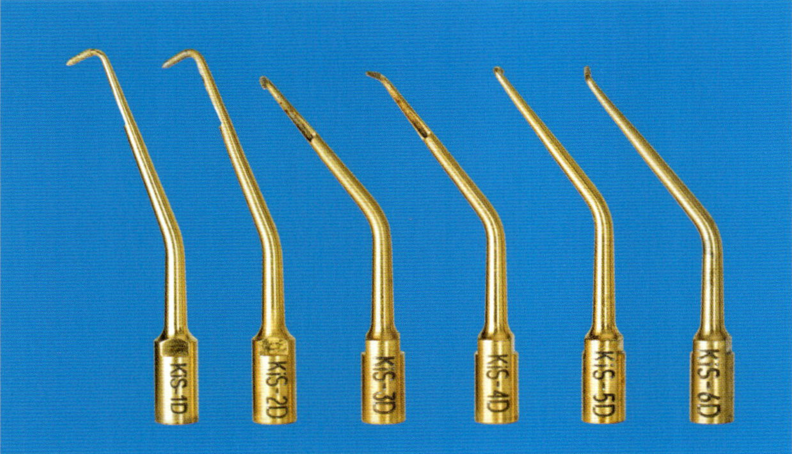

3.16 The Kim Surgical ultrasonic tips (KiS, by Spartan/Obtura).

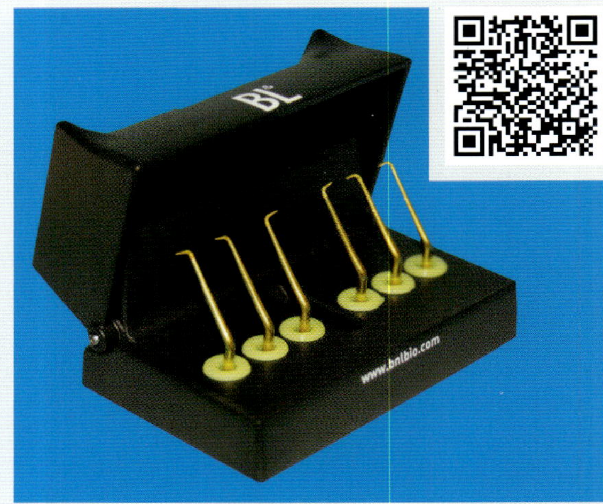

3.17 The Jet Tips (B&L Biotech).

Ultrasonic Tips

The first ultrasonic tips were those designed by Gary Carr at the end of the 80s and were known as Carr tips or CTs. They were made of stainless steel and because they did not have any coating, they are not very efficient. At the end of the 90s Spartan/Obtura introduced the Kim Surgical (KiS) ultrasonic tips (3.16), coated with zirconium nitride and having the water port next to the working tip rather than in the shaft, like the CTs. The coating makes the tips more efficient with a smoother cut and the correct position of the water port causes fewer microsurgical fractures because of the improved cooling due to the irrigation. Recently B&L Biotech introduced the Jet Tips (3.17) which have a special feature represented by "microsurgical projections" of the cutting surface (11.14). Those microsurgical projections make these tips very efficient especially in the removal of gutta-percha from the root canal. These tips are also bendable and can be bent in the desired direction for better access (11.15). In case there is the need to prepare a root-end cavity deeper than just 3 mm, Acteon recently introduced 3 ultrasonic tips designed by Dr. Betrand Khayat, having the length of 3 mm, 6 mm and 9 mm (3.18). They are particularly useful in front teeth where a long portion of the root canal remained completely empty (see 11.18). The tips have a diamond coating and they must always be used in sequence, from the shortest to the longest one.

Stropko Irrigator

This device is extremely useful both in nonsurgical and in surgical endodontics (3.19). It fits on Adec air/water syringe and allows for direct air or irrigation in a very limited area. During the root-end preparation the cavity must be carefully inspected and in order to do so, it must be completely dry. This cannot be obtained using paper points, the way we used to do years ago. The Stropko irrigator can mount a blunt needle of the desired size (Vista Dental) (3.20), small enough to enter into the root-end preparation (3.21).

Retrofilling Materials

As it will be described in detail in Chapter 12, amalgam was the most commonly used root-end filling material for many years and now it has been abandoned for many reasons, so that there is no valid reason today to continue its use. The first material that successfully replaced the old amalgam, was SuperEBA. SuperEBA (12.2) is a zinc oxide eugenol cement reinforced with ethoxy benzoic acid. It has been used for many years, especially after the advent of the ultrasonic root-end preparation.[3] The main characteristic of this material is that it maintains its plasticity for several minutes before setting, which allows one to condense it in large spaces, like the main root canal and the lateral canal, as shown in 1.1. Today the material of choice is MTA and other bioceramic cements (3.22).

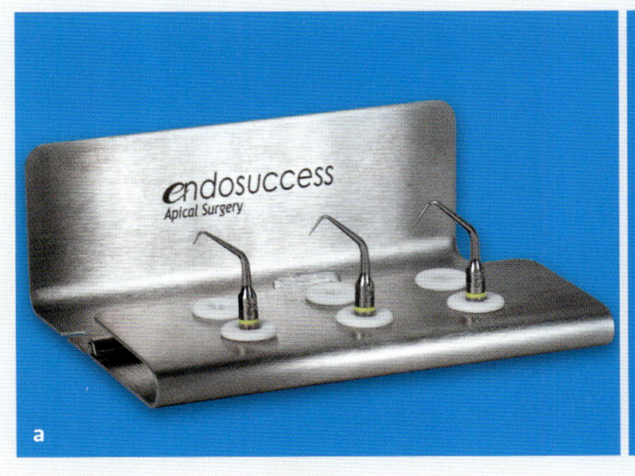

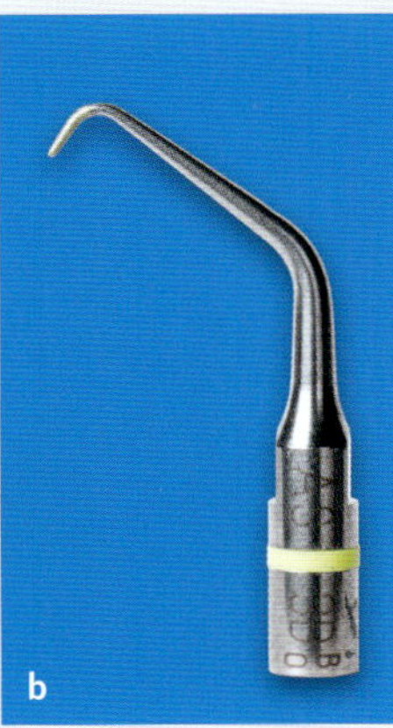

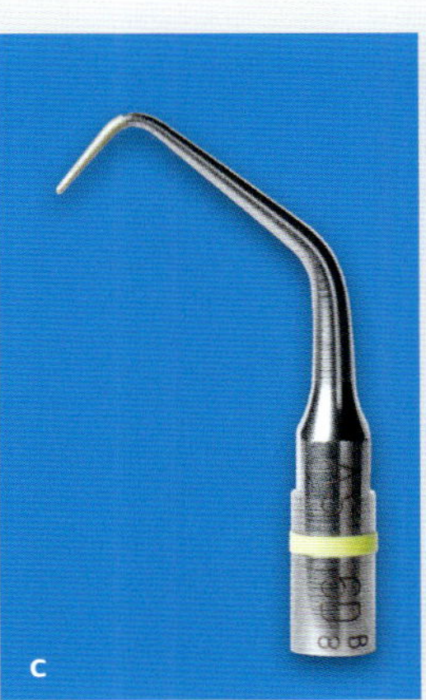

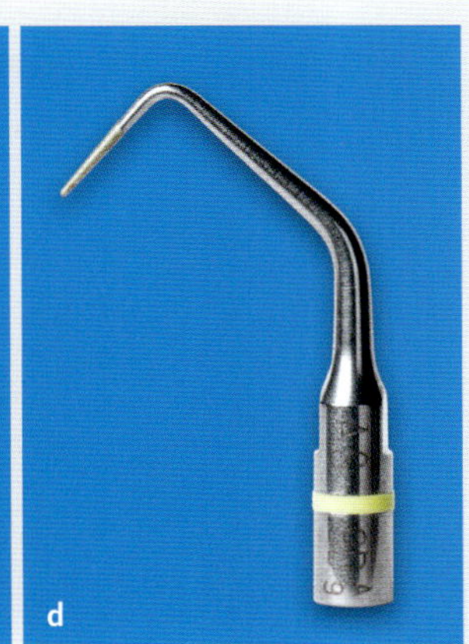

3.18 **a)** The Acteon ultrasonic tips designed by Dr. Betrand Khayat, having a length of 3 mm **(b)**, 6 mm **(c)** and 9 mm **(d)**.

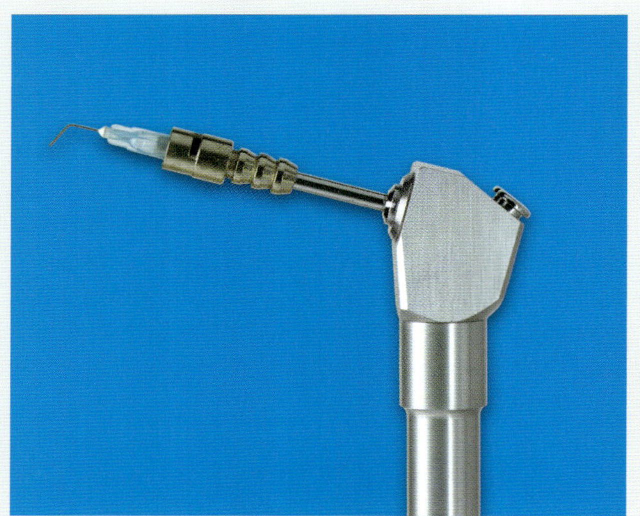

3.19 The Stropko irrigator mounted on the Adec Syringe.

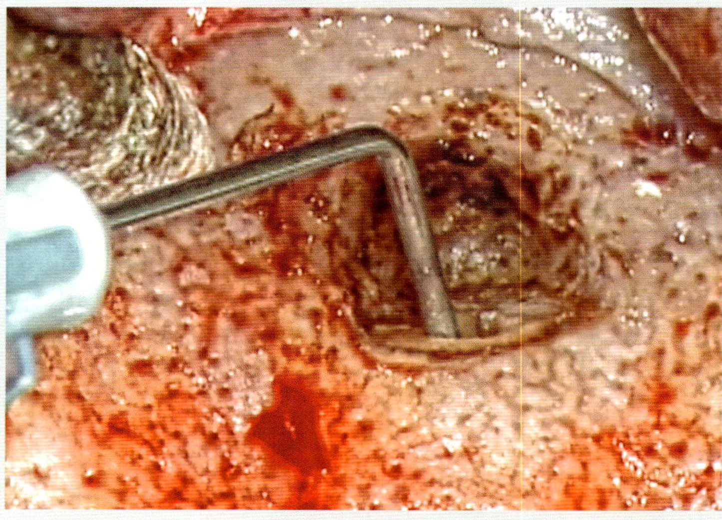

3.21 The Stropko irrigator is shown drying the root-end preparation.

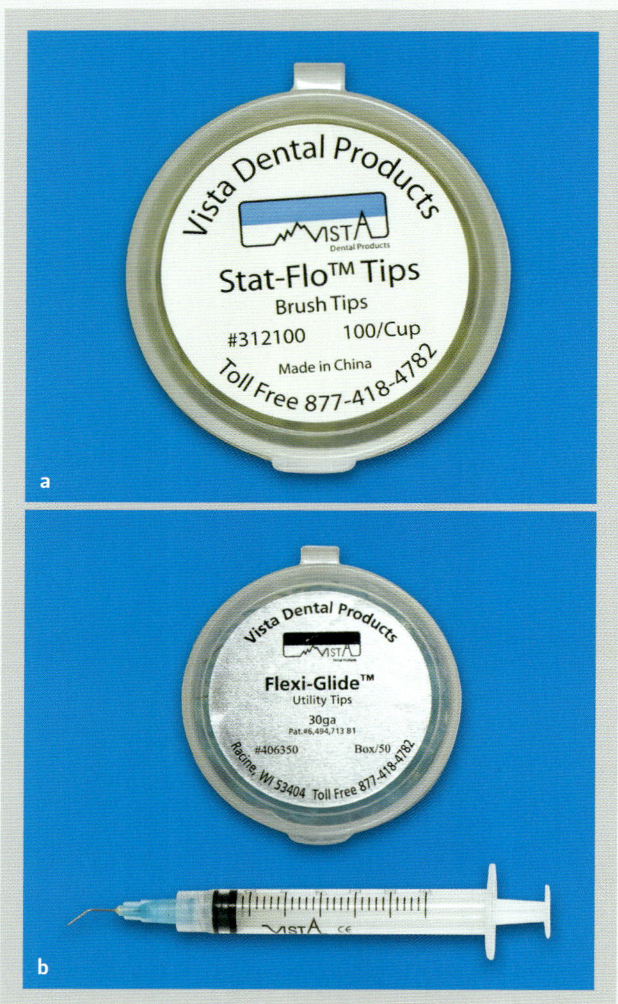

3.20 **a, b)** Different sizes of blunt needles to be mounted on the Stropko irrigator (Vista Dental).

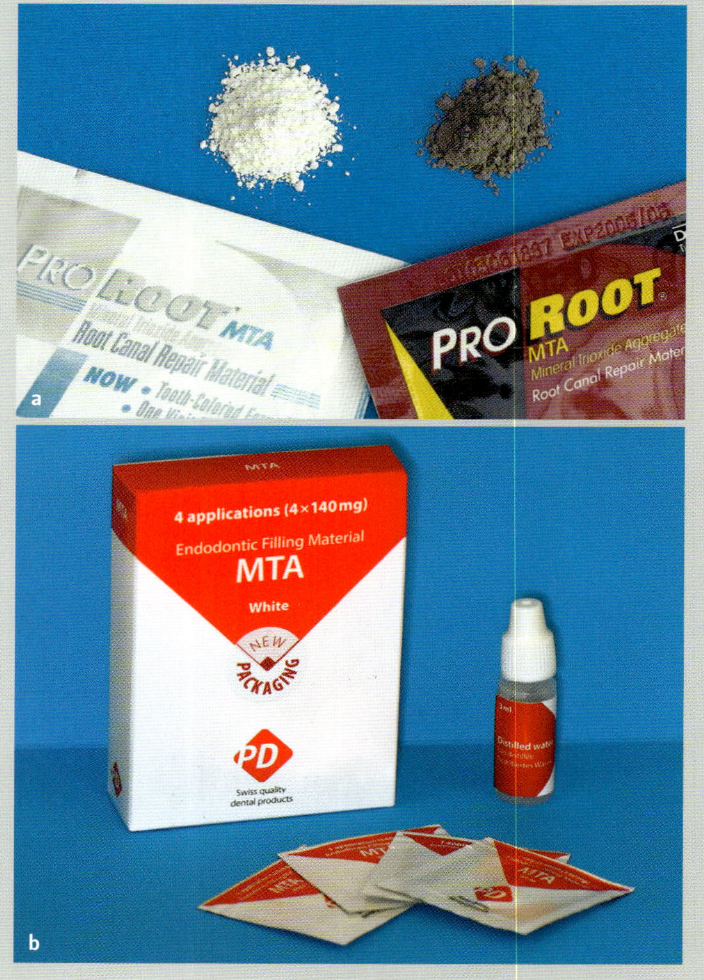

3.22 **a)** ProRoot® MTA Gray and White (Dentsply Sirona). **b)** PD White MTA (Produits Dentaires).

Retrofilling Carriers

When MTA was first introduced onto the market, there was no appropriate carrier to position it during different applications. The first carrier that became available was the Dovgan Carrier (Quality Aspirators) (12.12). However, even though the needles were bendable, the carrier was not comfortable for use during surgery. In 2000, another carrier was proposed by Dr. Edward Lee,[8] but its use was limited to surgery (12.13, 12.14). The Micro Apical Placement (MAP) System, a new universal carrier with special needles that can be used both in clinical and in surgical endodontics, was recently introduced by Produits Dentaires SA (3.23).[9,10]

The system consists of a stainless steel applicator with a bayonet catch (3.24) for several exchangeable applicator cannulas (needles). The straight and curved needles (3.25) are designed for nonsurgical endodontics, while the triple-bent needles (3.26), developed in cooperation with Dr. Bernd Ilgenstein are best indicated for surgical endodontics. The surgical needles are available in two variants, right-angled and left-angled, each with two external diameters, 0.9 mm (yellow) and 1.1 mm (red). The internal diameter of the cannulas is 0.6 mm (yellow) and 0.8 mm (red), which allows for sufficient portions of the retrofilling material to be applied successively. The intra-cannula plunger inside the needle is intentionally longer than the needle itself (3.27), so that it will not only deliver the MTA in the retropreparation but will also act as a plugger and thus begins to compact the material in the deepest portion of the prepared cavity.

The filling material can be taken from a dispenser/well (3.28). The intra-cannular plungers of the angled needles are made of a Polyoxymethylene (POM) material, which can easily navigate even a triple-bent needle (3.29). The residue of material inside the cannulas can easily be removed with a cleaning curette (3.30).

Microsurgical Pluggers

After positioning the root-end filling material inside the root-end preparation, the material needs to be carefully condensed using the specifically designed microsurgical pluggers. They are available in different length and different diameters (3.31), to completely fill the preparation. While the dental assistant is mixing the root-end filling material, the doctor fits the pluggers to select the ones that can enter deep enough to guarantee adequate obturation and a good seal.

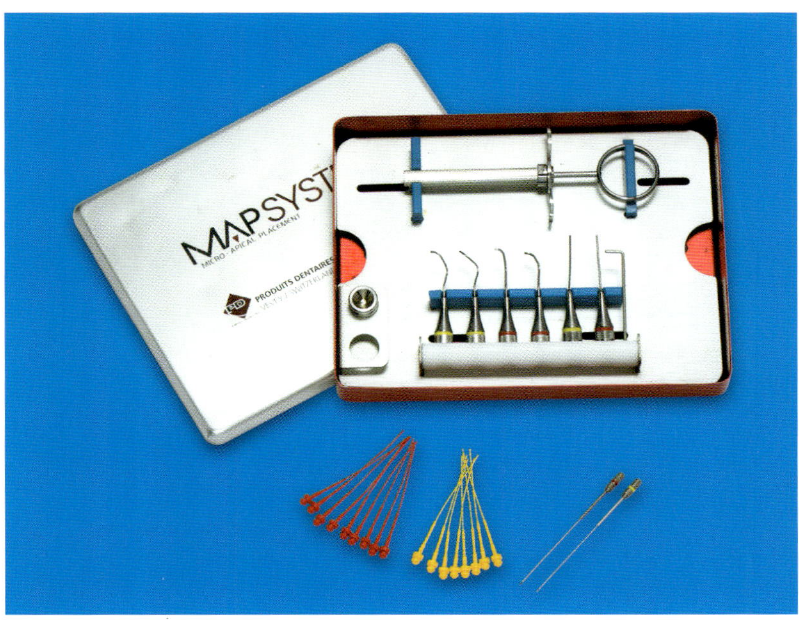

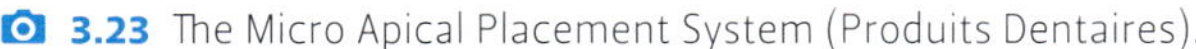
3.23 The Micro Apical Placement System (Produits Dentaires).

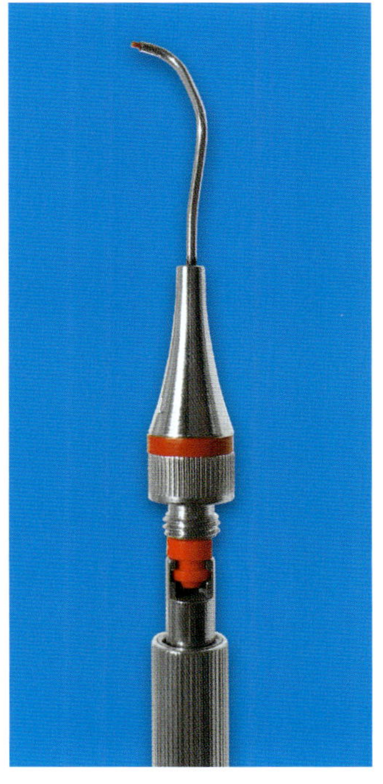
3.24 The bayonet catches to connect the interchangeable needles.

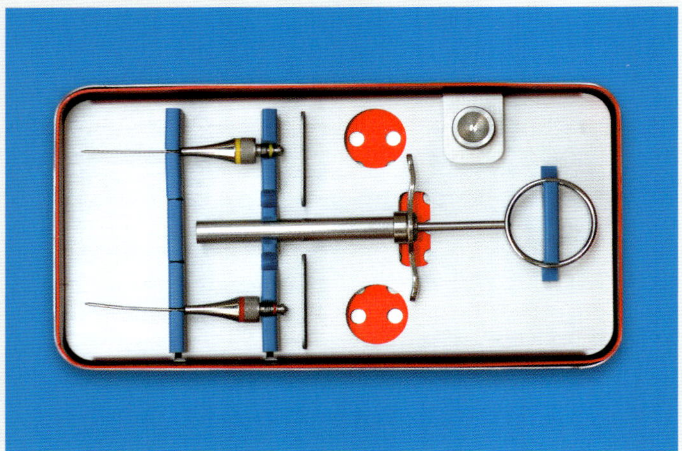

3.25 The straight needles for nonsurgical endodontics.

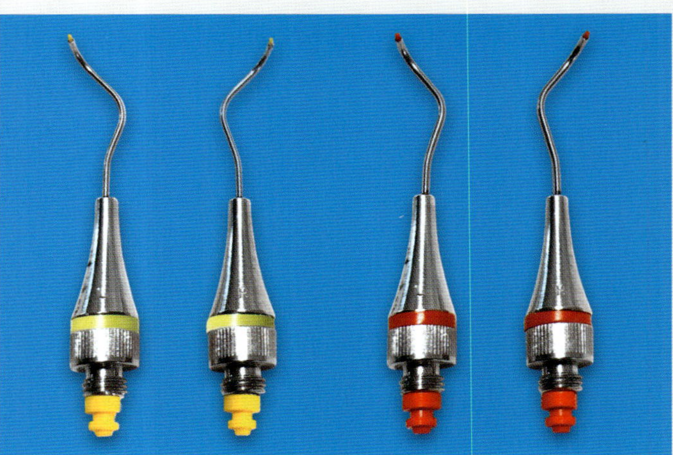

3.26 The triple-bent needles for surgical endodontics.

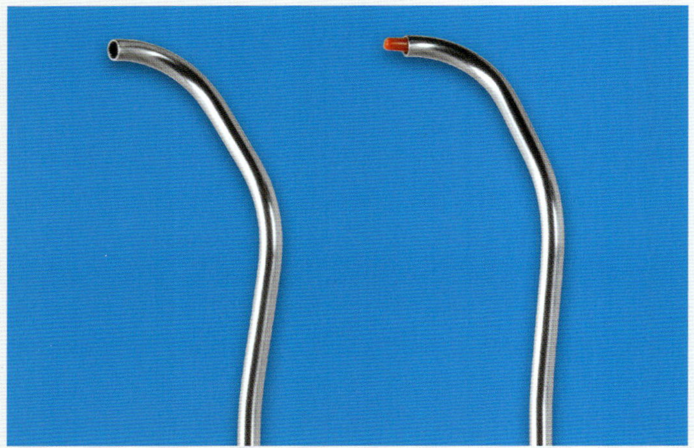

3.27 The intra-cannular plunger inside the needle is intentionally longer than the needle itself.

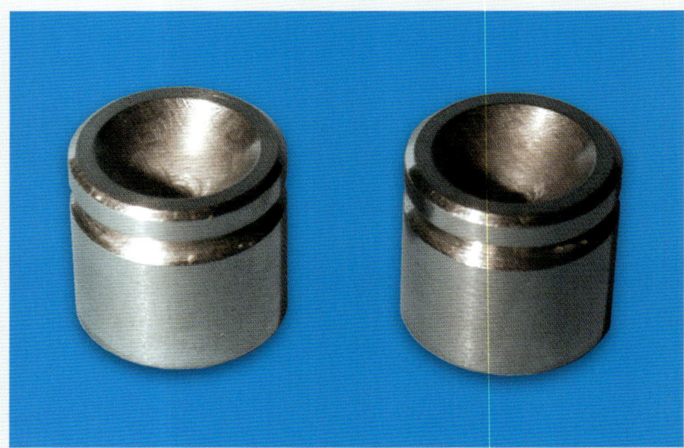

3.28 Dispenser (well) for filling material.

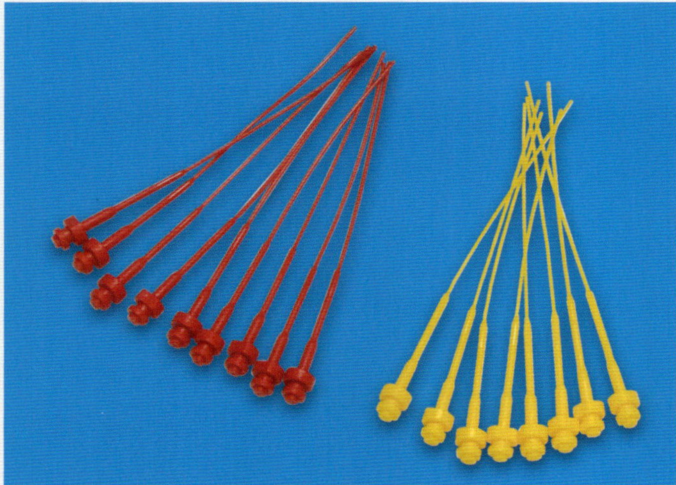

3.29 The intra-cannular plunger of the angled needles is made of Polyoxymethylene (POM) material.

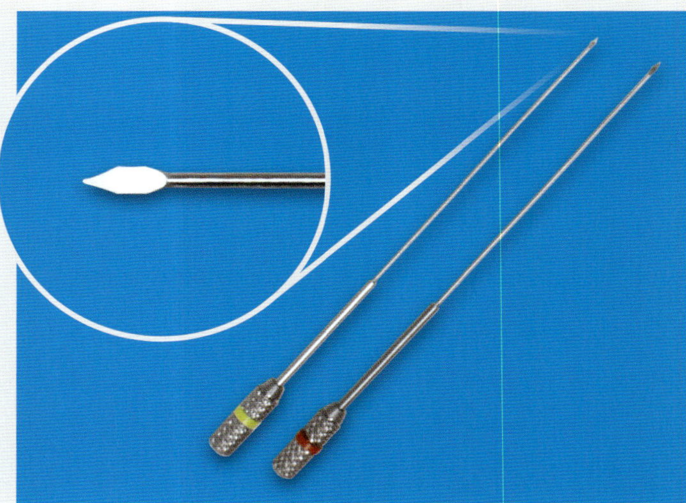

3.30 The cleaning curettes to remove the residue of material from inside the cannulas.

Sutures and Suturing Instruments

Once the root-end preparation has been filled and the radiograph confirms the good result, the bone cavity is full of blood, then the flap can be sutured. Several suture materials and sizes are available on the market. The black silk suture 4-0 or 5-0 is no longer recommended since, because of its braided nature, it very easily accumulates bacterial plaque (14.3), causing inflammation and delayed healing. The use of silk suture also requires great care during its removal, in order not to introduce bacteria under the wound margins. The most recommended suturing material today is the 6-0 monofilament nylon (Supramid, S. Jackson) or the 6-0 braided polyester suture-like Tevdek, composed of Polyethylene terephthalate, prepared from fibers of linear polyesters coated with Polytetrafluoroethylene (PTFE or Teflon) (Genzyme Corp. MA, USA), or the 6-0 polyester coated with a thin layer of wax (Omnia S.p.A. Italy) (3.32). The polyester sutures have the characteristic of not accumulating plaque, even when they remain in place longer than intended (3.33).

The selection of the suture should also take into consideration the needle, its curvature and its cross section. The most commonly used arc of the needle is 3/8 circle. It should allow the clinician to penetrate the tissue and pass from the flap to the attached tissue in one motion, just by rotating the needle holder on its long axis.

The body of the needle can be a "classic cutting needle", which enables the needle to be passed easily through the mucosa with little trauma. This needle has a triangular cross section, where the base of the triangle is towards the external or convex party of the arc, and the three cutting edges are two laterally and one superficially on its concave side. The risk of this cutting needle is that of cutting more tissue than necessary, due to the cutting edge of its blade on the concave side of the body. These cutting suture needles are not utilized in dentistry, since the cutting edge on the inside curvature of the needle tends to cause suture material to pull through the edge of the surgical flap.[11]

Unlike the classic cutting needle, "reverse cutting needles" have identical triangular section but with the base of the triangle towards the concave side and with the cutting edge towards the external, convex side of the needle. This shape has considerable advantages over the classic shape described above: it creates resistance to the suture material when tying the suture knot; the tissue is protected in the case of accidental traction being applied to the needle, since it is the needle's concave side, with no cutting edge, that meets the overlying tissues; it reduces excess trauma and the danger of "cutout": the suture material tearing through the tissues being sutured.[11]

This needle is particularly indicated for suturing the sulcular flap.

To suture the submarginal flap the most indicated needle is the so-called "taper point needle". This is superior to the reverse cutting type needle because there isn't the tendency to cut, or tear, the "entry" and "ex-

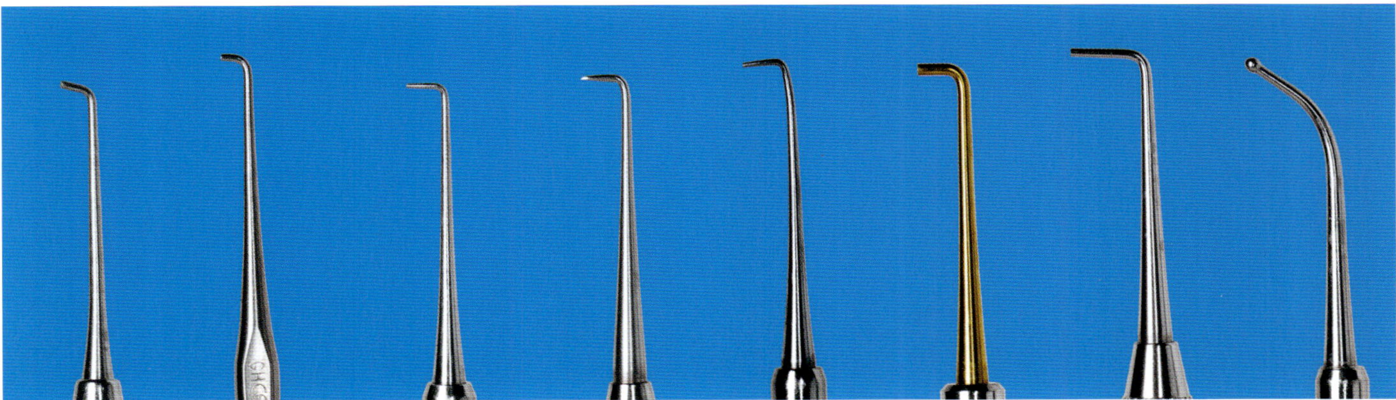

3.31 Microsurgical pluggers of different sizes and lengths.

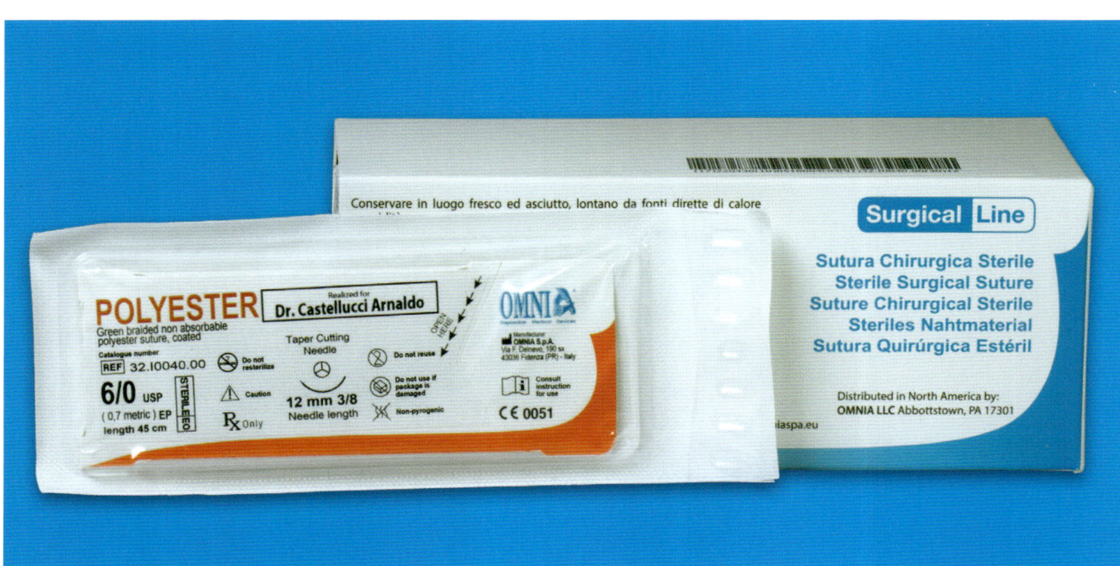

3.32 The 6-0 polyester suture coated with a thin layer of wax, so as not to accumulate bacterial plaque (Omnia S.p.A. Italy).

iting" needle points. As a result, the taper point needle is easier to guide through the tissues to a more accurate exit point when suturing the flap.[12]

Needle Holders

The needle holder is used to handle the suture needle and thread while suturing the surgical wound. It enables the surgeon to perform the procedure correctly and with great precision. The needle holders have a series of constituent parts, like the grip area, the shanks, and the catch mechanism at the working tip. The grip is the part by which the surgeon holds the instrument between his or her fingers and moves it during use. It may consist of two metal rings, which make this type similar to scissors. This kind of grip is quite uncomfortable since the surgeon needs to introduce the fingers inside each ring every time the needle holder is used: scissors hold. Much more comfortable are the needle holders where the grip is part of the shank, like the one designed by Castroviejo (3.34): palm hold.[13] In this instrument, the catch of the needle holder is included in the shank and this mechanism enables the surgeon to lock together the two parts of the instrument in a selected position, so as to hold the needle in the jaws of the working tip without having continually to exercise pressure.

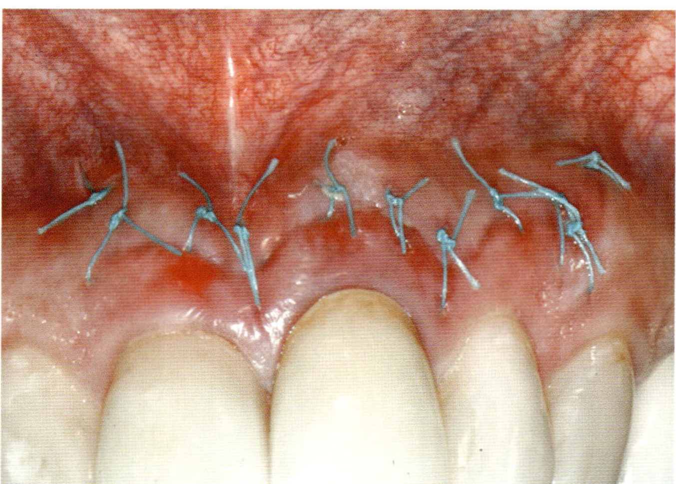

3.33 The patient could not come back for suture removal sooner than five days after surgery was completed. Note the complete absence of plaque around the 6-0 polyester suture.

On the other hand, some needle holders are without a catch and are known as open needle holders. In this case, the surgeon must continually exercise pressure on the instrument while suturing.[13]

The working tip forms the active part of the instrument and its function is to grasp, hold, guide and release the needle in a precise and controlled manner while performing the suturing procedure. The working tip should also be capable of grasping a very thin suture, like 6-0 or 7-0, to tighten the knot.

Scissors

Scissors are used to cut the suture thread, both when placing sutures and when removing them from the healing site. Just like for the needle holders, the scissors having two opposed metal rings, by means of which the instrument may be held and operated by the surgeon's fingers, are very uncomfortable. Much easier to use are the scissors that work by simple pressure of the shank (3.35), like the Castroviejo. The scissors of 3.35 also have the advantage of having blunt blades, which prevent cutting and damaging the oral soft tissue (3.36).

Regarding how and where to cut the sutures, they must be treated differently depending on the type. Resorbable sutures are cut off as short as possible, to avoid excess material having to be resorbed. Nonresorbable sutures should be shortened to a length that could allow easy removal, usually 3-4 mm from the knot. The surgeon's left hand holds the needle holder to grasp the suture while the right hand is holding the scissors to cut it. During the removal the operator must pay attention so that the portion of the suture that was exposed to saliva and bacteria will not pass through the soft tissue, carrying bacteria inside.

Recently, new scissors have been manufactured by Laschal (NY, USA) (3.37) which allows the surgeon to grab the suture, cut it and at the same time remove it (3.38) using just one hand. When using another kind of scissors, the surgeon needs to grasp the suture using the Castroviejo with one hand and the scissors with the other hand (3.39).

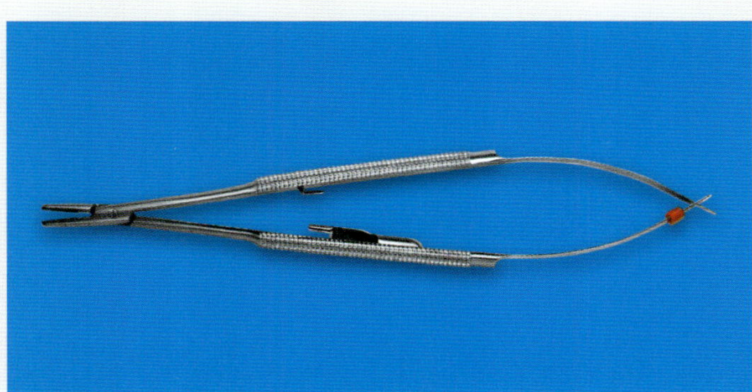

3.34 The Castroviejo needle holder.

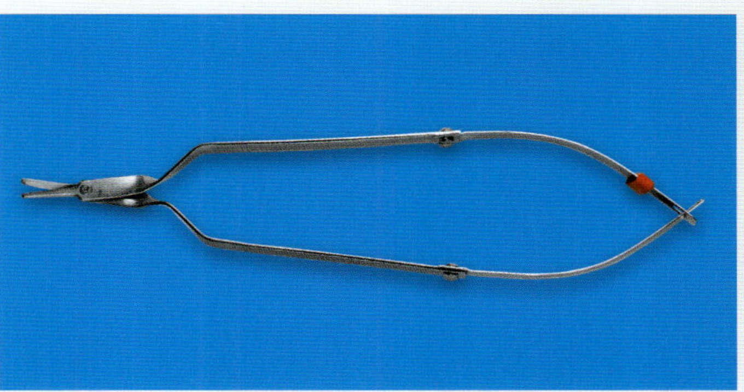

3.35 The scissors made by Laschal (NY, USA).

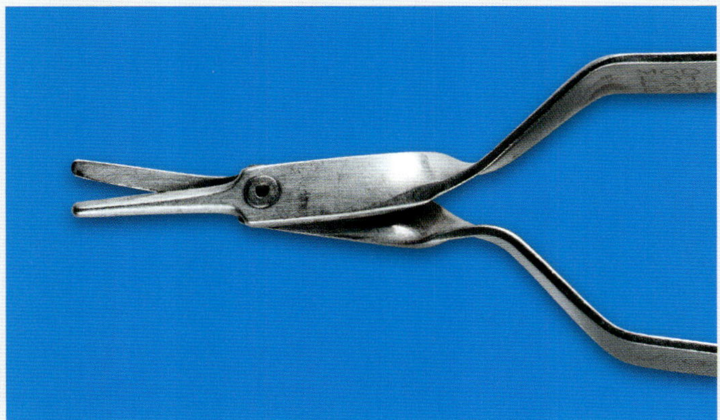

3.36 The scissors have blunt blades and sever the suture without cutting the soft tissue.

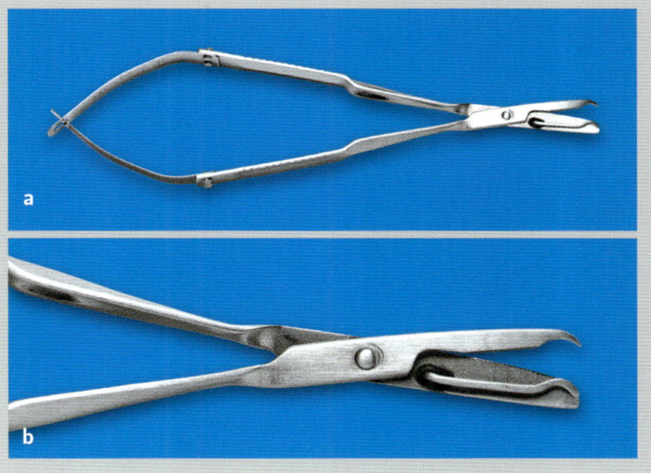

3.37 **a)** These scissors made by Laschal allow the surgeon to cut and grasp the suture using just one hand. **b)** The scissors at higher magnification.

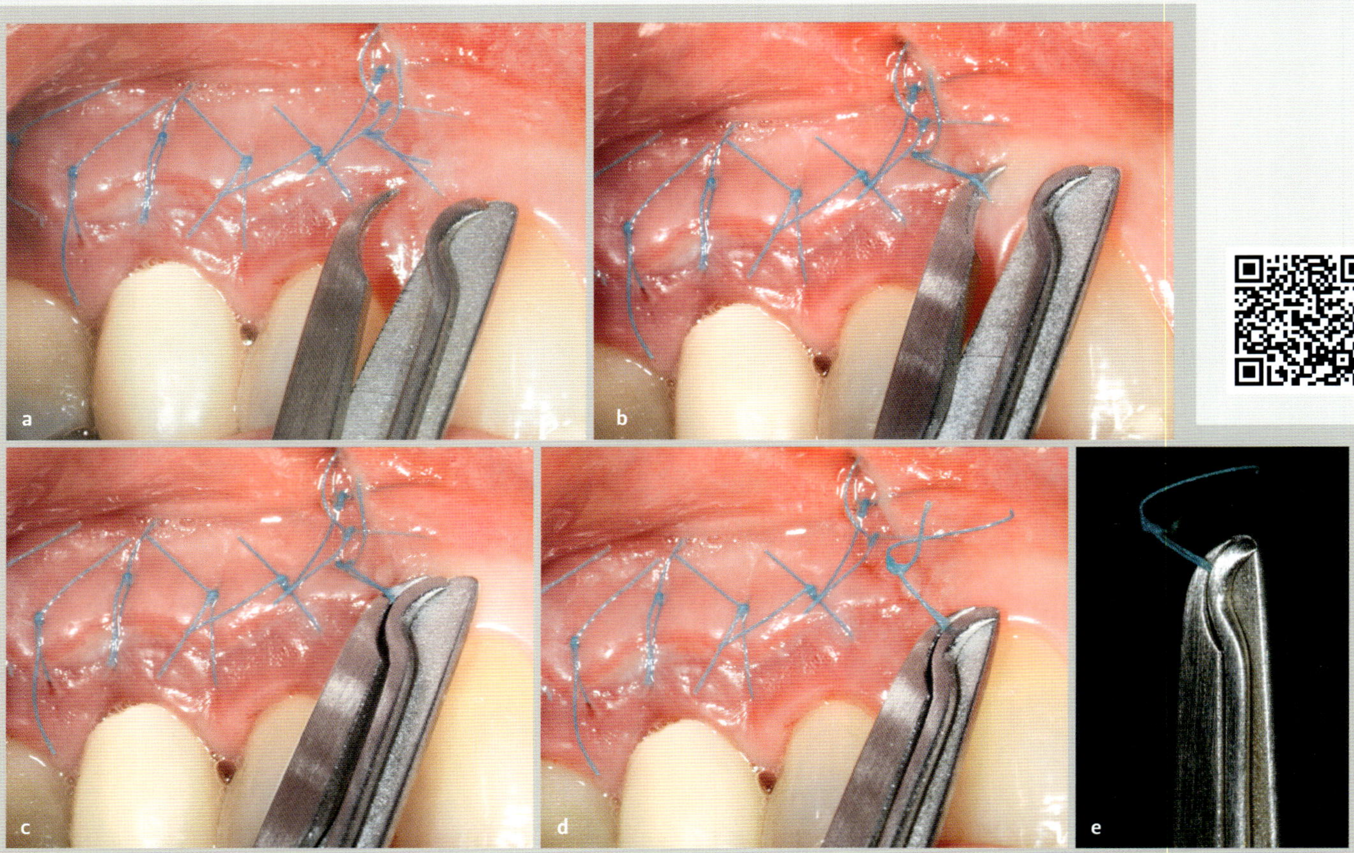

3.38 Suture removal 24 hours after surgery. **a)** The scissors are next to the suture. **b)** The scissors are ready to cut the suture. **c)** The scissors are now cutting the suture. **d, e)** The suture has been cut and removed.

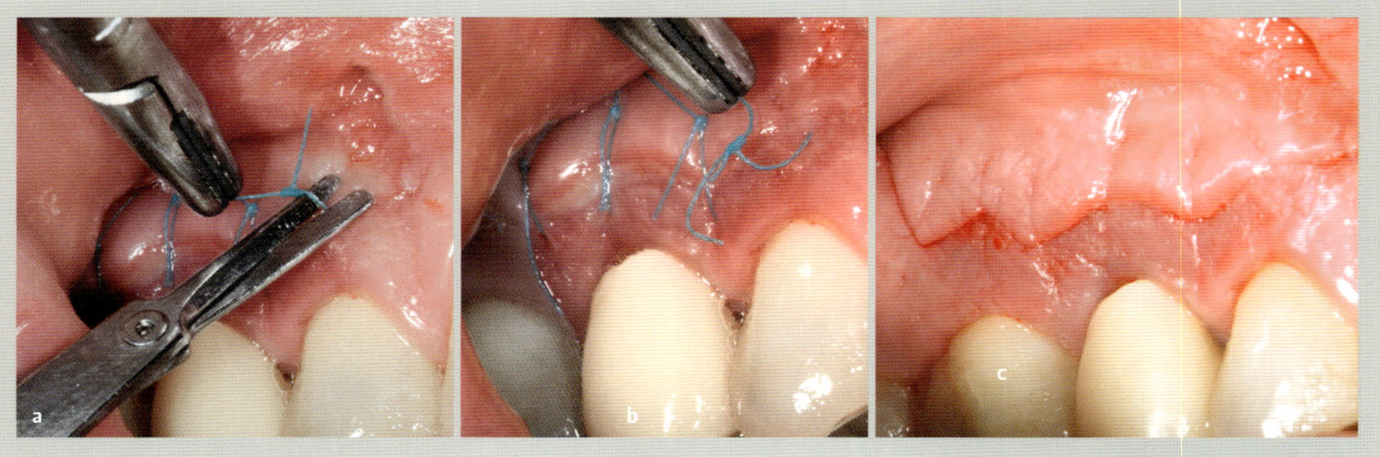

3.39 **a)** The left hand is holding the Castroviejo needle holder to grasp the suture while the right hand is holding the scissors. **b)** The suture has been cut and removed. **c)** The entire suture has been removed.

REFERENCES

1. **Kim S, Pecora G, Rubinstein R.** *Color atlas of microsurgery in endodontics.* Philadelphia: Saunders, 2001.
2. **Kim S.** *Principles of endodontic microsurgery.* Dent Clin North Am. 1997;41:481-497.
3. **Rubinstein RA, Kim S.** *Short-term observation of the results of endodontic surgery with use of a surgical operation microscope and Super-EBA as root-end filling material.* J Endod. 1999;25:43-48.
4. **Carr GB.** *Microscopes in Endodontics.* Calif Dent Assoc J. 1992;11:55-61.
5. **Carr GB.** *Surgical endodontics.* In: Cohen S, Burns R, eds. *Pathways of the pulp*, 6th ed. St. Louis: Mosby. 1994:531.
6. **Pecora G, Andreana S.** *Use of dental operating microscope in endodontic surgery.* Oral Surg Oral Med Oral Pathol. 1993;75:751-758.
7. **Kim S, Kratchman S.** *Modern endodontic surgery concepts and practice: a review.* J Endod. 52(7):601-623.
8. **Lee E.** *A new mineral trioxide aggregate root-end filling technique.* J Endod. 2000;26:764-766.
9. **Ilgenstein B, Jager K.** *Micro Apical Placement System (MAPS). A new instrument for retrograde root canal filling.* Schweiz Monatsschr Zahnmed. Vol. 116:1243-1252; 12/2006.
10. **Castellucci A, Papaleoni M.** *The MAP System: a perfect carrier for MTA in clinical and surgical endodontics.* Roots. 2009;3:18-22.
11. **Silverstein LH.** *Principles of dental suturing.* Montage Media Corporation. 1999;18-23.
12. **Stropko J.** *Micro-Surgical Endodontics.* In: Castellucci A. (Ed.) *EndodonticS.* Vol. III. Florence, Italy: Il Tridente. 2005:342-411.
13. **Siervo S.** *Suturing techniques in oral surgery.* Quintessence. 2008;73-81.

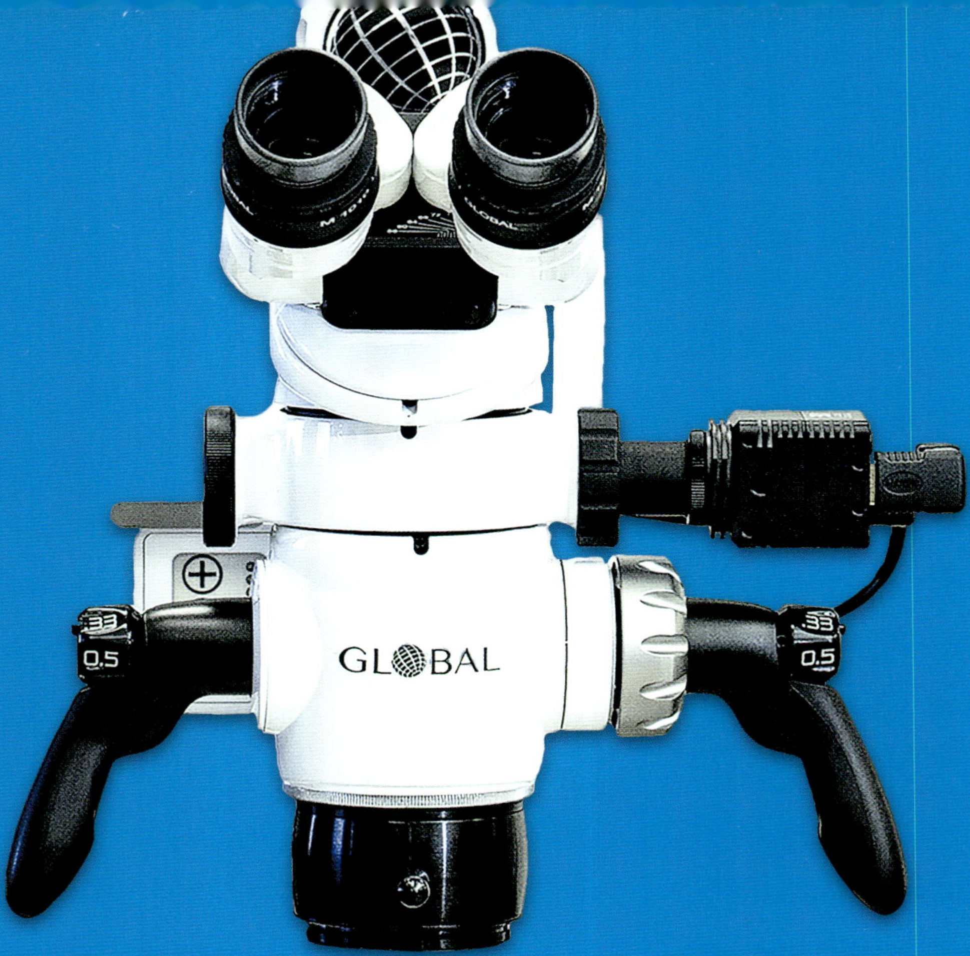

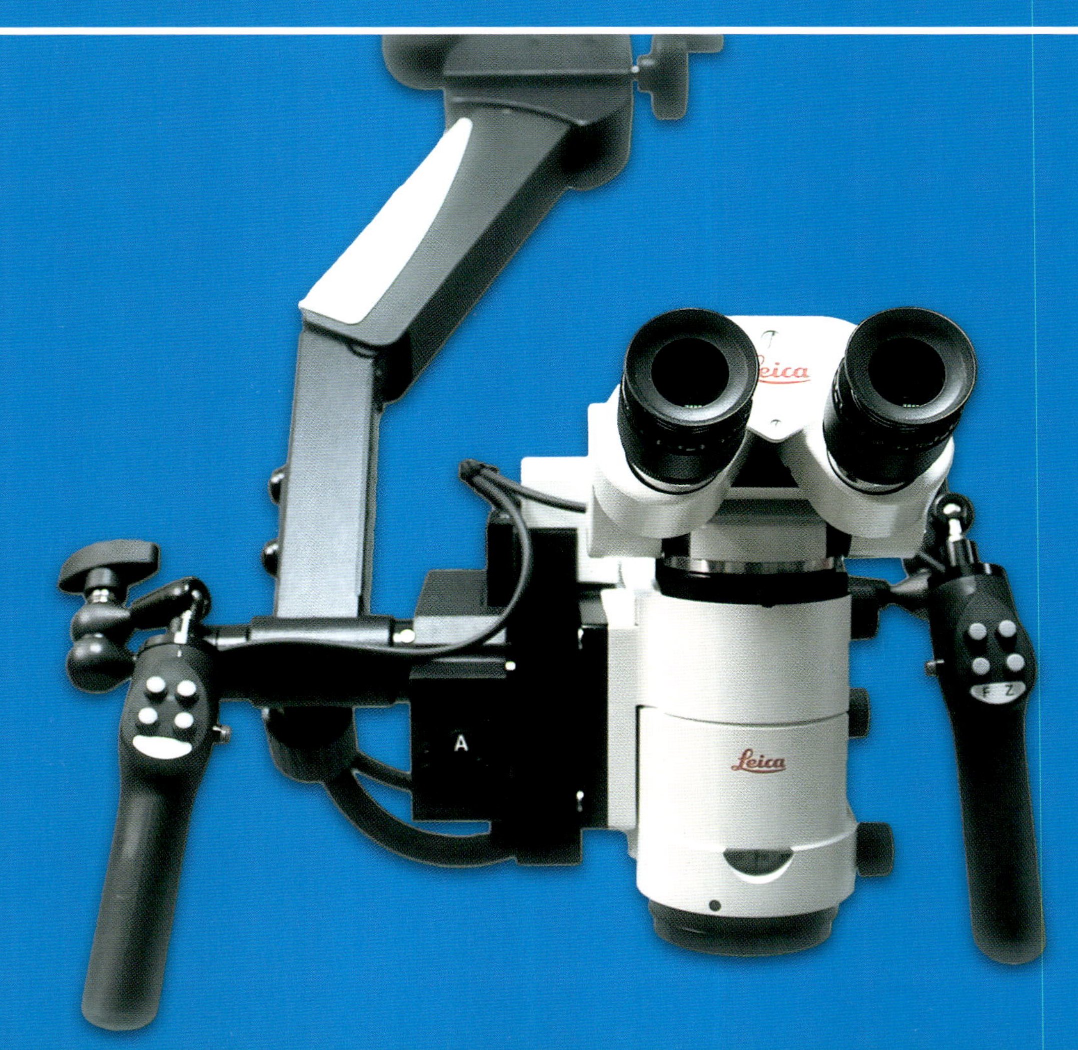
Leica
Leica

The Surgical Operating Microscope

Introduction to the Surgical Operating Microscope

One of the most significant developments in the past three decades in endodontics has been the use of the operating microscope (OM) for surgical endodontics.[1-6] The medical disciplines such as Neurosurgery, ENT, and Ophthalmology incorporated the microscope into practice 20 to 30 years ahead of Dentistry. It is now inconceivable that certain medical procedures would be performed without the aid of the microscope.[7]

In the early 90s, operating microscopes were introduced into Endodontics (4.1) and endodontic residency programs in the United States. By providing both intensely focused light as well as a high degree of magnification, the OM has become an important part of the armamentarium for many endodontists. The OM enables endodontists to resolve previously unrecognized or untreatable treatment challenges. Since the early 1990s, training in microscopes has become an important component of endodontic education, and their use is now universally taught at the graduate level in all Commission on Dental Accreditation-approved endodontic specialty programs. Since 1998, all postgraduate endodontic

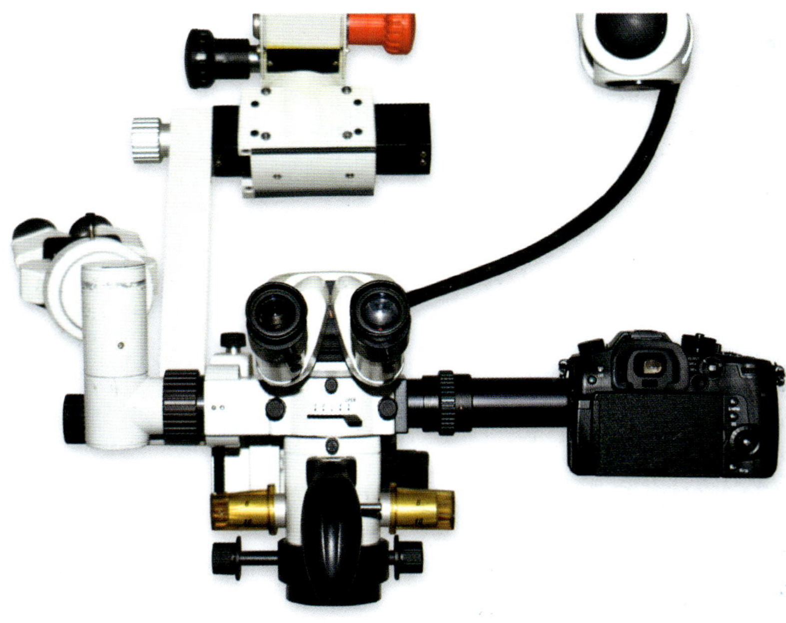

4.1 Leica microscope, fitted with the inclinable binocular, beam splitter (50/50), documentation adaptor, digital still camera (Panasonic Lumix 5), and assistant scope.

programs must teach the use of magnification in accordance with the American Dental Association Accreditation Standard for endodontic graduate programs.[8]

Microscopes are now also widely used in private practice. A 2007 survey of 1,091 endodontists indicated that 90% of endodontists in the U.S. have access to and use the OM in their practice, a dramatic increase from 52% in use in 1999. The American Association of Endodontists (AAE) anticipates that over the next 10 years, as endodontists trained without microscopes retire, the percent of endodontists using microscopes in private practice will approach 100%. Universal adoption of the OM is a function of time.[9]

The introduction of the surgical operating microscope represents a very important development in nonsurgical as well as in surgical endodontics.[4,10] For many years periapical surgery was performed without any magnification, using the dental light as the only light source to illuminate the surgical field. Surgery at that time, and until recently, was performed with inadequate lighting, no magnification, and a limited armamentarium (4.2). Frank et al.[11] reported that the success rate in apical surgeries sealed with amalgam, which had been considered a successful procedure for many years, dropped to 57.7% after 10 years. No surprise therefore if until recently the success rate after surgery was much lower compared to nonsurgical endodontics.[11] It is well recognized today that performing apical surgery without magnification is no longer adequate or defensible.[7]

Magnification. Loupes and Microscope

Loupes

Some clinicians may claim that using a 3× or 4× loupe is sufficient, but they should understand that loupes do not provide enough magnification and, even more important, they do not provide coaxial illumination. Using

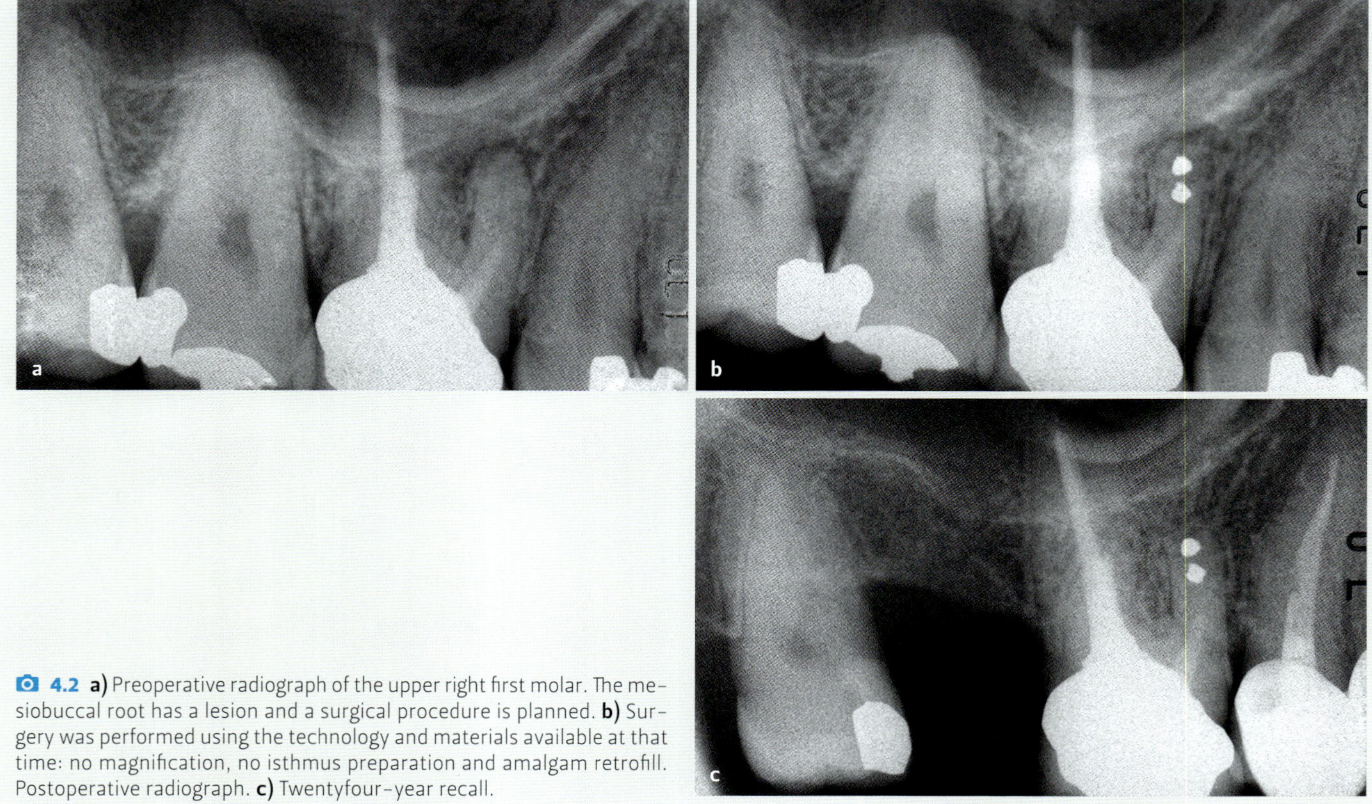

4.2 a) Preoperative radiograph of the upper right first molar. The mesiobuccal root has a lesion and a surgical procedure is planned. **b)** Surgery was performed using the technology and materials available at that time: no magnification, no isthmus preparation and amalgam retrofill. Postoperative radiograph. **c)** Twentyfour-year recall.

loupes is the first step and a welcome change from unaided vision, but effective magnification and illumination requires an operating microscope.[7]

Historically, dental loupes have been the most common form of magnification used in apical surgery. Loupes are essentially two monocular microscopes with lenses mounted side by side and angled inward (convergent optics) to focus on an object.[12]

Loupes are available in a variety of configurations and magnifications, starting from 2× up to 6×, with Galilean optics or prismatic optics.

Loupes are classified by the optical method in which they produce magnification. There are three types of binocular magnifying loupes:

1. a diopter, flat-plane, single-lens loupe
2. a surgical telescope with a Galilean system configuration (two-lens system)
3. a surgical telescope with a Keplerian system configuration (prism roof design that folds the path of light).

Galilean and Keplerian surgical telescopes produce an enlarged viewing image with a multiple-lens system positioned at a working distance between 11 and 20 inches (28-51 cm). The most used and suggested working distance is between 11 and 15 inches (28-38 cm).

The Galilean system provides a magnification range from 2× up to 4.5× and is a small, light and very compact system (4.3).

Prism loupes (Keplerian system) use refractive prisms and they are actually telescopes with complicated light paths, which provide magnifications up to 6× (4.4).

At the same magnification, prism loupes provide a more expanded field of view.

Both systems produce superior magnification, correct spherical and chromatic aberrations, have excellent depth of field, and are capable of increased focal length (30-45 cm), thereby reducing both eyestrain and head and neck fatigue. Both these types of loupes offer significant advantages over simple magnification eyeglasses.

The disadvantage of loupes is that the practical maximum magnification is only about 4.5 diameters. Loupes are available with higher magnification, but they are heavy and unwieldy with a limited field of view. Using computerized techniques, some manufacturers can provide magnifications from 2.5× to 6× with an expanded field. Nevertheless, such loupes require a constrained physical posture and cannot be worn for long periods of time without producing significant head, neck, and back strain. The biggest disadvantage of using loupes is that the eyes must converge to view an image. This convergence over time will create eye strain and fatigue, and as such, loupes were never intended for lengthy procedures.[12]

When a fiber optic headlamp is added to a loupe a coaxial light is projected into the surgical field, enhancing both magnification and illumination (4.5).

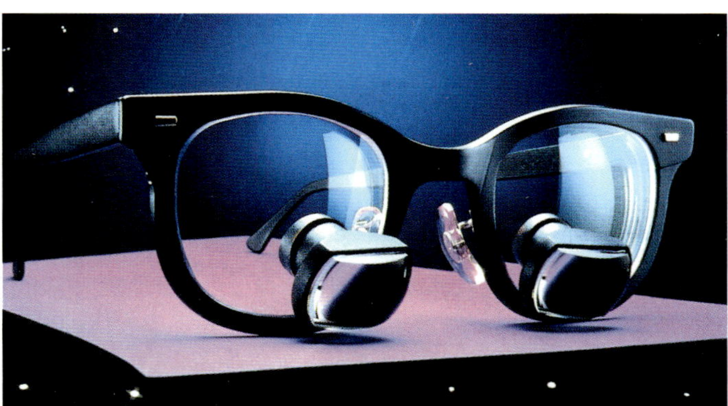

4.3 Compound loupes. Two separate lenses separated by air. These are preferable to simple magnifying eyeglasses (*Courtesy of Designs for Vision, Inc. Ronkonkoma, NY, USA*).

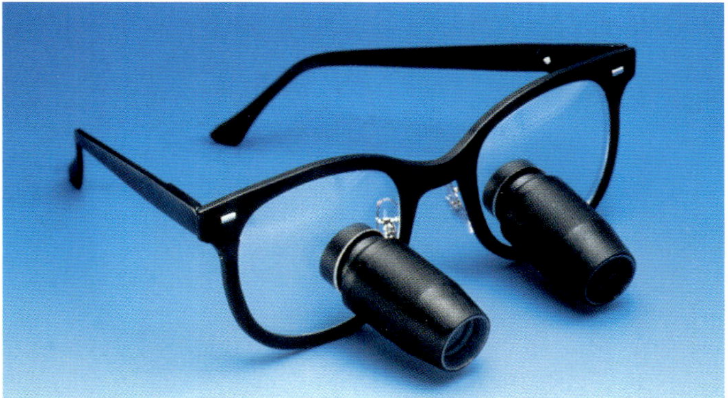

4.4 Prisms loupes. These loupes have sophisticated optics that rely on internal prisms to bend the light Compared to compound loupes, they provide an expanded field of view at the same magnification (*Courtesy of Designs for Vision, Inc. Ronkonkoma, NY, USA*).

Microscope

Clinicians who have benefited from the use of loupes and headlamps soon understand the limitations of this system. 6× magnification becomes, sooner or later, no longer sufficient and the headlamp is not capable of sending the light deep into the canal in surgical and nonsurgical endodontics. The next step, therefore, is to switch to an operating microscope, the normal reaction to which is "How could I possibly have managed without it in the past?"

Apotheker introduced the dental operating microscope in 1981.[13] The first operating microscope was poorly configured and ergonomically difficult to use. It was capable of only one magnification (8×), was positioned on a floor stand and poorly balanced, had only straight binoculars, and had a fixed focal length of 250 mm. This microscope used angled illumination instead of confocal illumination. It did not gain wide acceptance and the manufacturer ceased manufacturing them shortly after they first came out. Their market failure was more symptomatic of their very poor ergonomic design rather than their optical properties, which were actually quite good.

Howard Selden was the first endodontist to publish a paper on the use of the operating microscope in endodontics.[14] His article discussed their use in conventional tooth treatment, not in surgical endodontics. In 1991 Gary Carr introduced an operating microscope with Galilean optics, ergonomically configured for dentistry with several advantages that allowed for easy use of the scope for nearly all endodontic and restorative procedures.[15] This microscope had a magnification changer that allowed for five discrete magnifications (3.5–30×), had a stable mounting on either the wall or ceiling, had

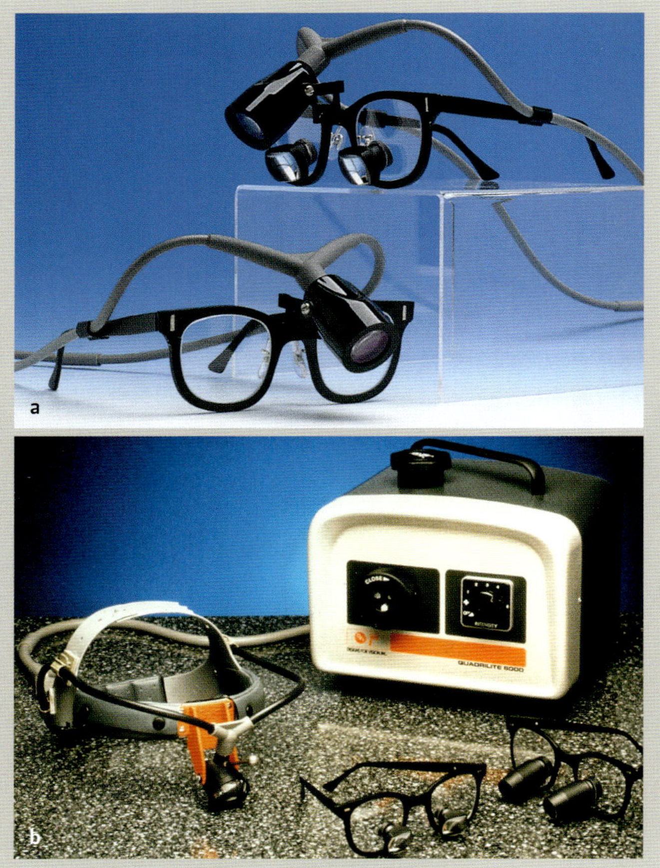

4.5 **a, b)** Surgical headlight and loupes. Together, these devices can greatly increase a clinician's resolution (*Courtesy of Designs for Vision, Inc. Ronkonkoma, NY, USA*).

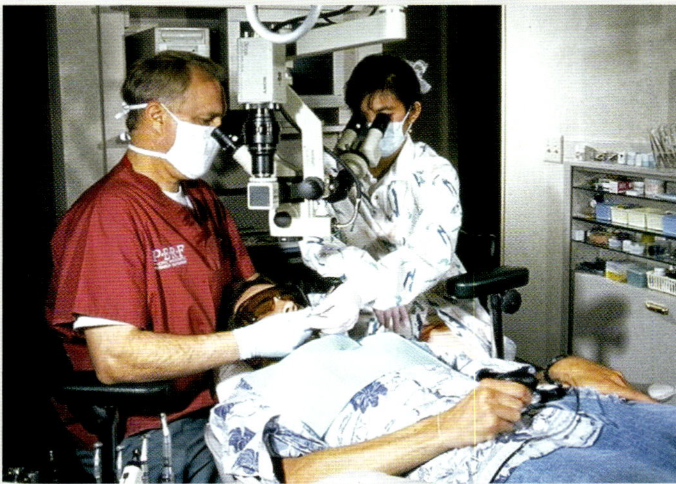

4.6 Today's dental microscope allows both the doctor and assistant to view the same field. This microscope is fitted with a 3CCD video camera (*Courtesy of Dr. Gary Carr, San Diego, CA*).

angled binoculars allowing for sit-down dentistry, and was configured with adapters for an assistant's scope and video/35 mm cameras (4.6). It used a confocal illumination module so that the light path was in the same optical path as the visual path and this gave far superior illumination than the angled light path of the earlier scope. This microscope gained rapid acceptance within the endodontic community and is now the instrument of choice not only for endodontics but for periodontics and restorative dentistry as well. The optical principles of the dental microscope are seen in 4.7.

The surgical operating microscope has a range of magnifications from 2.5× to 25× and the illumination is coaxial with the line of sight.

Coaxial illumination has two advantages:

1. the clinician can look into the surgical field without any shadows (which means for example that it is possible to examine the cleanliness of the retro-preparation during surgical endodontics);
2. Since coaxial illumination is made possible because the operating microscope uses Galilean optics, and since Galilean optics focus at infinity and send parallel beams of light to each eye, the operator's eyes are also focusing at infinity and every procedure can be performed without any eye fatigue.

As far as the magnification is concerned, there is no need to go beyond 20-25×. Lower-range magnifications (2.5× to 8×) are used for orientation to the surgical field and allow for a wide field of view. Mid-range magnifications (10× to 16×) are used for operating. Higher-range magnifications (18× to 25×) are used only for observing fine details. Working at high magnifications means having a very limited depth of field and limited illumination, and therefore is not practical.[15]

Experience suggests that maximum magnification is of little value in microsurgical endodontics, because the slightest movement by the patient, sometimes even breathing, moves the field out of view and out of focus. The clinician then must repeatedly recenter and refocus the microscope, wasting valuable time.[7]

The use of the surgical operating microscope has several advantages in surgical endodontics:

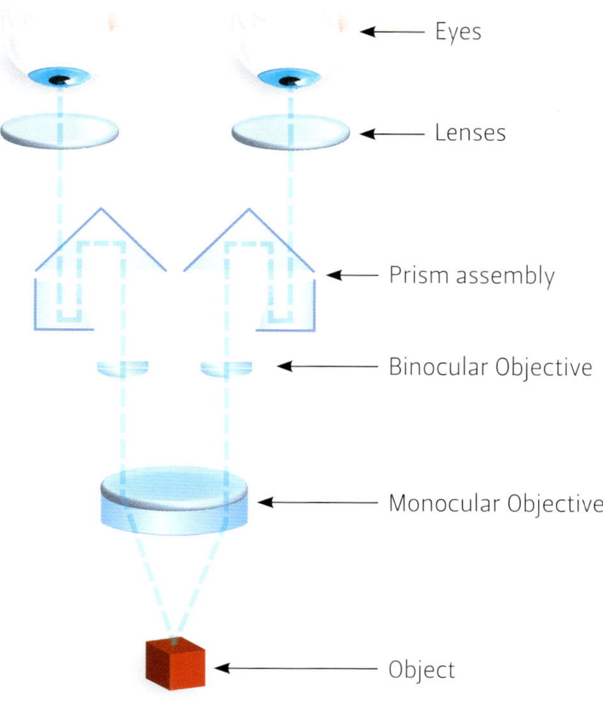

4.7 Galilean optics. Parallel optics enables the observer to focus at infinity, relieving eyestrain.

1. better visualization of the surgical field
2. better evaluation of the surgical technique
3. greater accuracy during the entire procedure
4. greater predictability of long term results.

For these reasons, the author is firmly convinced that surgical endodontics should **not** be performed without the use of a microscope, from the injection of anesthesia to the removal of sutures. Because vision is enhanced, cases can be treated with a high degree of confidence and accuracy.

Under a microscope, the incision made with the microsurgical scalpel is more accurate, with less trauma to the soft tissue, a more passive flap elevation and subsequent reapproximation is simplified. At minimum magnification, the entire surgical field can be observed (4.8), looking for the mental nerve (4.9), for instance. The size of the osteotomy is usually small (usually less than 5 mm), big enough to accommodate the ultrasonic tips,

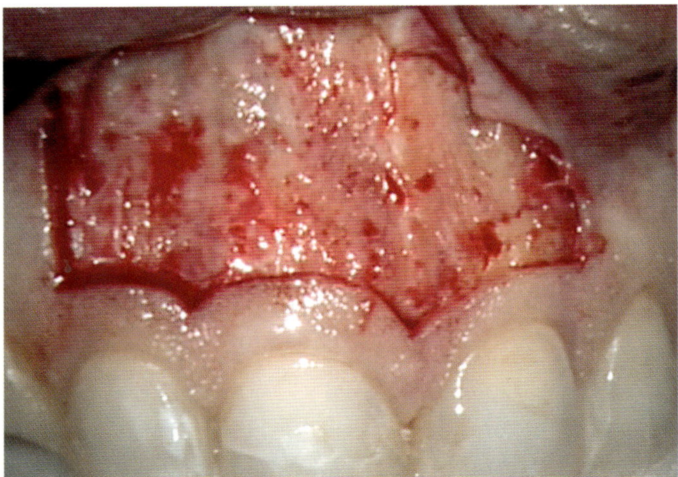

4.8 The entire surgical field can be observed working at minimum magnification.

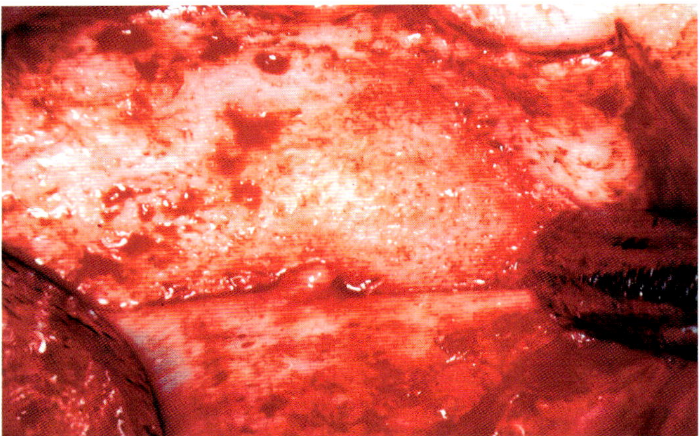

4.9 In order to avoid damaging the mental nerve, its location must be determined at the beginning of surgery.

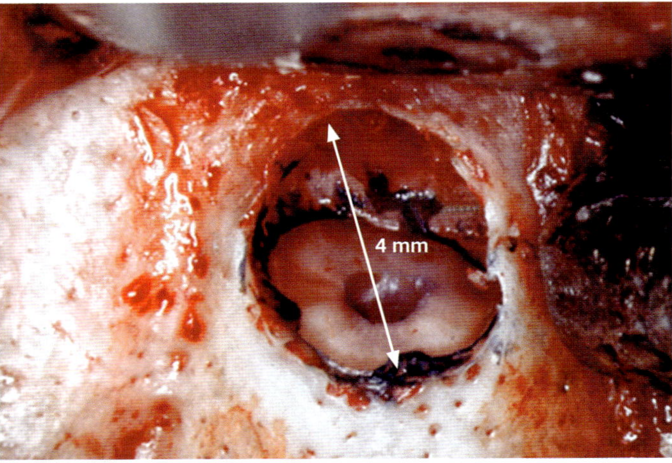

4.10 The bony crypt should be large enough to accommodate an ultrasonic retrotip.

which have a tip length of 3 mm (4.10). Working at 10× to 20× magnifications, the small osteotomy allows perfect control of the entire surgical procedure.

Moreover, from an ergonomic perspective, the microscope allows the clinician to maintain an upright position, which can help avoid long-term back and neck problems that may range from general discomfort to disability.[16]

Root Canal Anatomy and Anatomical Complexities

In 1925 Walter Hess[17] published a famous textbook on Root Canal Anatomy, after injecting vulcanized rubber in the root canals of 2,790 teeth and making these teeth transparent. The images showed how complex and bizarre the root canal anatomy is, and of course, this was very discouraging, since the enormous difficulty of taking care of all the complexities became clear. A few decades later, however, clinicians like Herbert Schilder started to seek more effective ways to clean, shape and obturate the root canal system, in order to address all the existing complexities (4.11).[18,19] West looked at the relationship between failed endodontic treatments and unfilled or underfilled portals of exit.[20] Using a centrifuged dye, he identified that 100% of the failed specimens studied had at least one underfilled or unfilled portal of exit (4.12). Kim et al.[1] demonstrated that 93% of the canal ramifications occur in the apical 3 mm. It is therefore clear that the clinician should attempt to treat the root canal system to the full extent of the anatomy, both nonsurgically and surgically. Failure to address these anatomical concerns will leave the etiology of failure unremoved, and reinfection, even after the removal of the periapical lesion, may reoccur.[12] When performing nonsurgical and surgical endodontic therapies, the pulpal anatomy, such as accessory canals and isthmuses, must be considered. Acceptance of the importance of the existing anatomical complexities and the necessity to eliminate all of them may have influenced the modern approach to periapical surgery and stimulated the necessity to work under magnification.

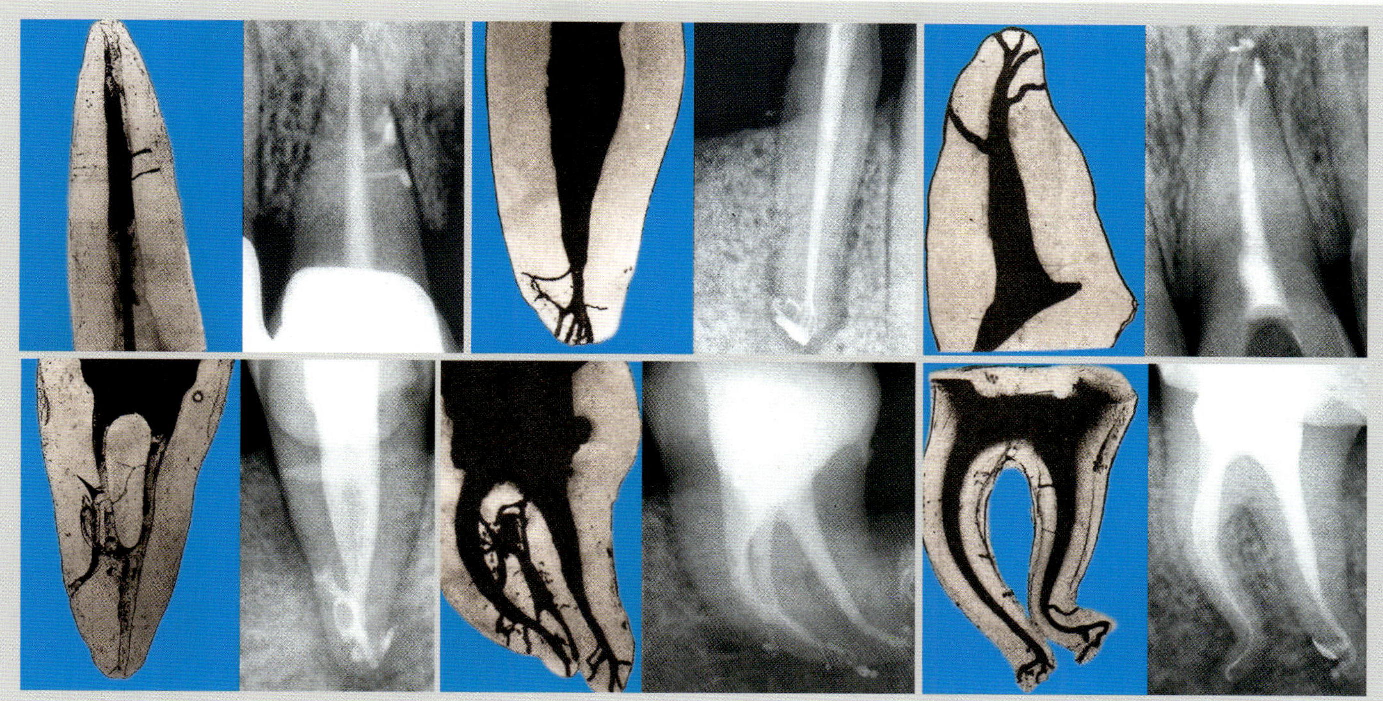

4.11 Hess's work next to postoperative radiographs showing the same anatomy. The teeth have been obturated with the Vertical Compaction of Warm Gutta-Percha.

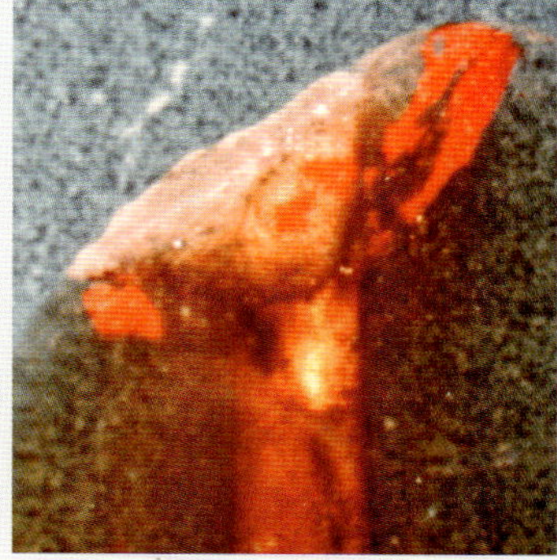

4.12 The retrofill has been positioned without completely resecting through the root: the apical delta remained untouched, leaving three portals of exit unsealed (*Courtesy of Dr. John West, Tacoma WA*).

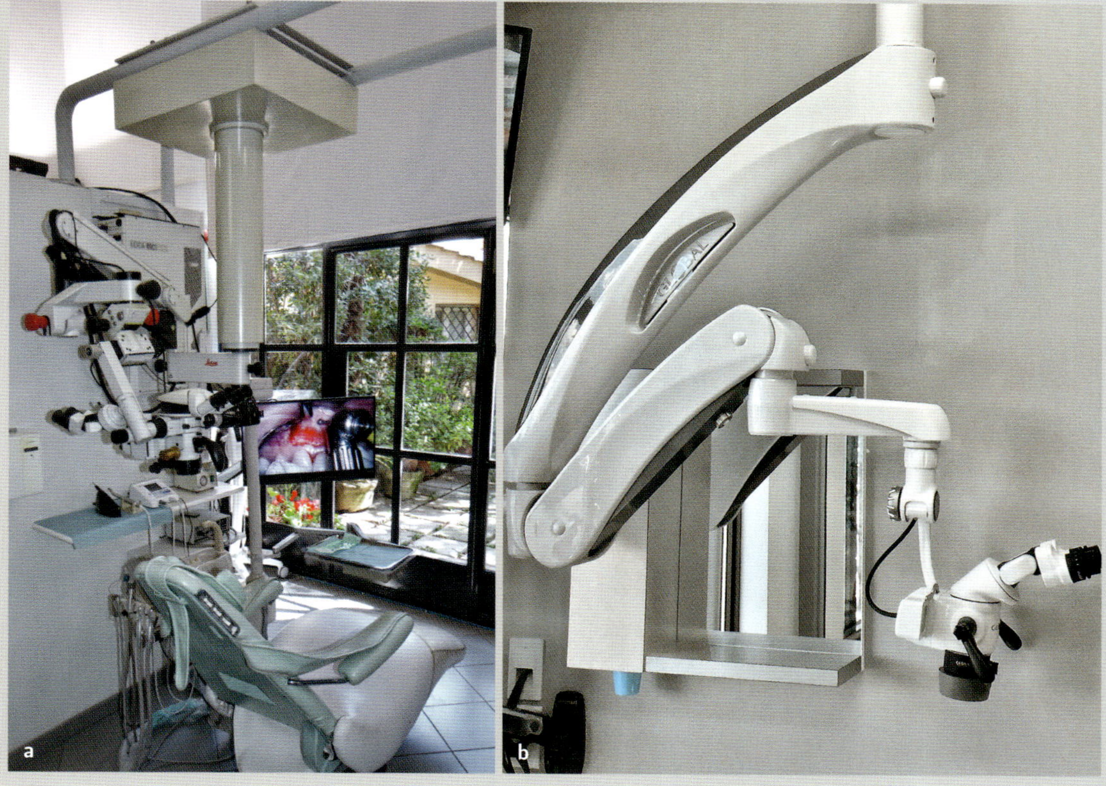

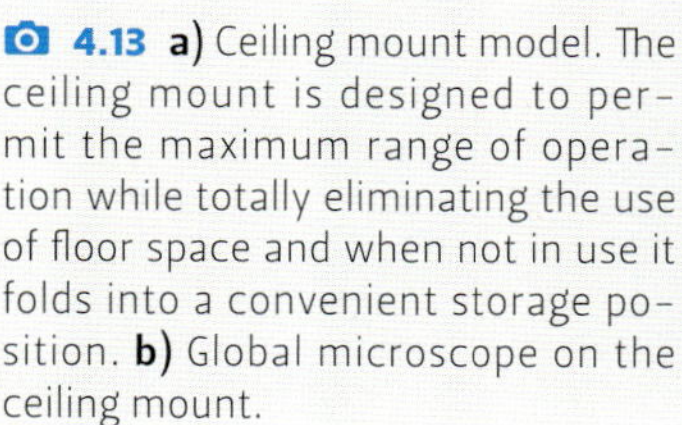

4.13 **a)** Ceiling mount model. The ceiling mount is designed to permit the maximum range of operation while totally eliminating the use of floor space and when not in use it folds into a convenient storage position. **b)** Global microscope on the ceiling mount.

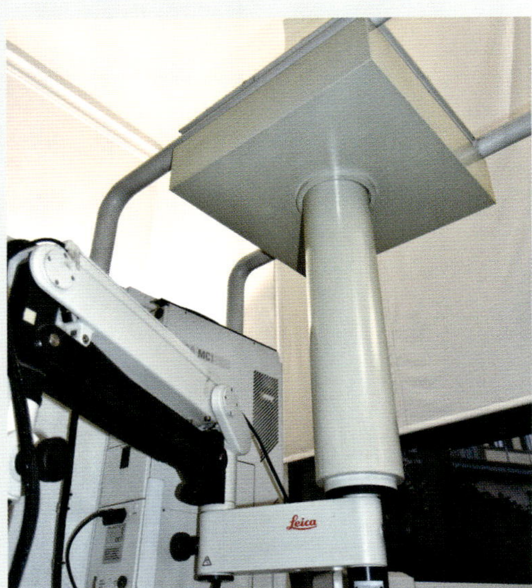

4.14 In case of a very high ceiling, a strong iron beam can be mounted wall-to-wall to attach the ceiling mount in a very stable way.

4.15 **a, b)** Wall mount model. The extension arm and oblique coupler allow greater maneuverability. Leica microscope, fitted with the inclinable binocular, beam splitter (50/50), documentation adaptor (Designs for Vision), 3CCD video camera (Sony DXC-C33P), digital still camera (Canon EOS 80D), and assistant scope. **c)** Global microscope on the wall mount.

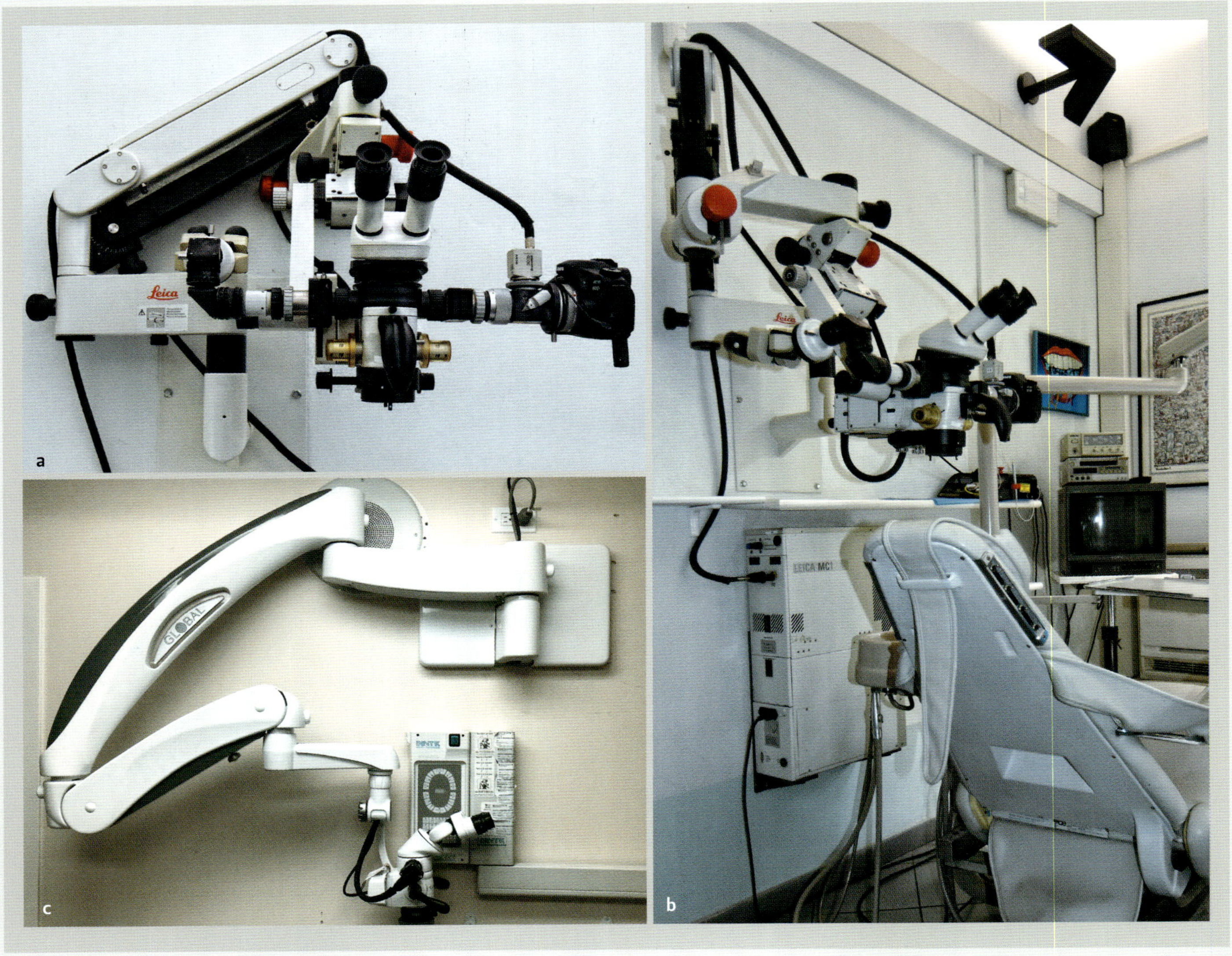

Anatomy of the Surgical Operating Microscope

The operating microscope consists of three primary components: the supporting structure, the body of the microscope, and the light source.

The Supporting Structure

The supporting structure can be mounted on the ceiling (4.13, 4.14), on the wall (4.15) or the floor (4.16). The ceiling mount is the preferable and most used method unless the ceiling is too high. As an alternative, a wall mount can be selected. The only advantage of the floor mounting is that it allows the microscope to be moved from one operating room to another, but usually it is too heavy to be moved and it will only be used in one room.

It is absolutely essential that the microscope is easy to reach, not in the way of the patient or the assistant and that it is completely stable, especially when working at high magnification.[21]

The Body of the Microscope

The body of the microscope is the most important component of the instrument (4.17), and it contains the lenses and prisms responsible for magnification and stereopsis. The body of the microscope is made of eyepieces, binoculars, magnification changer factor, and the objective lens.

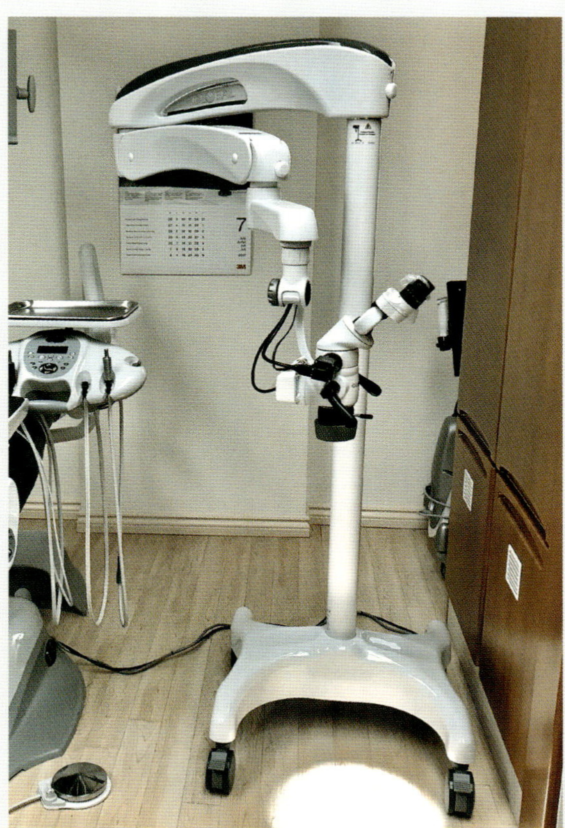

4.16 Global microscope on the floor mount.

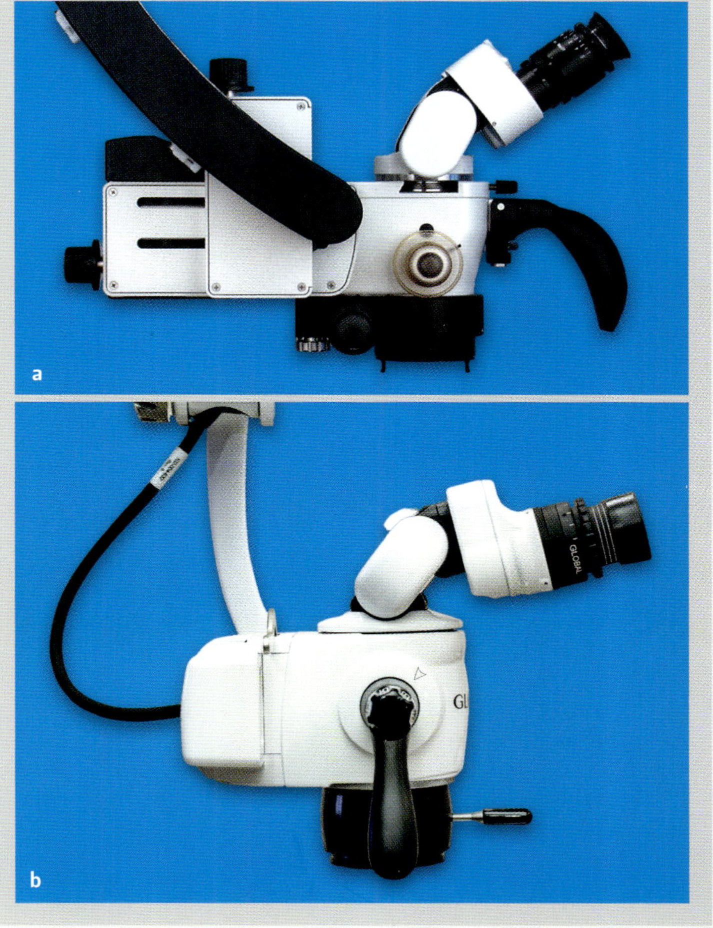

4.17 **a)** Body of the Leica microscope. **b)** Body of the Global microscope.

- **Eyepieces.** Eyepieces are generally available in powers of 10×, 12.5×, 16×, an d 20× (4.18). The most commonly used are 10× and 12.5×. The end of each eyepiece has a rubber cup that can be turned down for clinicians who wear eyeglasses. Eyepieces also have adjustable diopter settings. Diopter settings range from −5 to +5 and are used to adjust for accommodation, which is the ability to focus the lens of the eyes (4.19). Diopter setting is necessary in order to remain in focus when changing magnification and it is particularly important when an assistant scope and documentation equipment are used, so that everything is uniformly in focus (parfocalled). If documentation accessories are used, the eyepiece on the same side of the accessory should be provided with a "reticule" that will help to keep the images well centered in the field.
- The **binoculars** contain the eyepieces and allow adjustment of the interpupillary distance (4.20). Their focal length is 125 or 160 mm. They are aligned manually or with a small knob until the two divergent circles of light combine to a single focus. Once the diopter setting and interpupillary distance adjustments have been made, they should not have to be changed until the microscope is used by a surgeon with different optical requirements.[22] Binoculars are available with straight, inclined, or inclinable tubes. Straight tube binoculars are oriented so

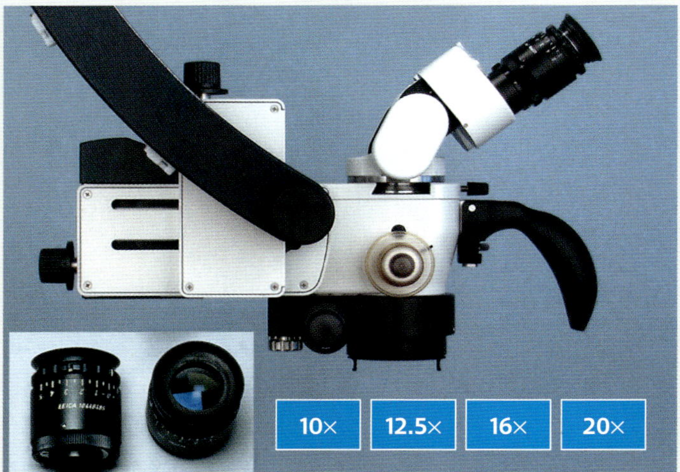

4.18 Depending on the final magnification desired, different eyepieces can be mounted on the binocular.

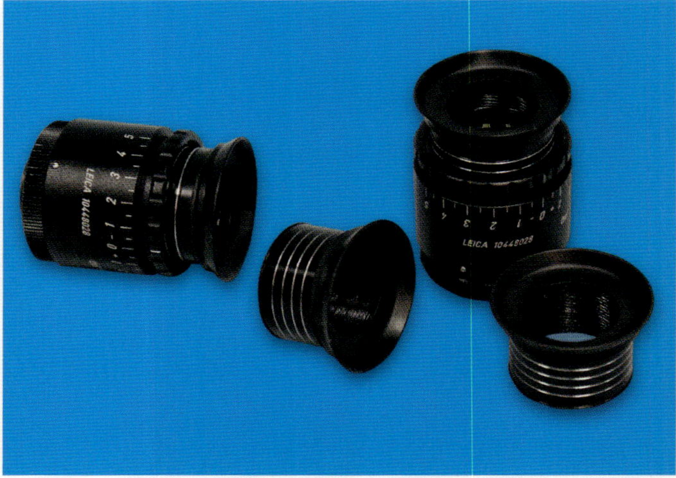

4.19 Eyepieces for the Leica microscope.

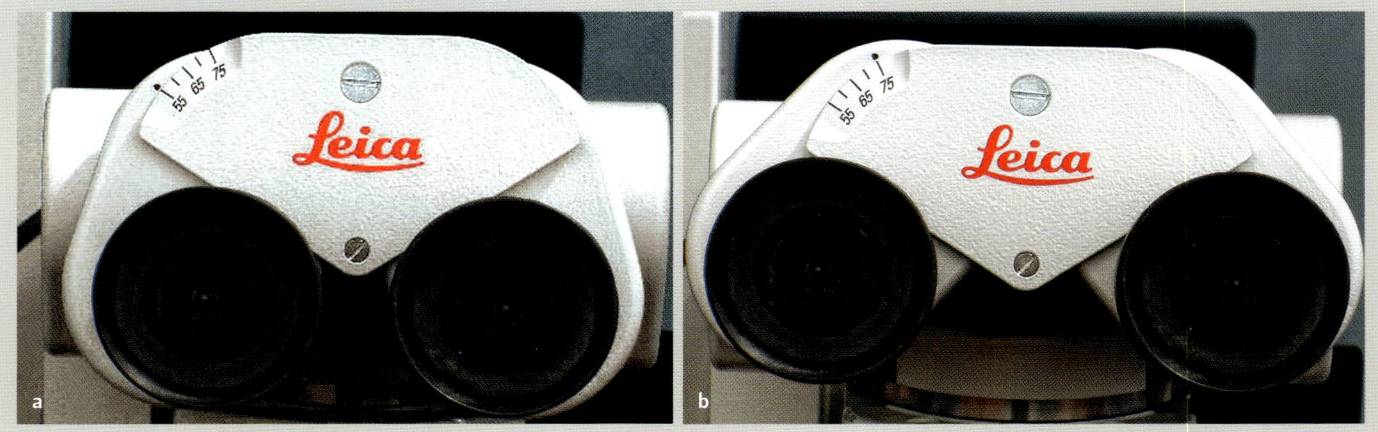

4.20 a, b) The binoculars allow the interpupillary distance to be changed at a range of 55–80 mm.

that the tubes are parallel to the head of the microscope. They are generally used in otology (4.21) and are not well suited for dentistry. Inclined tubes are fixed at a 45° angle to the line of sight of the microscope (4.22). The inclinable tubes are adjustable (4.23) through a range of angles and allow the clinician to always establish a very comfortable working position. Therefore, even if they are more expensive, inclinable binoculars are always preferred.

- **Magnification changers** are available as 3-, 5-, or 6-step manual changers, or a power-zoom changer. They are located within the head of the microscope. Manual step changers consist of lenses that are mounted on a turret that is connected to a dial located on the side of the microscope. The magnification is altered by rotating the dial (4.24). A power zoom changer is a series of lenses that move back and forth on a focusing ring to give a wide range of magnification factors. Focusing with a power zoom microscope is performed by a foot control or by a manual override control knob located on the head of the microscope (4.25). The advantage of power zoom changers is that they avoid the momentary visual disruption or jumping that occurs with manual step changers as the clinician rotates the turret and progresses up or down in magnification. The disadvantages are the following: moving from the minimum

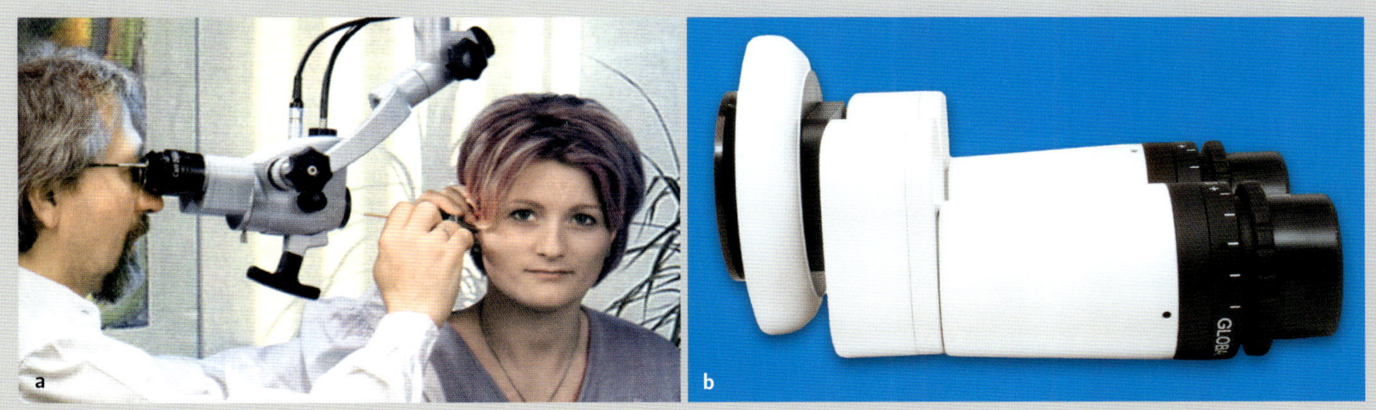

4.21 a) Straight tube binoculars are orientated so that the tubes are parallel to the head of the microscope. They are generally used in otology. **b)** Global straight tube binoculars.

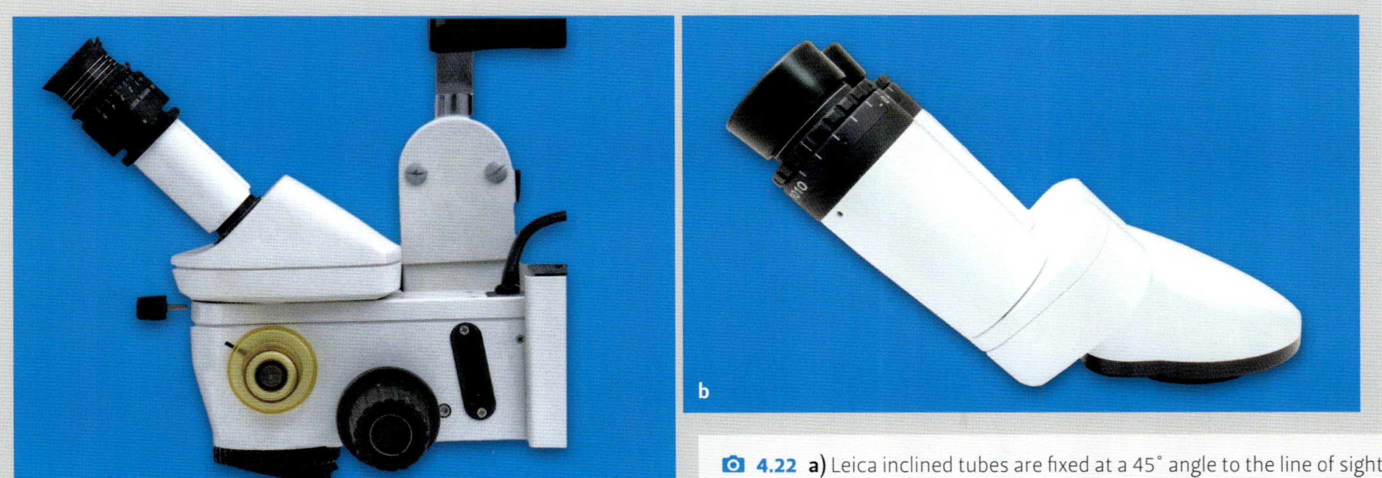

4.22 a) Leica inclined tubes are fixed at a 45° angle to the line of sight of the microscope. They are inexpensive but quite uncomfortable. **b)** Global inclined tube binoculars.

to the maximum magnification is quite slow, while it is much faster with manual step changers, the number of lenses is much higher compared to manual step changers, and this means a greater absorption of light; power zoom changers are much more expensive.

- The **objective lens** is the final optical element, and its focal length determines the working distance between the microscope and the surgical field (4.26). The range of focal length varies from 100 mm to 400 mm. A 200 mm focal length allows approximately 20 cm (8 inches) of working distance, which is generally adequate for use in endodontics. There is adequate room to place surgical instruments and still be close to the patient. A 400 mm lens focuses at about 16 inches. In periodontics, a 250 mm lens is suggest-

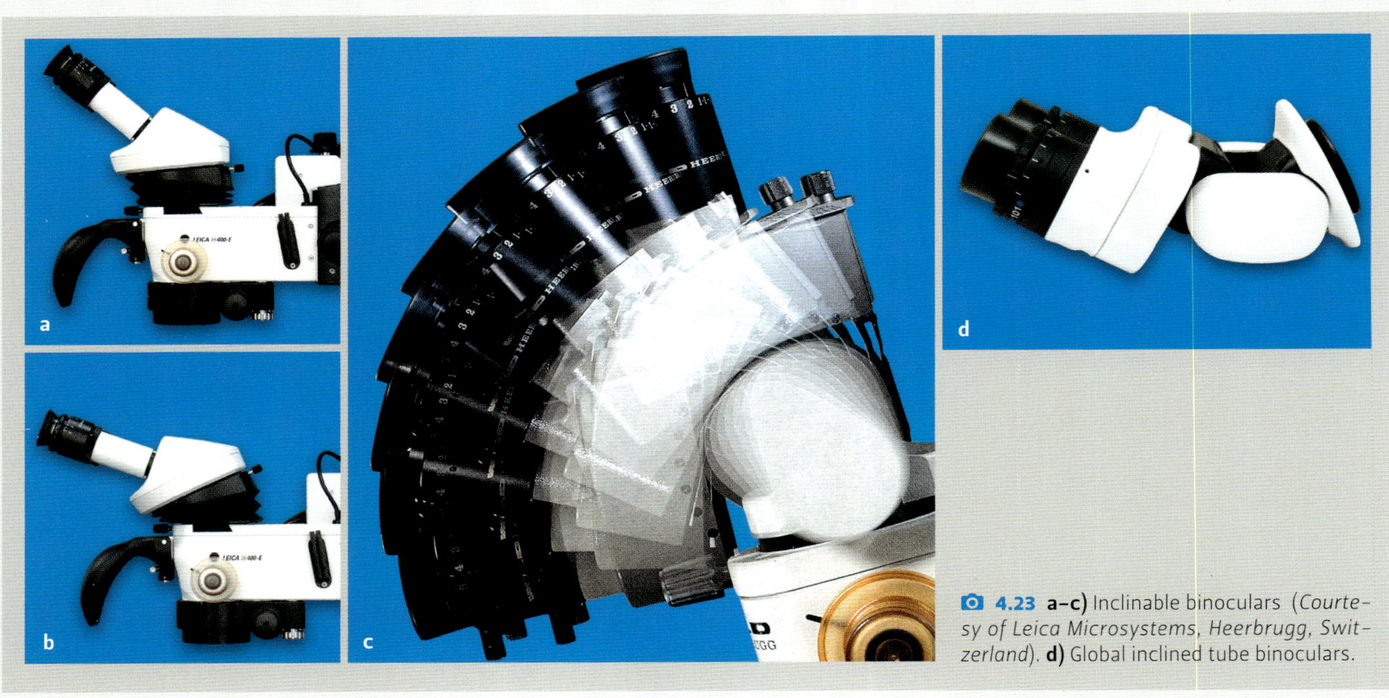

4.23 **a–c)** Inclinable binoculars (*Courtesy of Leica Microsystems, Heerbrugg, Switzerland*). **d)** Global inclined tube binoculars.

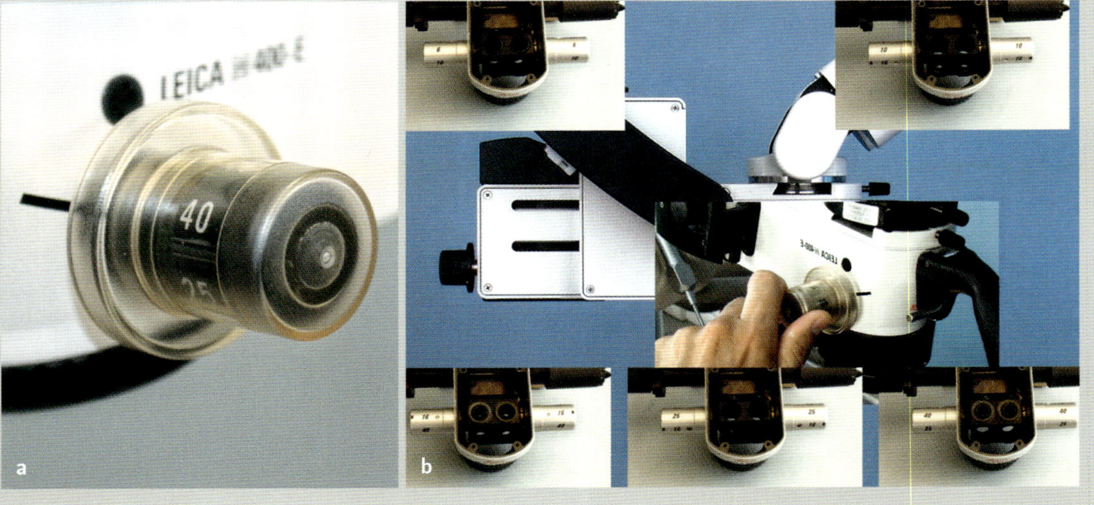

4.24 **a, b)** Manual step changers have a dial located on the side of the microscope connected to a turret where the different lenses are mounted. The magnification is altered by rotating the dial.

ed to give more room for the clinician to work both on the buccal and palatal side of the same quadrant and to rotate the patient's head. The objective lens, as well as all the other microscope lenses (eyepiece lenses, magnification turret lenses, camera attachment lenses, etc.), all have several layers of an anti-reflective coating on both surfaces, which reduces return light loss from the normal 2% per lens surface to just 0.5% per lens surface. In other words, the coating is used to absorb only a minimum amount of light in order not to decrease the illumination of the operative field.

The total magnification (TM) of a microscope depends on the combination of the four variables:

1. focal length of binocular (FLB)
2. focal length of the objective lens (FLOL)
3. eyepiece power (EP)
4. magnification factor of the changer (MF).

The total magnification can be represented by the following formula:

$$\text{TM} = (\text{FLB} / \text{FLOL}) \times \text{EP} \times \text{MF}$$

For example:

- Binocular focal length = 125 mm
- Objective lens focal length = 250 mm
- Eyepiece magnification = 10×
- Magnification factor = 0.5

$$\textbf{Total Magnification} = 125/250 \times 10 \times 0.5 = 2.5\times$$

Looking at this formula carefully, we can come to the following conclusions:

- increasing the power of the eyepieces increases magnification and decreases the field of view
- increasing the focal length of the binoculars increases magnification and decreases the field of view
- increasing the magnification factor increases magnification and decreases the field of view
- increasing the focal length of the objective lens, decreases magnification and increases the field of view. In addition, the illumination also decreases because we are farther away from the surgical field
- each time the magnification is increased, the depth of field and the illumination decrease.

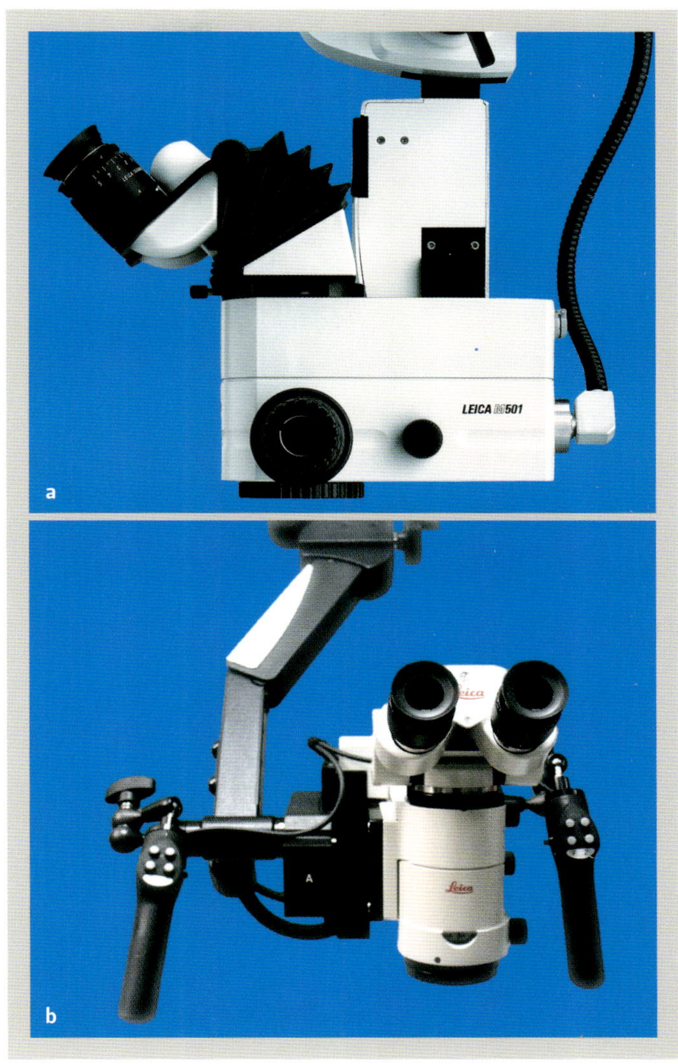

4.25 **a)** Manual zoom microscope. **b)** Microscope with power zoom changer.

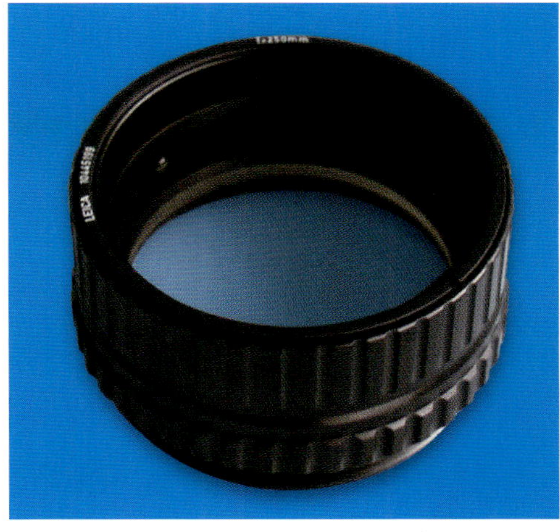

4.26 Objective lens.

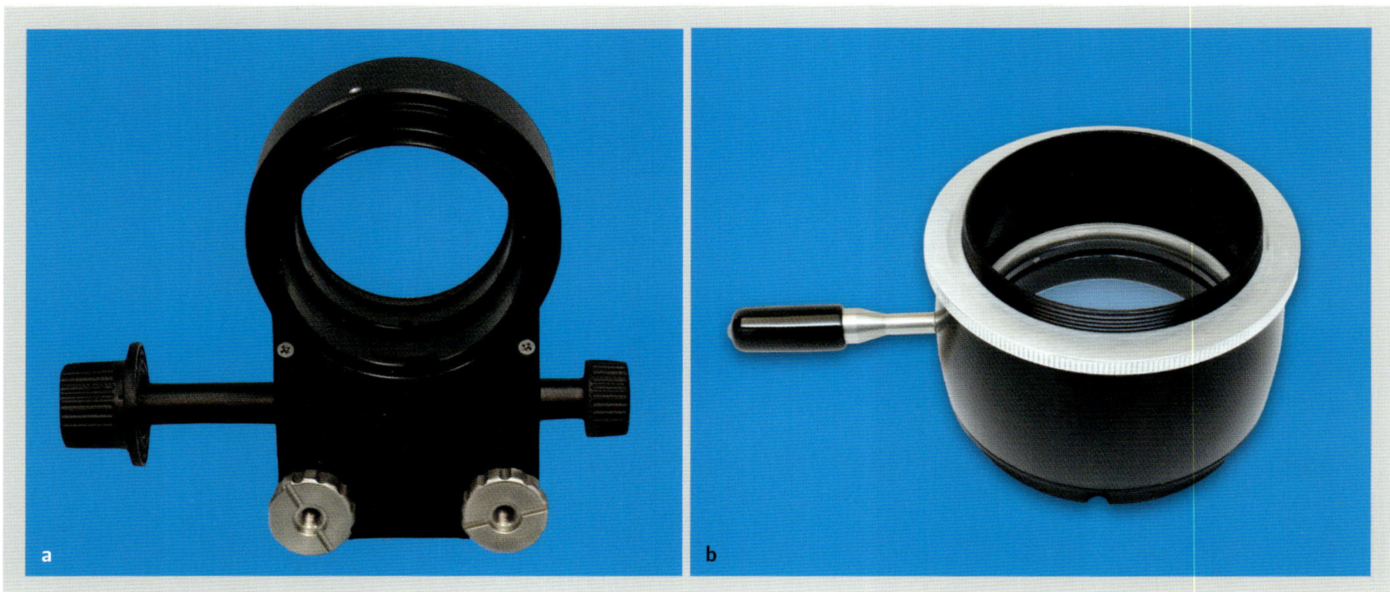

4.27 **a)** The fine focus can be done manually using the device integrated in the objective lens of Leica. **b)** The fine focus is integrated in the objective lens of Global.

As for the use of different magnifications, it is important to keep in mind that maximum magnification is used for checking, and most of the procedures are made at minimum or medium magnification. In endodontics, we do not need microscopes that can provide 20 or even greater magnifications since it is almost impossible to work at such high power. As already stated above, working at high magnification the operative field, the illumination, and mainly the depth of field decrease. In other words, at maximum magnification the area is extremely reduced, the illumination may be insufficient, and more importantly, it is very difficult to keep the operative field constantly in focus. A little movement on the part of the patient or sometimes just their breathing can be enough to be completely out of focus. Fine focus can be done manually using the device integrated into the objective lens (4.27), or by rotating a fine focus knob, which raises the entire body of the microscope, or by an electric foot control.

One might think that constantly working under a microscope may cause eyestrain and eye fatigue. Not only is this not true, but just the opposite is true. As a matter of fact, operating microscopes possess the additional benefit of Galilean Optics, as they focus at infinity and send parallel beams of light to each eye.[21,22] With parallel light, the operator's eyes are at rest, as though looking off into the distance, permitting performance of time-consuming procedures without inducing eye fatigue, as we would have if we were working with the naked eye at a small distance from the patient requiring convergent optics.

The Light Source

The light source is one of the most important features of an operating microscope.[21] Besides optics, the light source is responsible for operating in operative fields that are small and deep such as a root canal. This is possible because the microscope provides a powerful coaxial illumination, which means that the light is coaxial with the line of sight and eliminates the presence of any shadows.

Three light source systems are commonly available: halogen light, xenon light (4.28) and LED light.

Halogen light displays a yellowish hue (3,300 °Kelvin) and frequently does not provide enough illumination for quality documentation especially at higher powers.

Xenon light is much more powerful and provides a brighter light at about 5,500 °Kelvin approximating daylight. This ensures the best illumination for fine anatomical details and allows shorter documentation ex-

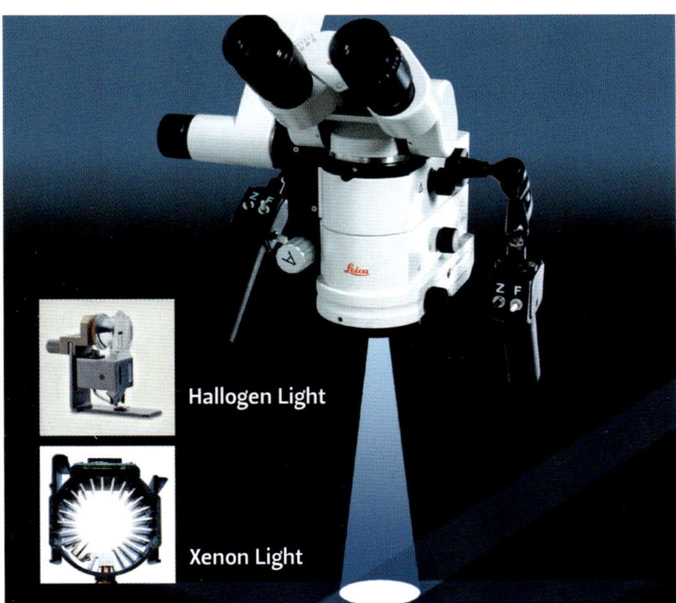

4.28 The xenon light source is much more powerful.

posure times, which will provide sharper images and higher depth of field.

LED light sources are similar to xenon light in color temperature (5,700 ˚K) and are almost as powerful as xenon light and much less expensive.

In all cases, light intensity is controlled by a rheostat and cooled by a fan. After the light reaches the surgical field, it is reflected back through the objective lens, through the magnification changer lenses, and through the binoculars and then exits to the eyes as two separate beams of light. This separation of the light beams is what produces the stereoscopic effect that allows the clinician to see the depth of field.[10]

Accessories

Some microscopes are built with fixed components and do not allow for the addition of any accessories. Others can be customized with accessories such as the assistant scope and documentation tools, like a digital DSLR camera (Digital Single-Lens Reflex) and a video camera.

BEAM SPLITTER

To supply light to such accessories, a beam splitter must be inserted in the path of light as it returns to the operator's eyes between the binoculars and the magnification changer. The beam splitter divides each path of light into two parts (50:50) (4.29); one goes to the operator's eye and the other goes to the accessory. Usually, half of

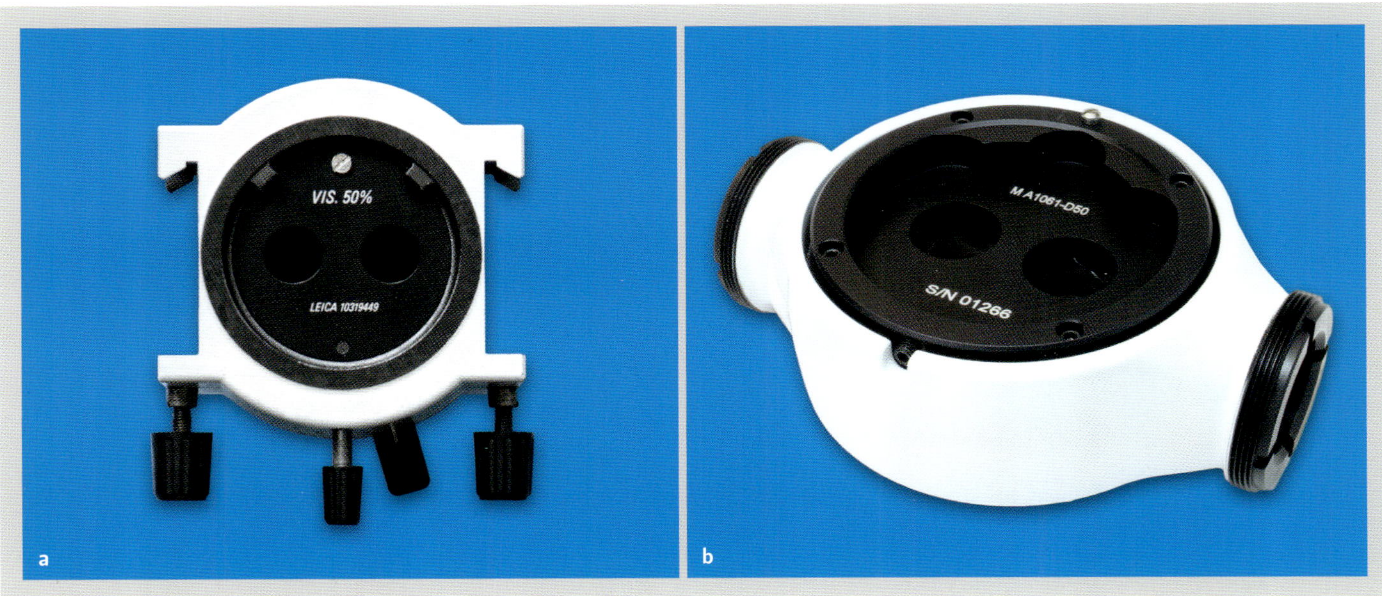

4.29 **a)** The Leica 50:50 beam splitter. **b)** The Global 50:50 beam splitter.

the light of the right beam goes to the documentation accessories (4.30), half of the light of the left beam goes to the assistant scope (4.31). In other words, this means that our dental assistant will see what we see with our left eye, and we will document what we see with our right eye. Furthermore, even though the dental assistants have their binoculars, they cannot have a stereoscopic view because they will be looking at the visual field from just the left port of the beam splitter with both eyes.

DOCUMENTATION

The accessories for documentation are the video camera and the digital SLR camera. They can be mounted separately or combined, through specifically designed photo or video adaptors connected to the beam splitter. Should one want to use both, it is important to keep in mind that the 50% of the light that goes to the documentation accessories will be once again divided by another prism into two parts, one for the video camera and one for the digital SLR camera, unless the adaptor is using a mirror instead of a prism. In this case, the entire 50% of the light can go either to the video camera or to the SLR camera so that both the documentation accessories receive more light. The disadvantage is that it will be impossible to take photos while the clinician is taking a video.

The digital still cameras available today allow excellent pictures and video to be taken. Should the operator want to have more light for still images, a strobe can be mounted over the objective lens (4.32). The video camera and the digital still camera can be connected to a monitor, a video tape recorder, and a video printer. The digital camera can also download the images directly onto a computer, allowing rapid organization of a rich database of images. The digital SLR camera can also take video of excellent quality.

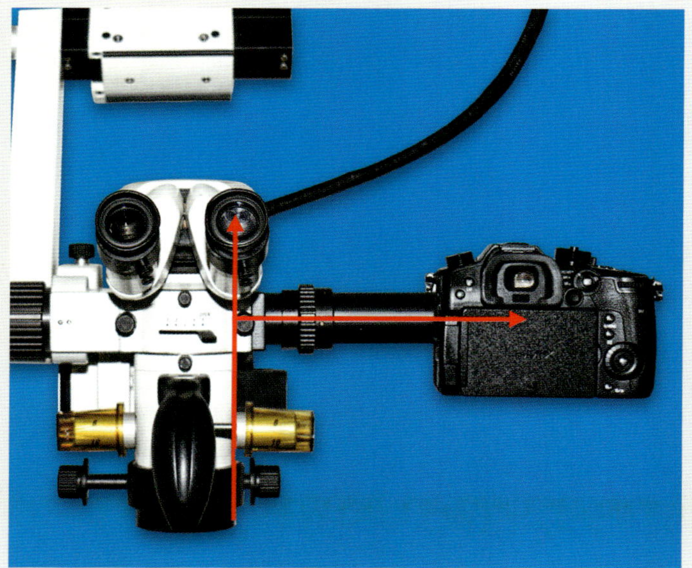

4.30 Using a 50:50 beam splitter, half of the light from the right beam goes to the documentation accessories.

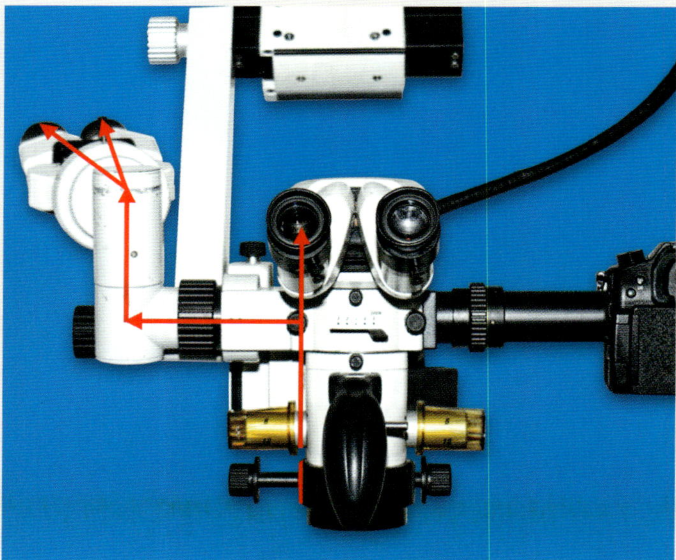

4.31 Using a 50:50 beam splitter, half of the light of the left beam goes to the assistant scope.

The video camera and the digital SLR can also be connected to a computer (4.33a), to a monitor (4.33b), a digital videocassette recorder and a video printer. The monitor can be used not only to motivate the patient, who can see the entire videotaped procedure, but it can also and primarily be used by the second surgical assistant, who can follow the surgical procedure and give the operator the right instruments at the right moment. Looking at the monitor, the dental assistants can also work as a video director and pause the recording if they think the picture is off center or out of focus.

RETICULE

The eyepiece on the same side of the documentation accessories should be provided with a reticule. This reticule can prove an invaluable aid for alignment during videotaping and photography because it helps the operator center the surgical field during documentation.

ASSISTANT SCOPE

The assistant scope (4.34) is very useful, as it allows the assistant to assist the operator during the entire procedure. The advantages of adding assistant articulating binoculars are numerous. The assistant becomes optically important to the surgical team and develops a keener understanding, not only of what is expected during surgery but also of why it is expected. They see exactly what the operator sees. The first assistant of the surgical team only has to keep the operative field free of bleeding, holding the surgical suction device during the entire procedure (4.35). Through the assistant scope, placement of the suction tips is more accurate, the assistant can visually anticipate the surgeon's next step in the procedure and can do their job much more precisely looking through the assistant scope, compared to just looking at the monitor. Most clinicians have found that bringing the assistant into the visual sphere increases job satisfaction significantly.[12]

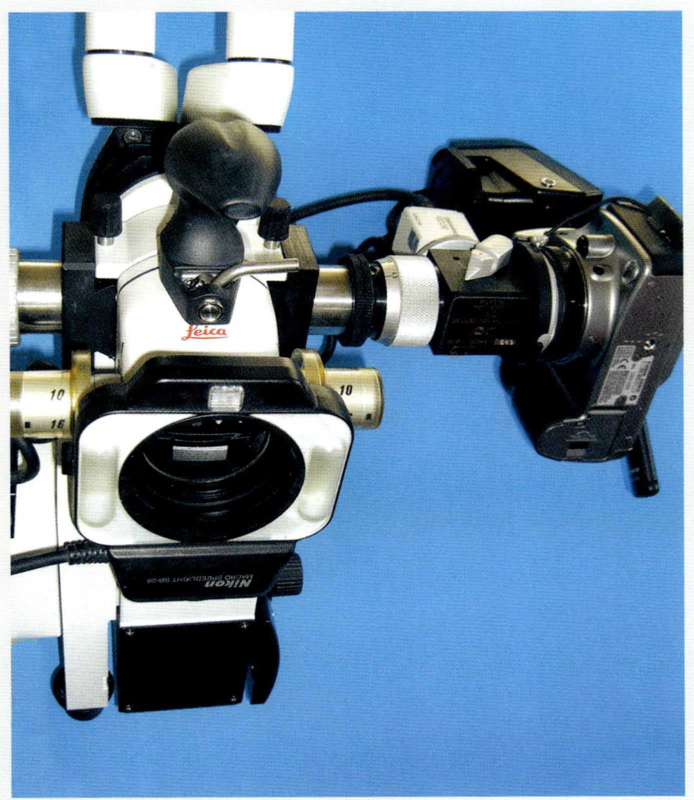

4.32 The digital camera is connected with a strobe.

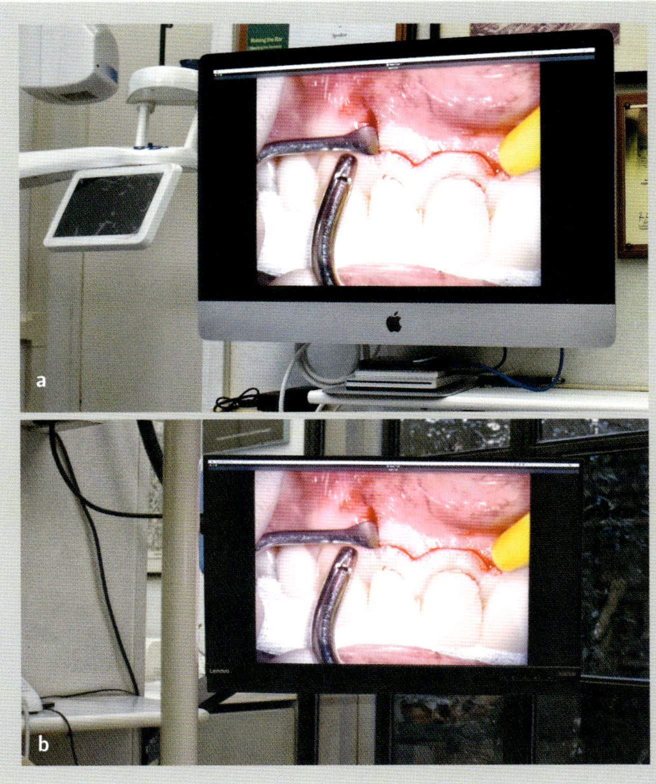

4.33 The video camera and the digital SLR can also be connected to a computer (**a**) and a monitor (**b**).

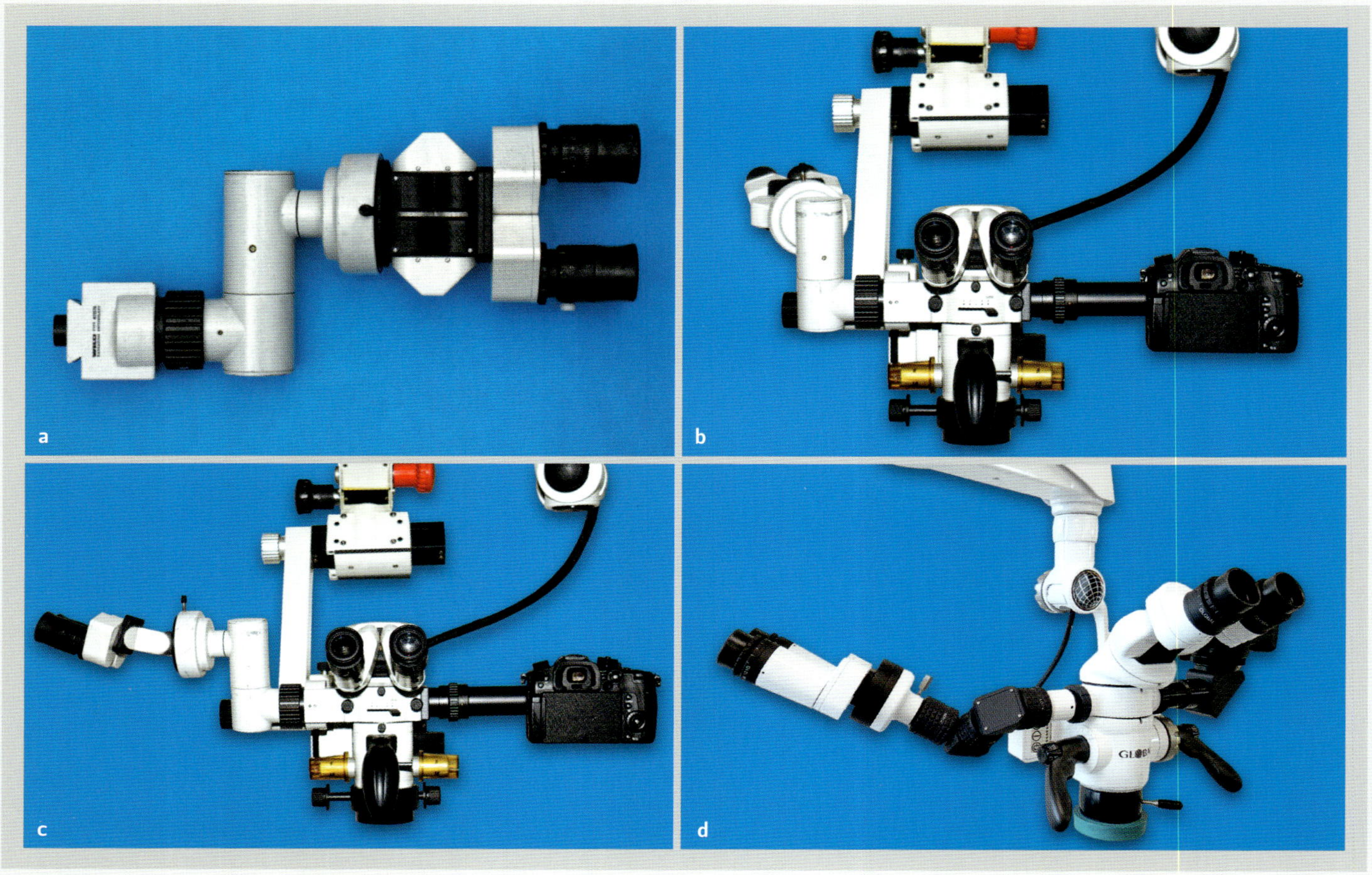

4.34 a) Leica assistant scope. The assistant scope can be oriented, depending if the doctor is working at a 9 o'clock position **(b)** or a 12 o'clock position **(c)**. **d)** Global assistant scope.

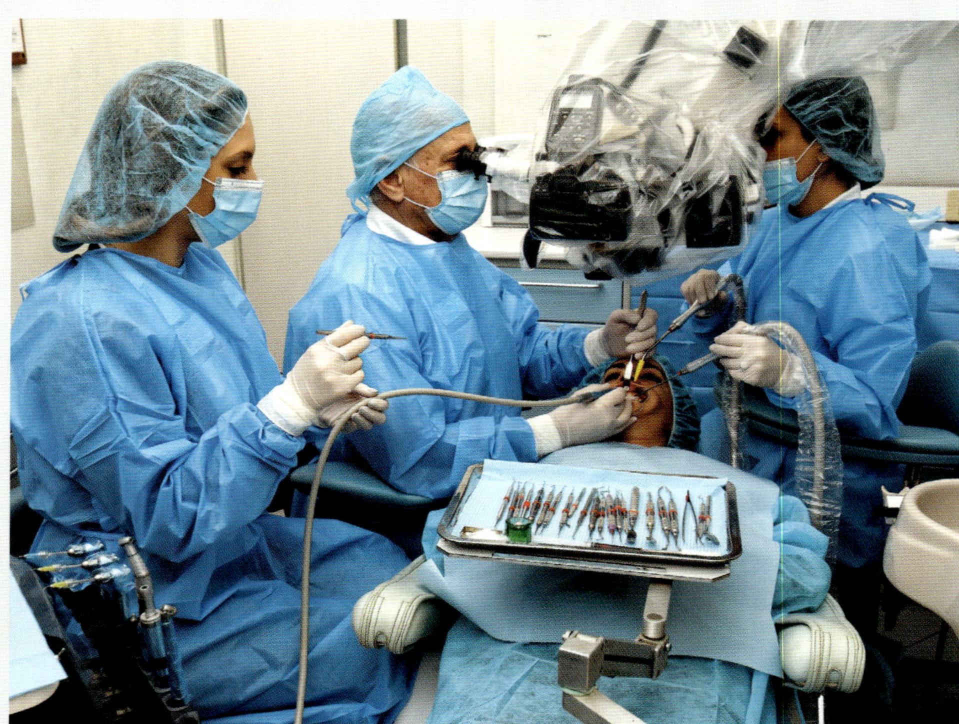

4.35 Through the assistant scope, the first assistant sees exactly what the operator sees and very carefully keeps the operative field free of bleeding, holding the surgical suction device during the entire procedure. The second assistant is ready to give the doctor the next instrument needed.

Positioning the Microscope

In chronological order, the preparation of the microscope involves the following maneuvers:[15]

1. Operator Positioning
2. Rough Positioning of the Patient
3. Positioning of the Microscope and Fine Focus
4. Adjustment of the Interpupillary Distance
5. Fine Positioning of the Patient
6. Parfocal Adjustment
7. Fine Focus Adjustment
8. Assistant Scope Adjustment

Operator Positioning

Many operators work directly behind the patient at the 11 or 12 o'clock position. Others prefer to work at 9 o'clock. They are both efficient positions and there is very little difference. How to select the right position depends on the position that the dentist used perhaps even for years before installing the microscope. The suggestion is **not** to change position: if the operator is used to working at the 9 o'clock position and feels comfortable, after installing the microscope, there is no reason to change working position. Working at higher magnification requires a learning curve and at the beginning may not be so easy. If the operator changes working position, everything becomes more difficult and changing perspective can be confusing. In surgical endodontics, the suggested position is, however, different depending on the arch or quadrant being worked on. For the upper arch, the author prefers the 8 or 9 o'clock position (4.36), while for the lower arch the preferred position is at 12 or 1 o'clock (4.37).

The operator should adjust the seating position so that their hips are 90° to the floor, their knees are 90° to the hips and their forearms are 90° degrees to the upper arms.[22] The operator's forearms should lie comfortably on the armrest of the operator's chair and their feet should be placed flat on the floor (4.38). The back should be in a neutral position, erect, perpendicular to the floor, with the natural curve of the back supported by the lumbar support of the chair, with the eyepiece inclined so that the head and neck can be held at an an-

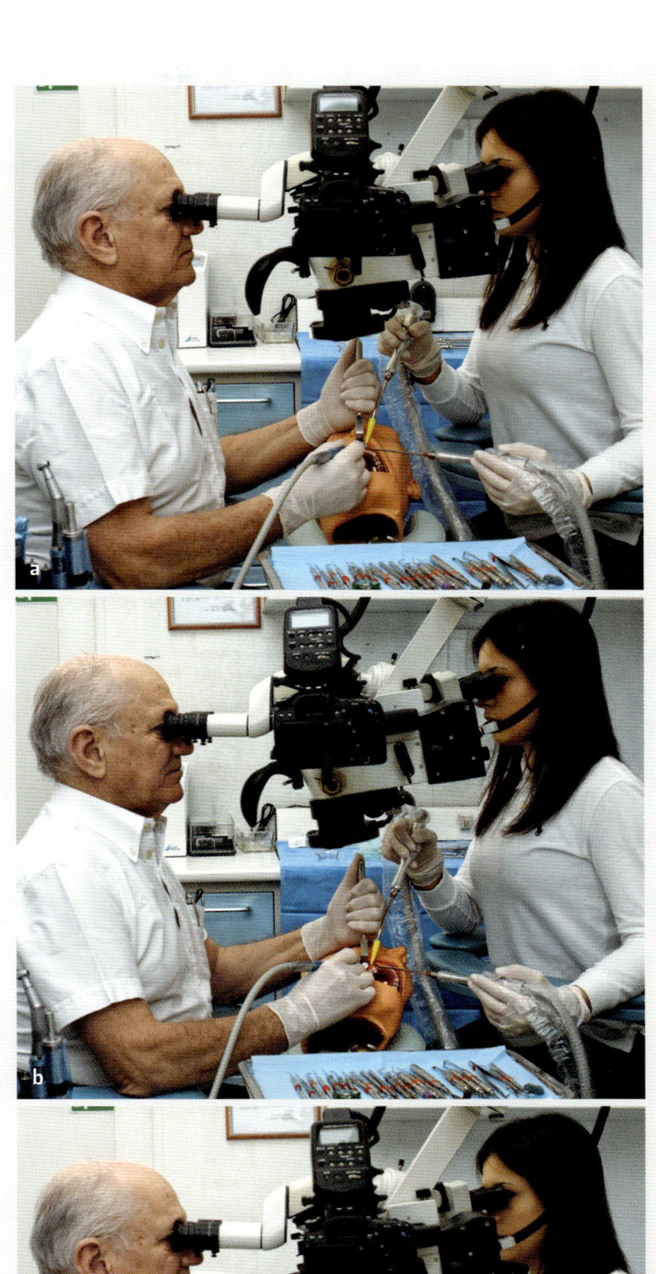
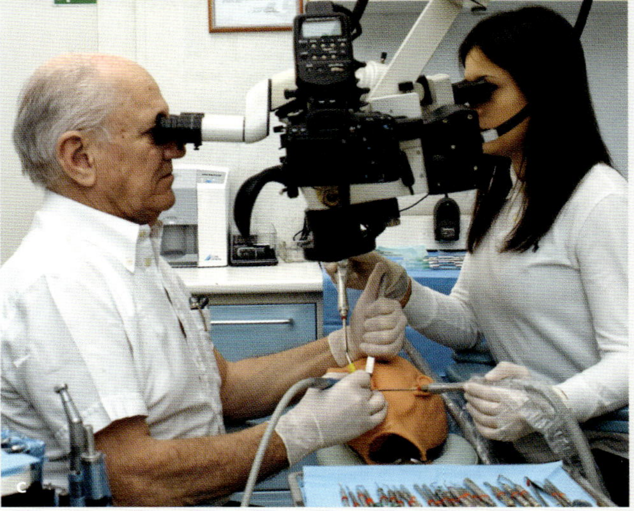

4.36 Working positions when performing surgery in the upper arch. **a)** Front teeth. **b)** Right quadrant. **c)** Left quadrant.

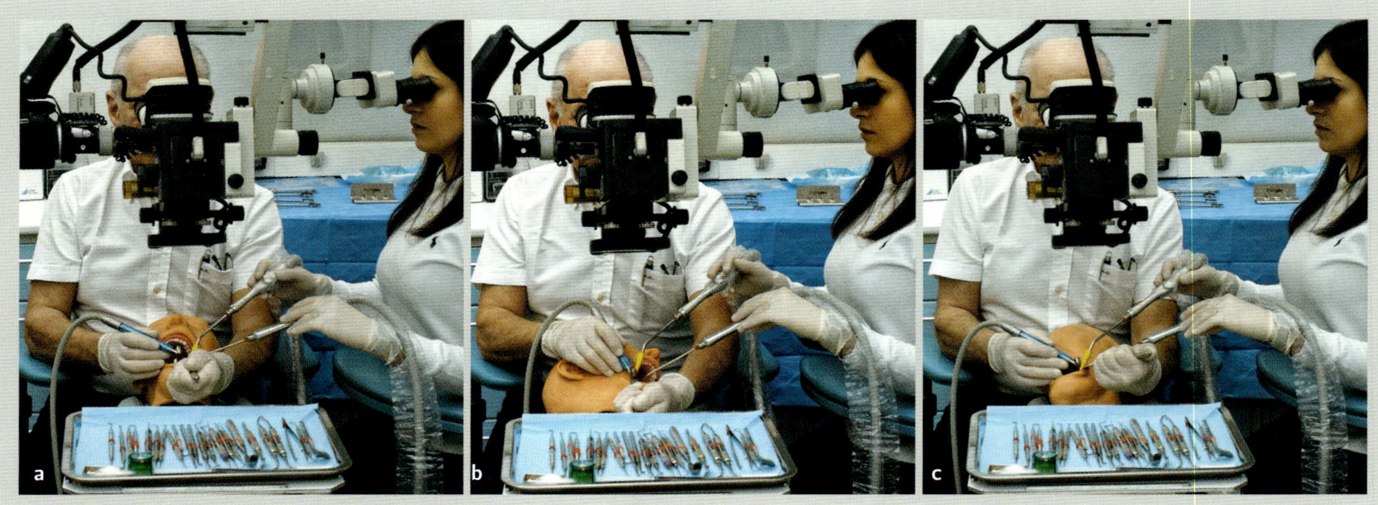

4.37 Working positions when performing surgery in the lower arch. **a)** Front teeth. **b)** Right quadrant. **c)** Left quadrant.

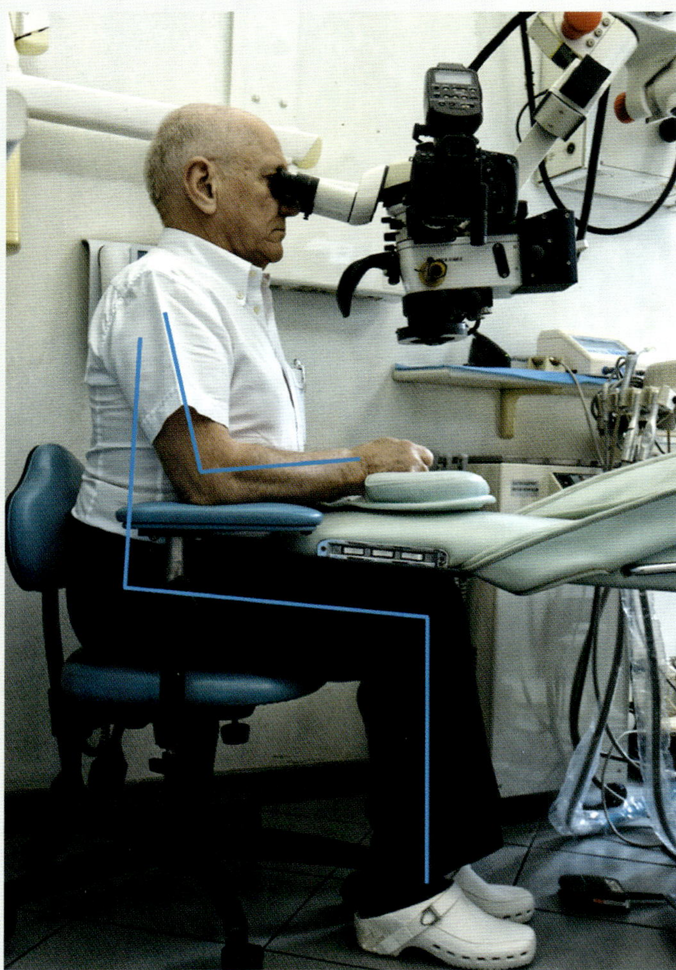

4.38 The correct position of the operator at the microscope. Each angle should be a 90° angle.

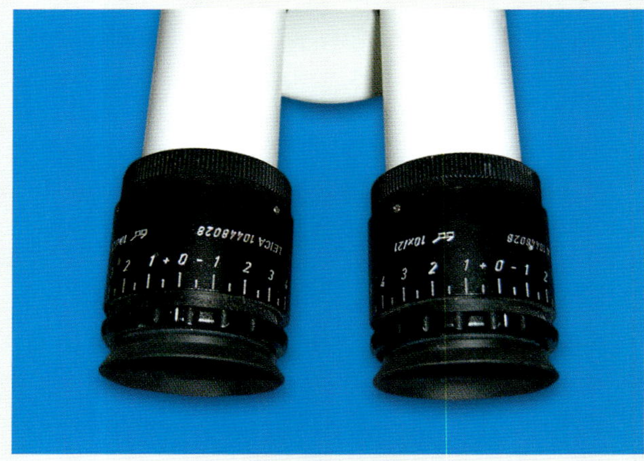

4.39 The rubber cups of each eyepiece are positioned in a lower position if the operator wears glasses.

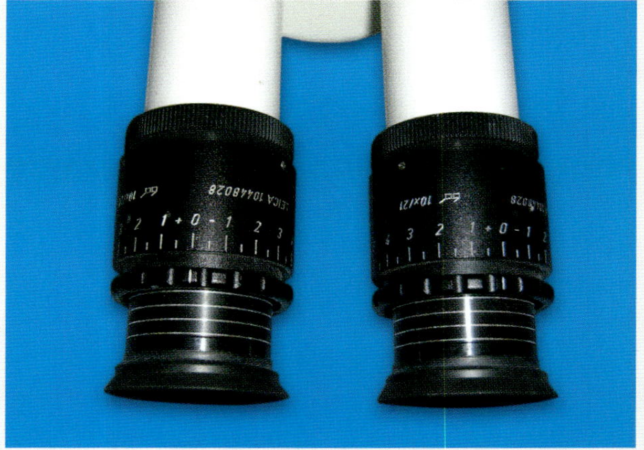

4.40 The rubber cups of each eyepiece are positioned in a raised position if the operator is not wearing glasses.

gle that can be comfortably sustained. This position is maintained regardless of the arch or quadrant being worked on. It is the patient who is moved to accommodate this position.

Rough Positioning of the Patient

The patient is placed almost horizontally if the operator works in the upper arch and the Trendelenburg position if the operator works in the lower arch. The chair is then raised until the patient is in focus.

Positioning of the Microscope and Fine Focus

After turning on the light of the microscope, the microscope should be maneuvered so that the circle of light shines on the working area. Knowing the focal length of the objective lens, the operator moves the body of the microscope approximately to the working distance and then, looking through the eyepiece, moves the microscope up and down until the working area comes into focus. During this maneuver, which is made at minimum magnification, the fine focus device of the objective lens should be in an intermediate position in order to allow a wide range (20 mm) during the fine focusing of the operative field. The inclinable eyepiece is now adjusted so that the operator's head and spine can maintain a comfortable position with the working area in focus.

Adjustment of the Interpupillary Distance

Looking through the binocular, each eye sees a small circle of light. The interpupillary distance should be now adjusted by taking the two halves of the binocular head of the microscope (see 📷 4.20) and moving them apart and then together until the two circles are combined and only one illuminated circle is seen. With some microscopes, this maneuver is made by moving a knob located on the binocular. Adjustable rubber cups extend from the ends of the eyepieces. Glasses wearers should have the cups in the lowered position (📷 4.39) and those who work without glasses should work with the cups in the raised position (📷 4.40).

Fine Positioning of the Patient

Now small movements need to be made to the back of the dental chair in order to position the patient in the final position. While 100% of the microscope work in nonsurgical endodontics is performed in indirect vision through the mirror, which means that the operator has to consider the angle that the light makes with the mirror to enter inside the root canal, in surgical endodontics everything is performed by means of direct vision. Therefore, the positioning of the patient is much easier and the operator position is also much more comfortable.

Parfocal Adjustment

The process of parfocaling is important because it allows the focused view of the working area to stay sharp as the magnification setting is changed and maintains everything in focus including for the assistant scope and the documentation accessories. This is achieved by individually adjusting the eyepieces (📷 4.41).

These are the steps to follow for parfocal adjustment:

1. Position the microscope above a flat, stationary surface.
2. Using a pen or pencil, make an X on a piece of white paper to serve as a focus target and place it within the illumination field of the microscope.
3. Set both the eyepiece diopter settings to 0. Also set assistant's eyepieces (if any) to 0.
4. Set the microscope near the middle of its focus range.
5. Position the microscope vertically at a convenient

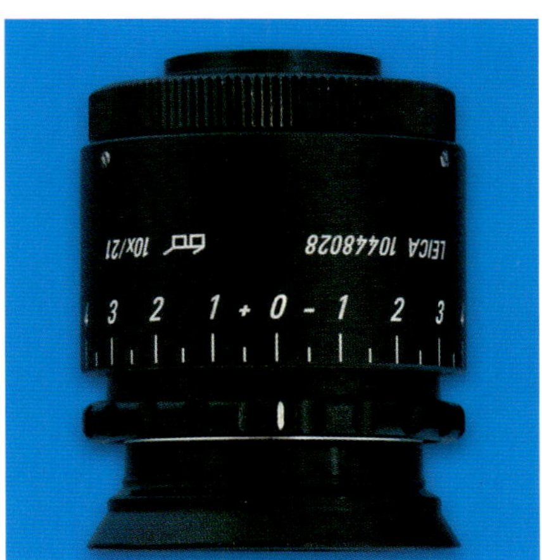

📷 **4.41** Each eyepiece has several settings for parfocal adjustment.

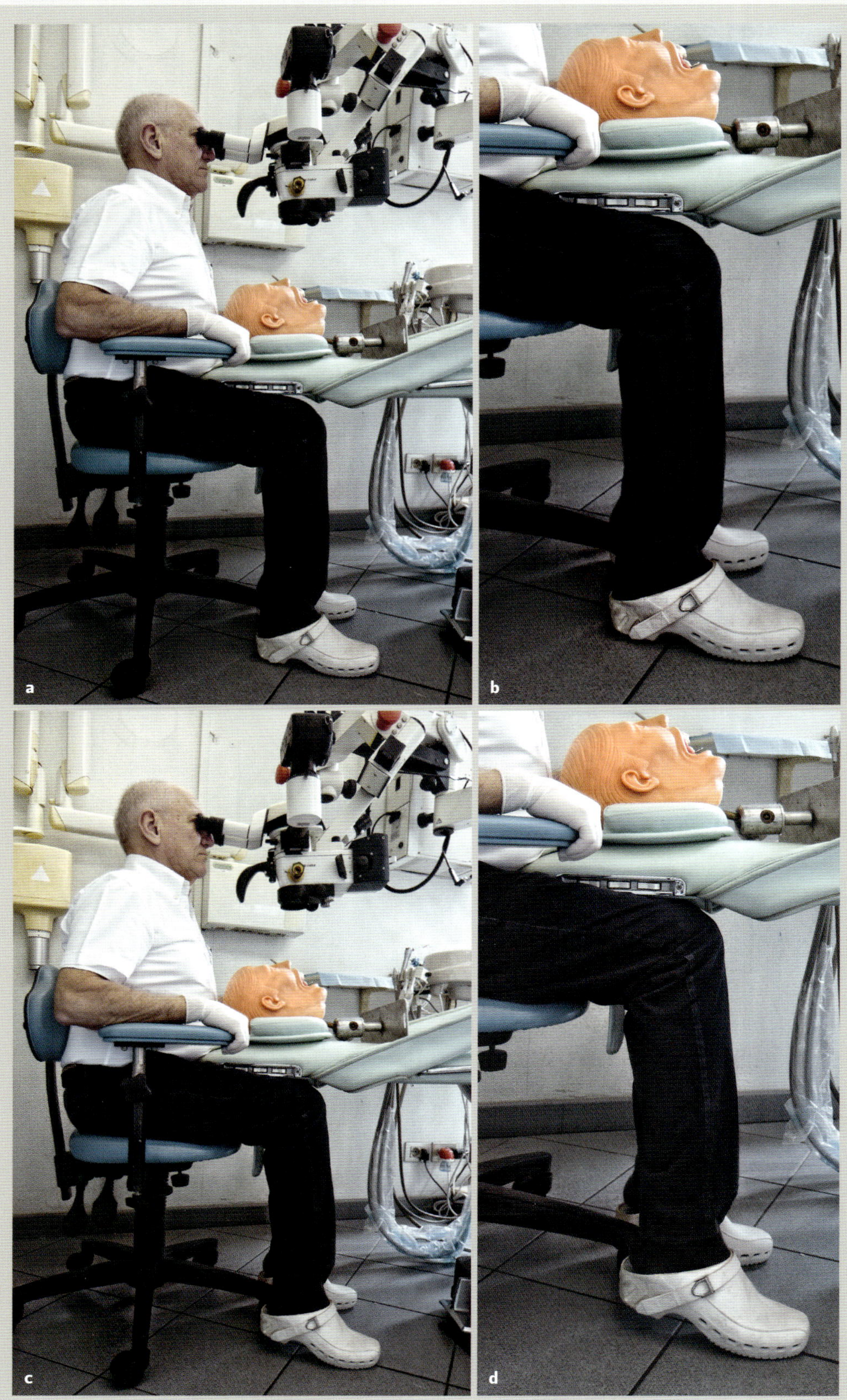

4.42 **a–d)** Fine focus is done by lifting the entire back of the dental chair a few millimeters with the operator's knee.

view height and so that the target is within the view range.

6. Set the microscope on its highest magnification setting (zoom in), and focus using the fine-focus control until a sharp image is obtained.
7. Being careful not to physically shift the microscope position, change the magnification setting to its lowest position (zoom out). Focus left and right eyepieces, one at a time, by turning the diopter ring until the image is clear and sharp. Tighten the diopter lock button to lock in this position and record the setting for future use.
8. Each operator will have their own particular setting that is to be dialed in whenever that particular operator uses the microscope.

This procedure does not have to be repeated by the same operator each time the microscope is used, but rather the diopter settings noted the first time the parfocaling procedure was performed by that operator should be used. Due to changes in eye correction associated with time, however, it is recommended that this procedure be repeated by the operator once or twice per year.

Fine Focus Adjustment

Some microscopes are provided with an electric fine focus adjustment while in some other microscopes this can be done by hand. In both cases, the operator has to let go of any instruments they are holding to adjust the fine focus. To avoid this, it is extremely easy to adjust the fine focus or to change the focused area (for instance, during surgery, focus on the surface of the bevel and then focus on the deepest point of the retropreparation) by just lifting the entire back of the dental chair a few millimeters with the operator's knee (📷 4.42). This way the focused area will change without the operator using their hands and without moving the hands from the working area. The dental chair should, therefore, have a back thin enough to allow the operator to position their legs underneath. Lifting the entire back of the dental chair by just a few millimeters with the operator's knee will allow the operator to make the fine focus and if needed to change the focused area from one plane to another deeper inside the root canal, without letting go of what they are holding.

Assistant Scope Adjustment

Once the clinician has completed all the above procedures, the dental assistant will perform the same adjustments on the binocular and on the eyepieces, without changing the position of the microscope.

Usually, adjustment 4, 6 and 8 are made only once, while the others are made each time the operator starts a new endodontic procedure.

Ergonomics and the Microscope

Preparation of the Patient

The patient is seated in the dental chair and a small foam pillow is positioned under the neck as a headrest, to make them as comfortable as possible (📷 4.43).

The surgical procedure is performed by the surgical team, made up of three people: the doctor and two dental assistants, and uses a six hands approach (📷 4.44). The surgical assistant sits next to the doctor, uses the assistant scope so that they can see exactly what the doctor sees and their job is to keep the operative field free of bleeding, holding two high volume aspirator tips (📷 4.45). The second assistant sits next to the doctor, follows the surgical procedure directly through the monitor and is in charge of placing instruments in the doctor's fingers.

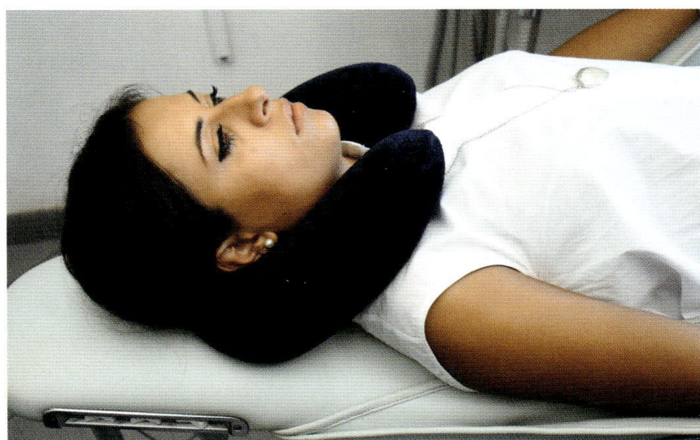

📷 **4.43** The use of the soft foam pillow positioned under the neck will make the patient much more comfortable.

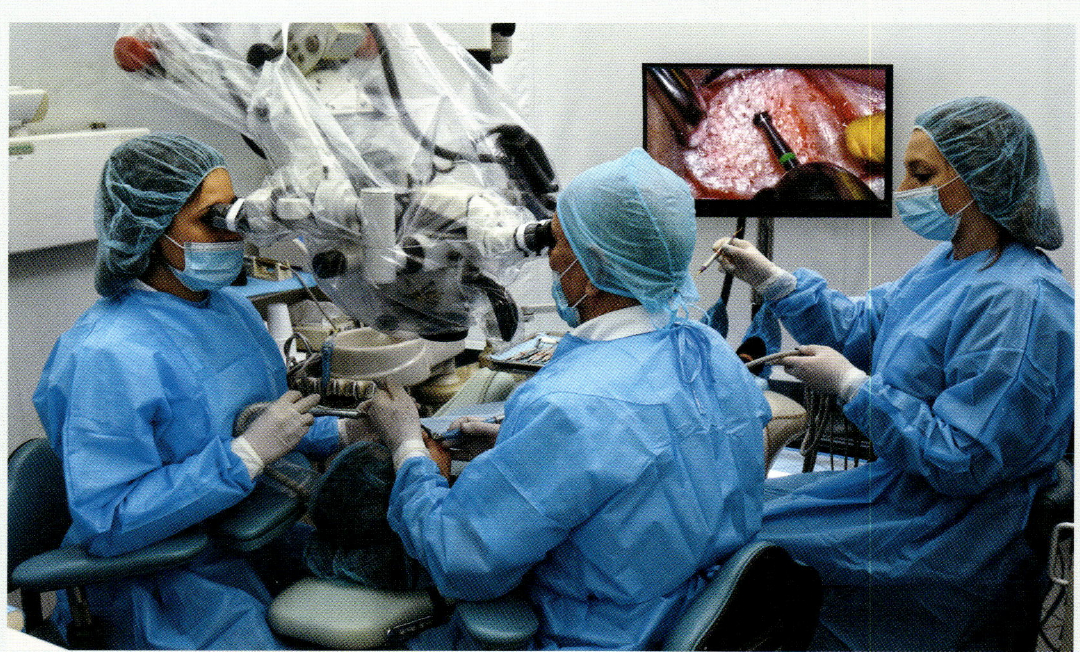

4.44 The surgical team.

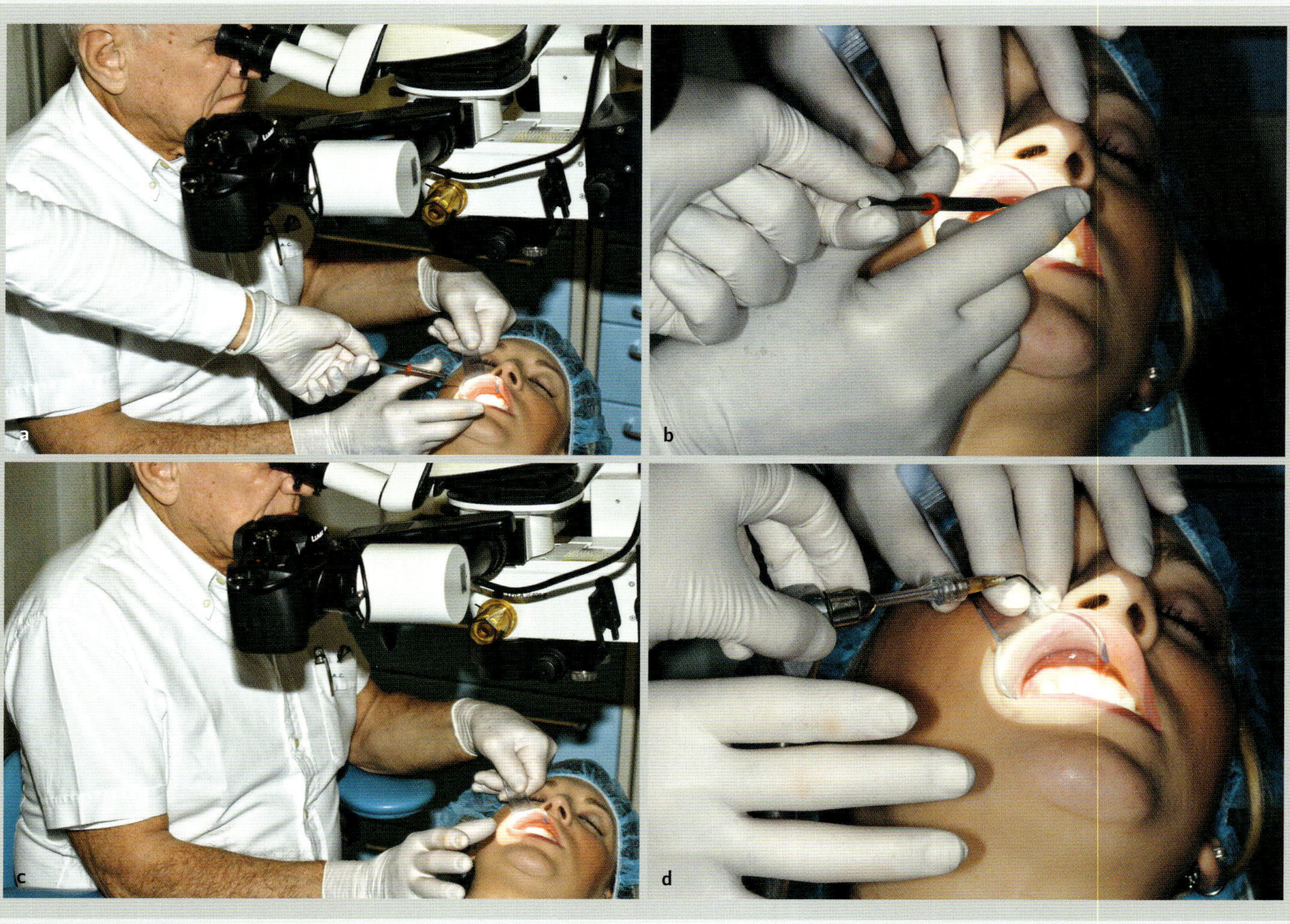

a

b

c

d

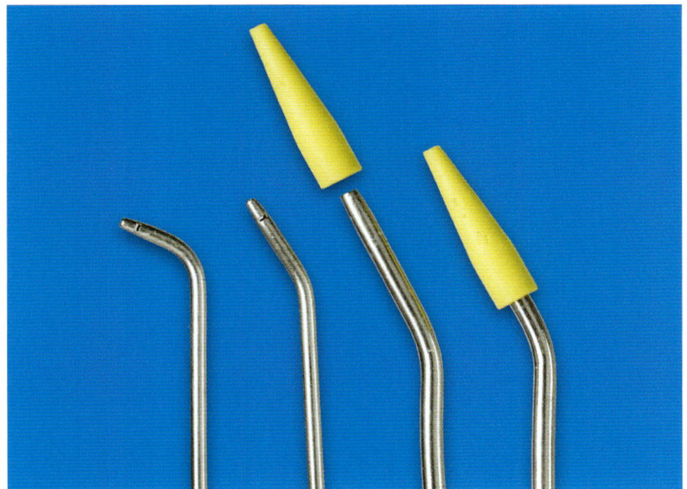

4.45 The aspirator tips (Quality Aspirators, Duncanville, Texas USA). The large one has a silicon tip so as not to damage the soft tissues during suctioning.

To develop the highest efficiency, the surgical procedure should be performed by the doctor without removing their eyes from the binocular of the microscope and without increasing the distance between their hands and the patient's mouth and each instrument should be placed by the second dental assistant not just in their hands, but onto their fingers. During surgery, the *operator* will *always* hold the retractor with the left hand and every instrument should be firmly placed in the right hand by the second dental assistant. All the operator does is open his/her fingers, without losing contact with the patient's cheek (4.46).

The instruments have been previously positioned on the tray in the order of use and each time an instrument is given to the doctor it is put back in the same place af-

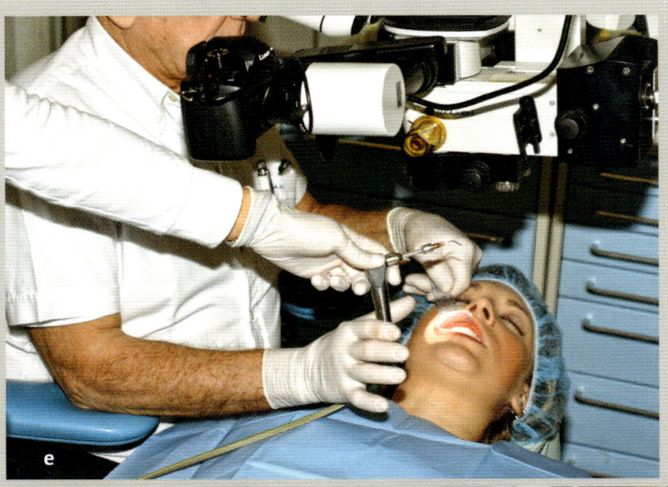

4.46 **a, b)** When receiving an instrument from the second assistant, the operator will simply open his or her fingers, without losing contact with the patient's cheek. **c–g)** When the operator needs the Stropko, he or she opens his or her hand; the dental assistant puts the syringe in the operator's hand and then guides it until the tip of the syringe is in the operative field.

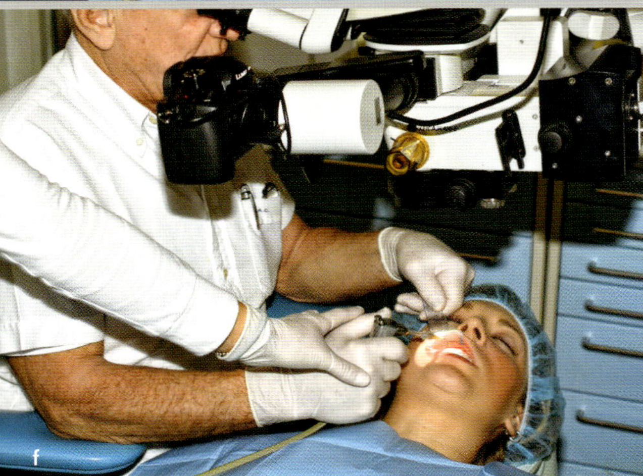

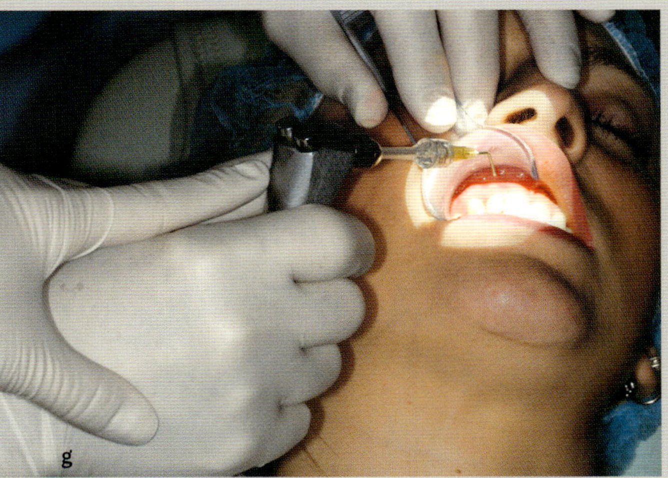

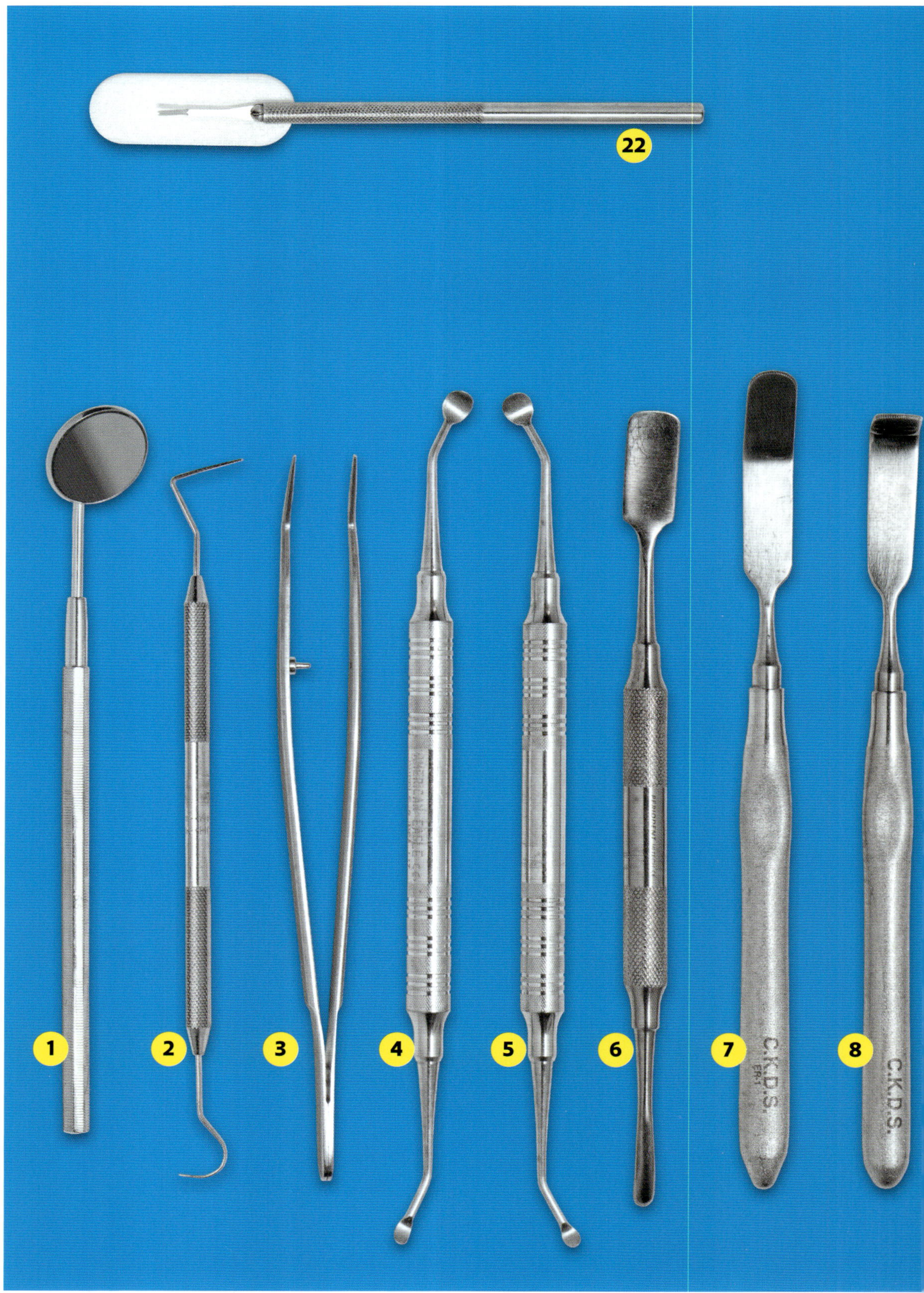

4.47 Microsurgical instruments tray set-up.

1. Mirror Front surface.
2. Periodontal probe.
3. Pliers
4. Periosteal elevator right
5. Periosteal elevator left
6. Prichard elevator
7. Carr retractor 45°
8. Carr retractor 90°.
9. Micro explorer
10. Carr Explorer CX1.
11. Spoon excavator small
12. Spoon excavator medium
13. Curette
14. Micromirror oval
15. Micromirror round
16. Microplugger small
17. Microplugger medium
18. Microplugger long
19. Ball burnisher
20. Finishing spatula
21. Cutting spatula
22. Microsurgical blade
23. Methylene blue
24. Micro brush
25. Ferric sulfate
26. Gingi Pak pellets

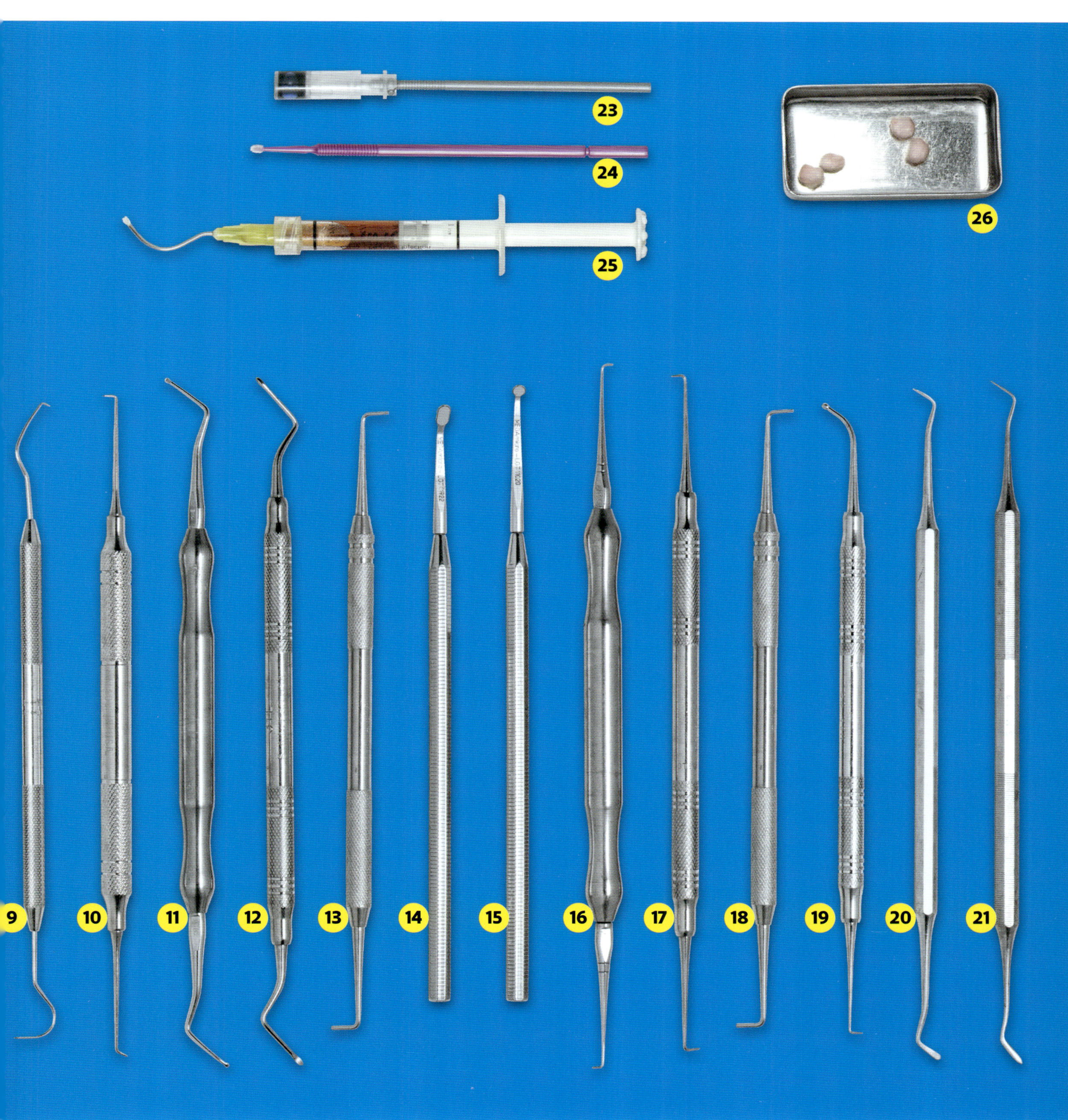
23
24
25
26
9
10
11
12
13
14
15
16
17
18
19
20
21

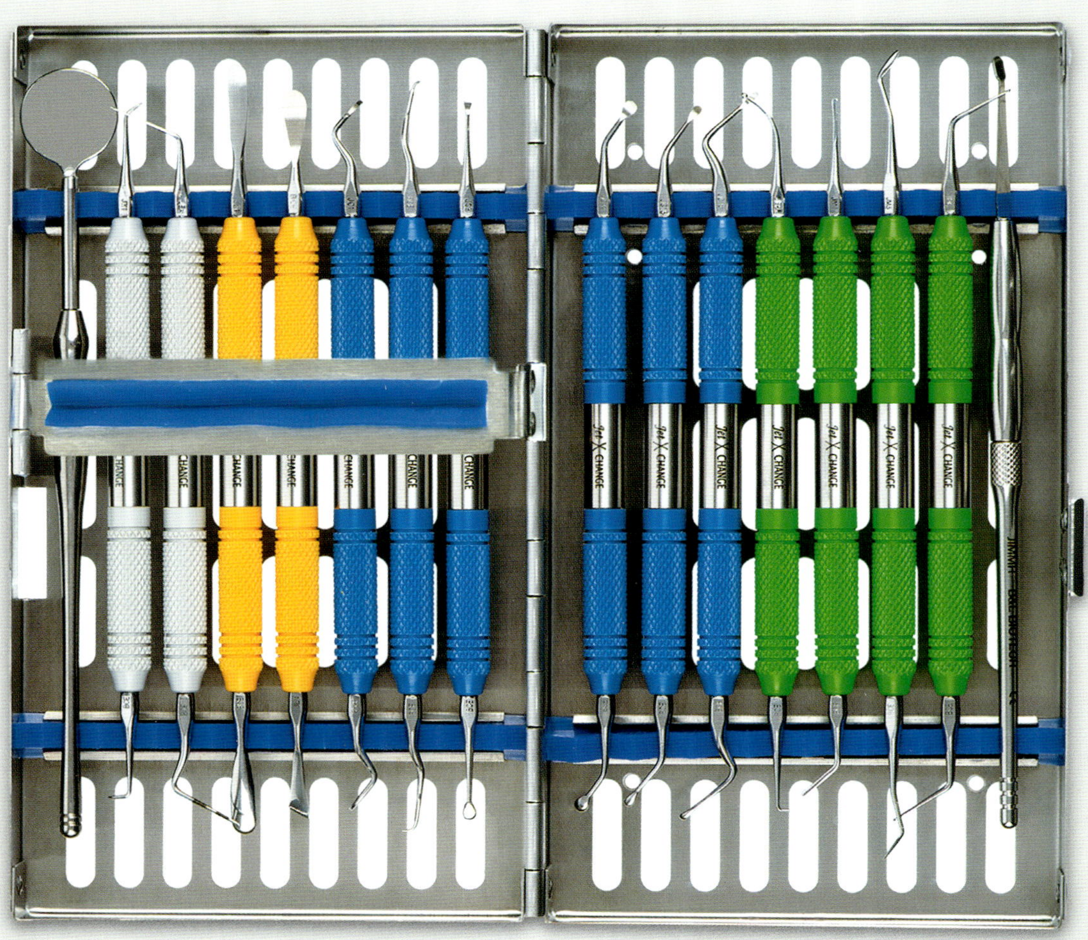

4.48 Jet XChange Basic Micro-Surgical Basic Set (B&L Biotech).

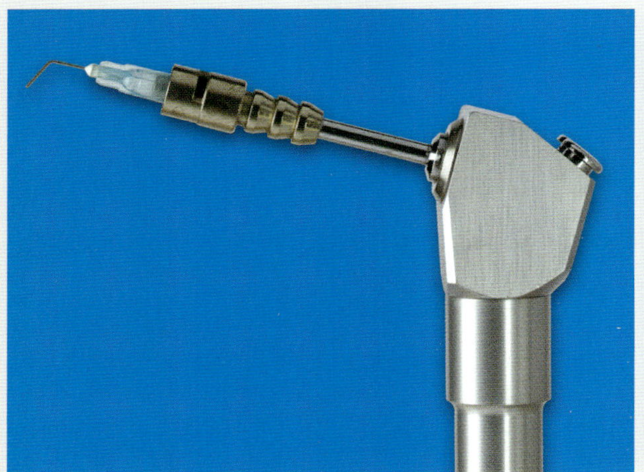

4.49 Adec syringe with Stropko irrigator and a microtip.

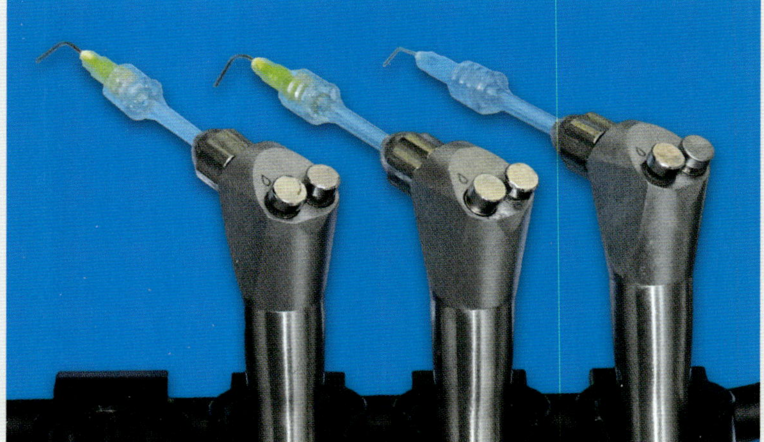

4.50 The Stropko on the left is connected only to air at high pressure and is contraindicated during surgery. The Stropko in the middle has air and water for irrigating. The Stropko on the right is connected only to air at very low pressure and is used during surgery to dry the retroprep.

ter use so that it is easy to find it and give it back to the doctor for further use (4.47, 4.48).

Once in a while, the doctor will need to irrigate or dry the surgical field and for this purpose, it is best to have two dedicated Stropko irrigators with microsurgical tips[23] (4.49):

- Dedicated "air-only" Stropko for drying
- Dual Stropko with air and water for irrigating (4.50).

When using Stropko irrigators, it is mandatory that the air and water supply pressure be regulated down so that the force of air and water expelled is much lower than normal to prevent unwanted splashing during irrigation or emphysema or air embolism beneath the flap when drying the retropreparation.

Selection of Different Magnifications (4.51)

Minimum magnification (3×) is used for the incision (4.52) and for the initial osteotomy (4.53), as well as for the accurate location of the root apex. During these initial steps, the operator needs a wide field of view, in order to have a better perspective of the surgical area.

Medium magnification (5× – 8×) is used for the elevation of the flap (4.53), for the osteotomy (4.54), for the apical resection (4.55), for the curettage of the granulation tissue (4.56), and for the initial inspection of the resected root surface (4.57).

Intermediate magnification (8× – 12×) is used for a more accurate inspection of the root surface, for

4.51. The five different magnifications of a one-dollar bill as seen through a Global 5-step microscope. The spaces between the lines on George Washington face are .20 mm apart. The squares on the background behind his face are .10 mm wide.

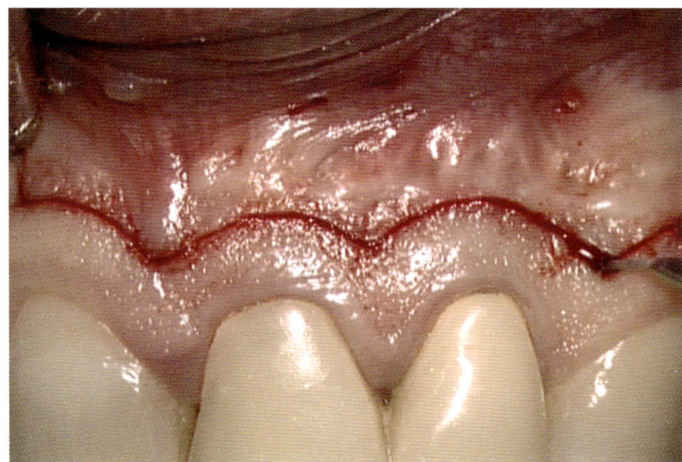

4.52. The submarginal incision (3x).

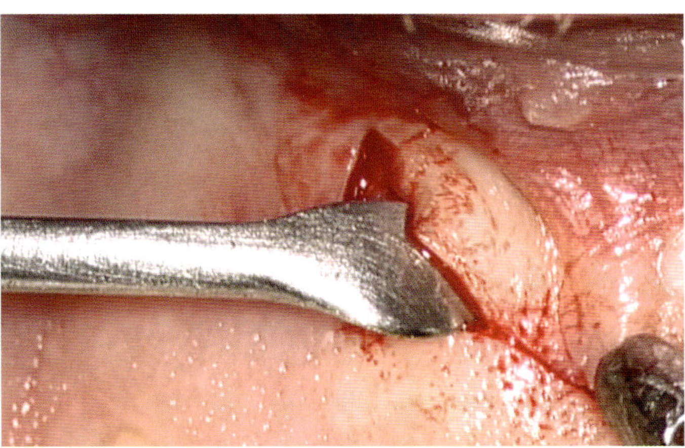

4.53. The elevation of the flap (3x).

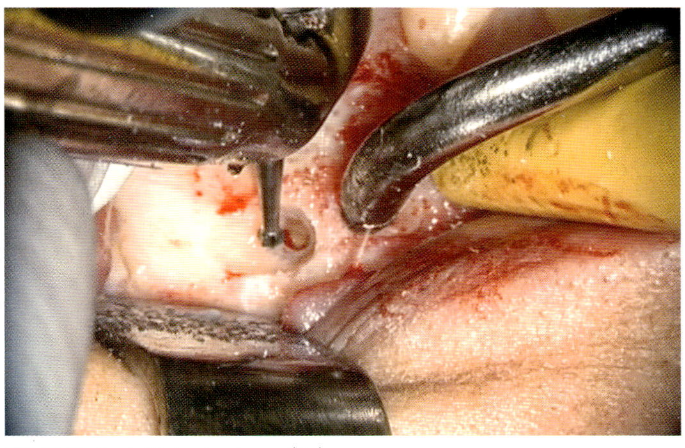

4.54. The initial osteotomy (3x).

identifying a fracture, an isthmus or a missed canal (4.58), and for the ultrasonic root-end preparation (4.59).

Maximum magnification (18×) is used for a more accurate inspection of the resected root surface (4.60), of the root-end preparation (4.61) and of the root-end obturation (4.62).

Minimum magnification is also use for suturing (4.63), and medium magnification is used for the removal of the sutures (4.64).

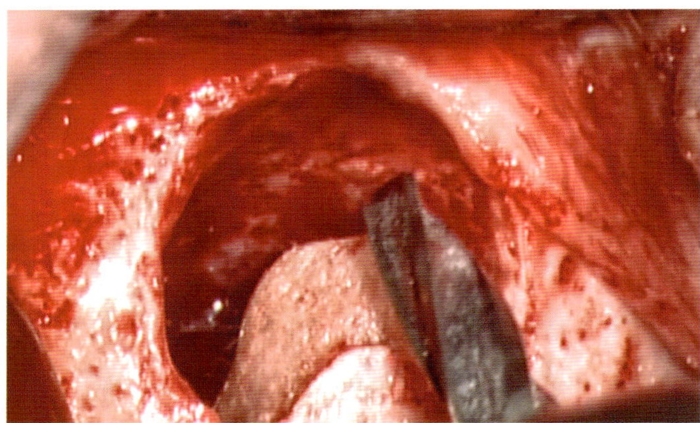

4.55. The apical resection (8x).

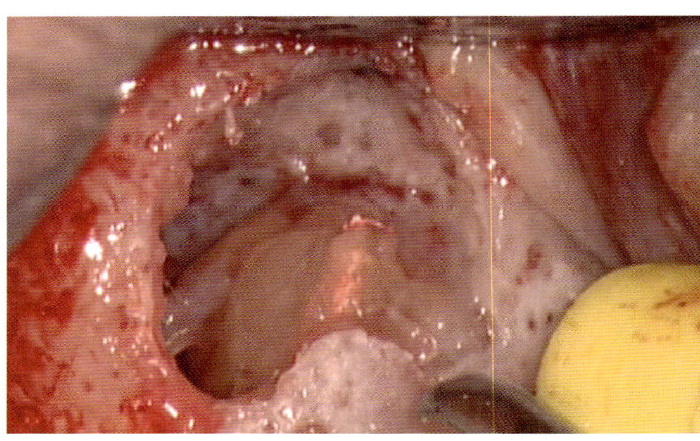

4.56. The curettage of the granulation tissue (8x).

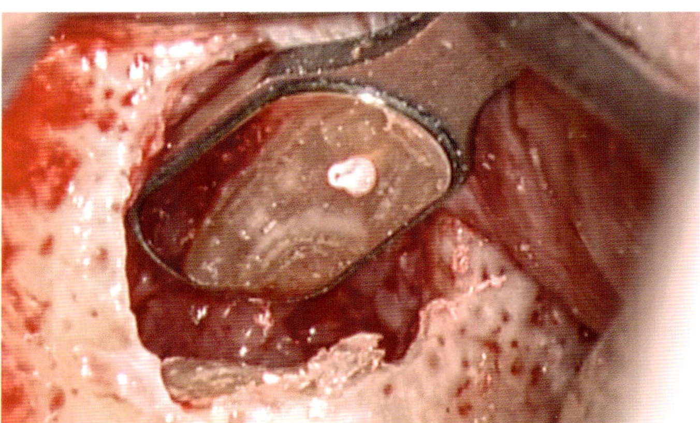

4.57. The initial inspection of the resected root surface (8x).

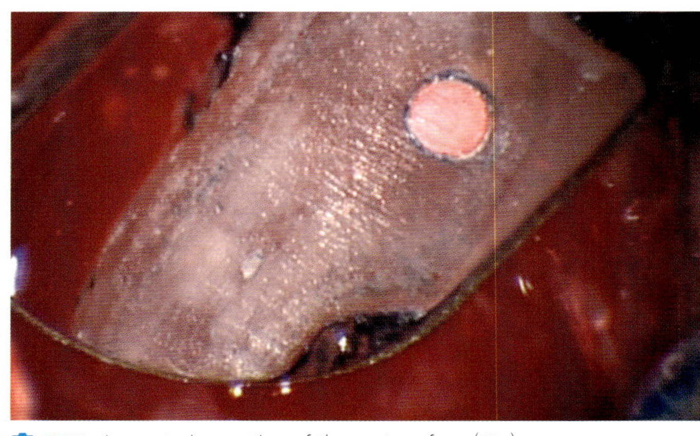

4.58. Accurate inspection of the root surface (12x).

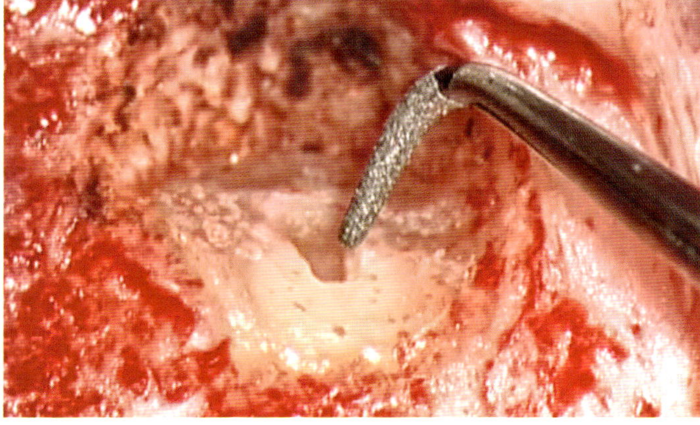

4.59. The ultrasonic root end preparation (12x).

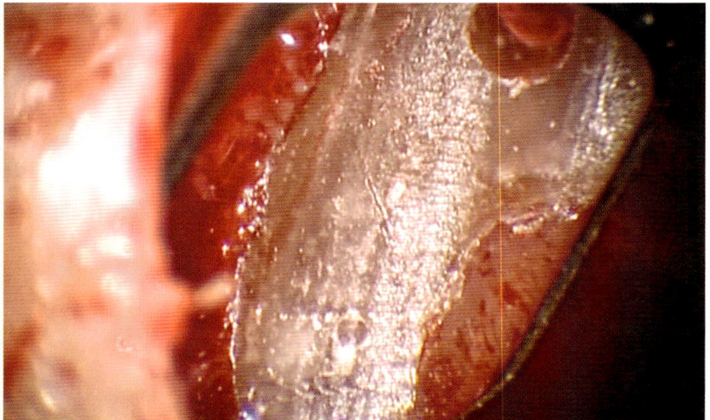

4.60. A more accurate inspection of the resected root surface (18x).

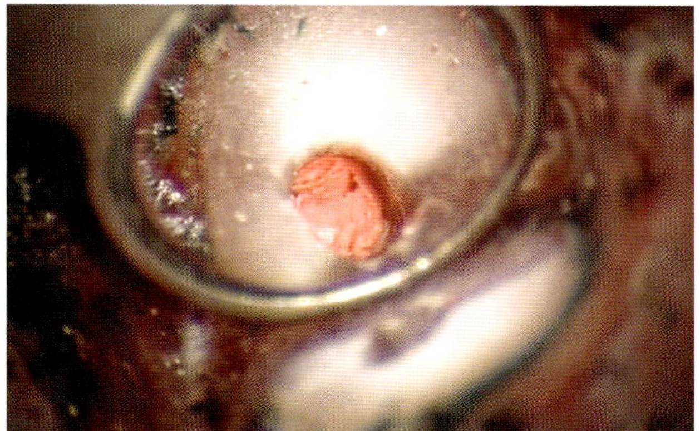

4.61. Accurate inspection of the root end preparation (18x).

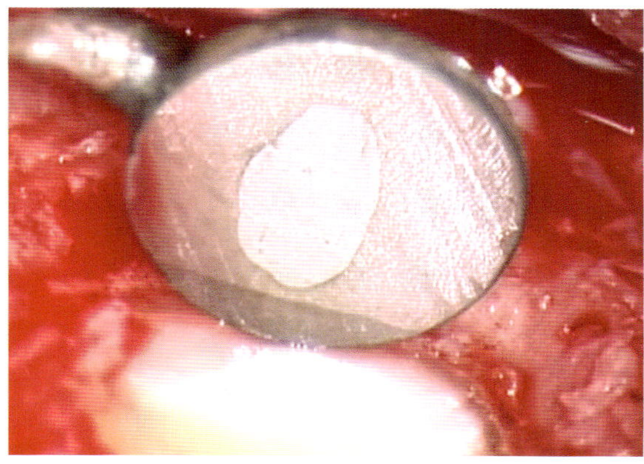

4.62. Accurate inspection of the root end obturation (18x).

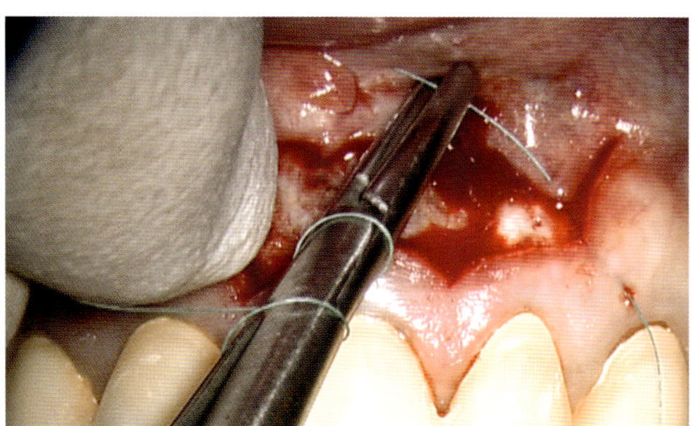

4.63. Suturing (3x).

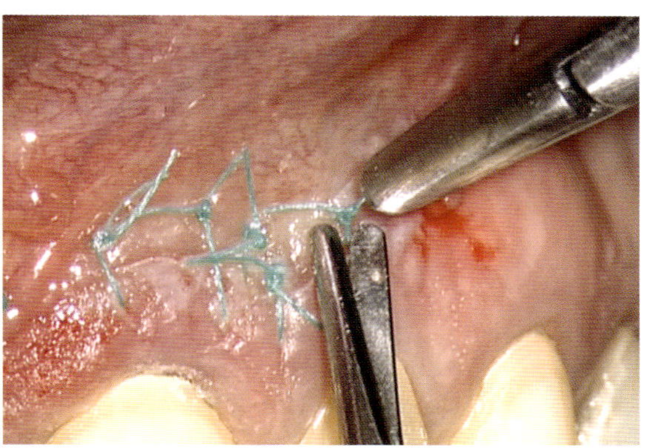

4.64. The removal of the sutures (3x).

REFERENCES

1. AAE Special Committee to Develop a Microscope Position Paper. *AAE Position Statement. Use of Microscopes and Other Magnification Techniques.* J Endod. 2012;38(8):1153-5.
2. Carr GB. *Microscopes in Endodontics.* Calif Dent Assoc J. 1992;11:55-61.
3. Rubinstein RA. *The anatomy of the surgical operating microscope and operating positions.* In: Kim S. ed. *The Dental Clinics of North America. Microscopes in Endodontics.* Philadelphia, USA: W.B. Saunders Company Vol. 41, N° 3, July 1997:391-414.
4. Frank AL et al. *Long-term evaluation of surgically placed amalgam fillings.* J. Endod. 1992;18:391.
5. Rubinstein R. *Magnification and illumination in apical surgery.* In Torabinejad M, Rubinstein R. eds. *The art and science of contemporary surgical endodontics.* Quintessence Publishing Co, Inc. 2017:113.
6. Apotheker H. *A microscope for use in dentistry.* J. Microsurg. 1981;3:7.
7. Selden HS. *The role of the dental operating microscope in Endodontics.* Pa Dent J (Harrisb) 1986;53(3):36.
8. Carr GB, Castellucci A. *The use of the operating microscope in endodontics.* In: Castellucci A. ed. *EndodonticS.* Vol. III. Florence, Italy: Il Tridente, 2005:222-263.
9. Setzer F. *The dental operating microscope.* In: Kim S, Kratchman S, ed. *Microsurgery in Endodontics.* Wiley Blackwell, 2018.
10. Hess W, Zurcher E. *The anatomy of the root canals of the teeth of the permanent dentition. The anatomy of the root canals of the teeth of the deciduos dentition and of the first permanent molars.* London: J. Bale Sons & Danielsson, 1925.
11. Schilder H. *Filling root canals in three dimensions.* Dent Clin North Amer. 1967; 723-44.
12. Schilder H. *Cleaning and shaping the root canal.* Dent Clin North Am. 1974;18(2):269-96.
13. West JD. *The relationship between the three-dimensional endodontic seal and endodontic failures.* Thesis, Boston University, 1975.
14. Kim S, Pecora G, Rubinstein R. *Color atlas of microsurgery in endodontics* Philadelphia: Saunders, 2001.
15. Khayat BG. *The use of magnification in endodontic therapy: the operating microscope.* Pract Periodont Aesthet Dent. 1998;10(1):137.
16. Michaelides PL. *Use of the operating microscope in dentistry.* J Calif Dent Assoc. 1996;24(6): 45.
17. Stropko J. *Micro-Surgical Endodontics.* In: Castellucci A. ed. Endodontics. Vol. III. Florence, Italy: Il Tridente, 2005:342-411.

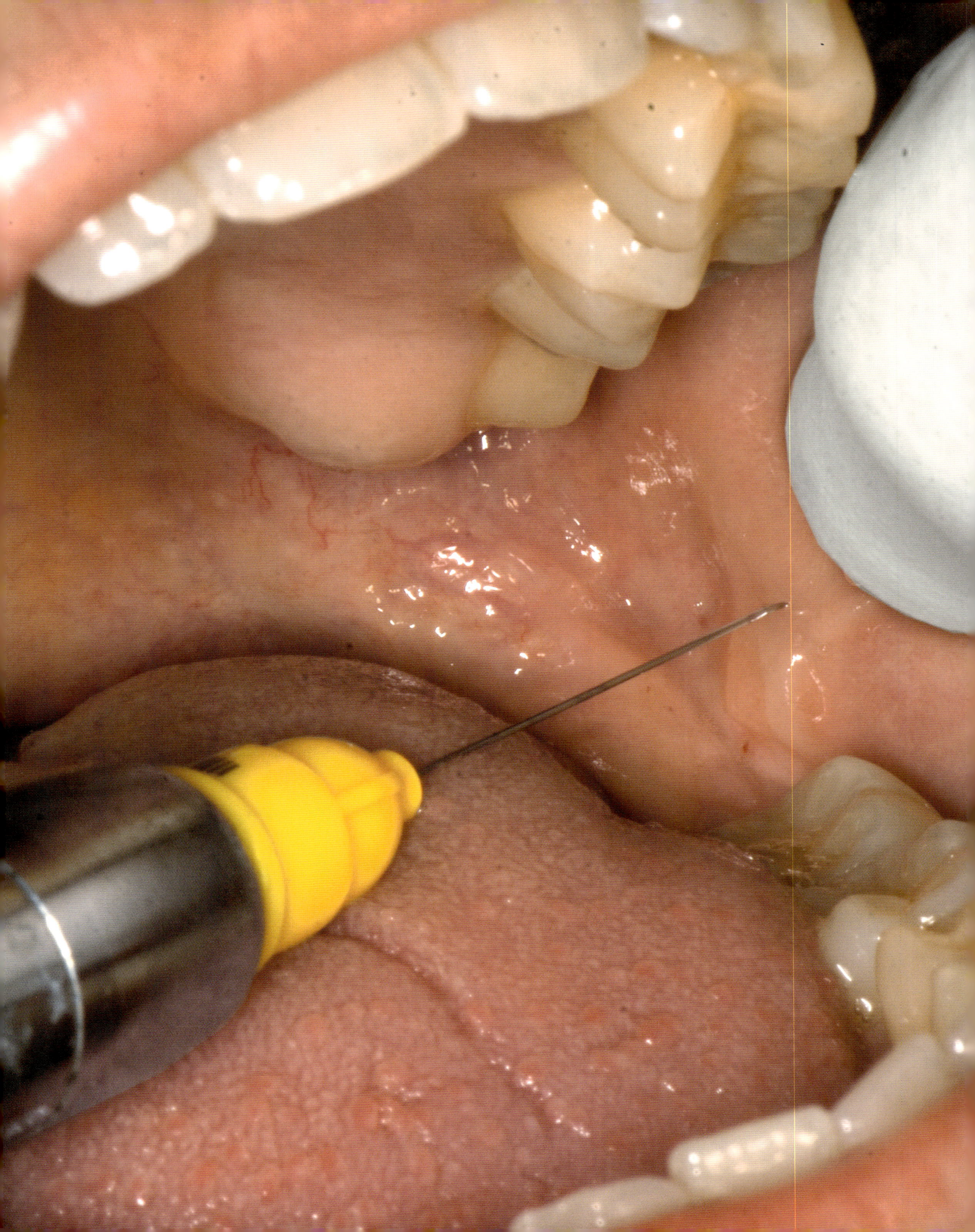

Local Anesthesia

The Role of Vasoconstrictors in Surgical Endodontics

In microsurgical endodontics the anesthetic solution used has two purposes:

- to provide effective and long lasting anesthesia
- to provide effective hemostasis.

In order to be successful, the clinician needs to work on having the patient perfectly anesthetized and the operative field free of bleeding, in order to have a proper visualization of the area, precise placement of the root-end filling materials, accurate inspection for possible accessory foramina or apical root fractures. Furthermore, adequate hemostasis will reduce the time of the surgical procedure, reduce the blood loss and guarantee less postoperative bleeding and swelling.

For all the above reasons, the local anesthetic solution must contain a vasoconstrictor, and the preferred choice is epinephrine. This is because epinephrine binds alpha- and beta-adrenergic receptors. However, we should keep in mind that epinephrine can cause both vasoconstriction or vasodilation, depending with which receptors it binds. Alpha-1, alpha-2 and beta-1 are responsible for vasoconstriction, while beta-2 receptors trigger vasodilation. For this reason, the area where the solution is injected is very important in order to involve the right receptors and to obtain the desired result. Beta-2 receptors are prevalent in blood vessels that supply muscles; however, they are relatively rare in mucous membranes, oral tissues and skin. Ideally, for the purpose of microsurgical endodontics, an adrenergic vasoconstrictor would be a pure alpha-agonist. Fortunately, the predominant receptors in the oral tissues are alpha-receptors, and the number of beta-receptors is very small.[1] However, for the above mentioned reasons, it is important to inject the solution in the oral mucosa, avoiding a deep insertion of the syringe needle that will involve the blood vessels supplying muscles and thereby cause vasodilation.

The vasoconstrictor causes constriction of the blood vessels and thereby controls the tissue perfusion. This will allow the local anesthetic to be effective for a longer period of time and decreases bleeding during the surgical procedure, which means an improvement of visibility.

Regarding the systemic effect of epinephrine when used in relatively small amounts for local anesthesia, to avoid any damage to the cardiovascular system, an aspirating syringe should always be used, to make sure that epinephrine is not accidentally injected into the bloodstream. The adverse effects are also dependent on the dose. The recommended maximum dosage of anesthetic solution with a concentration of epinephrine 1:50,000 used for surgery is 10 ml, which means 5.5 cartridges. As will be explained later, it is also important to inject local anesthetic with vasoconstrictor very, very slowly. Some patients could show a transitory, statistically insignificant increase in pulse rate, but within a few minutes, the pulse rate will return to normal.[2] In conclusion, the use of 1:50,000 epinephrine with 2% lidocaine is recommended for local anesthesia in the majority of cases. With severe cardiac patients, a consultation with his/her physician before the surgery is highly recommended and should be a routine part of the surgical protocol.[1]

Technique

The technique and the choice of anesthetic solution will differ depending on whether the surgery is in the upper or lower arch.

When treating teeth in the upper arch, only infiltration with local anesthetic having vasoconstrictor 1:50,000 is to be used in the area of surgery.

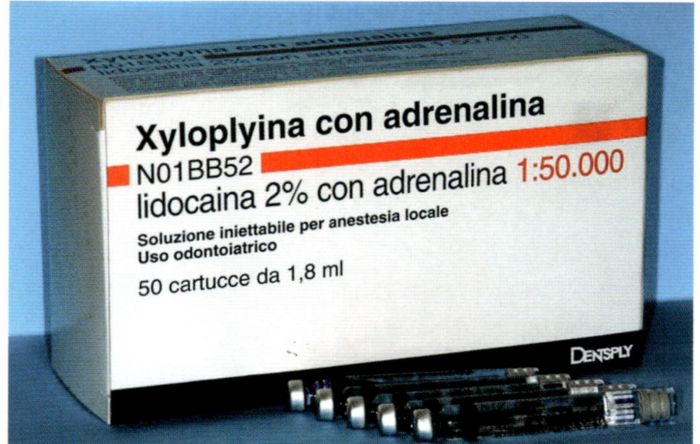

5.1 Lidocaine 2% with epinephrine 1:50,000.

When treating teeth in the lower arch, after obtaining the inferior alveolar nerve block, use anesthesia without any vasoconstrictor, then subsequently local anesthetic with vasoconstrictor 1:50,000 is injected in the entire area that will be involved in the surgical procedure.

The first anesthesia is performed using mepivacaine without any vasoconstrictor and it is used just to provide a profound anesthesia for the patient. The local anesthetic is then used mainly and only to provide a good vasoconstriction in order to have good control of the bleeding as well as excellent visibility for the surgical team. For this reason, the second anesthetic solution used, as already stated, is 2% lidocaine with epinephrine 1:50,000 (5.1). This is a *conditio sine qua non* to perform the surgical procedure. When a vasoconstrictor is not used, the anesthesia is less deep and of short duration. Also, hemostasis is not well-controlled, resulting in extremely difficult crypt management, poor visibility and unnecessary stress on the entire surgical team.[3] If for some reason epinephrine cannot be used on a patient, hemostasis will be compromised enough to jeopardize the quality of the procedure. The same is true for lower concentrations of vasoconstrictor. In the Author's personal experience, having "had" to use epinephrine 1:80,000 once and 1:100,000 another time, the conclusion was made that it was such a bad experience – never again! Therefore the use of epinephrine 1:50,000 is the *conditio sine qua non* , which in other words means: "No epinephrine, no surgery"!

Mandibular Anesthesia

Inferior Alveolar Nerve Block

This is usually called the "mandibular nerve block". It serves to anesthetize all the mandibular nerves of the same quadrant.

Adequate anesthesia is indicated by tingling and numbness of the lower lip and, when the lingual nerve is affected, the tip of the tongue. This technique does not achieve anesthesia of the vestibular mucosa or periosteum associated with the molars, which are innervated by the long buccal nerve. This is one of the two reasons why, in endodontic surgery, this kind of anes-

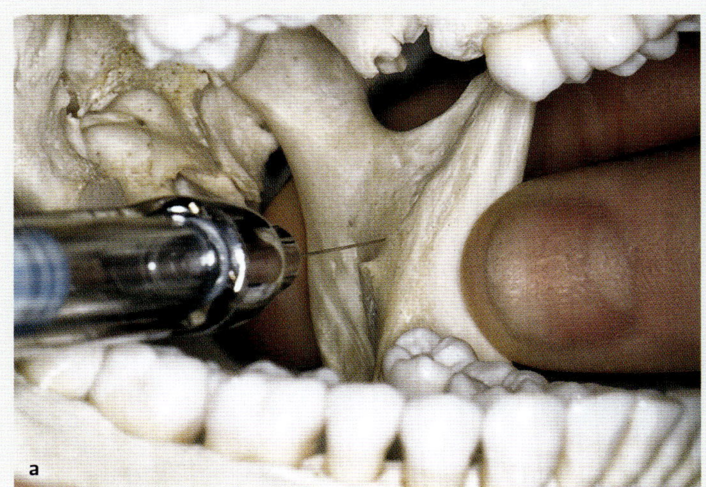
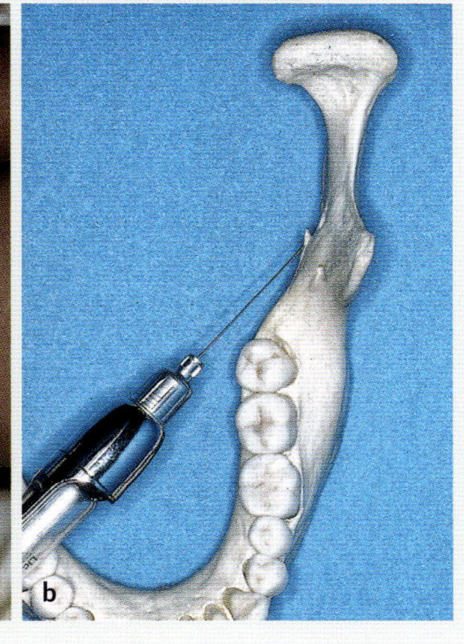

5.2 **a, b)** Block of the inferior alveolar nerve, using a short needle and the direct technique.

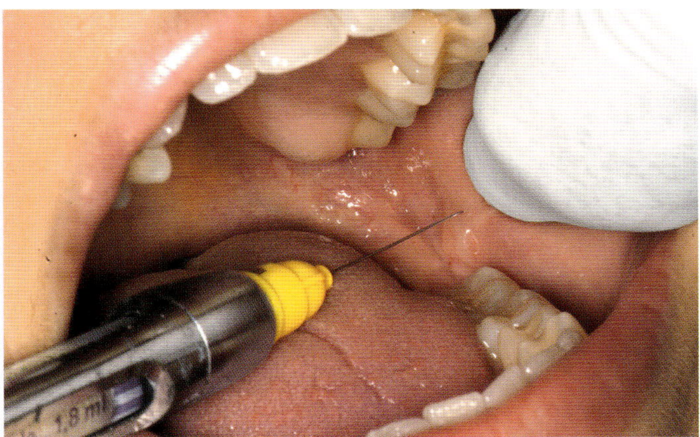

5.3 The thumb is used to identify the anterior margin of the mandibular ramus.

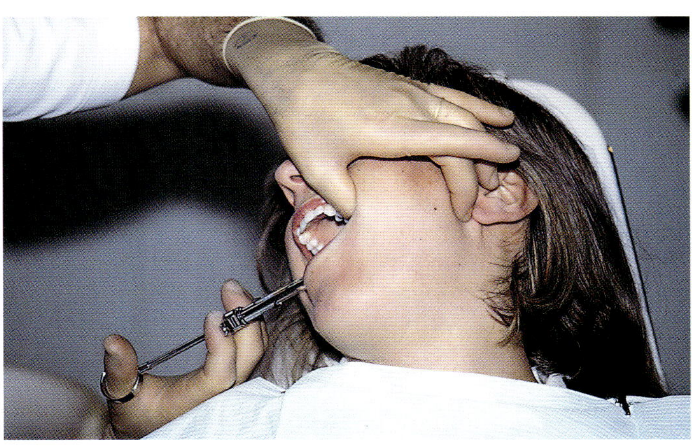

5.4 The middle finger is used to support the posterior margin of the mandibular ramus.

thesia is not sufficient. The other reason is that this anesthesia doesn't provide any vasoconstriction.

Anesthesia of the long buccal nerve is performed by inserting the needle into the mucosa distal and buccal to the last molar.

To anesthetize the inferior alveolar nerve, the anesthetic solution must be deposited in the vicinity of the nerve before it enters the mandibular ramus at the level of the mandibular spine; the most popular and fastest technique is the "direct technique".

A short 30-gauge needle is used to penetrate as close as possible to the mandibular spine (5.2). With the patient's mouth wide open, the dentist places the thumb into the patient's mouth to identify the anterior border of the mandibular ramus (5.3). The middle finger supports the posterior border, outside the mouth (5.4).

With the syringe directed along an imaginary line passing above the contralateral premolars, one penetrates the mid-point between the thumb and middle finger, and after aspirating to avoid injecting the anesthetic directly into the bloodstream, the solution is injected. The point of insertion of the needle is just lateral to the pterygomandibular raphe, which is midway between the two hemiarches, to a depth of about 1 cm. During this procedure, it is important to ask the patient to keep the mouth wide open.[4]

This type of anesthesia is the principal means of anesthetizing the teeth of the lower arch, since local anesthesia would not be efficacious, given the high bone density of the mandible.

Local Infiltration

Once the lower lip of the patient is numb, then now is the moment to use the second kind of anesthesia to provoke a good vasoconstriction. As already stated, for this purpose the anesthesia of choice is 2% lidocaine with epinephrine 1:50,000.

Local infiltration may be defined as a technique by which an anesthetic solution is deposited within the treatment area.[4]

The needle must be inserted near the apices of the teeth that will be involved in the surgical site, approximately 2-3 mm apical to the mucogingival line. The insertion of the needle should be just 1 or 2 mm in the alveolar mucosa without going too deep into the muscle or muscle attachment. This is because, in general, the smaller peripheral blood vessels in the oral mucosa have a high concentration of alpha2-receptors, whereas the blood vessels supplying skeletal muscles have a high concentration of beta2-receptors. The alpha2-receptors cause vasoconstriction, allowing better visibility during surgery. On the other hand, the beta2-receptors will cause vasodilation, which will decrease the operator visibility (5.5). Good visibility provided by a good hemostatic effect is the most important requisite for a successful surgical procedure. Another important factor for a good hemostasis is the time used for the injection. A few drops are injected at each insertion of the needle and they must be injected **very, very slowly** (5.6). Usually, two cartridges are used and this will take at least several minutes! After the injections are completed, a common mistake is to discard the syringe

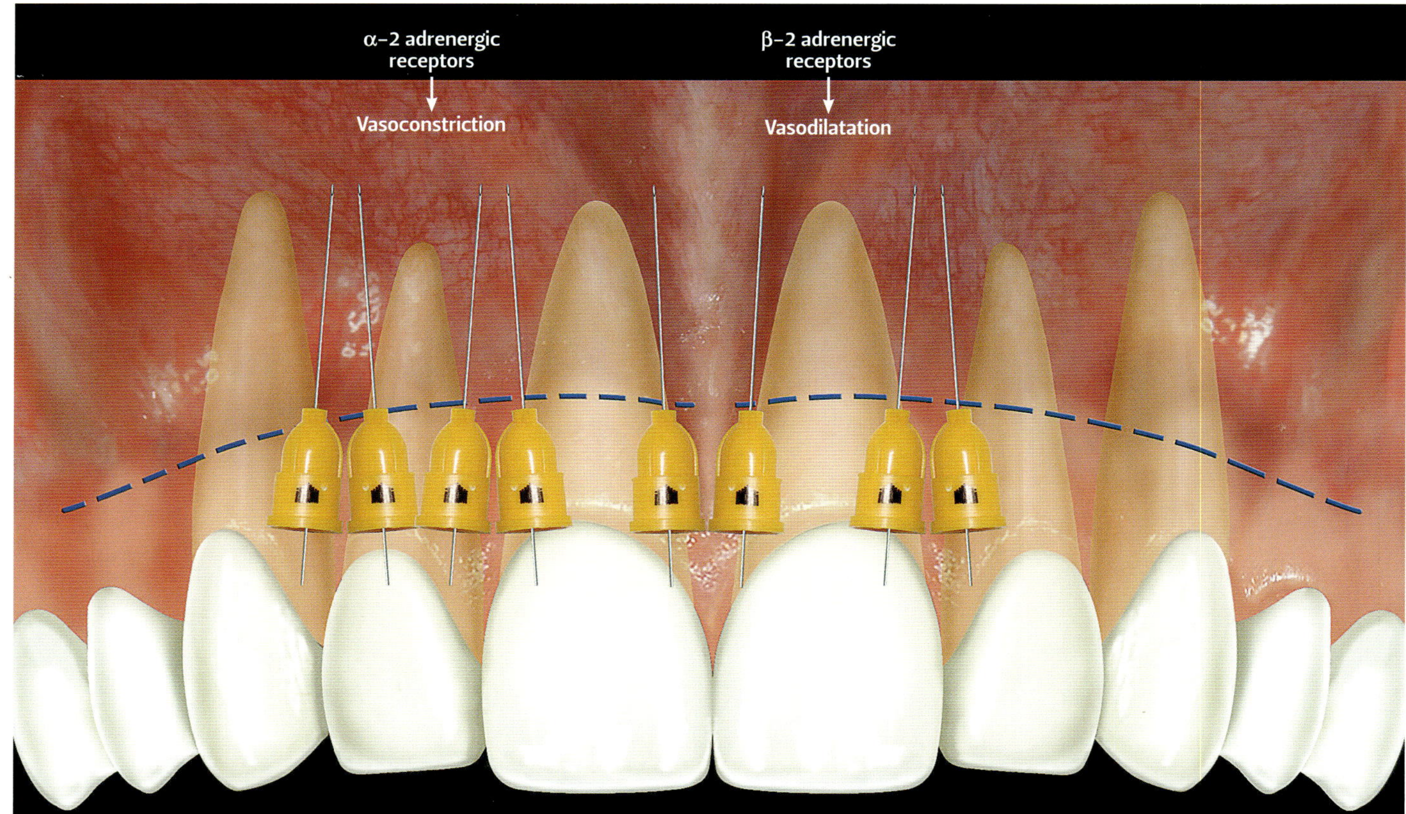

5.5 The short needle should be inserted into the alveolar mucosa near all the apices of the teeth that will be involved in the surgical site, entering only 1 or 2 mm and slowly depositing only a few drops of solution at a time.

and start the incision. In order to have a good vasoconstriction, it is mandatory to *wait* at least 15 or 20 minutes. After this amount of time the oral mucosa will be ischemic, pale and not pink anymore, and this is the time to start the surgery.

Maxillary Anesthesia

Local Infiltration

The local anesthesia for endodontic surgery in the upper arch follows exactly the same principles used in the lower arch. The short 30-gauge needle should be inserted only a few millimeters into the alveolar mucosa next to the apices of the teeth that will be involved with the incision, which means usually one tooth mesial and one tooth distal to the tooth or teeth to be treated. Usually one or maybe two cartridges of 2% lidocaine with 1:50,000 epinephrine is enough to provide both anesthesia and vasoconstriction. As already stated for the lower arch, the anesthetic solution must be injected very slowly, a few drops at a time, injecting in the vestibular fold and avoiding the more apically positioned muscle attachments in order to avoid vasodilation. It is also important to wait 15 or 20 minutes before making the incision for the vasoactive agent in the anesthetic solution to constrict the blood vessels in the soft tissues as well as in the hard tissues. This way the vasoconstriction will have enough time to take place.

In case of surgery on upper premolars and molars, and when we are dealing with large lesions that most probably involve the palatal mucosa as well, it is important to use a palatal injection along with the same anesthetic solution. Palatal infiltration is quite painful. Therefore, it should be performed slowly by steadily depositing a small amount of anesthetic (0.5 ml) under adequate pressure. Before performing the palatal infiltration, it is advisable to achieve anesthesia of the mucosa, for example, by cooling (5.7).[5]

A useful strategy to provide increased postoperative analgesia is to administer a long-acting local anesthetic at the end of the surgical procedure, prior to dismissing the patient.[6,7]

Local Hemostatic Agents

As already stated, the local anesthetic infiltration is used not only to provide long lasting anesthesia, but also and mainly to ascertain effective hemostasis. A common mistake in microsurgical endodontics is to start the procedure and to make the incision too soon after the anesthetic is administered. It is absolutely important to wait at least 15 to 20 minutes, in order to give the solution enough time to penetrate into the medullary space, and to constrict the blood vessels and establish hemostasis. This is important not only when dealing with soft tissues, but also during the osteotomy and inside the bony crypt. It is possible that one might have good hemostasis with excellent visibility until the root apex is reached and the osteotomy made with subsequent bleeding. In such a case, local hemostatic agents should be considered.

Many different kinds of topical hemostatic agents are available, but the most commonly used and highly recommended are ferric sulfate and epinephrine pellets.

FERRIC SULFATE

Ferric sulfate (Cut-Trol, Mobile, AL; Astringedent, Ultradent Products, Inc., UT) is a chemical agent that was first introduced in restorative dentistry to help control bleeding from the gingival sulcus before taking impressions (5.8a). Ferric sulfate effects hemostasis through a chemical reaction with blood proteins. It provokes agglutination of blood proteins, which then forms plugs that occlude the capillary orifices.[2] It can be easily applied with a specific syringe having a little brush at the end of the needle (5.8b). The brush should not be dripping, but just wet and should be delicately used to literally brush the bony crypt for a few seconds. A dark brown or greenish brown coagulum forms immediately on contact with blood. The bleeding will stop immediately and the rest of the surgical procedure can be completed working in a dry field. Although ferric sulfate is known to be cytotoxic and to cause tissue necrosis, systemic absorption of ferric sulfate is unlikely, because the coagulum isolates it from the vascular supply.[1]

There are only two contraindications to the use of ferric sulfate: it should not be used on the cortical bone plate

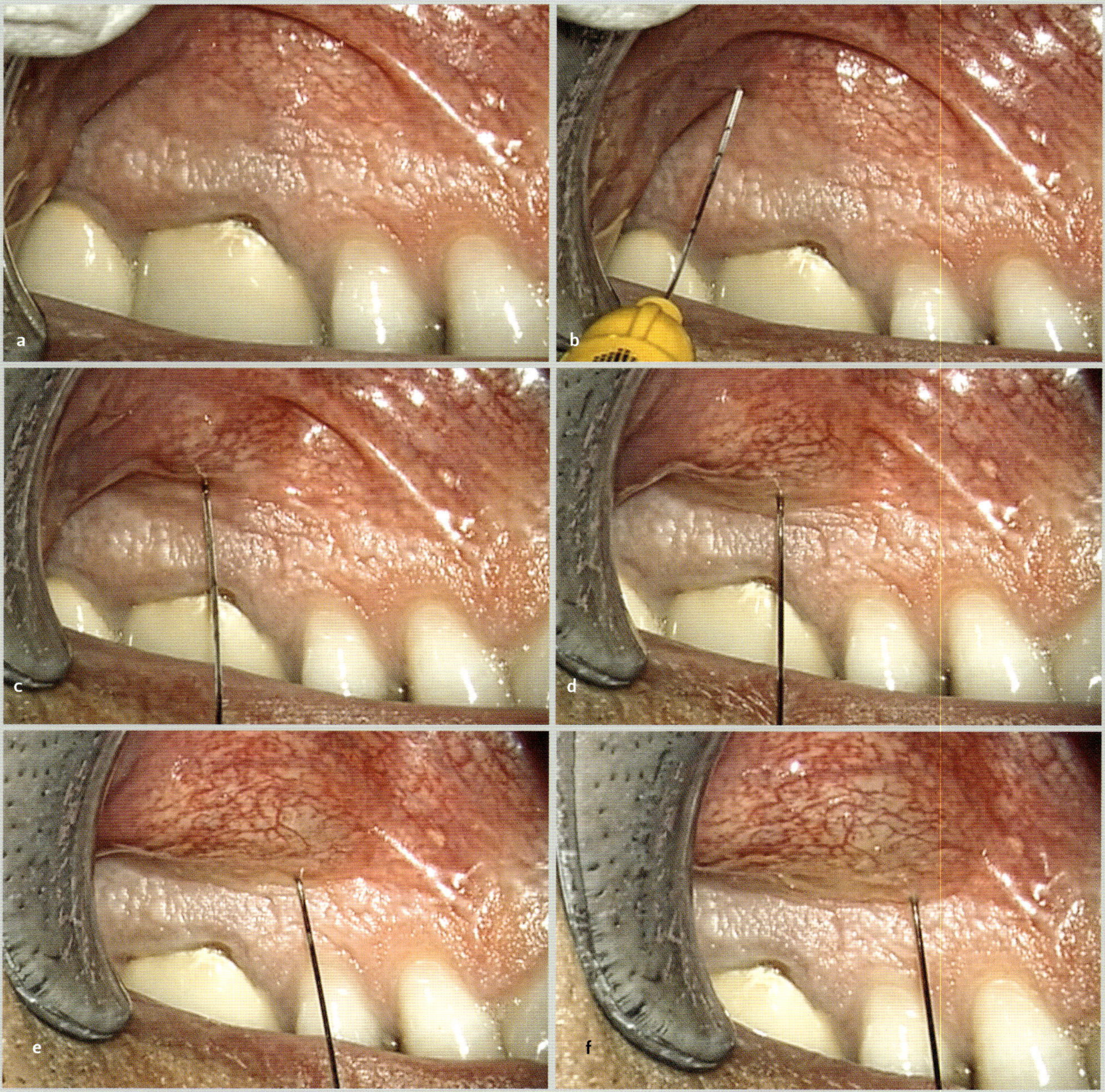

5.6 Anesthesia in preparation of the surgical procedure on the upper right first molar. **a)** Aspect of the mucosa before injecting the anesthetic solution. **b)** First introduction of the needle in the alveolar mucosa next to the mesiobuccal root of the second molar. **c)** Second introduction of the needle in the alveolar mucosa next to the distobuccal root of the first molar. **d)** Third introduction of the needle in the alveolar mucosa next to the mesiobuccal root of the first molar. **e)** Fourth introduction of the needle in the alveolar mucosa between the first molar and the second premolar. **f)** Fifth introduction of the needle in the alveolar mucosa next to the second premolar. **g)** Sixth introduction of the needle in the alveolar mucosa next to the first premolar. **h)** Seventh introduction of the needle in the alveolar mucosa between the first and the second premolar. The injection of the anesthetic solution took almost 2 minutes. **i)** After about 20 minutes the vasoconstriction took place and the attached gingiva appears ischemic and the procedure can start. **j)** Note the absence of bleeding after completing the submarginal incision.

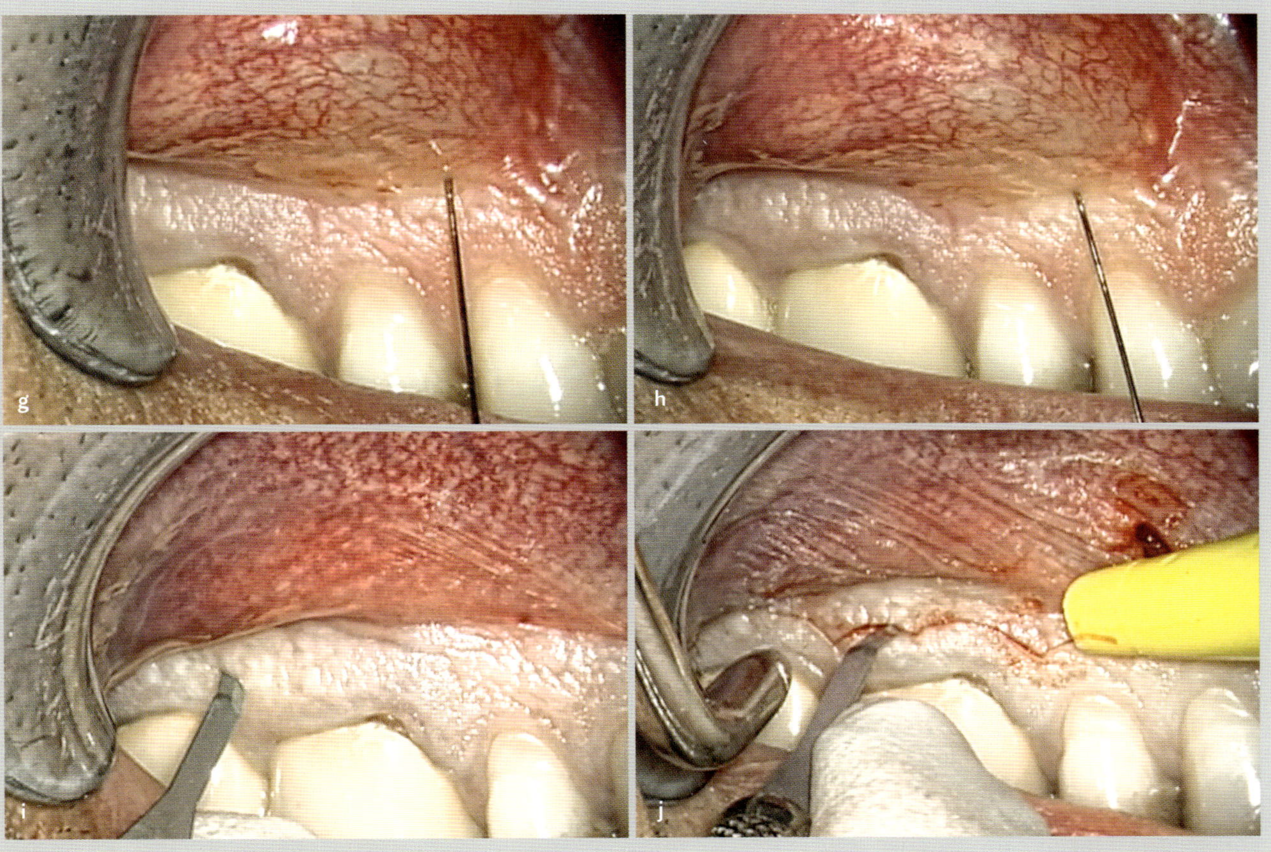

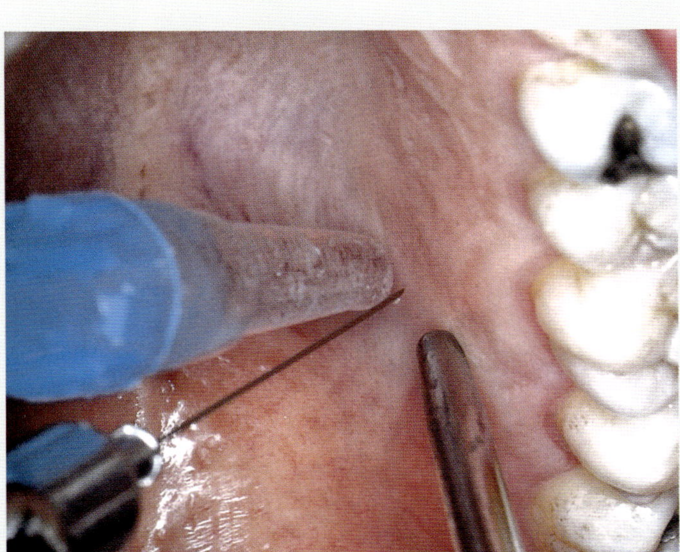

5.7 An ice stick achieves anesthesia by cooling the palatal mucosa. This allows painless introduction of the needle.

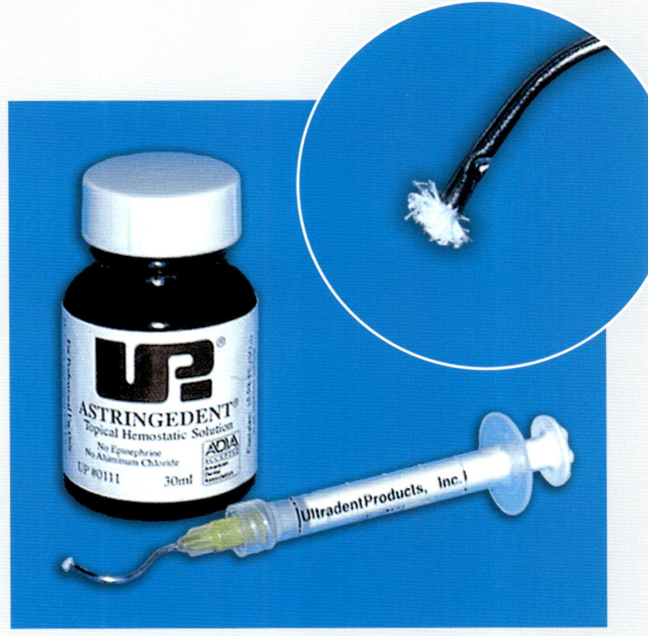

5.8 Ferric sulfate 12,7%. The needle has a little brush to be used inside the bony crypt.

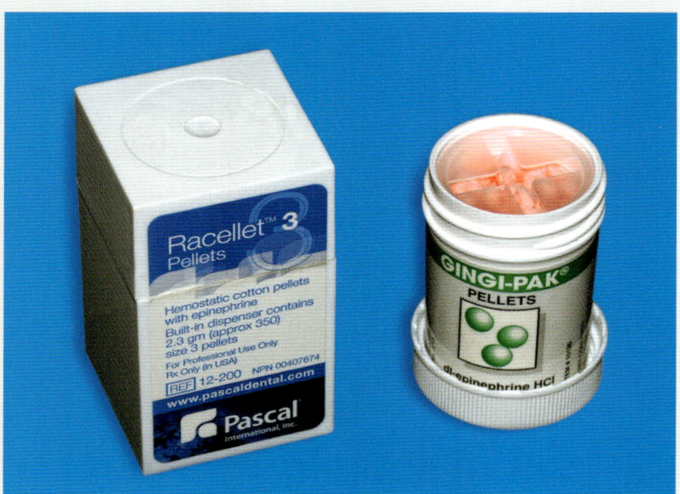

5.9 Epinephrine pellets.

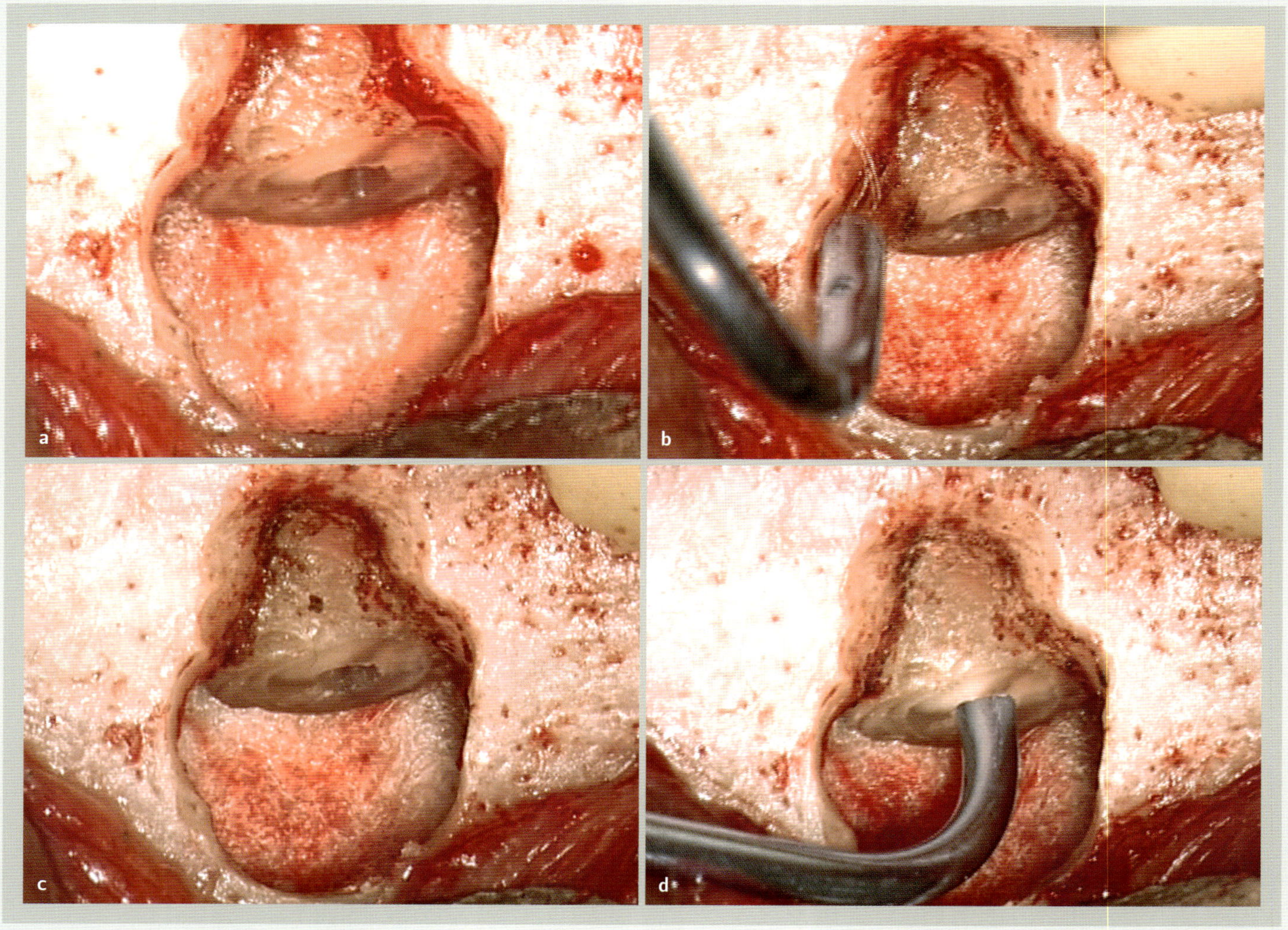

5.10 **a)** One epinephrine pellet remains in the bony crypt during the retrofilling. **b)** The little brush is carrying ferric sulfate to stop the bleeding coming from the periodontal ligament. **c)** Now the bleeding is under control and the procedure can be completed working in a "dry" field. **d)** The MAP System is carrying MTA into the retroprep.

and it should not be used on the soft tissue, like the mucosal flap, where it can cause tissue necrosis. No adverse effects are described after its use, as long it is used in small quantities and as long as it is removed at the end of the procedure with careful curettage and irrigation with saline solution, in order to stimulate new bleeding. If left *in situ*, can cause damage to the bone and delay in healing.[8,9]

EPINEPHRINE PELLETS

Racellets (Pascal Co, Bellevue, WA) are little cotton pellets containing racemic epinephrine hydrochloride (📷 5.9). The amount of vasoconstrictor contained in each pellet varies depending on the number on the box. Racellet #3 pellets contain 0.55 mg of racemic epinephrine and Racellet #2 pellets contain 1.15 mg of racemic epinephrine.[1] The epinephrine cotton pellets are mechanical/chemical agents. The pellets should be pressed against the bone of the bony crypt, and, for this reason, the granulation tissue must be removed prior to placement of the pellets. After placing the first one, several more pellets are placed on top of it and pressure is applied for about 2 to 4 minutes. The epinephrine and the pressure will provide a profound vasoconstriction so that the procedure can be completed with excellent visibility, working in a dry field. Epinephrine causes local vasoconstriction by acting on the alpha-1 receptors present in the blood vessels wall, and the pressure augments this hemostatic potential.[1]

After a few minutes, the cotton pellet can be removed, leaving just one, the first one positioned, still in contact with the bone of the crypt (📷 5.10). This cotton pellet is also used to prevent debris from getting lodged into the bony crypt during root end preparation and root end filling. At the end of the procedure, this will be removed, the bony crypt will be gently irrigated with saline solution and curetted, in order to stimulate bleeding and particular attention must be given to avoid leaving any cotton fiber in the lesion, which could interfere with the healing (📷 5.11). The use of the microscope and careful irrigation with saline solution will prevent this from happening. Even though the amount of epinephrine of these pellets is much higher compared to the amount contained in the anesthetic solution, the systemic effects seem to be minimum when used as described.[10] It has been shown that when Racellet #2 was used in periapical surgery, the pulse rate of patients did not change with the application of pressure to the bone cavity.[11]

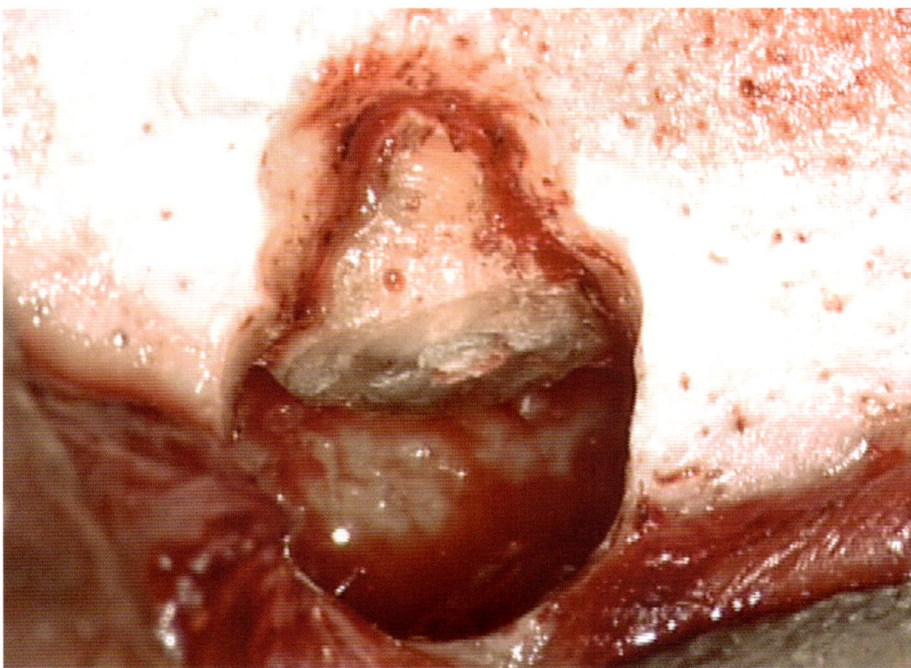

📷 **5.11** The cotton pellet has been removed, the ferric sulfate has been curetted, the bleeding is slowly filling the bony crypt and now is time for suturing.

BONE WAX

Another local hemostatic solution used in surgical endodontics is bone wax, first introduced by Horsley in 1892.[12] Selden described its efficacy when used in periapical surgery.[13] Bone wax is composed of beeswax and isopropyl palmitate and its hemostatic mechanism has essentially a tamponade effect. The wax, when placed under moderate pressure, plugs all vascular openings and its method of action is purely mechanical and does not affect the blood clotting mechanism.[1] However, more recent studies have shown that bone wax causes a foreign body reaction if left in the surgical site and, for this reason, it is not recommended anymore, since it can impair healing and decrease clearance of microorganisms.[14–16]

Systemic Medications

Anticoagulant Therapy

Anticoagulant therapy is prescribed for a variety of medical conditions and microsurgical endodontics is usually possible even in patients having this kind of therapy. However, considering the wide variety of drugs currently used for anticoagulation, a medical consultation is usually advisable.[17]

Bisphosphonates

Patients affected by osteoporosis are commonly treated with bisphosphonates, which can cause adverse response to surgical procedures, including osteonecrosis of the jaw.[18] The potential association between bisphosphonate use and osteonecrosis of the jaw was first reported in 2003.[19,20] The current preferred term for this condition is bisphosphonate-associated osteonecrosis (BON).[21]

Osteonecrosis can occur spontaneously but is more commonly associated with dental procedures that involve bone trauma, including extractions or surgical endodontics. Patients at high risk of necrosis are those who make chronic use of bisphosphonates for more than 2 years, especially patients on intravenous therapy (IV) (e.g., zoledronic acid and pamidronate).[22] The risk for osteonecrosis with commonly prescribed oral bisphosphonates appears to be very low. The estimated incidence of osteonecrosis in patients taking oral bisphosphonates ranges from 0 to 1 in 2260 cases, although dental extractions may quadruple the risk.[21,23] Any attempt should be used to manage apical periodontitis conservatively to reduce the risk of osteonecrosis. Nonsurgical retreatment should usually be considered the first choice. On the other hand, when the only viable treatment options for managing persistent periradicular inflammation are surgical root canal therapy or extraction, the question as to which option is more or less likely to lead to osteonecrosis in at-risk patients remains unanswered. In general, the procedure that could most predictably eliminate the peri-radicular inflammation with the least amount of surgical trauma would be preferred (📷 5.12).[22] However, it is always highly recommended to have a consultation with the physician who is treating this kind of pathology.

Postsurgical Recommendations

It is important that the hemostasis is maintained after surgery and, for this reason, after suturing the flap, a moist sterile gauze is positioned on top of the suture and maintained with gentle pressure for several minutes. This is done also to reduce the thickness of the blood clot that will form underneath the flap and to allow for stabilization of the initial fibrin stage of the blood clot.[16] The patient is also advised to apply an ice pack to the cheek for 15 minutes every hour for the rest of the day, to maintain hemostasis and to reduce the postoperative swelling that the patient will have on the second or third day after surgery. Sometimes in case of capillary vessel fragility, an ecchymosis could appear on the skin correspondent to the same area as the surgical procedure (📷 5.13) or on the lip (📷 5.14). There is no complication associated with this phenomenon and it always disappears in a couple of weeks.

For further discussion of postoperative instructions, *see* chapter 14.

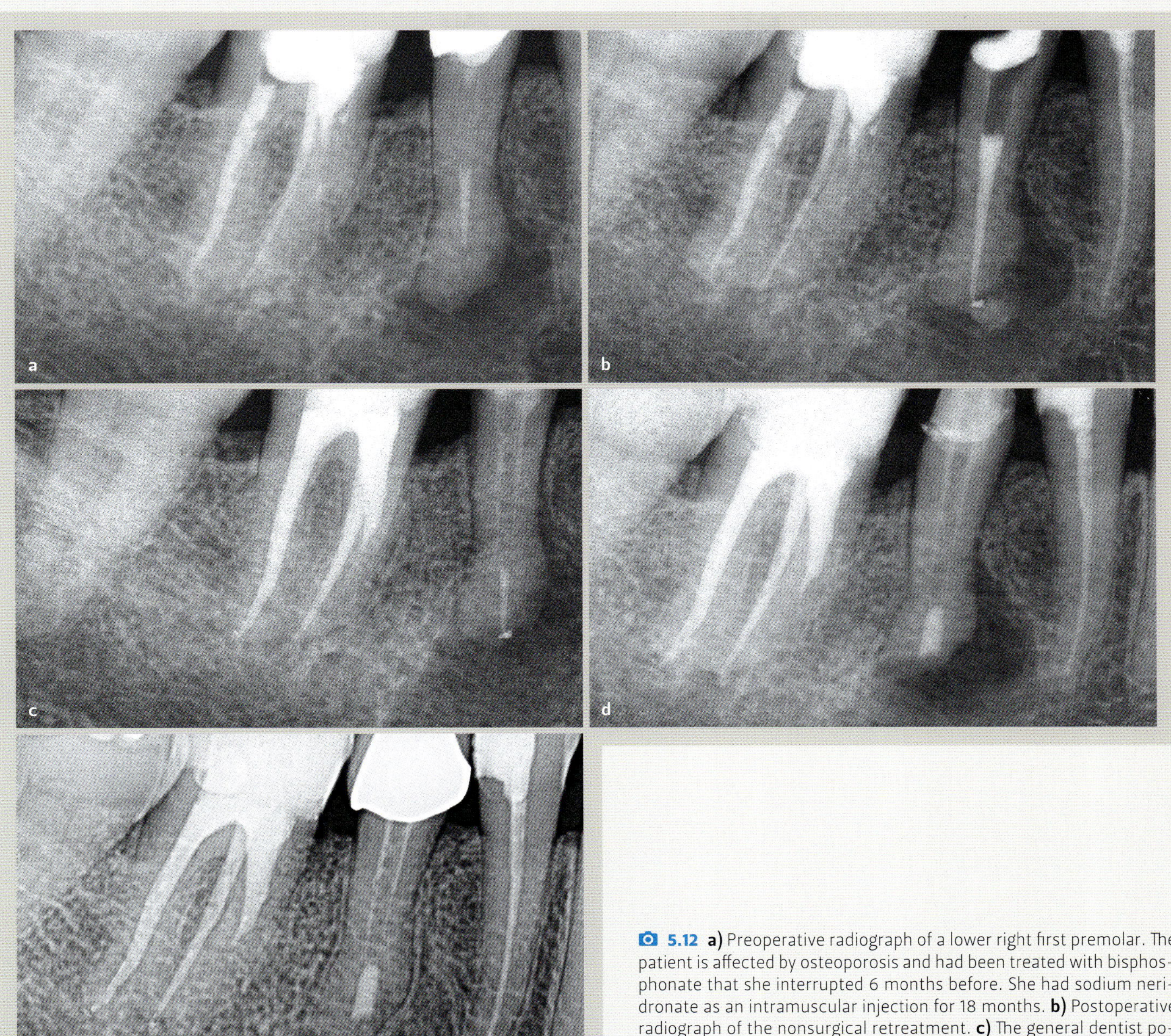

5.12 **a)** Preoperative radiograph of a lower right first premolar. The patient is affected by osteoporosis and had been treated with bisphosphonate that she interrupted 6 months before. She had sodium neridronate as an intramuscular injection for 18 months. **b)** Postoperative radiograph of the nonsurgical retreatment. **c)** The general dentist positioned a carbon fiber post too deep in the canal, removing too much obturating material and the tooth became symptomatic. Surgical retreatment now became strictly necessary. **d)** Postoperative radiograph. **e)** One-year recall.

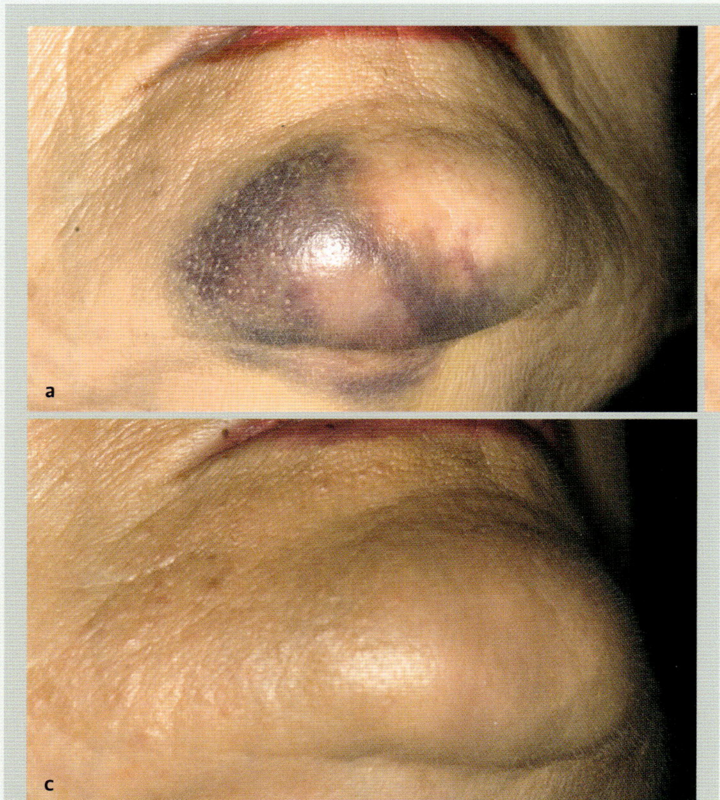

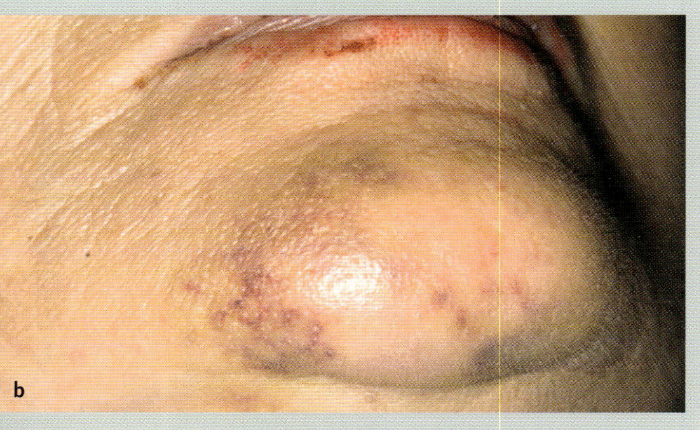

5.13 **a)** Ecchymosis two days after surgery on the lower right cuspid. **b)** One week after surgery. **c)** Two weeks after surgery.

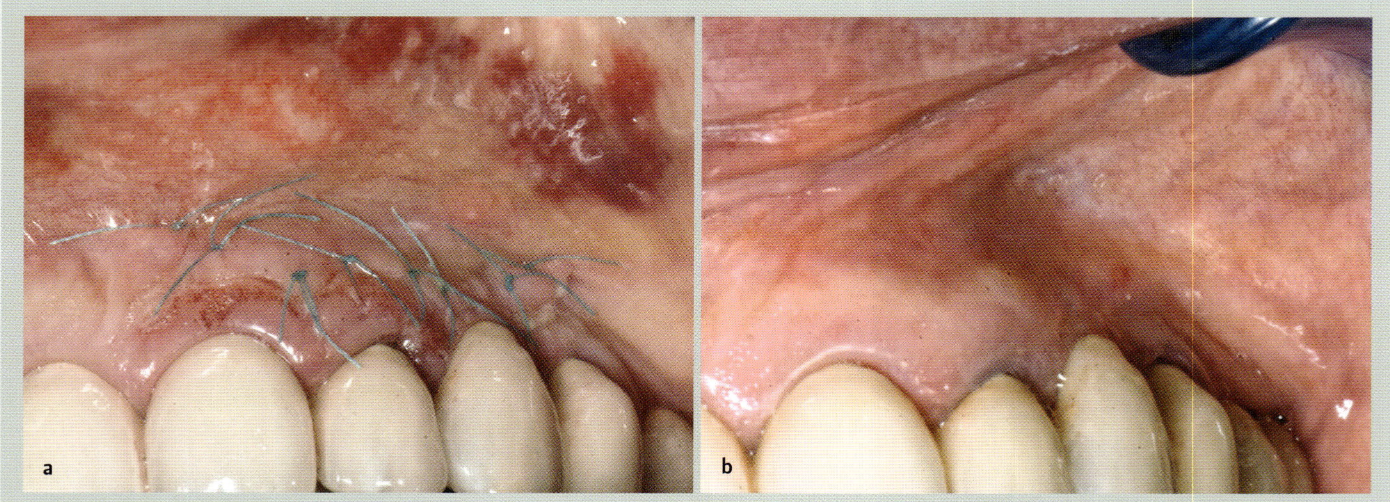

5.14 **a)** Ecchymosis on the lip two days after surgery on the upper left lateral incisor. **b)** One week after surgery.

REFERENCES

1. Kim S, Kratchman S. *Modern endodontic surgery concepts and practice: a review.* J Endod. 2006;32(7): 601-623.
2. Rethnam-Huag S, Iofin A, Kim S. *Anesthesia and Emostasis.* In: Kim S, Kratchman S. eds. *Microsurgery in Endodontics.* Wiley Blackwell. 2018:39-48.
3. Stropko J. *Micro-Surgical Endodontics.* In: Castellucci A. Ed. *EndodonticS.* Vol. III. Florence, Italy: Il Tridente. 2005:342-411.
4. Malamed SF. *Handbook of local anesthesia,* 6th ed. St. Louis, MO: Elsevier Mosby. 2011:225-252.
5. Harbert H. *Topical ice: a precursor to palatal injections.* J Endod. 1989;15:27.
6. Danielsson K, Evans H, Holmlund A, Kjellman O, Nordenram A, Persson NE. *Long-acting local anesthetics in oral surgery: Clinical evaluation of bupivacaine and etidocaine for mandibular nerve block.* J Oral Maxillofac Surg. 1986;15:119-126.
7. Gordon SM, Dionne RA, Brahim J, Jabir F, Dubner R. *Blockade of peripheral neuronal barrage reduces postoperative pain.* Pain 1997;70:209-215.
8. Lemon RR, Steele PJ, Jeansonne BG. *Ferric sulfate hemostasis: effect on osseous wound healing. Left in situ for maximum exposure.* J Endod. 1993;19:170-3.
9. Jeansonne B, Boggs WS, Lemon R. *Ferric sulfate hemostasis: effect on osseous wound healing. II. With curettage and irrigation.* J Endod. 1993;19:174-6.
10. Vickers FJ, Baumgartner JC, Marshall G. *Hemostatic efficacy and cardiovascular effects of agents used during endodontic surgery.* J Endod. 2002;28:322-323.
11. Besner E. *Systemic effects of racemic epinephrine when applied to the bone cavity during periapical surgery.* Va Dent J. 1972;49:9-12.
12. Horsley V. *Antiseptic wax.* BMJ. 1892;1:1165.
13. Selden HS. *Bone wax as an effective hemostat in periapical surgery.* Oral Surg Oral Med Oral Pathol. 1970;29:262-264.
14. Aurelio J, Chenail B, Gerstein H. *Foreign-body reaction to bone wax. Report of a case.* Oral Surg Oral Med Oral Pathol. 1984;58:98-100.
15. Johnson P, Fromm D. *Effects of bone wax on bacterial clearance.* Surgery. 1981;89:206-209.
16. Johnson BR, Abedi H. *Local anesthesia and hemostasis.* In: Torabinejad M, Rubinstein R. eds. *The art and science of contemporary surgical endodontics.* Quintessence Publishing Co, Inc. 2017;129-140.
17. Klammerer PW, Frerich B, Liese J, Schiegnitz E, Al-Navas B. *Oral surgery during therapy with anticoagulants- A systematic review.* Clin Oral Invest. 2015;19:171-180.
18. Jurosky K. *Wound healing.* In: Torabinejad M, Rubinstein R. eds. *The art and science of contemporary surgical endodontics.* Quintessence Publishing Co, Inc. 2017;237-259.
19. Marx RE. *Pamidronate (Aredia) and zoledronate (Zometa) induced avascular necrosis of the jaws: a growing epidemic.* J Oral Maxillofac Surg. 2003;61:1115.
20. Migliorati CA. *Bisphosphanates and oral cavity avascular bone necrosis.* J Clin Oncol. 2003;21:4253.
21. Aframian DJ, Lalla RV, Peterson DE. *Management of dental patients taking common hemostasis-altering medications.* Oral Surg Oral Med Oral Pathol Oral Radiol Endod. 2007; 103(Suppl):S45 e1.
22. Johnson BR, Fayad MI. *Periradicular surgery.* In: Hargreaves KM, Berman LH, eds. *Pathways of the Pulp.* 11th ed. St. Louis, MO: Elsevier. 2016; 387-446.
23. Mavrokokki T, Cheng A, Stein B, Goss A. *Nature and frequency of bisphosphonate-associated osteonecrosis of the jaws in Australia.* J Oral Maxillofac Surg. 2007;65:415.

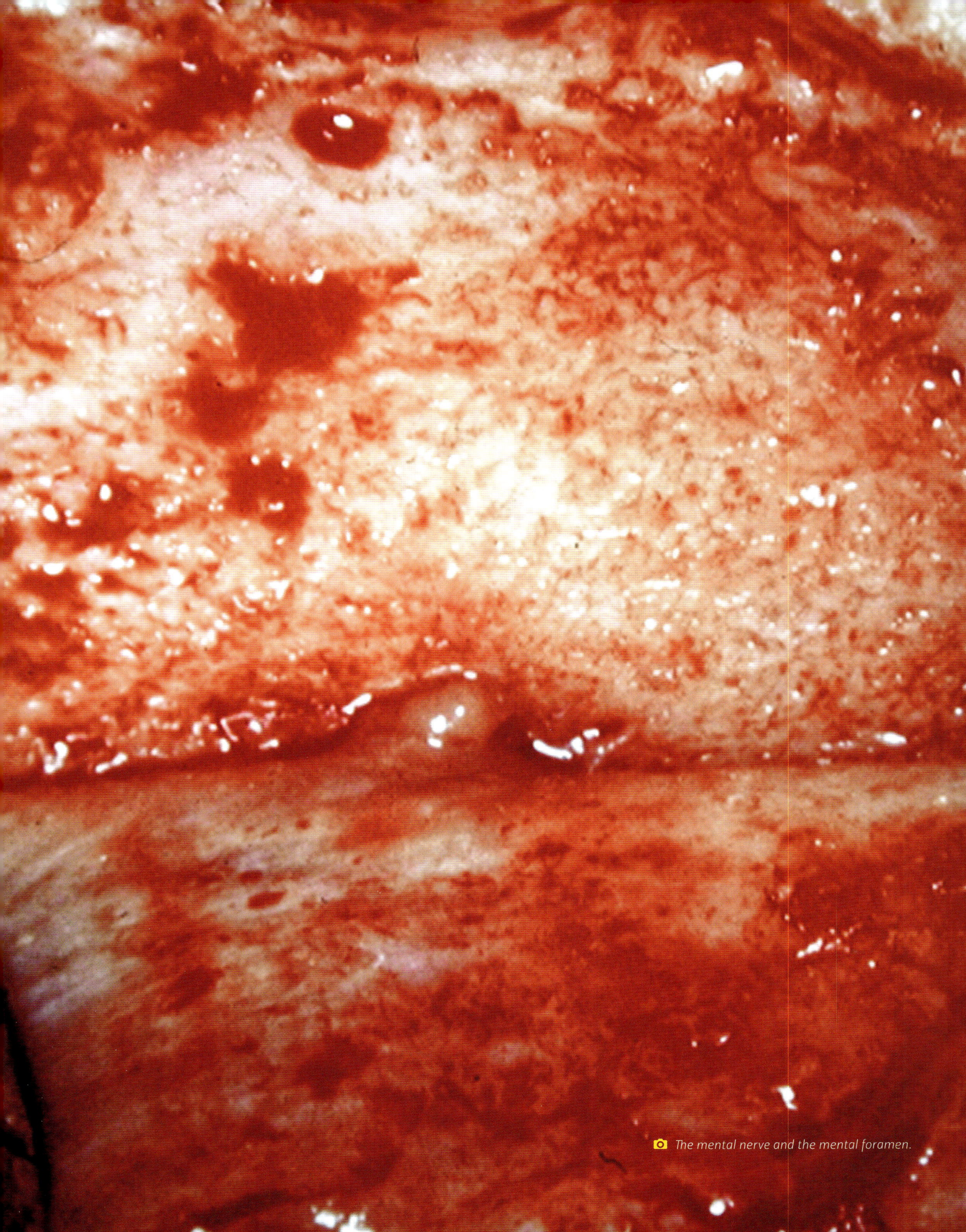

The mental nerve and the mental foramen.

Anatomic Considerations and Danger Zones

Access to Surgical Site

In case selection for microsurgical endodontics it is extremely important to evaluate the access to the surgical site. For this reason, during the first visit the patient will be clinically and radiographically examined, the periodontal probe will inform about the periodontal conditions of the teeth that will be involved in the surgical procedure and, most important, the patient will be positioned in the dental chair exactly in the same position that will be used during the surgical procedure so that the operator can accurately examine the access to the surgical site. A small oral opening, thick facial muscles, a thick buccal alveolar bone, a shallow vestibule, a limited retractability of the cheek, all can significantly increase the difficulty of the procedure, even in cases that may appear easy on radiographic examination (2.60).

Danger Zones

When performing surgical endodontics, the clinician is in proximity or in contact with a number of anatomical and neurovascular structures that are vulnerable and could be temporarily or even permanently damaged. It is therefore imperative to have a perfect knowledge of the anatomy associated with the areas adjacent to the teeth involved in the procedure.

MAXILLARY SINUS AND GREATER PALATINE ARTERY

Perforation of the sinus during surgery is quite common and sometimes can be intentional, when it is necessary to remove some foreign material (6.1). A reported incidence of perforation is of about 10% to 50% of cases.[1-3] On the other hand, perforation of the Schneiderian membrane very rarely results in long-term postoperative problems.[4] Usually the membrane regenerates and a thin layer of new bone often forms over the root apices.[1,5,6]

Sometimes colleagues are afraid of the maxillary sinus and they refer patients saying that the root apex of the involved tooth on the radiograph appears to be completely submerged in the sinus. This is a common mistake of radiographic interpretation, especially when dealing with upper first or second premolars. The root

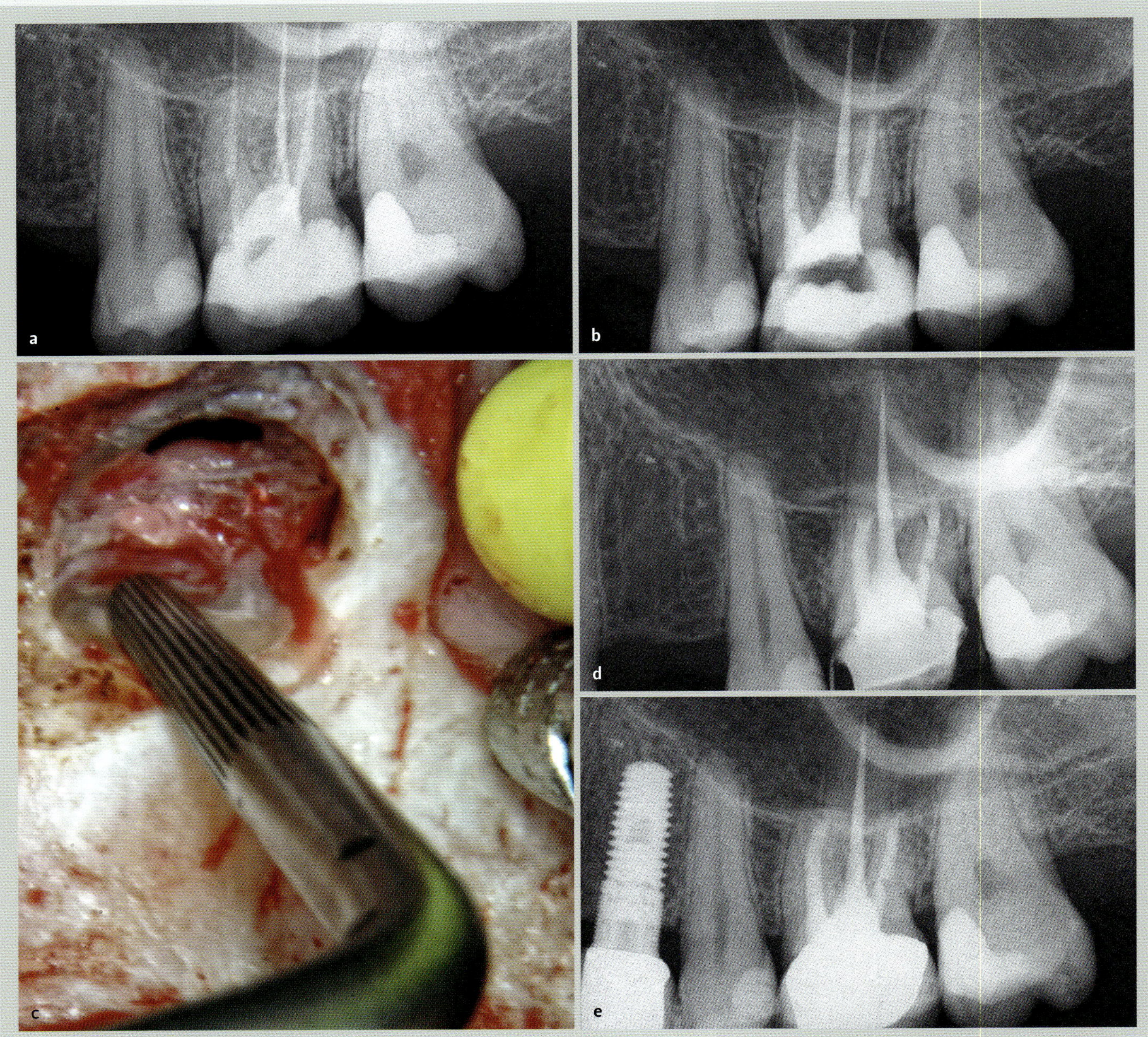

↑ 6.1 **a)** Preoperative radiograph of the upper left first molar. Two long pieces of gutta-percha points have been pushed inside the maxillary sinus. **b)** After the nonsurgical retreatment, the two pieces of gutta-percha remained inside the sinus and the patient remained uncomfortable. **c)** During the surgical retreatment an intentional perforation of the Schneiderian membrane was made to pull out the gutta-percha. In order not to damage the membrane more and not to push debris into the sinus, the bevel of the root apices has been made using an ultrasonic tip, having two suction tips close to the bony crypt during the retropreparation and retrofill. **d)** Postoperative radiograph. The retropreps of the buccal roots have been filled with white MTA. **e)** Two-year recall.

→ 6.2 **a)** The upper left first molar already had surgery but the lesion is not healing and the tooth is sensitive. A surgical retreatment has been planned. Preoperative radiograph. **b)** After elevating the flap, an attempt is made to lift the Schneiderian membrane. **c)** The delicate membrane has been perforated. **d)** A sterile gauze is introduced into the sinus to collect debris. **e)** The ultrasonic retrotip is being used to prepare the cavity. **f)** The retro-cavity has been prepared in the disto-buccal root. A piece of gutta-percha has been collected by the sterile gauze. **g, h)** The MB1, MB2 and the isthmus have been filled with white MTA. **i)** The disto-buccal retroprep has also been filled with white MTA. **j)** The full thickness flap is now sutured. **k)** The suture. **l, m)** The suture removal after 48 hours. **n)** Postoperative radiograph. **o)** One-year recall.

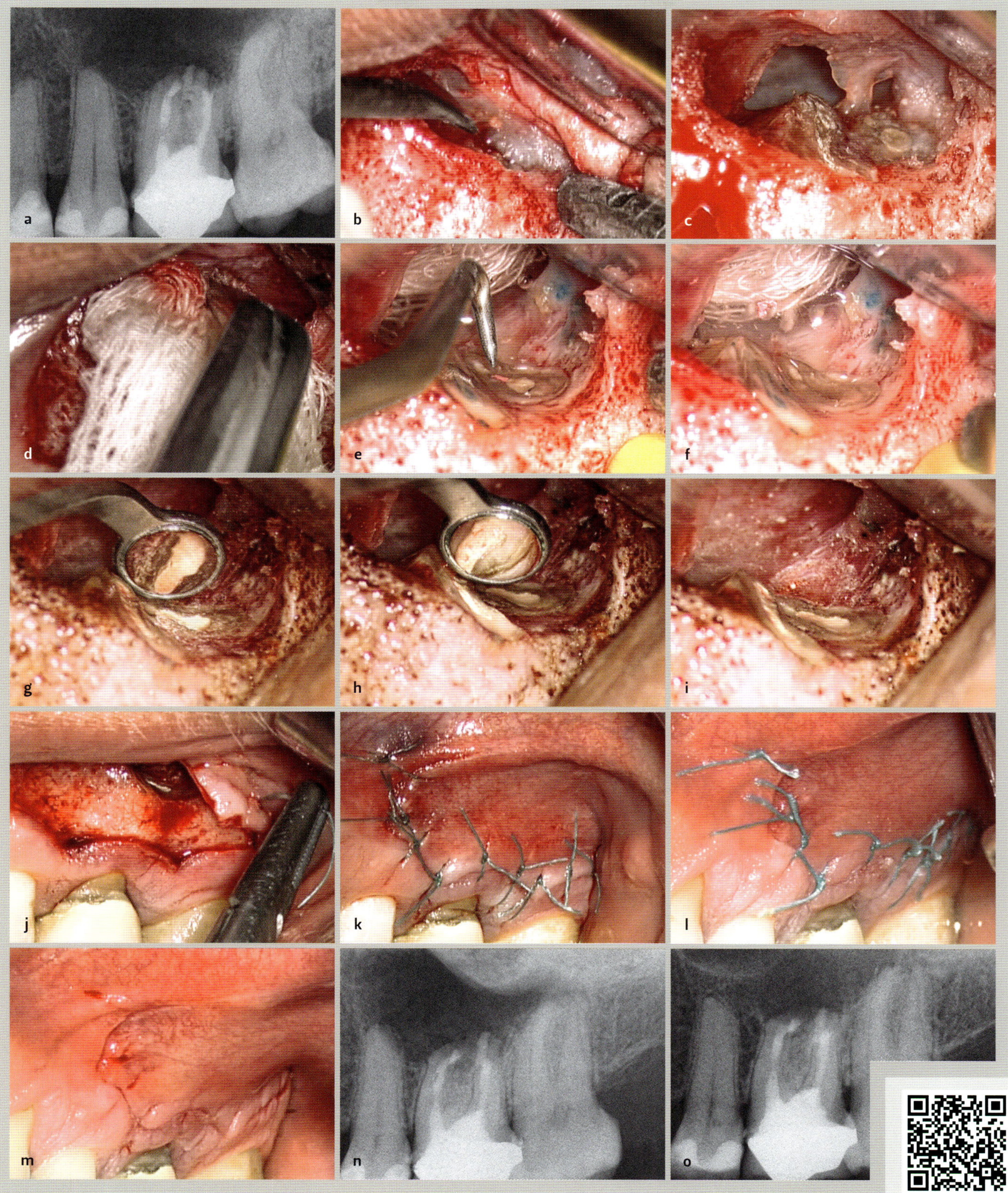
a
b
c
d
e
f
g
h
i
j
k
l
m
n
o

apex seems to be "inside" the sinus, but actually the sinus is always palatal to the root apex. In more than 40 years of experience, it has never happened to the author, that to reach the root end of an upper premolar, required crossing the maxillary sinus. The only teeth that could be more easily involved with the sinus are the upper molars. The membrane can lie exactly over the buccal root ends (in this case it can be delicately lifted), or the same membrane can be present between the two buccal and the palatal roots. In this case, if the palatal approach is selected to surgically treat the palatal root (transantral approach), the intentional perforation of the membrane cannot be avoided. The surgeon must be very careful to prevent infected root fragments and debris from entering the sinus. The sinus may be packed with a moist sterile gauze to catch debris and then should be carefully irrigated with saline solution before suturing (6.2). Usually, the root resection technique involves grinding

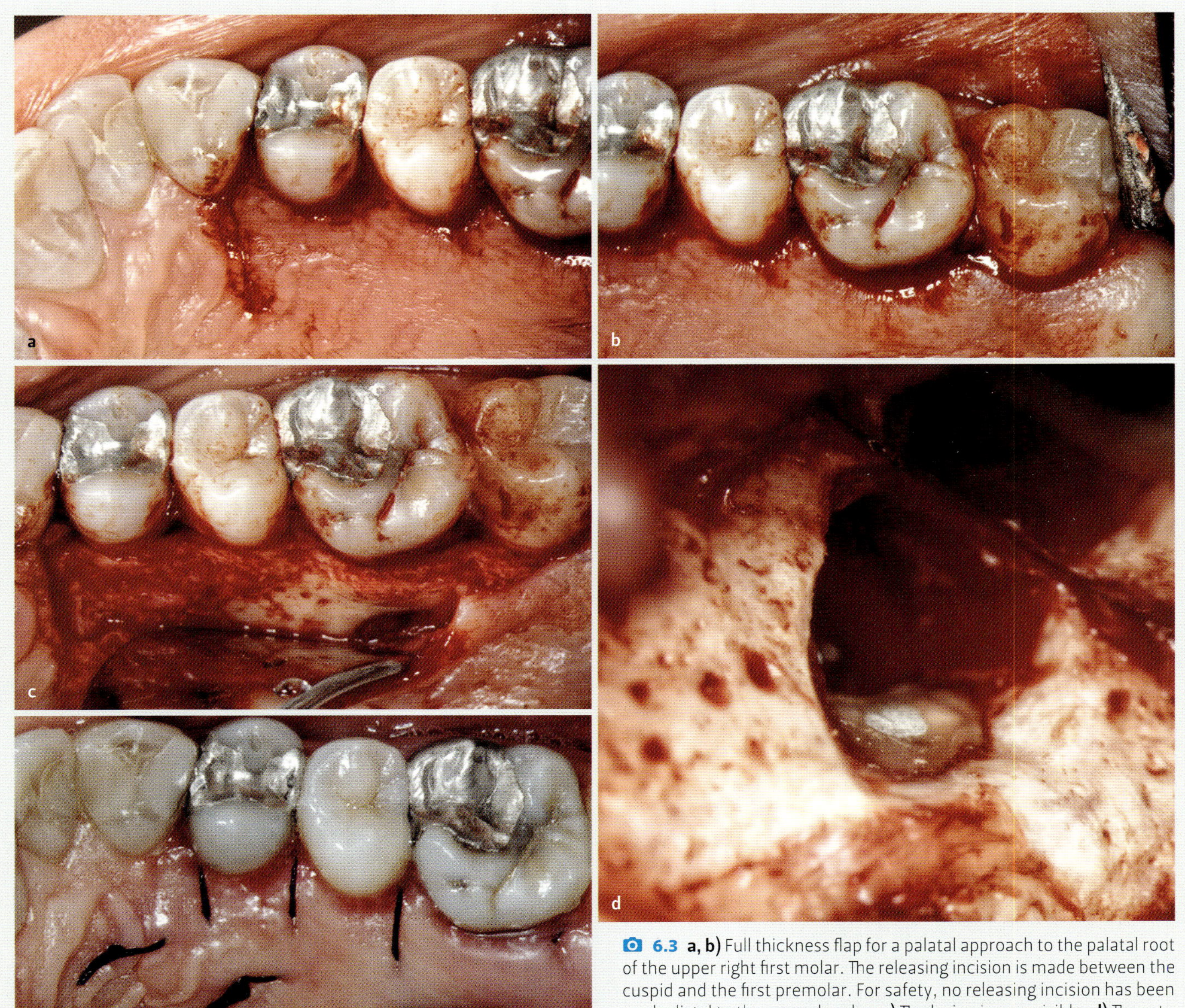

6.3 a, b) Full thickness flap for a palatal approach to the palatal root of the upper right first molar. The releasing incision is made between the cuspid and the first premolar. For safety, no releasing incision has been made distal to the second molar. **c)** The lesion is now visible. **d)** The retrofill has been made using amalgam. **e)** The flap has been sutured using 5.0 silk. The case was treated in 1983.

the root apex with a high-speed drill for about 3 mm in an apical to coronal direction. The concomitant spray of water could be responsible for pushing debris into the sinus and the aggressive tip of the drill could make the perforation even larger. To avoid this, the root resection can be made using specific ultrasonic tips, always having the suction tips very close the site of the perforation. This way the resection of the root apex will be slower and more time consuming, the ultrasonic tip will cause no further damage to the sinus membrane (it is well known that ultrasonic tips are efficient when in contact with hard tissue and they are completely inert when they are used in contact with soft tissue) and the clinician will be able to avoid pushing any debris into the sinus (6.1). The enhanced illumination and magnification provided by the operating microscope of course is essential in this kind of surgery.

On the other hand, the palatal approach to the palatal root of the maxillary molars in the author opinion is extremely more complicated and fraught with difficulties. Different from the surgery performed in any other area, where the patient is instructed to maintain the mouth closed (biting on a folded gauze) all the time during the procedure (7.1), while using the palatal approach the patient is asked to keep the mouth "wide open". From time to time he/she gets tired and start to close the mouth little by little, limiting our visibility. The attached gingiva is quite difficult to elevate and to retract. The releasing incision for safety can only be done mesially (6.3), and if it is also needed distally, it must be very short, in order not to section the anterior palatine artery.

This artery emerges from the greater palatine foramen distal to the maxillary second molar at the junction of the maxillary alveolar process, and the palatine bone and continues anteriorly (6.4). A vertical releasing incision can be placed between the maxillary first premolar and canine (6.3a), where the artery is relatively thin and branches off into smaller arteries. If needed, a short distal vertical releasing incision may be made distal to the second molar, but it should not approach the junction of the alveolar process and roof of the palate. If the anterior palatine artery is severed, local clamping and pressure may not stop the hemorrhage, and ligation of the external carotid artery may be necessary.[7]

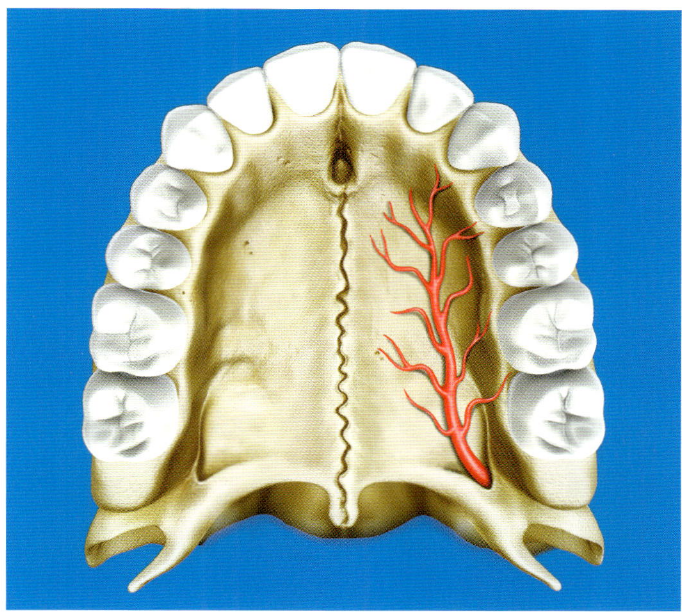

6.4 The anterior palatine artery emerges from the greater palatine foramen.

INFERIOR ALVEOLAR NERVE AND MENTAL NERVE

From a careful examination of the preoperative radiograph the clinician can evaluate the distance between the apices of the molar and the inferior alveolar nerve. More precise information can be obtained from the three-dimensional exam provided by a CBCT (6.5). However, usually the inferior alveolar nerve is more apical and more lingual relative to the apices of the lower first molar and even more lingual compared to the apices of the second molar. Therefore, it is extremely rare to damage the nerve when doing surgery on these teeth. The only situation when the nerve can be damage is when a large lesion is present and the surgeon unnecessarily attempts to curette the bone around the entire lesion to make sure of the complete removal of the granulation tissue or the cystic wall (2.5a). One important concept should never be forgotten. When we perform a surgical endodontic treatment, we are still treating a "lesion of endodontic origin", it doesn't matter if it is a granuloma or a cyst, and it could have healed completely with a nonsurgical therapy. If this is true as it is true, there is no need to remove the entire mass of the lesion, especially if doing so there is a risk of damaging important anatomical structures. For this reason, in case of a large lesion, it is enough to remove part of the lesion, enough to have access to the root to be treated (2.15d). This is done to avoid sectioning the blood supply of the adjacent vital teeth, perforating the nasal floor or the maxillary sinus, damaging the inferior alveolar nerve or the mental nerve.

The mental nerve exits the mental foramen at or near the apices of the lower premolars (6.6). However, there are several anatomical variations; therefore, the clinician must examine each patient very carefully to determine its location (6.7). Vertical location of the mental foramen may vary even more than horizontal location. When a vertical releasing incision is indicated, usually is made mesially to the cuspid and it should be long enough in order to allow the atraumatic elevation of a long flap and to visualize the mental foramen (6.8). This is done in order to avoid damaging the

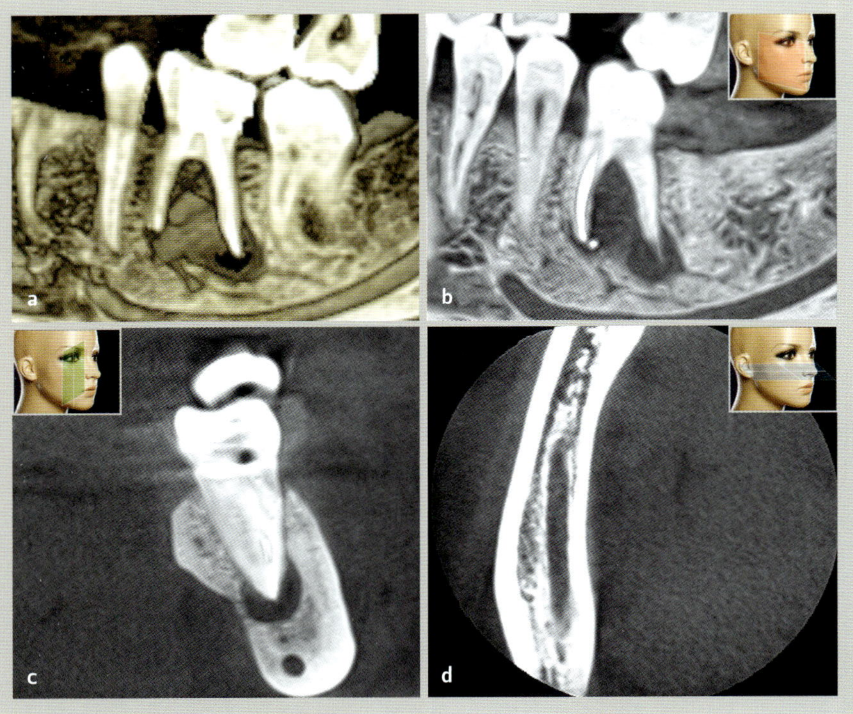

6.5 a, b) The CBCT is showing the inferior alveolar nerve. **c, d)** The nerve is always more apical and more lingual compared to the apices of the lower first molar.

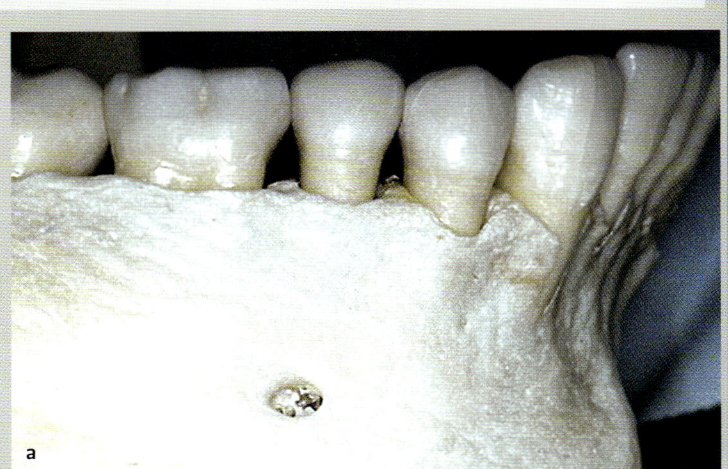

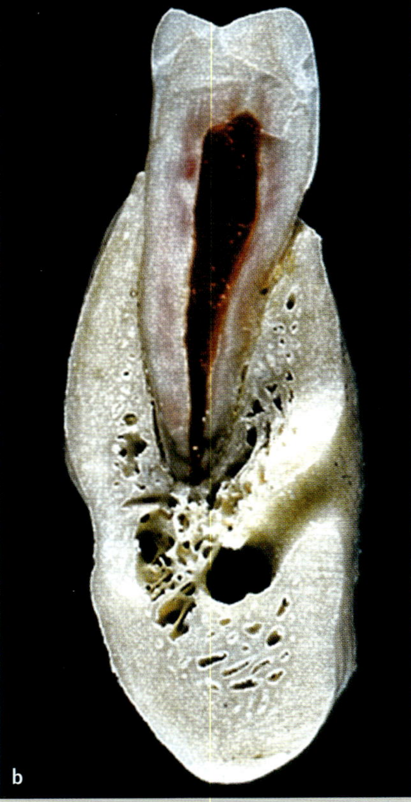

6.6 a, b) The mental foramen.

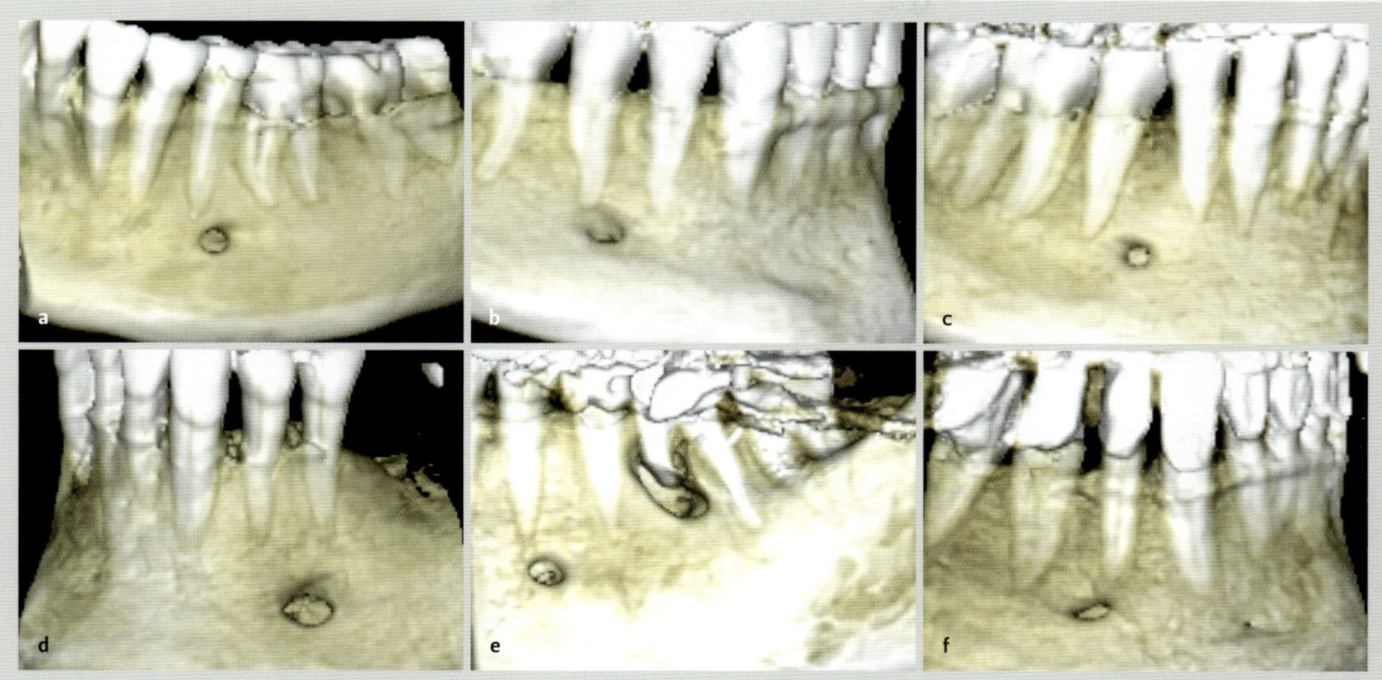

6.7 **a)** The mental foramen here is distal to the apex of the second premolar. **b)** The mental foramen here is exactly over the apex of the second premolar. **c)** The mental foramen here is mesial to the apex of the second premolar. **d)** The mental foramen here is exactly between the first and the second premolar. **e)** The mental foramen here is distal to the apex of the first premolar. **f)** The mental foramen here is exactly over the apex of the first premolar.

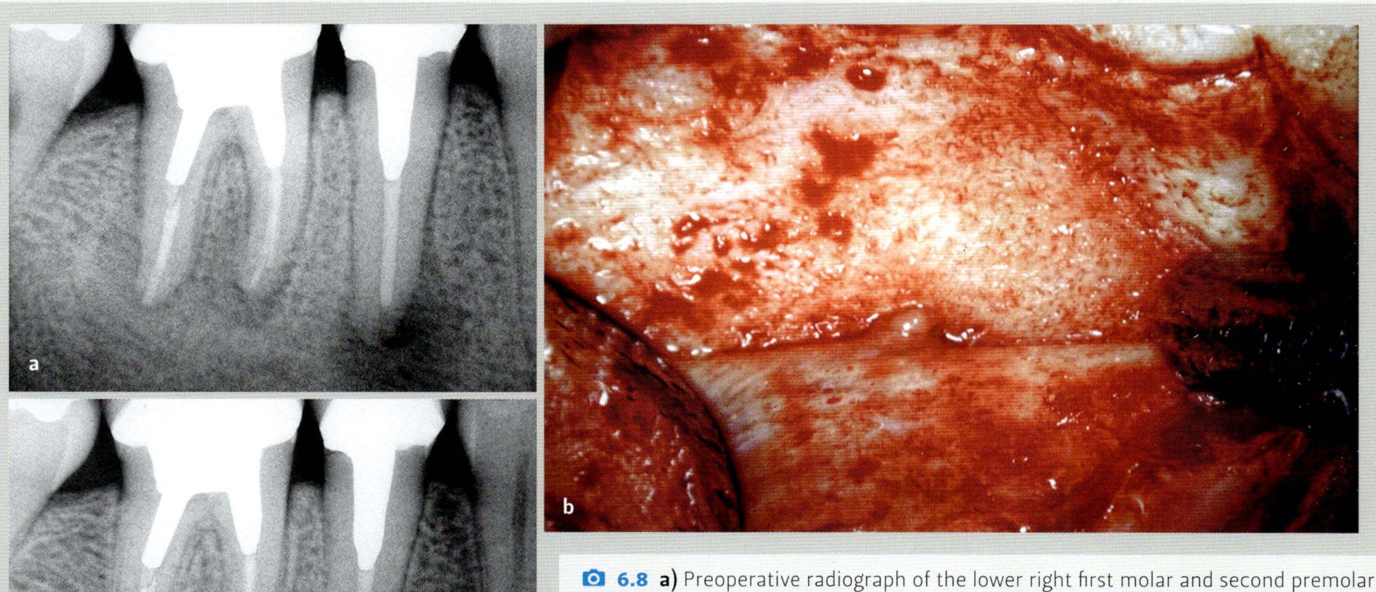

6.8 **a)** Preoperative radiograph of the lower right first molar and second premolar. **b)** The full thickness flap had two long vertical incisions in order to expose the mental foramen. The retractor will be positioned elsewhere. **c)** Two-year recall.

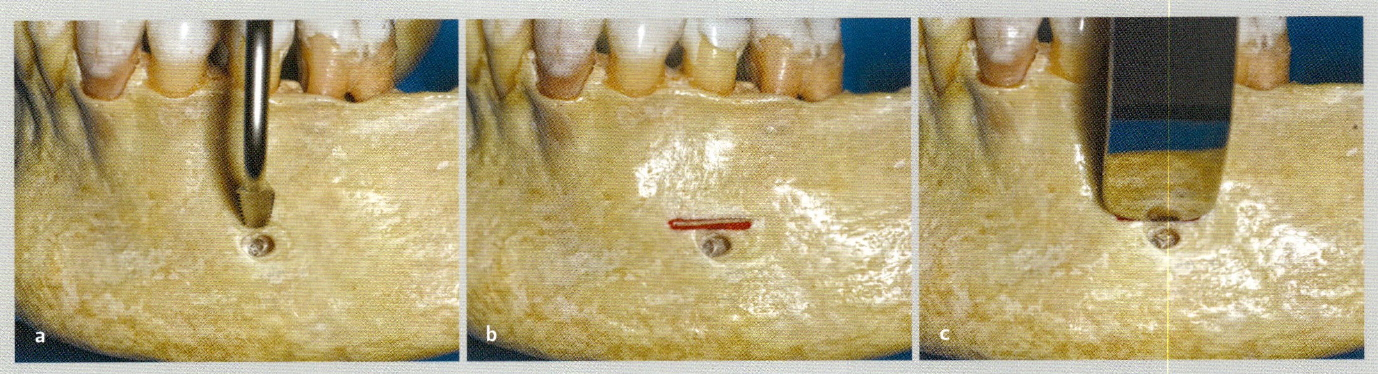

6.9 **a, b)** The Groove Technique as suggested by S. Kim. A small narrow horizontal groove is made just above the mental foramen. **c)** The retractor is firmly seated in the groove protecting the nerve during the osteotomy.[8]

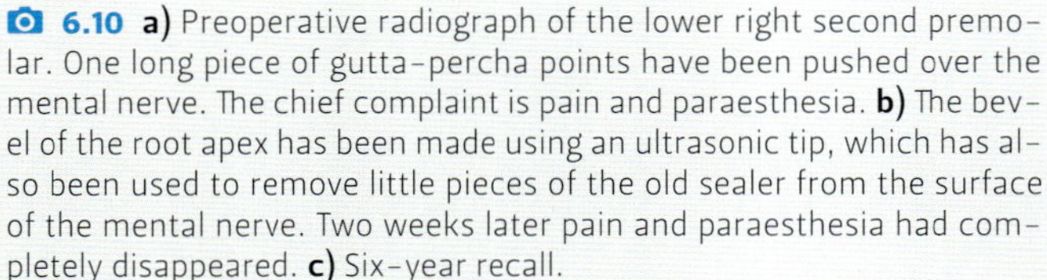

6.10 **a)** Preoperative radiograph of the lower right second premolar. One long piece of gutta-percha points have been pushed over the mental nerve. The chief complaint is pain and paraesthesia. **b)** The bevel of the root apex has been made using an ultrasonic tip, which has also been used to remove little pieces of the old sealer from the surface of the mental nerve. Two weeks later pain and paraesthesia had completely disappeared. **c)** Six-year recall.

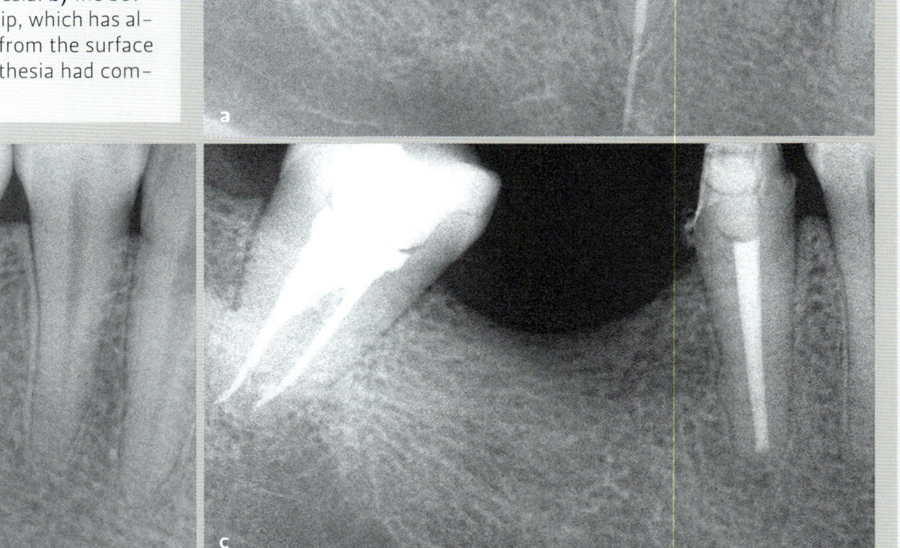

mental nerve with the retractor. Once we know where the foramen is, then we also know where **not** to position the retractor. Serious damage to the nerve can be done not only by sectioning the nerve itself with the scalpel, but also compressing the nerve with the retractor during the entire time of the surgical procedure. In the case where the foramen is very close to the apex of the premolar and to avoid the retractor from slipping continuously over the mental nerve, Kim suggests to make a groove with a high speed bur or even better still with piezosurgery (piezotome blade) to stabilize the retractor which can then rest in the groove (6.9).[8]

In the case when the root apex to be beveled during the surgical procedure is exactly over the mental foramen, instead of grinding the root surface with an aggressive bur, it is much safer to use an ultrasonic tip, which will be efficient against the hard structure of the root but absolutely innocuous and inefficient when in contact with soft tissue, like the mental nerve (6.10).

The unusual location of the mental foramen coronal to the apex of the premolar that needs surgery is an obvious contraindication for the surgical procedure (6.11), as well as the unusual location of the disto-buccal root of the upper first molar (6.12).

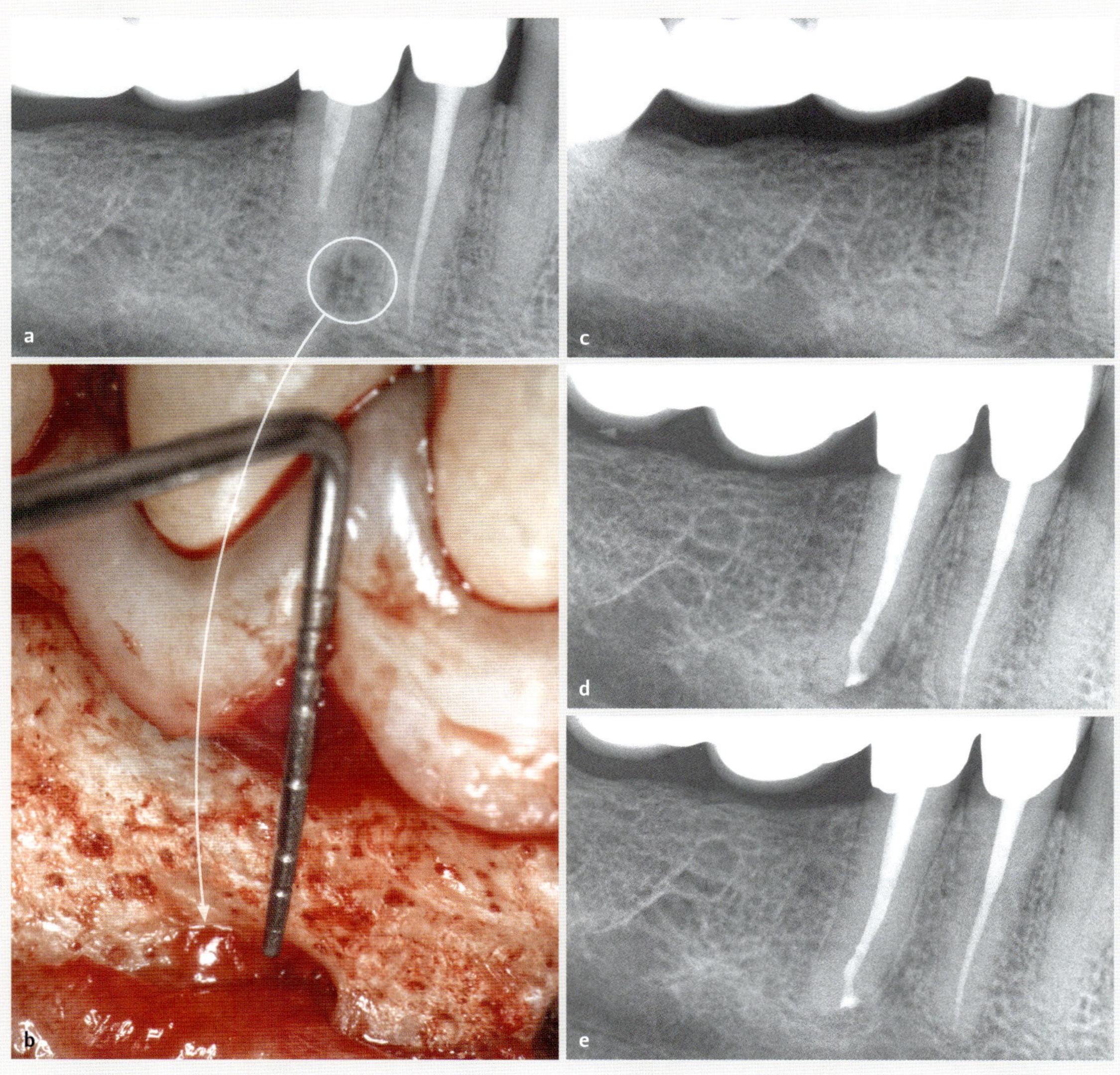

6.11 **a)** Preoperative radiograph of the lower right second premolar. The patient is referred with the specific request to do surgery and not to make an access cavity, in order not to ruin the "brand new" porcelain crown. **b)** Once the flap is partially elevated, the mental foramen appeared to be coronal to the apex that needed periapical surgery. The surgical procedure was interrupted in order not to section the mental nerve and the patient was scheduled for a nonsurgical retreatment. **c)** The rubber dam has been positioned, the access cavity has been made and now the working length is checked. **d)** Postoperative radiograph. **e)** Two-year recall.

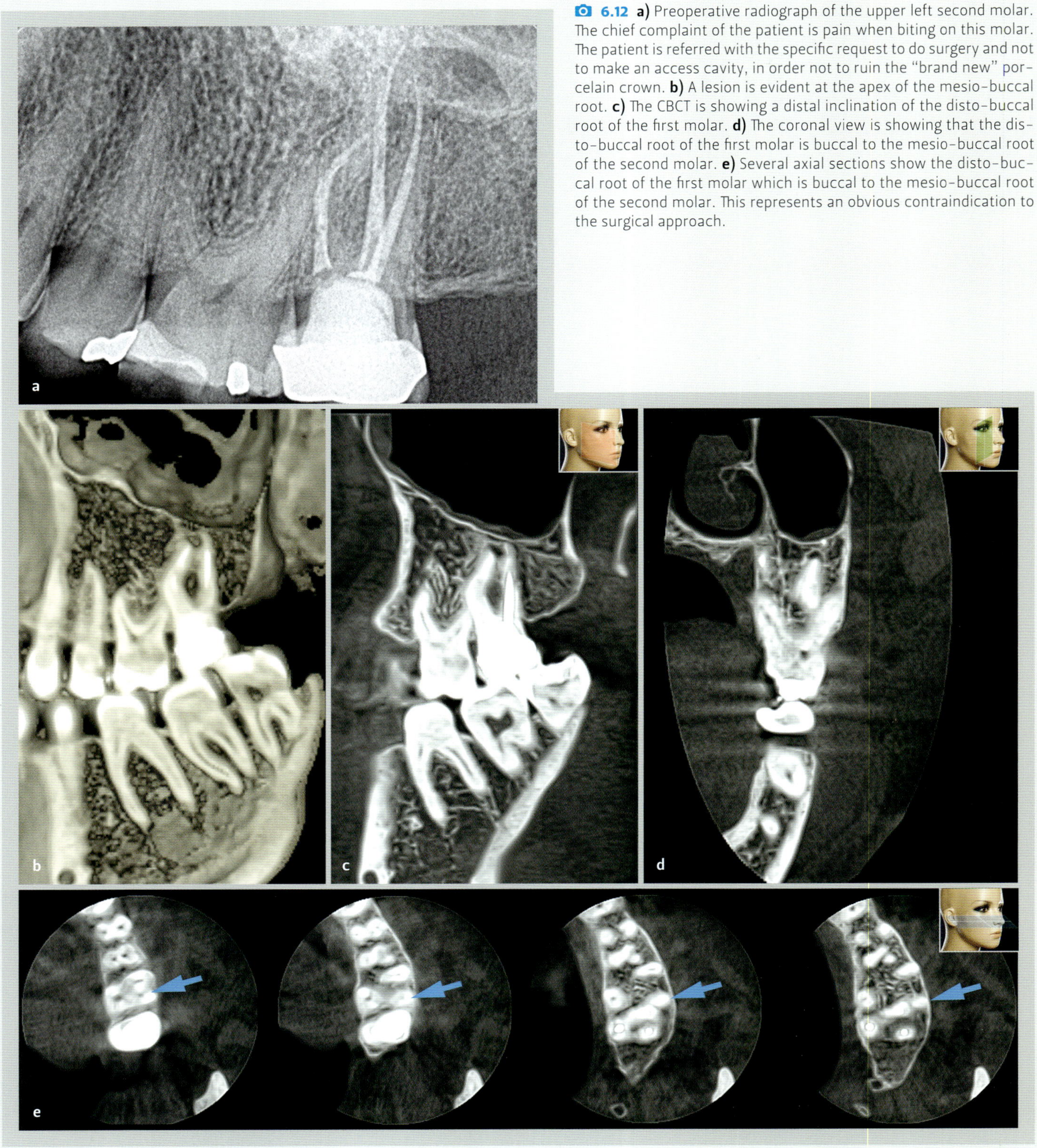

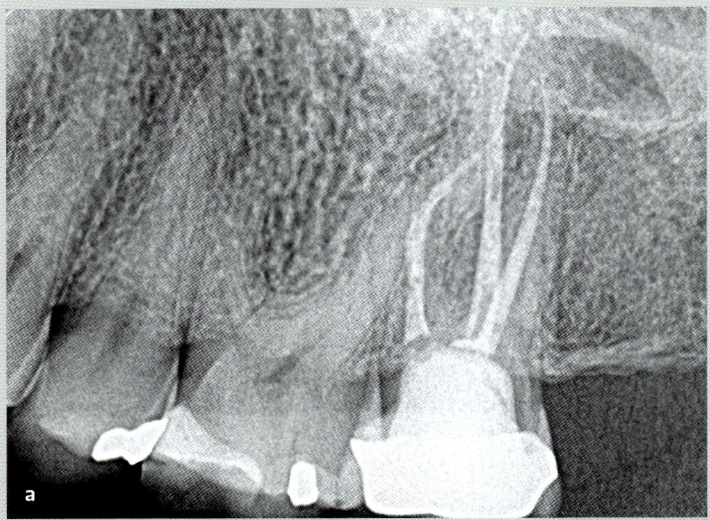

6.12 **a)** Preoperative radiograph of the upper left second molar. The chief complaint of the patient is pain when biting on this molar. The patient is referred with the specific request to do surgery and not to make an access cavity, in order not to ruin the "brand new" porcelain crown. **b)** A lesion is evident at the apex of the mesio-buccal root. **c)** The CBCT is showing a distal inclination of the disto-buccal root of the first molar. **d)** The coronal view is showing that the disto-buccal root of the first molar is buccal to the mesio-buccal root of the second molar. **e)** Several axial sections show the disto-buccal root of the first molar which is buccal to the mesio-buccal root of the second molar. This represents an obvious contraindication to the surgical approach.

REFERENCES

1. Ericson S, Finne K, Persson G. *Results of apicoectomy of maxillary canines, premolars and molars with special reference to oroantral communication as a prognostic factor.* Int J Oral Surg. 1974;3:386.
2. Freedman A, Horowitz I. *Complications after apicoectomy in maxillary premolar and molar teeth.* Int J Oral Maxillofac Surg. 1999;28:192.
3. Rud J, Rud V. *Surgical endodontics of upper molars: relation to the maxillary sinus and operation in acute state of infection.* J Endod. 1998;24:260.
4. Hauman CH, Chandler NP, Tong DC. *Endodontic implications of the maxillary sinus: a review.* Int Endod J. 2002;35:127.
5. Benninger MS, Sebek BA, Levine HL. *Mucosal regeneration of the maxillary sinus after surgery.* Otolaryngol Head Neck Surg. 1989;101:33.
6. Watzek G, Bernhart T, Ulm C. *Complications of sinus perforations and their management in endodontics.* Dent Clin North Am. 1997;41:563.
7. Johnson BR, Fayad MI. *Periradicular surgery.* In: Hargreaves KM, Berman LH, eds. *Pathways of the Pulp.* 11th ed. St. Louis Mo: Elsevier. 2016; 387-446.
8. Kim S, Kratchman S. *Modern endodontic surgery concepts and practice: a review.* J Endod. 52(7):601-623.

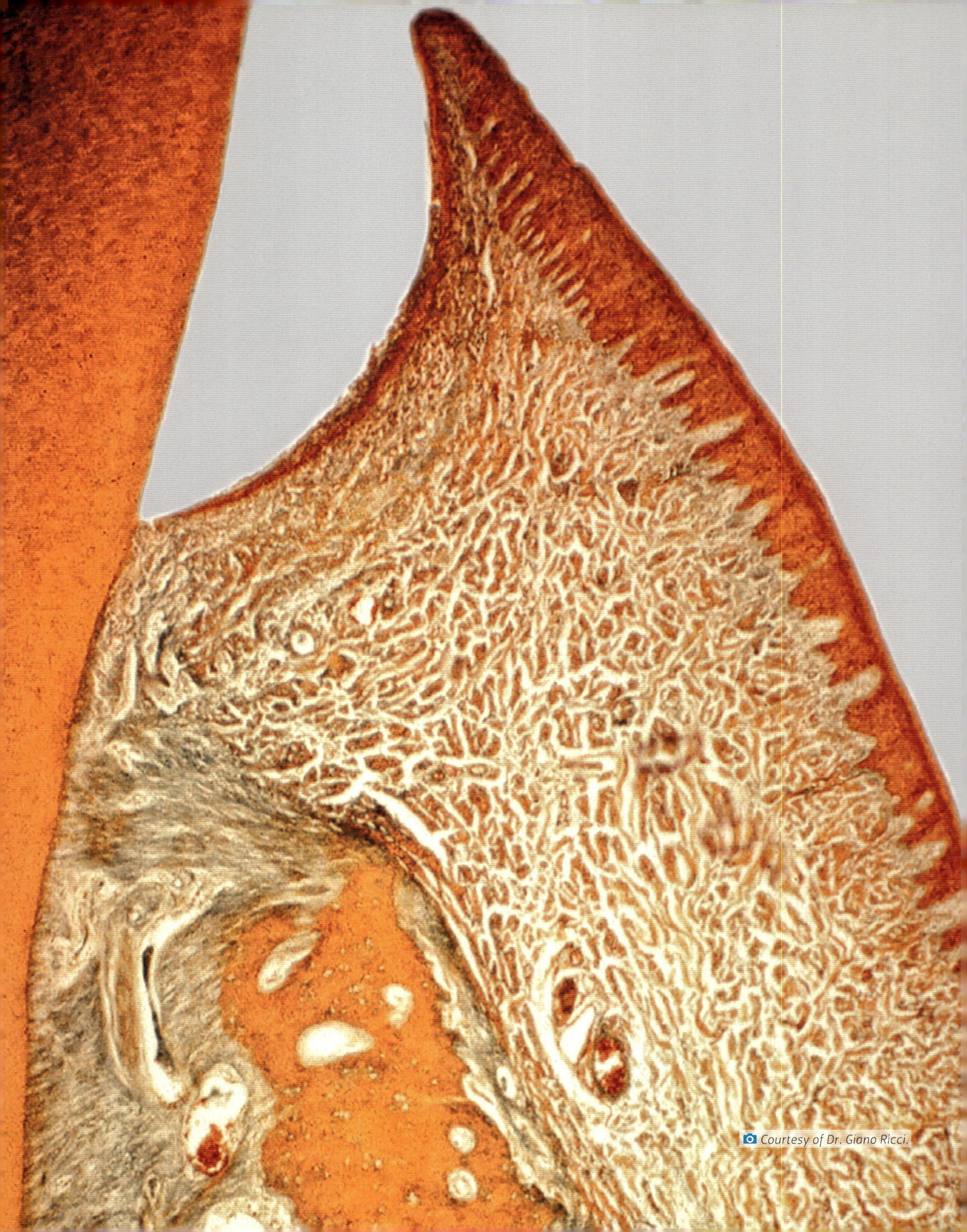

Courtesy of Dr. Giano Ricci.

Soft Tissue Management

Stabilization of the Surgical Site

It is desirable to begin the procedure with the surgical area as clean of debris and free of plaque as possible. For this reason, it is important, before the surgery appointment, to schedule an appointment for oral hygiene.

The day before surgery the patient is told to rinse with 12% aqueous chlorhexidine gluconate solution and before making the incision the surgical area is thoroughly cleaned with the same solution, to further reduce the pathogenic bacterial flora.[1]

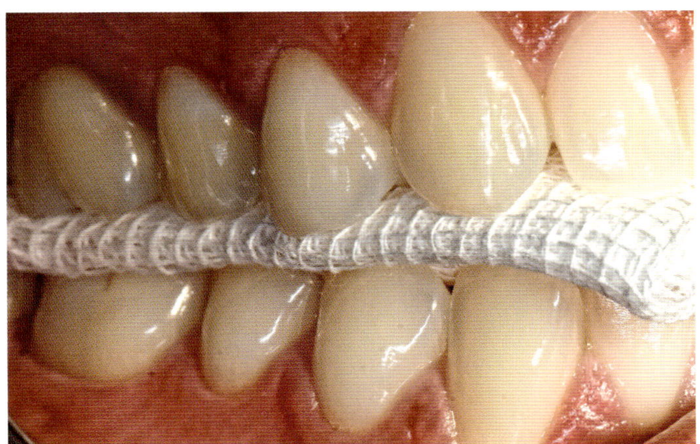

7.1 The patient is asked to bite on a gauze pad to stabilize the jaws and teeth and to maintain a comfortable position.

When everything is ready, the patient is instructed to close on a sterile folded gauze to help stabilize the jaws and maintain a comfortable position for the patient during the rather long surgery (7.1).[1] Approximately 8-10 thicknesses of 2'' by 2'' sterile gauze squares (4 or 5-2 × 2's folded over twice) are used so that just a small portion of the folded portion is protruding buccal to the line of occlusion. Now the cheek and the lips are relaxed so that they can be retracted and the surgical procedure can start.

The Incision

The incision is made with the microsurgical blade Surgistar (Micro-Mini Blade Surgistar USM6910, Vista, CA) which is much smaller then the BP # 15 and the BP # 15C (7.2). The blade has a round tip and double sided cutting edges and has several advantages compared to the much larger BP # 15. It will allow more precise and accurate incisions, which later will allow a more accurate repositioning and suturing of the flap resulting in better and faster healing. Another advantage particular-

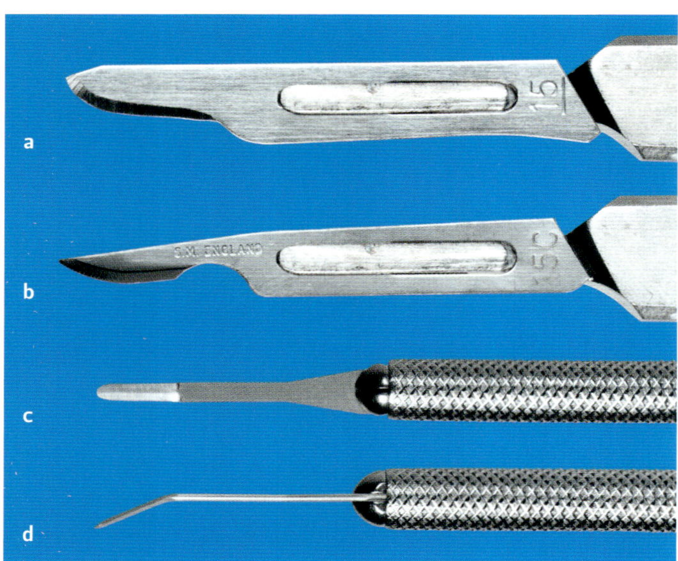

7.2 Comparison between a BP # 15 (**a**), BP # 15C (**b**) and a Surgistar microsurgical blade (**c**) (Surgistar Micro-Mini Blade USM6910, Kohler, Medizintechnik, Germany). **d)** Note the 10° angle of the microsurgical blade.

ly important for the submarginal flap is the possibility to cut on two sides. The first incision is made using one side of the blade and the cut involves the soft tissue only overlying the periosteum. Then the blade is used in the previous incision going in the opposite direction, making a deeper cut, in order to section the periosteum to make a full thickness flap. In this manner the incision of the periosteum is made with a "brand new" blade. As it will be described later in this chapter, when using the submarginal flap design the blade is used at 90° to the bone and the 10° angle of the blade will make the incision perpendicular to the bone much easier.

Regardless of the design, all flaps must be full thickness, involving the periosteum and the overlying mucosa. The split thickness flap should be avoided, because for this surgery it has several disadvantages: the periosteum keeps bleeding during the entire procedure, compromising visibility, and being the most traumatic, it also compromises the healing.[2]

The incision must always be made thinking of the later suturing. It must always be extended one tooth mesial and one tooth distal to the involved tooth or teeth.[3] It must be large enough to allow adequate vision, atraumatic elevation and retraction, passive repositioning and allow easy suturing. A small incision will force the operator to traumatize the flap with the retractor to improve visibility, which will cause postoperative discomfort, like pain and swelling.

One thing to always keep in mind is that all the postoperative discomfort of the patient is only related to the manner in which the doctor managed the full thickness flap. For this reason, the length of the flap should be large enough in order to be passively retracted and passively repositioned. The length of the flap will not influence the healing. Actually, it will influence the healing in a positive manner: the larger it is, the better it will be, meaning that the larger it is, the faster the healing and less the discomfort that the patient will have.

In the Author's experience, during suturing of a large incision, the patients often ask: «Doctor, how many stitches are you putting in my gingiva?» And my answer is: «As many as you need. Its in your best interest!»

Flap Design

The outcome of any surgical procedure depends among other factors upon the extent to which an adequate access is possible.[3] Surgical endodontics first requires exposure of the bone overlying the tip of the roots and then exposure of the root-ends per se (7.3). To access the bone, a full thickness flap must be raised. This comprises a soft tissue flap, which consists of gingival and mucosal tissue as well as periosteum. To mobilize the flap various types of incisions can be selected including horizontal, sulcular or submarginal, and vertical releasing incisions. The flap can in its entirety be a full thickness flap or a combination of a full and split thickness flap.[3]

- Before choosing an appropriate flap, several variables have to be considered, in order to select the best flap design for each case.
- Regional anatomical structures such as the location and the path of the blood vessels and nerves should be evaluated, protected and preserved during the surgical procedure.
- Position of the root within the mandible or the maxilla, its inclination and the thickness of the overlying bone between the surface and root structure.

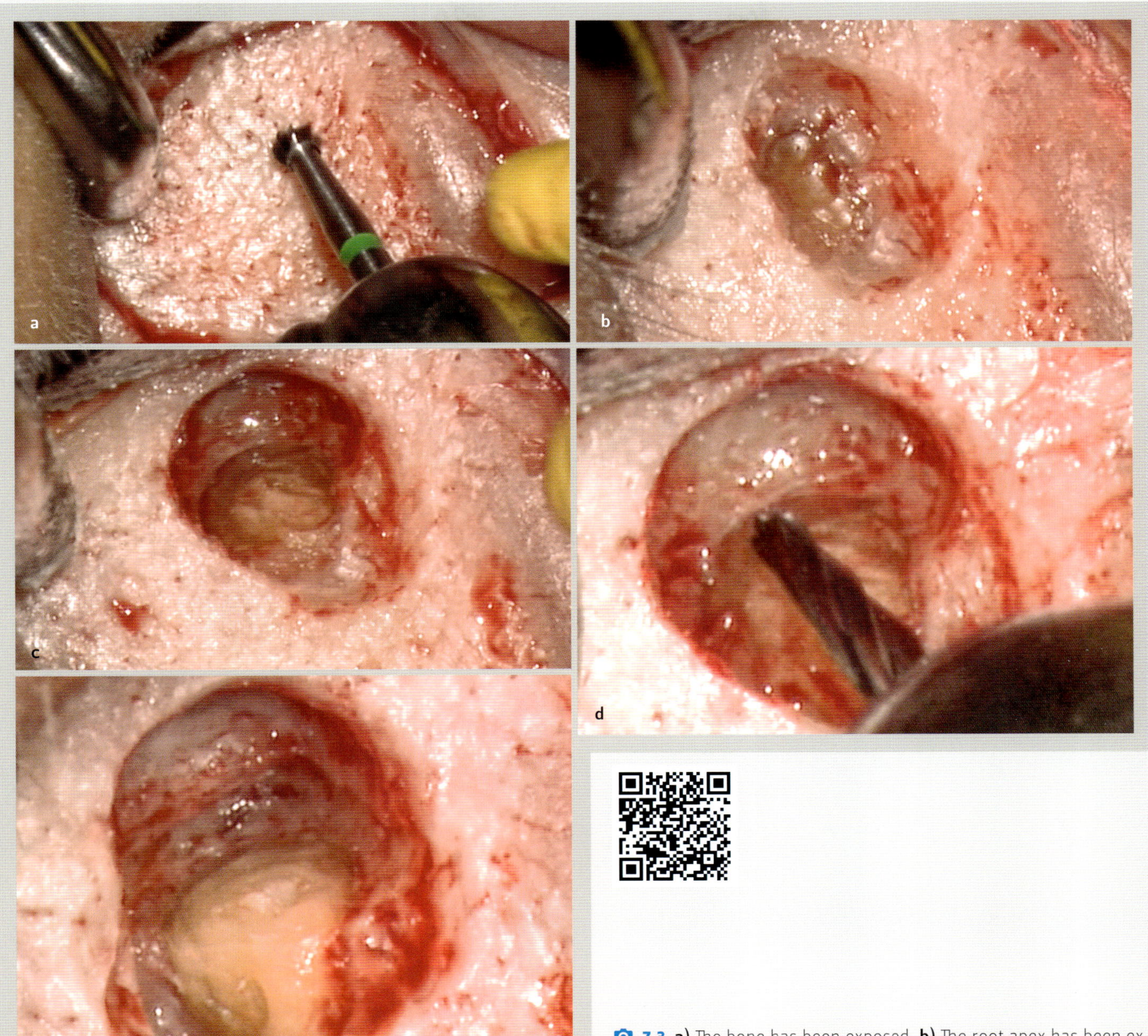

7.3 **a)** The bone has been exposed. **b)** The root apex has been exposed. **c, d)** The granulation tissue has been removed and the root apex can be shaved. **e)** The root apex is now ready for the root-end preparation.

- Periodontal conditions, probing depth, attachment loss, recessions and signs of periodontal inflammation.
- Width of the attached gingiva and location of the mucogingival junction.
- Presence, type and quality of restorations, position of the restoration margins relative to the gingiva.
- Size and position of the expected periradicular pathology in relation to the root, neurovascular structures and the sinus.
- Assessment of the local blood supply to the soft tissues.[3]

Various flap designs have been discussed in the literature.[2,4–6] Examples include marginal mucoperiosteal flaps with one (triangular flap) or two (trapezoidal or rectangular flap) releasing incisions, submarginal mucoperiosteal flaps with the horizontal incision within the attached gingiva and semilunar flaps.

The following discussion will review the pros and cons of the classic flaps used in microsurgical endodontics:

1. semilunar flap
2. submarginal flap
3. marginal flap.

Basically, the incision should provide a good access and protect the epithelial attachment. As already stated, the selection of the flap design depends on several factors, like the integrity of the bone over the roots, the amount and nature of the attached gingiva and the presence or absence of a fixed dental prosthesis.[1]

Semilunar Flap

This flap has either a straight or a curved horizontal incision, with the concavity towards the apex of the root (7.4). It is a full thickness flap and the incision is made entirely in the alveolar mucosa. This is the incision usually preferred by the oral surgeons and maxillofacial surgeons and the only advantages of this flap is the respect for the epithelial attachment and the absence of periodontal involvement: the marginal tissue remains untouched and thus no recession will occur. On the other hand, there are many disadvantages, such as limited access to the surgical area, poor visibility (the incision usually is not sufficiently large), difficult control of the bleeding (the incision involves blood vessels of a large diameter), the suture is not over healthy bone (because the incision is most often over the endodontic lesion), it is difficult to precisely reposition and suture the flap (because the incision is in the alveolar mucosa, very thin and rich in muscle attachments and elastic fibers, both of which exert pulling forces on the repositioned surgical wound margins), the healing could be by secondary intention (in case one of the sutures is lost and the bony lesion is in communication with the oral cavity), and quite often there are visible scars (7.5).

Because of the many drawbacks mentioned, a semilunar flap design is no longer recommended.[7]

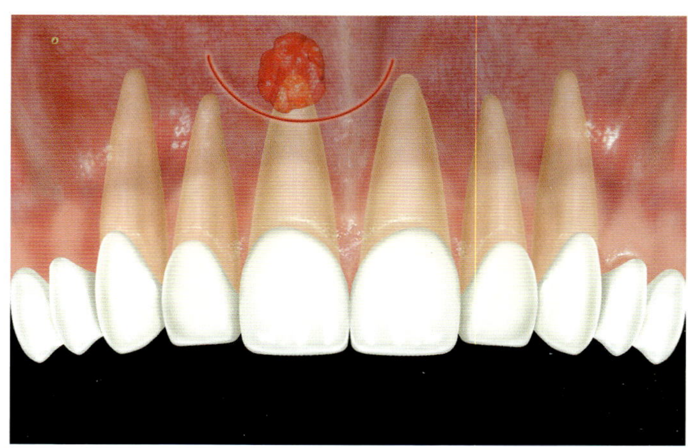

7.4 A semilunar flap, often used by oral surgeons and maxillofacial surgeons.

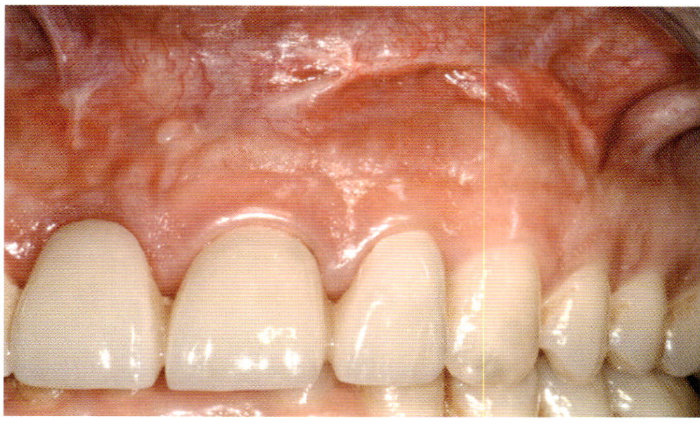

7.5 The scar of the semilunar flap is quite evident. The flap design here was convex instead of concave.

Submarginal Flap (Ochsenbein-Lubke)

The most popular paramarginal or submarginal flap is the one designed by Ochsenbein and Luebke.[8] This flap is most indicated when there is an adequate amount of attached gingiva, the expected apical lesion or surgical bony access will not involve the incision margins, and there is no periodontal involvement in the surgical area, if the probing is within normal limits. It is also especially indicated in case of the presence of dental restorations in the frontal area, in order not to interfere with the cervical tissue and avoid later aesthetic problems.

The flap is full-thickness and has one horizontal and two vertical components (📷 7.6). The horizontal is made about 1 mm coronal to the mucogingival junction, leaving at least 2 mm of attached gingiva at the coronal margin of the flap.[9] The incision has rounded scallops that follow the architecture of the teeth and later will allow an easy and passive repositioning and suturing. The two terminal scallops, the mesial and the

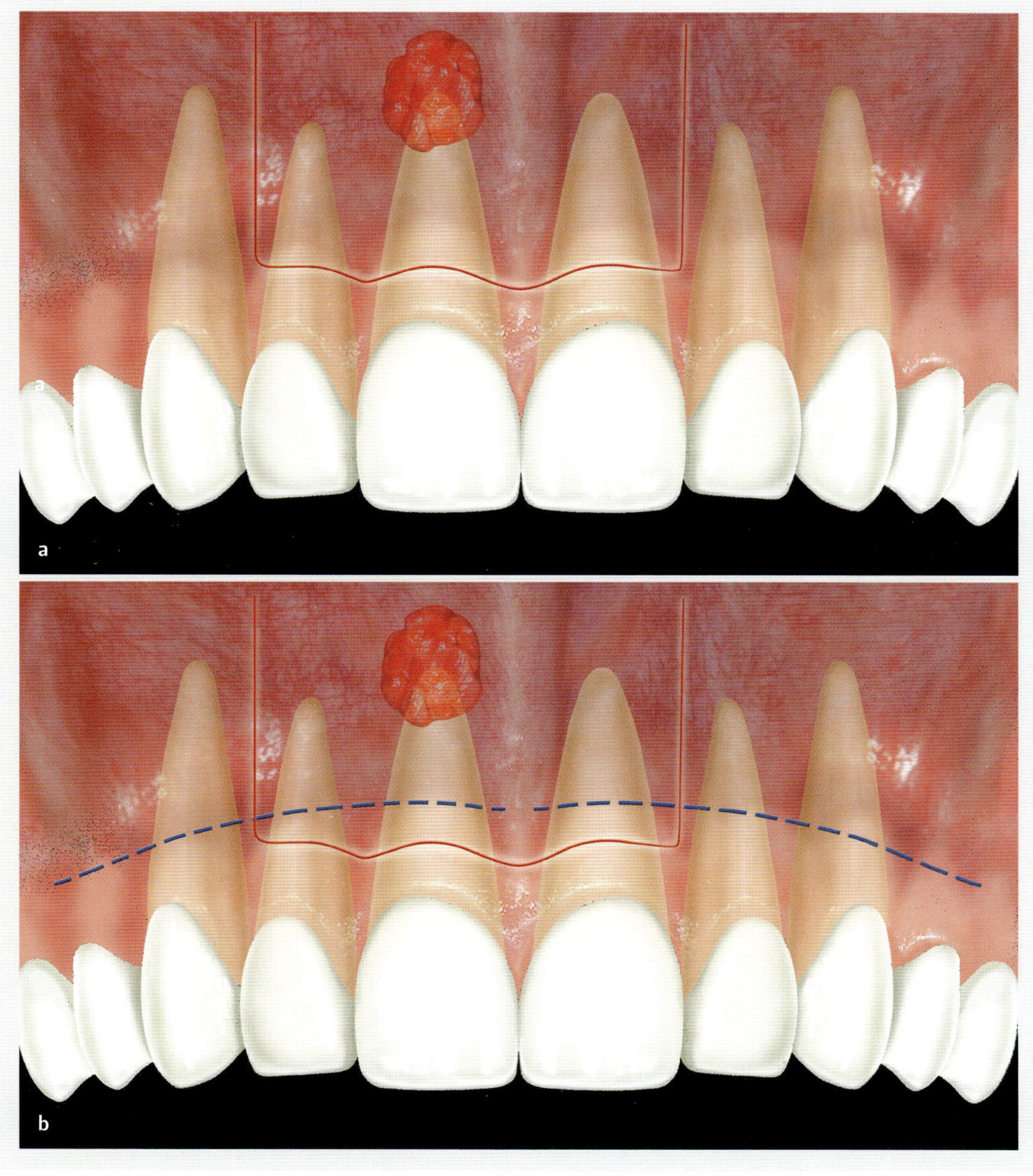

📷 **7.6 a)** A submarginal flap by Ochsenbein and Luebke. **b)** The horizontal incision is about 1 mm coronal to the mucogingival junction.

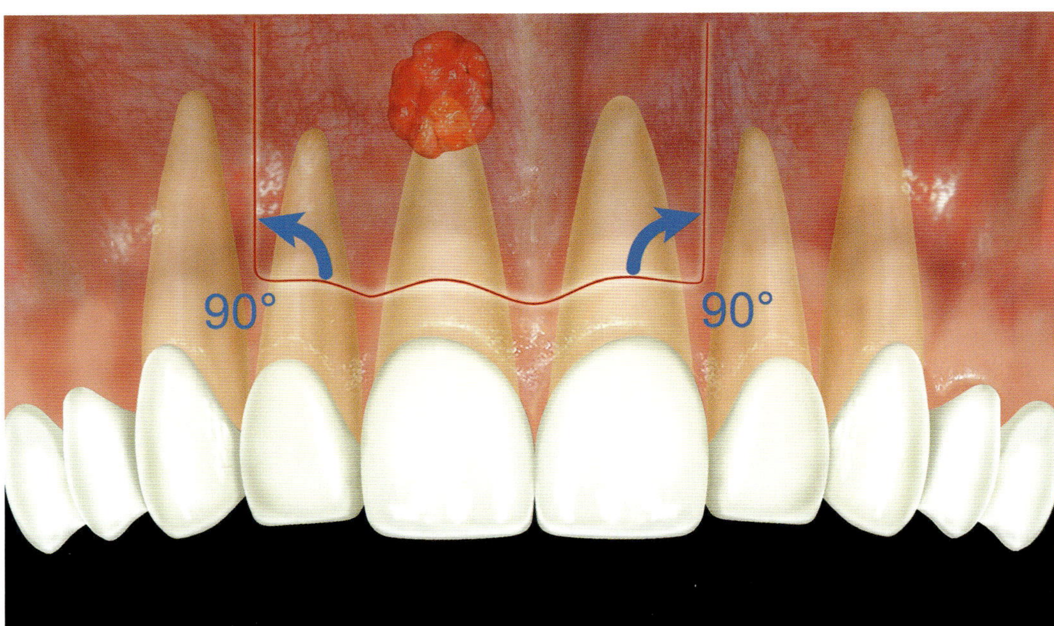

7.7 Both sides of the horizontal incision should make a 90° angle with the vertical incisions.

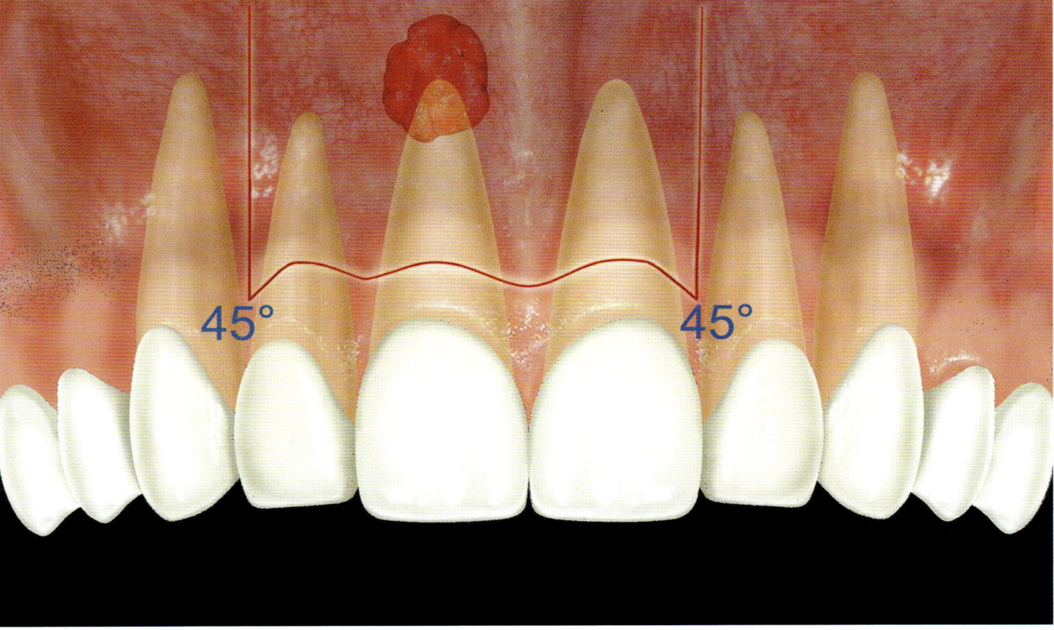

7.8 With this flap design, the flap can very easily fold in on itself during suturing.

distal, should terminate horizontally, in order to make a 90° angle with the vertical releasing incision (7.7). This will facilitate the repositioning and suturing of the flap, avoiding the flap from folding in on itself, as could happen if the angle is less than 90° (7.8). The incision must always involve one tooth mesial and one tooth distal to the one being operated on. The two vertical components at each end of the horizontal one are made as releasing incisions, in order to allow a passive and atraumatic reflection of the flap. The two vertical incisions should be placed directly over healthy bone and should always avoid bony eminences. The releasing incisions must be parallel and not divergent, so that the incision is rectangular and not trapezoidal, as it used to be years ago. They must have a 90° rounded angle with the horizontal component and must be parallel to the long axis of the teeth, in order not to section the blood vessels that are also parallel to the long axis

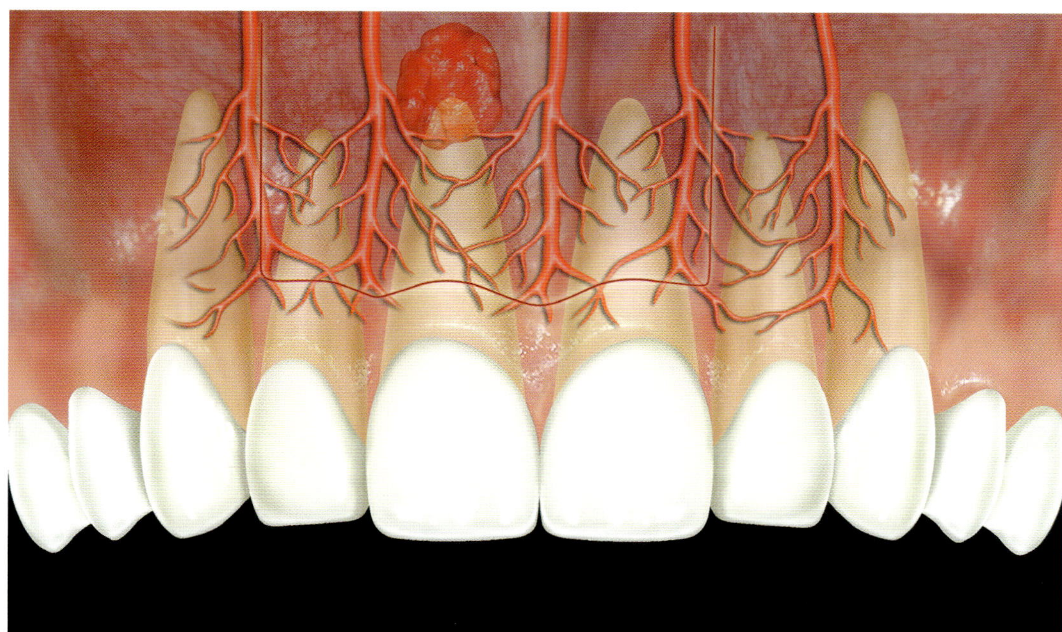

7.9 The blood supply is parallel to the long axis of the roots, and the vertical incisions should not section the blood vessels.

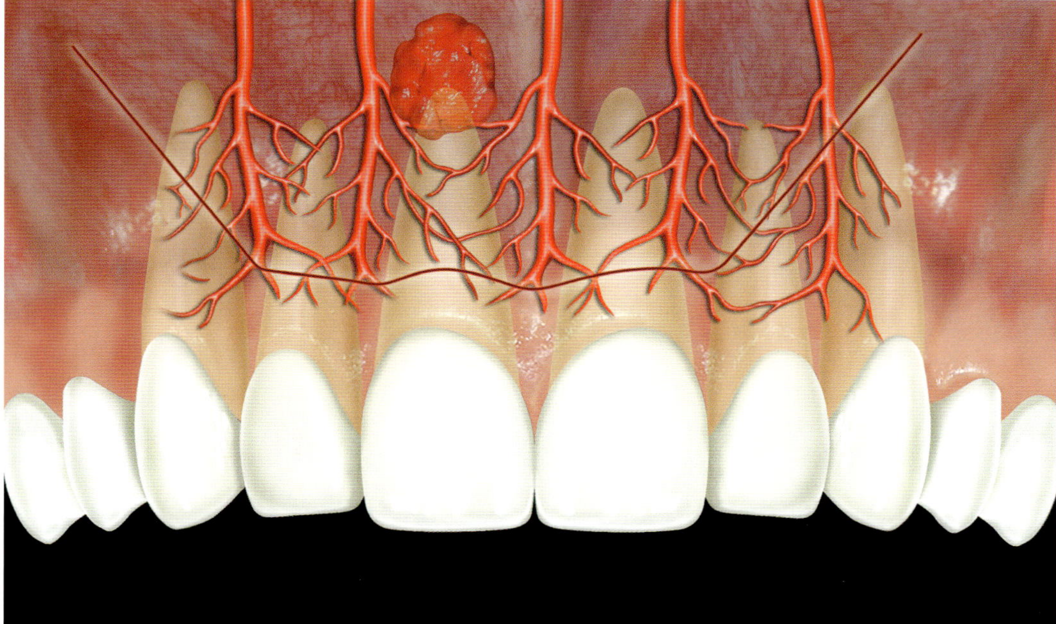

7.10 The "wide base" of the incision blocks some of the blood supply to the coronal tissue.

of the teeth (7.9). On the other hand, if the flap has a "wide base" (7.10), some of the blood supply to the coronal tissue is interrupted with consequent compromised healing. As blood vessels run mostly parallel to the long axis of the teeth from the apical to the coronal direction, one consideration is to disrupt the least number of vascular structures.[3,10,11] Previously, survival and blood supply of mobilized tissue appeared to be best, when the base was broader than the proximal end of the flap. On the other hand, blood supply to the unreflected tissues was often compromised by this approach,[10] therefore the wider base of the flap is considered an unnecessary procedure and it is no longer recommended.[11–134]

This flap design has the advantage of leaving the marginal gingiva untouched and it does not expose any restoration margins.

In case there is not an adequate amount of attached gingiva along the entire length of the horizontal component, the flap can be modified, by doing a sulcular flap where there is no attached gingiva and submarginal where there is attached gingiva. However, according to Kramper et al.,[12] the submarginal incision is the flap of choice in surgical endodontics, when not contraindicated by the anatomical location of the lesion or by insufficient attached gingival tissue.

The releasing incisions can be modified during the surgical procedure by increasing their length if the surgeon needs to eliminate any tension on the flap. Always remember that all the postoperative discomfort of the patient depends on how the flap was managed during the surgery: the reflection and retraction must be as passive and atraumatic as possible, and of course the retraction it is not the assistant's job. Only the surgeon knows where to position the retractor and how to manage the soft tissues (📷 4.35).

A disadvantage of the Ochsenbein and Luebke flap described in the literature is the risk of scarring (📷 7.11).[15,16] According to Lavagnoli and Carnevale,[16] the cause of the scar visible on the attached gingiva is the inclination of the blade to the underlying bone. If the blade is used at 90° to the bone, the incision will involve the epithelium and the periosteum and the two scars will be superimposed one on top of the other so that they become visible. On the other hand, according to the two authors, if the incision is beveled, the periosteal scar will be covered by healthy epitelium, which will hide the underlying scar. We know today that this is an old theory, based on the fact that the periodontists use beveled incisions and they don't have scars. However, we know today that scarring doesn't depend on the inclination of the blade, but rather on the correct repositioning of the flap, the precise suturing done under the operating microscope and the early removal of the sutures, as will be described later. In conclusion, the blade can be used at 90° to the bone and by following the above suggestions, there is no risk of scarring (📷 7.12).

Examples of submarginal incisions in different quadrants (📷 7.13).

Marginal Flap

This flap design is mainly indicated when there is not enough attached gingiva and where aesthetics is not a concern. Certainly, this is the flap design of choice when it is necessary to completely expose the buccal aspect of the root due to a vertical root fracture or when a perforation is suspected, since it provides excellent visibility of the root surface (📷 7.14).

Apart from the good visibility of the operative field, other advantages of this flap are: the incision and later suturing over healthy bone as well as the flap is easy to reposition and suture precisely with healing by primary intention.

The disadvantage of this flap is represented by the epithelial involvement, which as consequences could have a periodontal involvement. In case of the presence of a

Cont'd on page 148

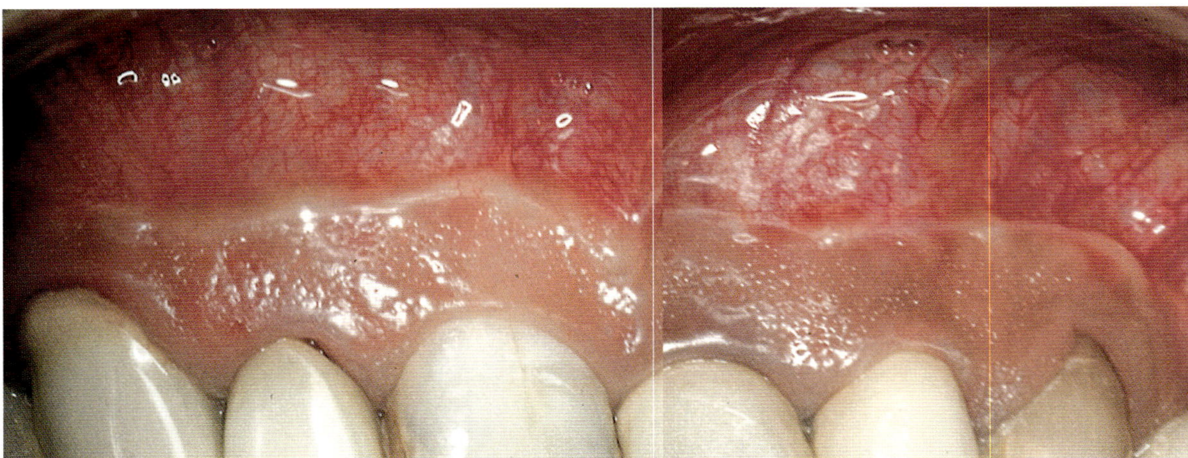

📷 **7.11** The unaesthetic scar is quite evident.

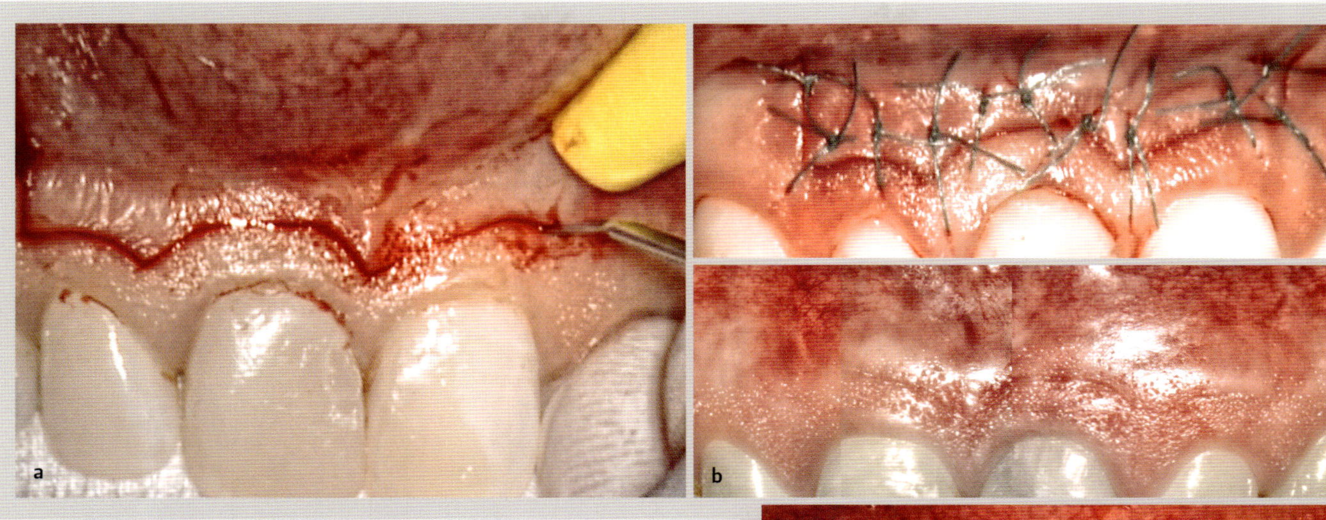

7.12 **a)** The microsurgical blade outlines the submarginal flap working at 90° to the bone. **b)** The flap has been accurately repositioned and sutured and after one month no scar is visible. **c)** Two-year recall.

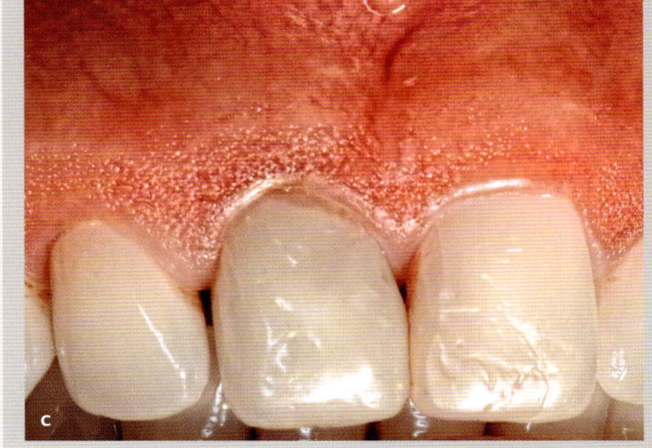

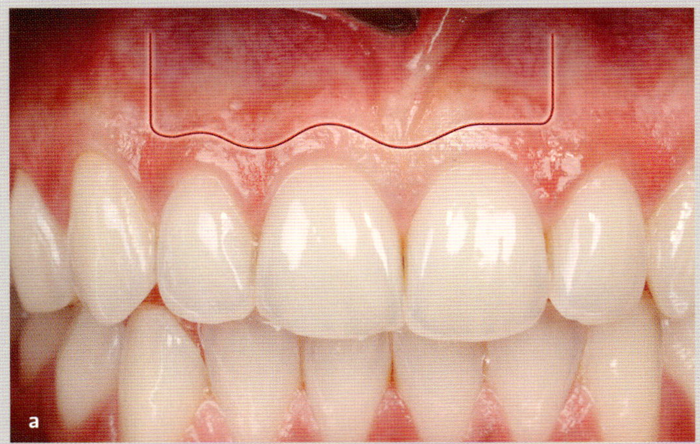

7.13 Examples of submarginal incisions in different quadrants. **a)** Upper right central incisor. **b)** Upper right first premolar. **c)** Upper right second premolar. **d)** Upper right first molar. **e)** Lower right central incisor. **f)** Lower right lateral incisor. **g)** Lower right cuspid. **h)** Lower right second premolar. **i)** Lower right first molar.

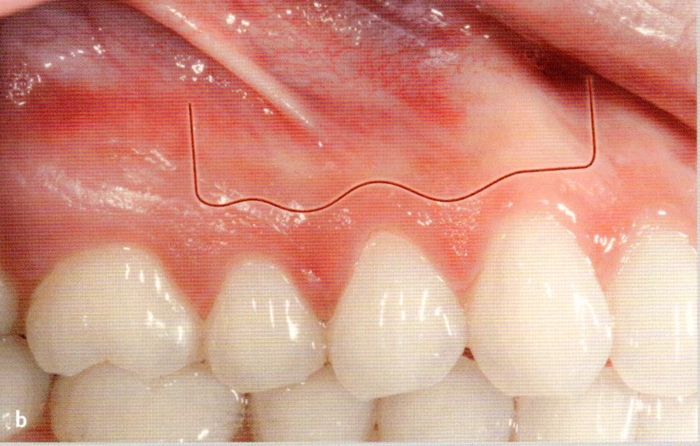

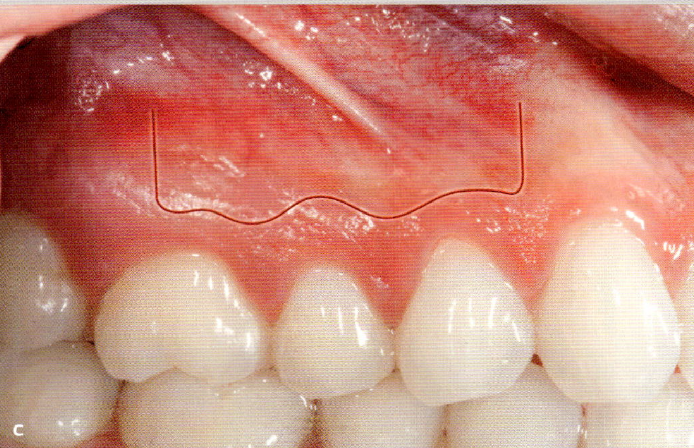

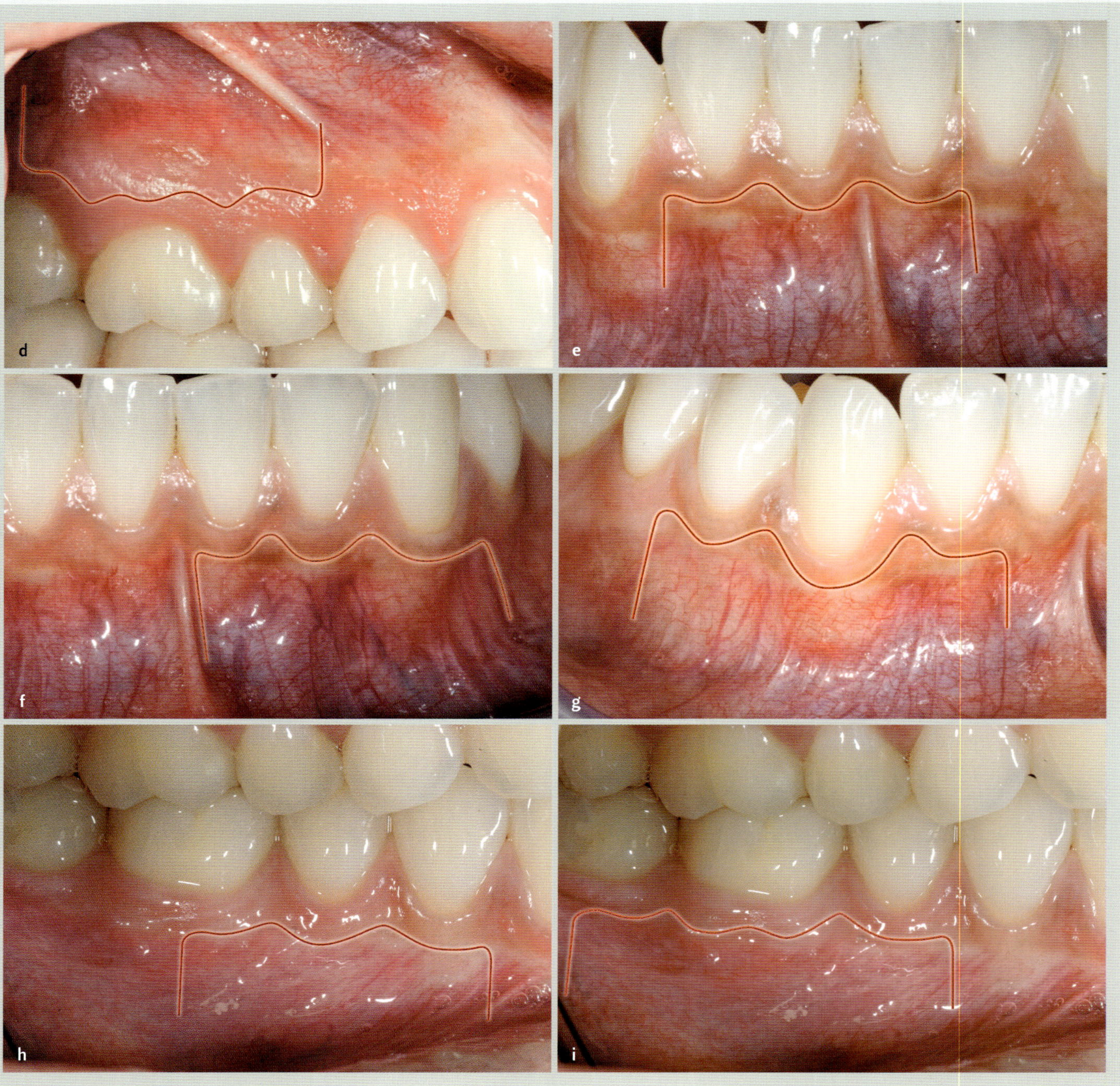

d e f g h i

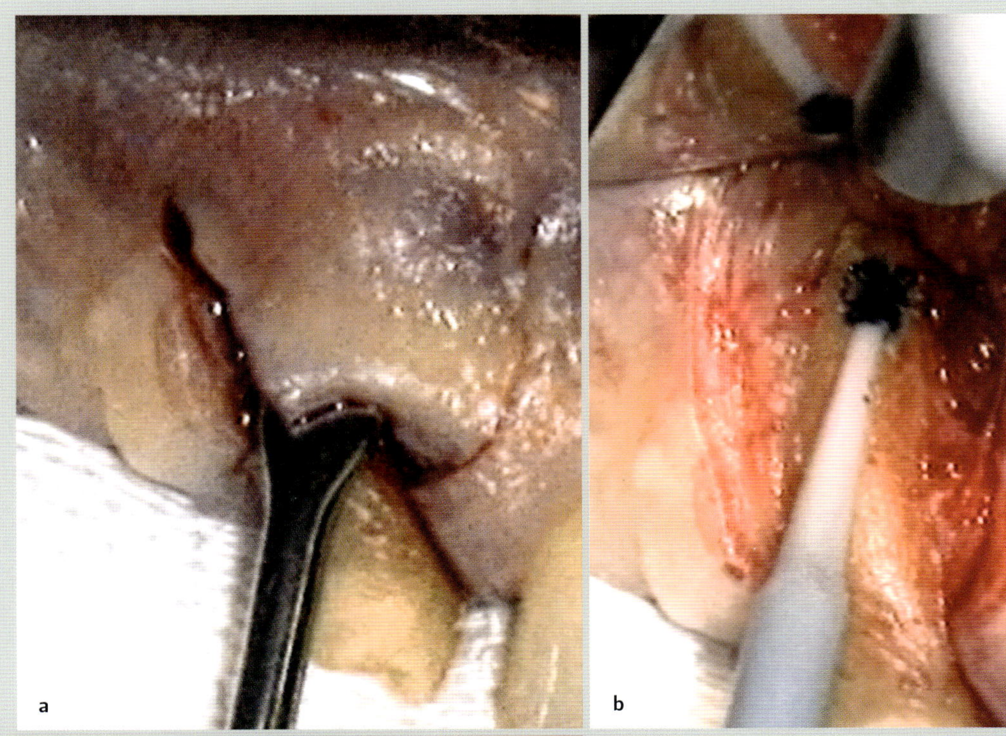

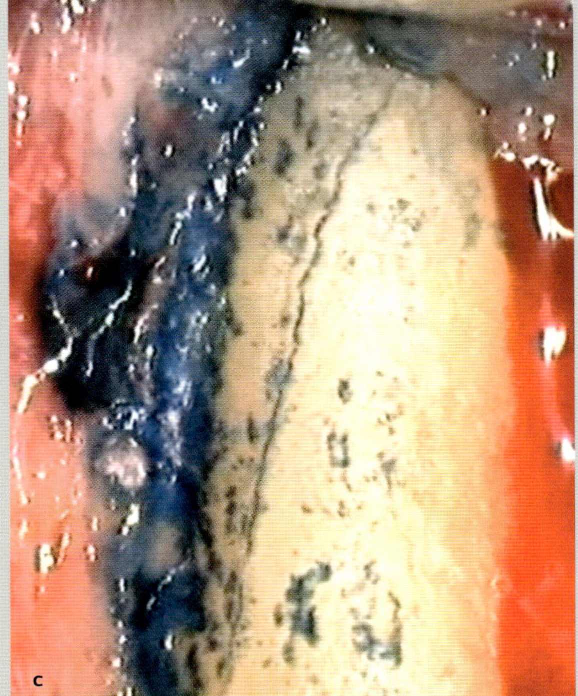

7.14 a) To confirm a vertical root fracture the instrument elevates a full thickness marginal flap. **b, c)** Methylene blue is used to make the fracture more visible.

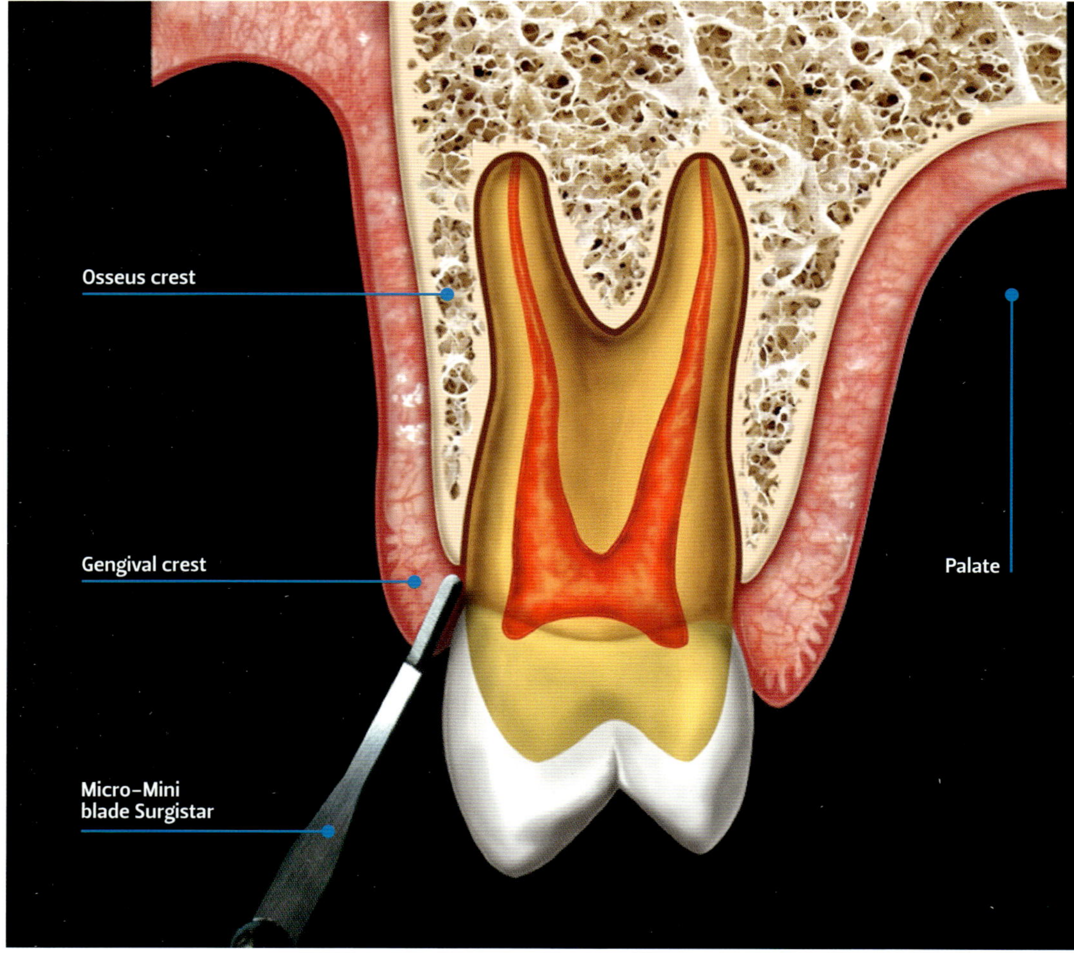

7.15 Full sulcular flap with the incision made to the osseous crest and the microsurgical blade held almost parallel to the long axis of the tooth.

fixed prosthesis involving subgingivally placed crown margins, a postoperative consequence could be recession, leading to aesthetically compromising exposure of the crown margins.

The incision is made inserting the blade into the gingival sulcus and cutting the fibers of the periodontal ligament all the way to the crestal bone, using the scalpel parallel to the long axis of the buccal surface of the tooth (7.15). The incision could be triangular if only one releasing incision is made on the mesial aspect of the flap, or rectangular or trapezoidal if a second releasing incision is made on the distal aspect of the flap.

- In case of a triangular incision, the flap comprises a horizontal incision extending at least one tooth mesially and one tooth distally to the involved area, combined with one releasing incision performed on the mesial part of the flap (7.16).[3] This flap technique exposes mostly marginal areas of the tooth in question and does not create enough access to the apical region. Therefore, it is mainly indicated for procedures in the cervical area and in the mid-root portions, for example in presence of cervical root resorptions, perforations and resections of very short roots. The main advantages of this flap design are minimal disruption of the blood supply to the mobilized tissue and easy repositioning of the wound edges. As in all intra-sulcular horizontal incisions, recession may result after the healing process.[3]
- In case there is a second vertical incision, the flap can be rectangular (7.17) or trapezoidal (7.18). In both cases the access to the apical area is excellent. The dif-

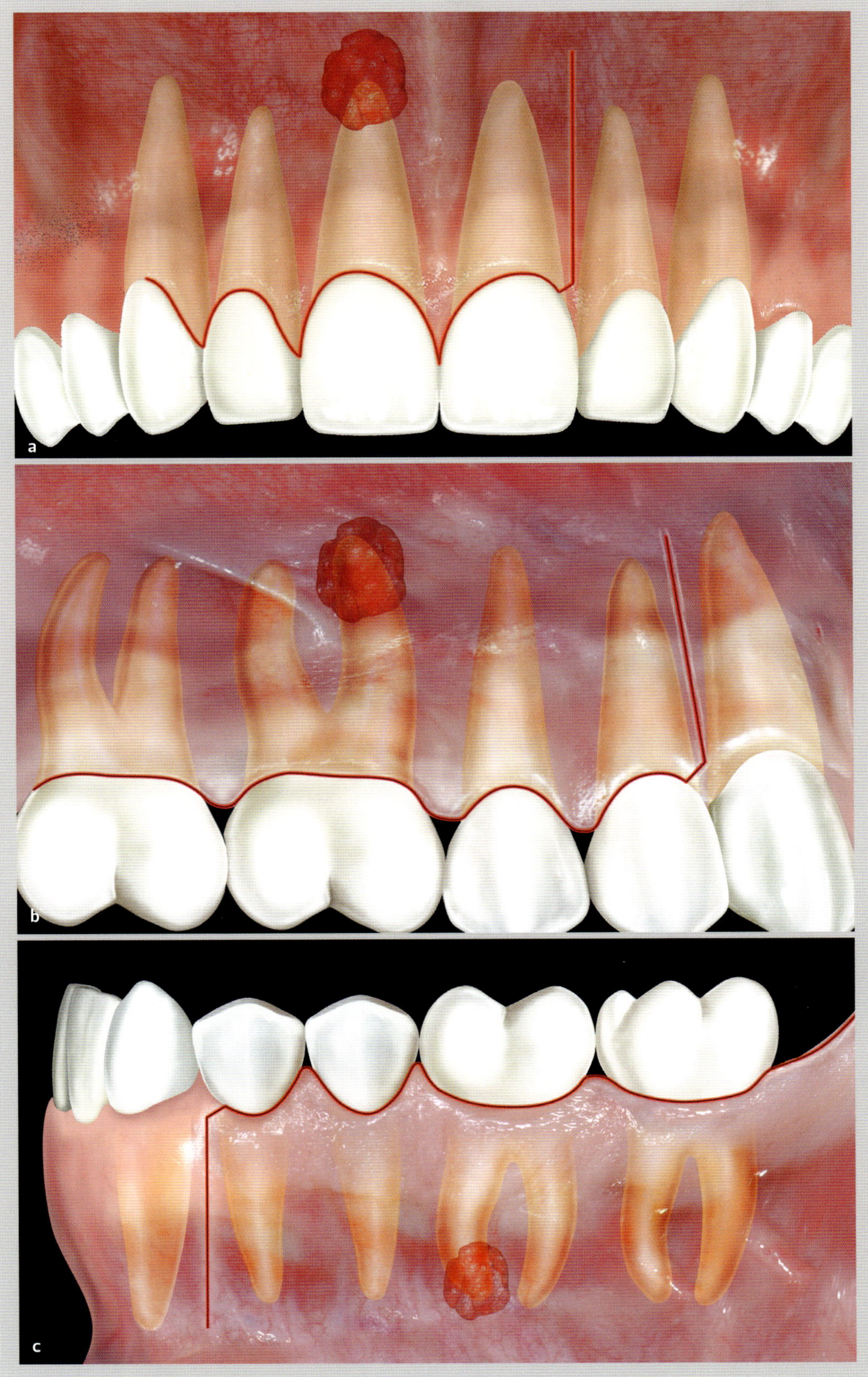

7.16 The triangular flap design, with a single releasing incision for the front maxillary teeth **(a)**, for the posterior maxillary teeth **(b)** and for the posterior mandibular teeth **(c)**.

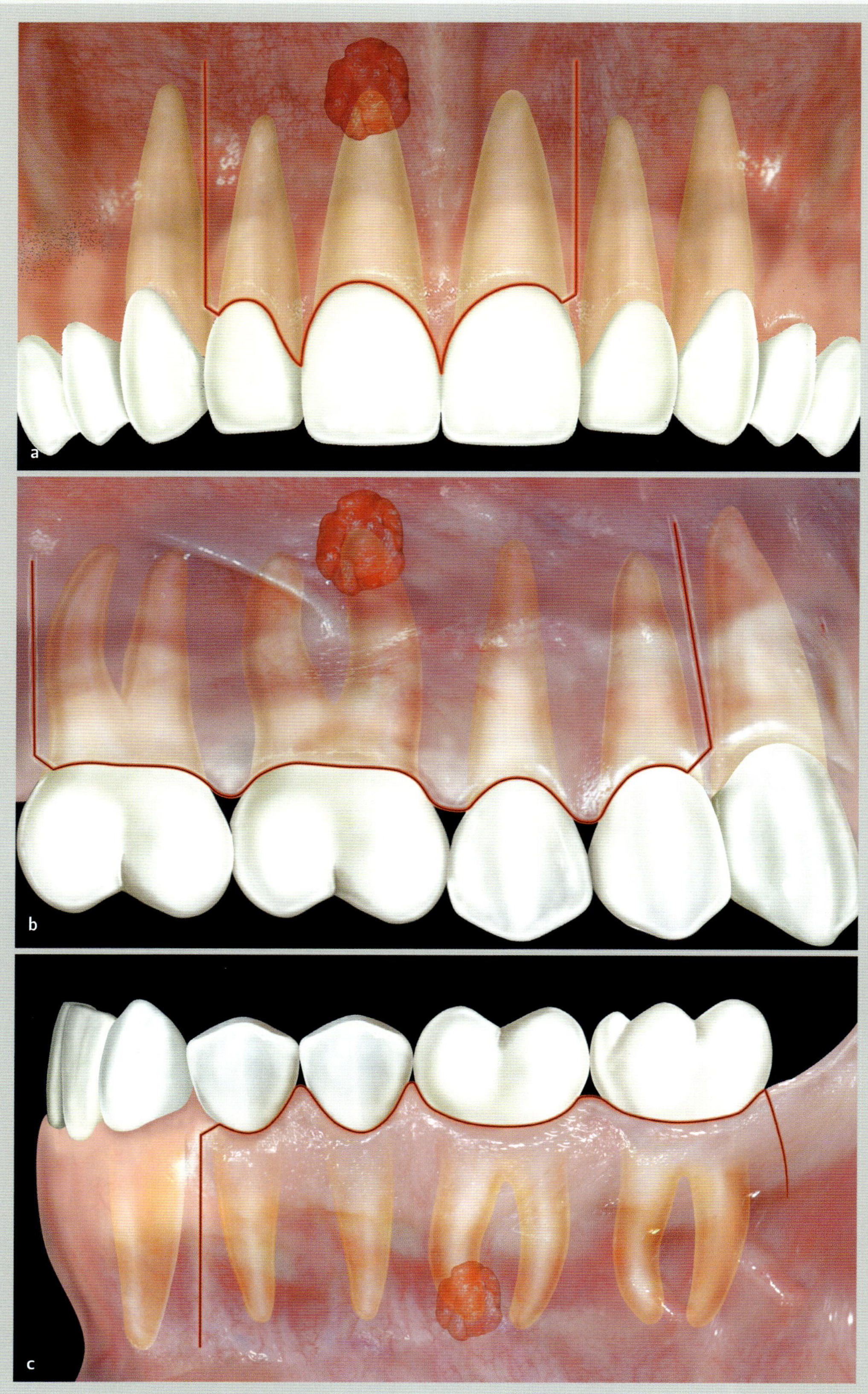

7.17 The rectangular flap design, with two releasing incisions for the front maxillary teeth **(a)**, for the posterior maxillary teeth **(b)** and for the posterior mandibular teeth **(c)**.

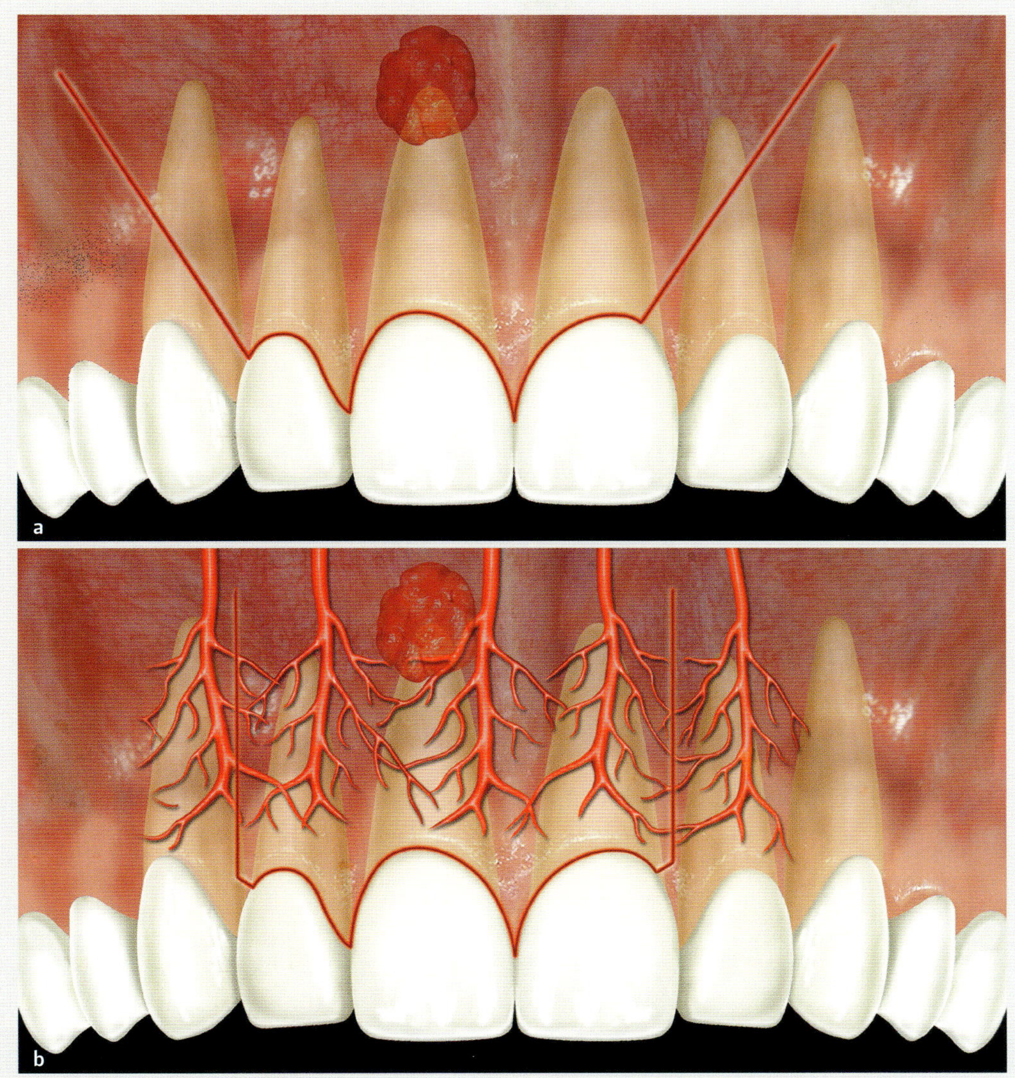

7.18 **a)** The trapezoidal flap design should be avoided in order not to section a large amount of blood supply to the coronal tissue. **b)** The vertical releasing incisions must be parallel to the long axis of the roots.

ference between the two flaps is the degree of divergence of the releasing incisions. Considering that the blood vessels run mostly parallel to the long axis of the teeth in an apico-coronal direction, the trapezoidal flap design will disrupt a larger amount of vascular structures and for this reason it should be avoided, in favor of the rectangular flap.[10,11] Years ago the trapezoidal flap was preferred, thinking of a broader blood supply of the mobilized tissue. Today we know that when using this approach, the blood supply to the unreflected tissues is compromised, therefore the trapezoidal flap as well as converging releasing incisions should be avoided.

For both the trapezoidal and the rectangular flaps the repositioning and wound closure is easy. However, in cases where the prosthetic restorations involve subgingivally placed crown margins, a postoperative consequence could be recession, leading to aesthetically compromising exposure of the crown margins.[3]

Papilla Base Flap

A sulcular full thickness flap is frequently used in periradicular surgery and a frequent complication is the shrinkage of the papilla during healing, that may initiate the ultimate loss of the papilla height. This has been demonstrated in a recent study by Zimmermann et al.[17] and becomes particularly evident 3 months after surgery. From this study we know today that a conventional sulcular flap results in a considerable retraction of papilla height, with consequent functional, phonetic and aesthetic problems. Complete and predictable restoration of lost interdental papillae remains one of the biggest challenges in periodontal reconstructive surgery,[18] therefore it is imperative to maintain the integrity of the papilla during restorative and surgical procedures.[19]

The interdental papilla is the portion of the gingiva between two adjacent teeth. The presence or absence of the interdental papilla depends upon the distance between the contact point to the crestal bone.[20]

In anterior periodontal surgery a papillary retention procedure is advocated to maintain the papillary height to maximize postoperative aesthetics.[21]

In surgical endodontics exposure of the bone covering the roots and the apices is required and to achieve this access a full thickness flap must be raised, which consists of gingival and mucosal tissue as well as periosteum. If the sulcular incision is selected, the clinician must be aware of the periodontal complications that quite often may arise.

To prevent marginal recession and an unpredictable shrinkage of the papilla during healing, the submarginal incision can be selected.[8] However, this flap design can only be used when there is a broad band of attached gingiva and the expected apical lesion or surgical bony access will not extend to the incision line. As has been already described, this flap design preserves the marginal gingiva and in maxillary anterior areas is preferred in situations with subgingivally placed margins of crowns and bridgework.

According to some authors,[22] the sulcular flap is the most frequently used in surgical endodontics. It is therefore important to adopt a new incision for the marginal mucoperiosteal flap, specifically designed to prevent loss of interdental papilla height. This new flap design involves the preservation of the entire papilla and is called the "papilla base incision".[19]

The papilla base flap consists of two releasing vertical incisions, connected by the papilla base incision and the horizontal intrasulcular incision. The vertical incisions start and end at a 90° angle to the gingival margin, resulting in a curved line at the base of the papilla (7.19). The marginal incision starts with the preparation of the papilla base incision using a 2.5 mm

Cont'd on page 156

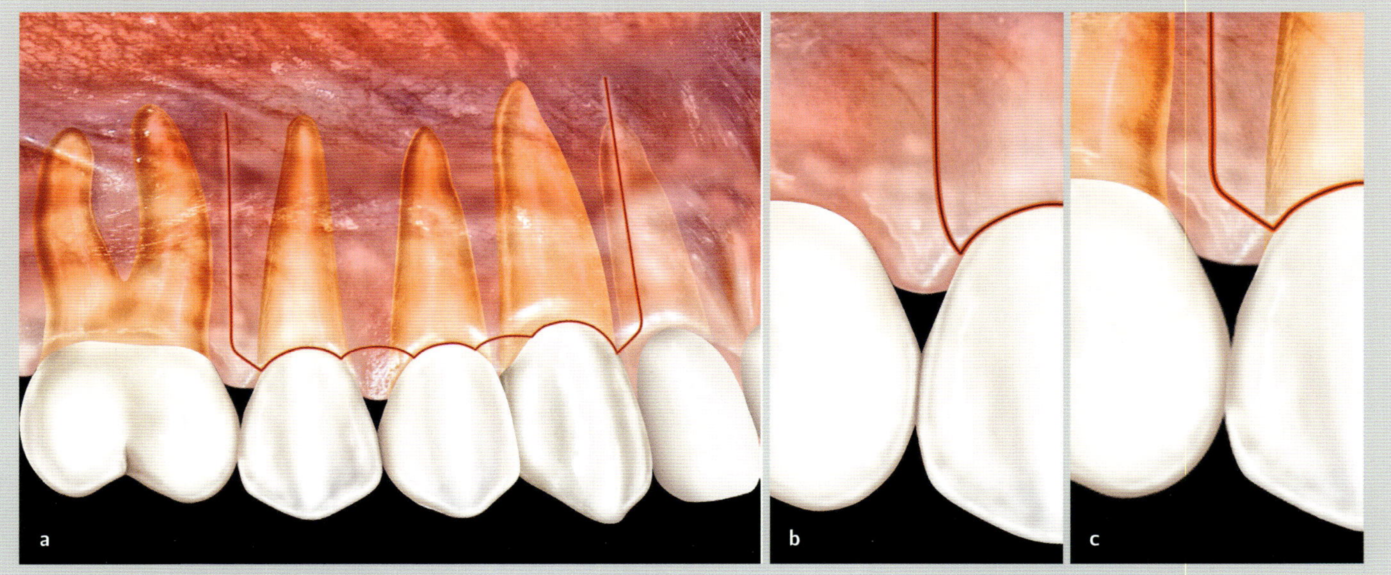

7.19 a) The curved incision must be perpendicular to the gingival margin. **b)** The vertical releasing incision creates a compromised tissue area. The proximal unreflected tissue portion could easily necrotize because of insufficient blood supply. **c)** The correct vertical incision begins perpendicular to the gingival margin.[3,15]

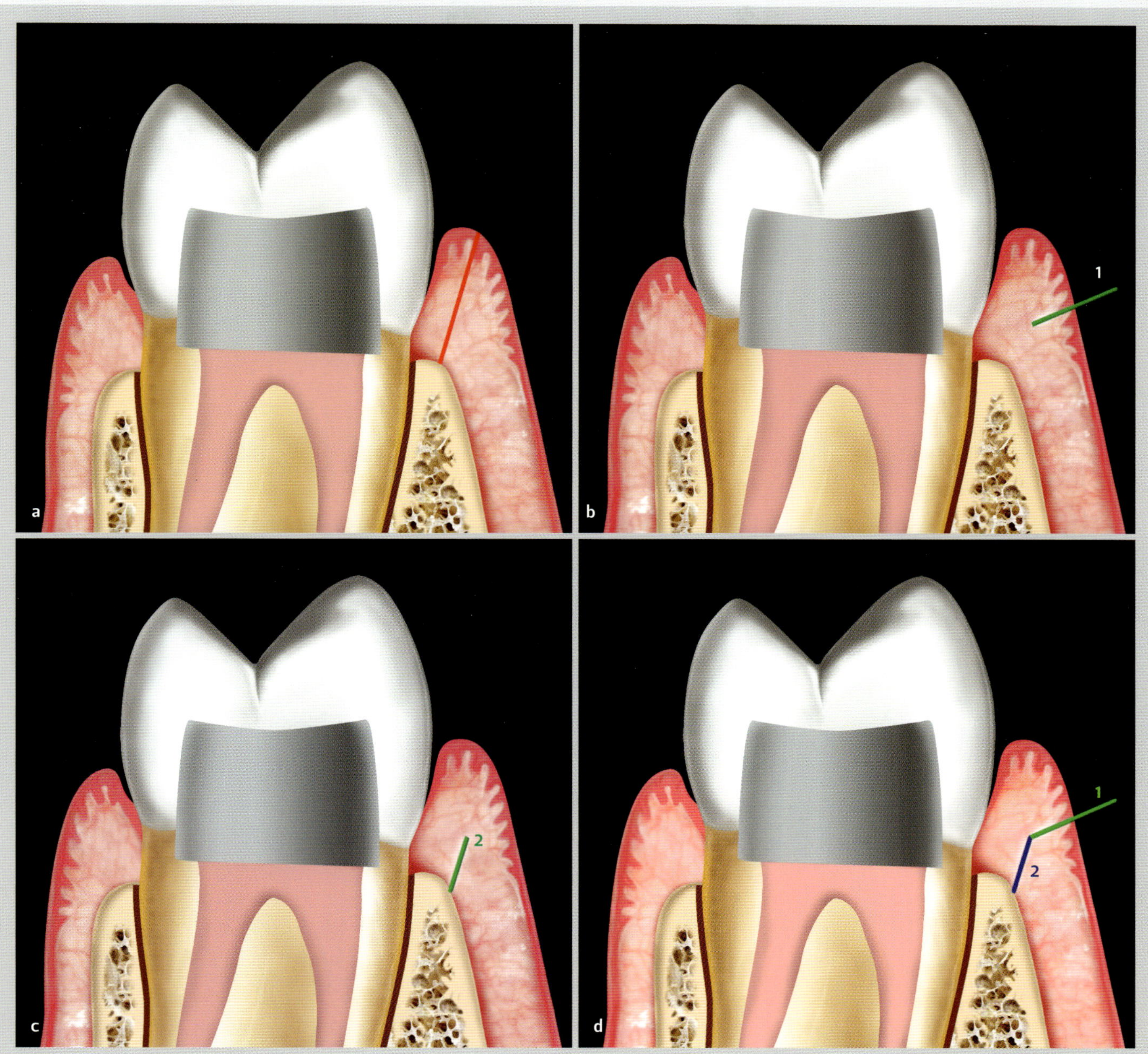

7.20 Schematic drawing of the incision design for the papilla base flap. **a)** Incorrect incision directed towards the crestal bone. **b)** Correct incision. The first shallow incision is placed at the level of the lower third of the papilla in a slightly curved line, connecting one side of the papilla to the other, perpendicular to the gingival margin (line #1). **c)** A second incision is placed at the base of the previously created incision, inclined apically, almost parallel to the long axis of the tooth and directed towards the crestal bone margin (line #2). **d)** The result is a split-thickness flap at the base of the papilla.[3,15]

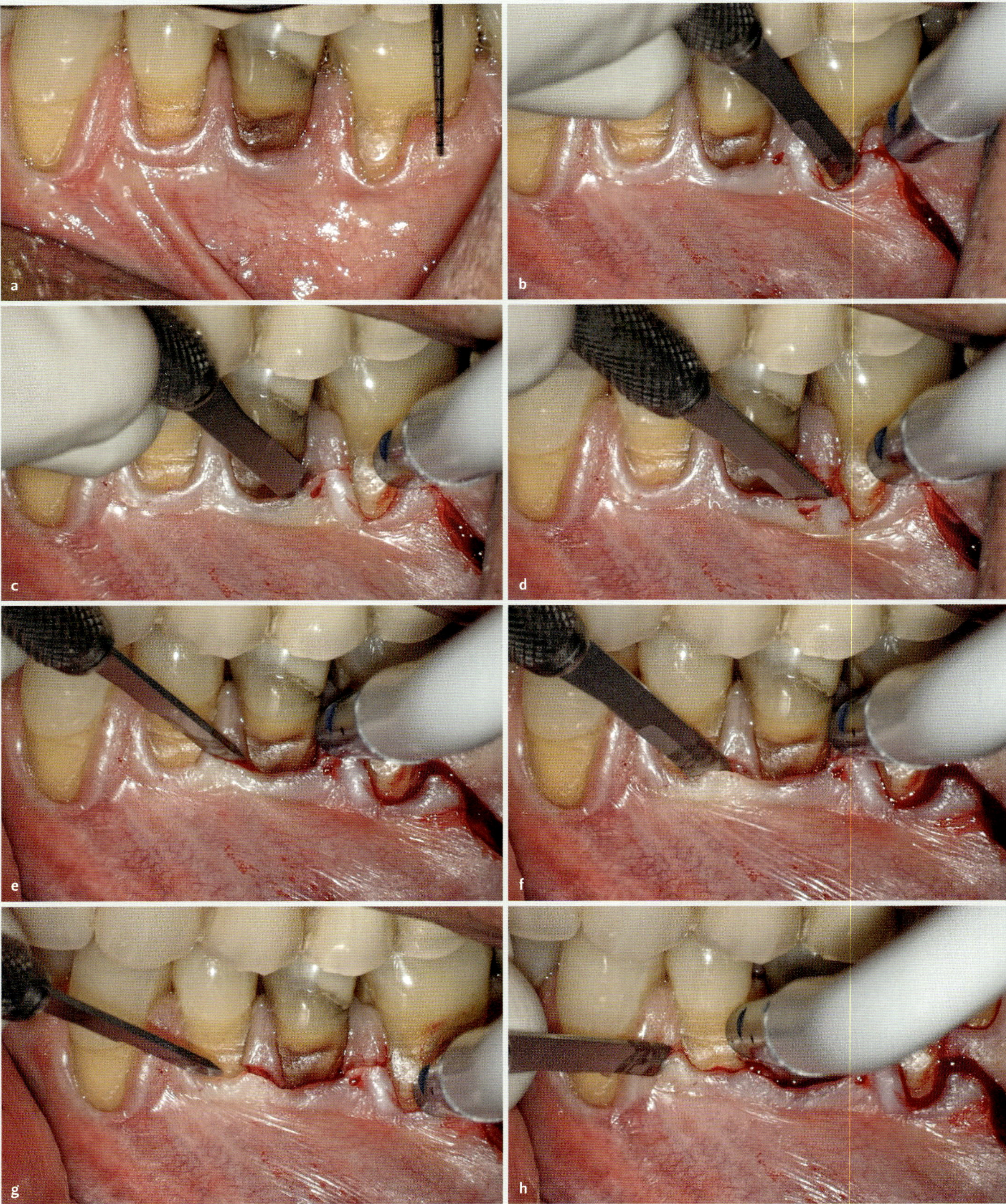
a
b
c
d
e
f
g
h

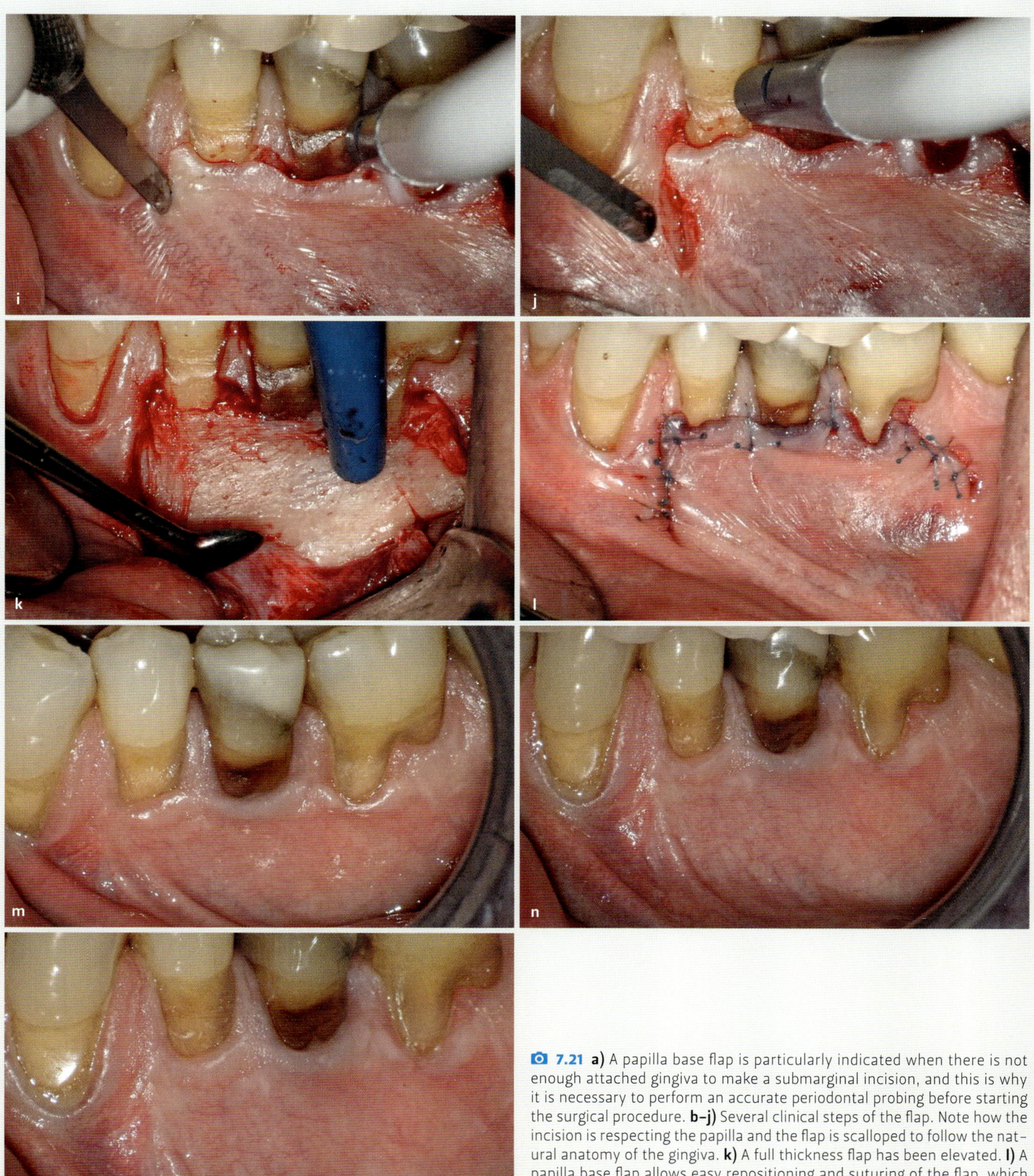

7.21 **a)** A papilla base flap is particularly indicated when there is not enough attached gingiva to make a submarginal incision, and this is why it is necessary to perform an accurate periodontal probing before starting the surgical procedure. **b–j)** Several clinical steps of the flap. Note how the incision is respecting the papilla and the flap is scalloped to follow the natural anatomy of the gingiva. **k)** A full thickness flap has been elevated. **l)** A papilla base flap allows easy repositioning and suturing of the flap, which will heal by primary intention and no scarring. **m)** Healing of the soft tissues after one month. **n, o)** Four months after surgery perfect healing is evident and no scarring is present (*Courtesy of Dr. Fabio Gorni, Milano, Italy*).

Cont'd from page 152

microsurgical blade Surgistar (Micro-Mini Blade Surgistar USM6910, Vista, CA) having a round configuration at the tip and cutting edges on both sides and all around the tip.[19]

The papilla base incision requires two different incisions at the base of the papilla.[3]

- The first shallow incision separates epithelium and connective tissue to the depth of 1.5 mm from the surface of the gingiva. The incision is placed at the level of the lower third of the papilla in a slightly curved line, connecting one side of the papilla to the other. The incision begins and ends in a 90° angle to the tooth and gingiva (7.20b). This shallow incision prevents thinning of the coronal aspect of the flap.
- For the second incision, the scalpel is placed at the base of the previously created incision and subsequently inclined apically, almost parallel to the long axis of the tooth, directed towards the crestal bone margin (7.20c). With this second incision, a split thickness flap is prepared in the apical third of the papilla base. The incision terminates at crestal bone level and separates the periosteum from the bone (7.20d). From this level on the preparation continues as a full thickness mucoperiosteal flap (7.21).

Buccally over the tooth the vertical incision and papilla base incision are joined by an intrasulcular incision. The scalpel is moved within the sulcus, dissecting the gingiva to the crestal bone. The sulcular incision stretches from the releasing incision to the start of the papilla base incision, or from one papilla to the next papilla. The flap now can be mobilized and retracted, during the root-end resection and filling.

Regarding the flap closure, an atraumatic and tension free suturing is a key factor to improve healing. The flap closure starts from the releasing incision, using a 6/0 suture, because of the close proximity to muscle insertion in the mucosa, which may exert some tension to the wound during mastication and speech.[3] The material of choice is a multifilament suture, with a coating providing a monofilamentous appearance with a smooth surface. The papilla base incision is best sutured with two or three 7/0 interrupted sutures, depending on the width of the papilla. The removal of the suture should be performed after 3 to 5 days to promote rapid healing and the recall evaluation after three months should reveal completely undetectable or only partially detectable incision lines and generally should demonstrate excellent healing.[3]

While the papilla base incision is challenging to perform, its use can lead to predictable results.[3]

Flap Elevation

The elevation of the flap must be done in an atraumatic manner, in order not to cause postoperative discomfort to the patient and to guarantee a fast and uneventful healing. For this pourpose a sharp periosteal elevator is used, like one of the Ruddle elevators (American Eagle, Missoula, MT) (7.22), by gently dissecting the periosteum from the osseous surface, without leaving fragments of the periosteum that later will cause continuous bleeding. The elevator should be inserted in the releasing incision at the junction of the submucosa and the attached gingiva and the full thickness flap should be gently undermined and dissected without any tearing, moving the instrument in an apico-coronal direction (7.23) and moving horizontally from mesial to distal. This approach has been referred to as *undermining elevation*.[23] The tendency is to introduce the elevator in the horizontal portion of the incision and push the tissue with a corono-apical movement. This

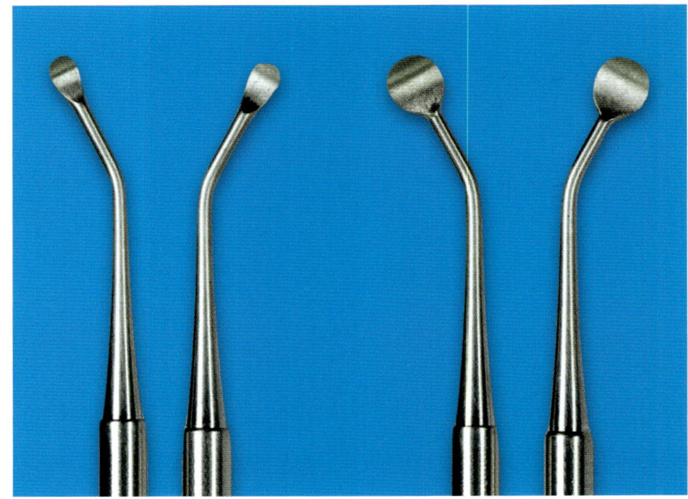

7.22 Ruddle elevators (American Eagle, Missoula, MT).

is contraindicated as it will easily cause tearing of the tissue and difficult management of the bleeding later.[11] In case of a chronic lesion and the presence of a sinus tract, the sectioning of the sinus tract with a scalpel could be necessary to complete the elevation process. After elevation of the gingival tissue, elevation is continued in an apical direction, lifting the alveolar mucosa and underlying periosteum from cortical bone to allow adequate surgical access to the periradicular tissues.[24] After reflecting a mucogingival flap, scaling of root-attached tissues and tissue tags on cortical bone should be avoided to allow rapid reattachment and protection from bone resorption.[24–26]

Flap Retraction

Once the elevation is completed, retraction of the tissue is necessary to provide surgical access to the apex of the involved tooth or teeth. The retractor must always rest on cortical bone with light but firm pressure directed against the bone, so that the instrument merely acts as a passive mechanical barrier to the reflected tissues. Impingement of the tissue during the retraction process must be avoided because this will cause postoperative pain and swelling.

The retraction of the flap must be done in an atraumatic manner, in order not to cause postoperative discomfort to the patient. If at the beginning of the retrac-

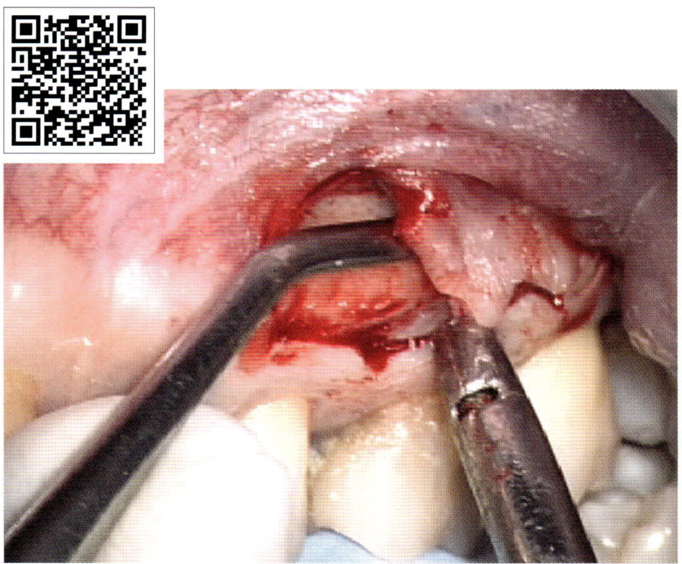

7.23 The elevator undermines the full thickness flap.

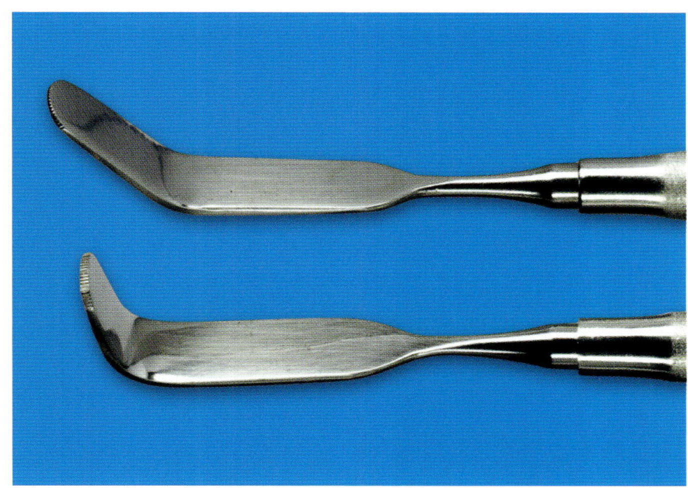

7.24 Carr retractors.

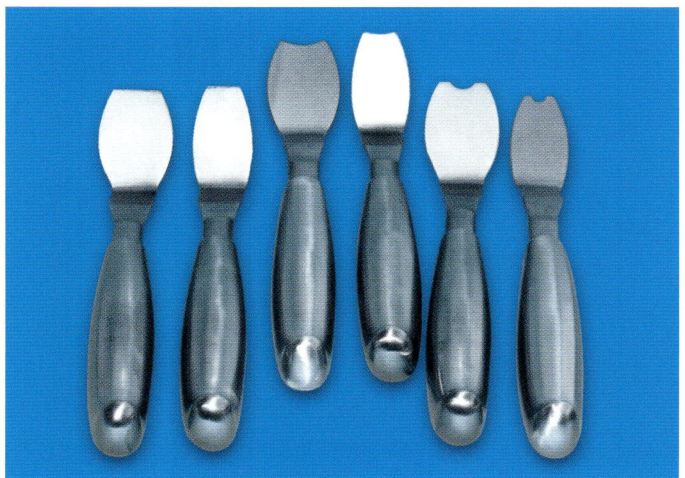

7.25 Rubinstein retractors.

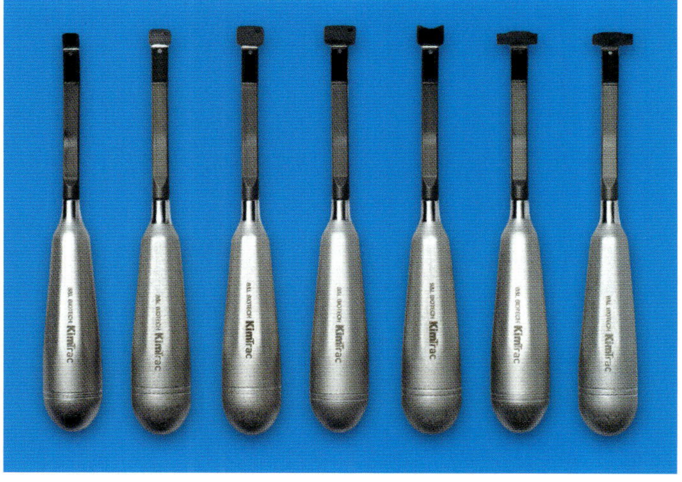

7.26 Kim retractors.

tion the operator realizes that there is too much tension on the flap, then this means that the releasing incisions are too short and need to be extended. To stabilize the retractor, a groove can be made on the osseous surface apical to the surgical site, using a high-speed bur.

A 15 mm long horizontal groove is cut into the bone with a Lindemann bur, beyond the apex to allow space for the osteotomy and subsequent apicoectomy. The groove permits secure anchoring of the serrated retractor tip and secure, steady retraction of the flap.[13]

This will prevent the slipping of the retractor and the impingement of the tissue. The groove is particularly necessary when the surgical procedure is performed in the lower quadrant and the retractor is very close to the mental foramen: serious damage to the mental nerve can be caused by the pressure of the retractor sometimes held for up to one hour over the nerve. To avoid this, after identifying the foramen, a groove is made above the mental nerve, then the nerve is protected with the retractor in the groove made just above it (6.9).[13]

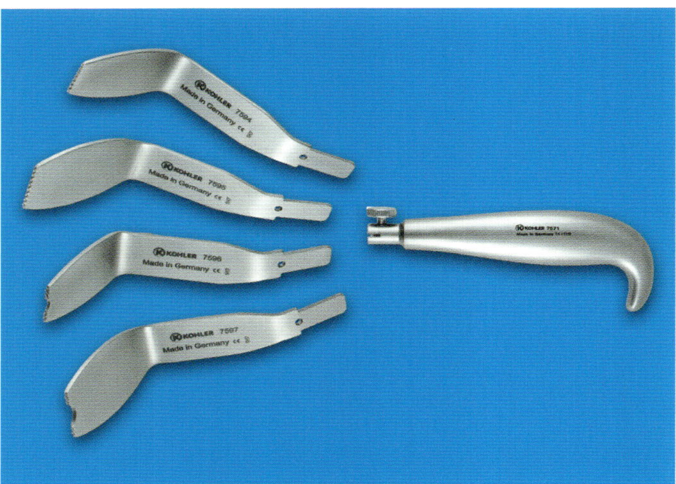

7.27 Rubinstein retractors modified by Kohler, with retractor blades interchangeable (Kohler Medizintechnik, Germany).

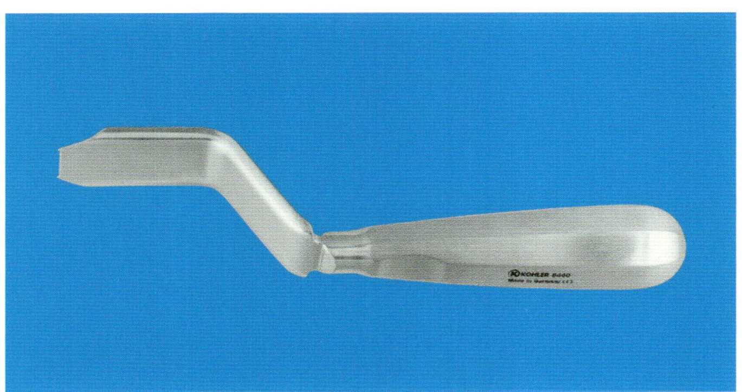

7.28 Han retractor with a reflective surface to allow indirect vision (Kohler Medizintechnik, Germany).

Many retractors are available on the market. The most popular are the Carr retractors (7.24), the Rubinstein retractors (7.25), the Kim retractors (7.26) and retractors manufactured by Khohler (7.27, 7.28).

Regarding the time of retraction, an axiomatic principle of surgery is that the longer the flap is retracted, the greater the complications following surgery. This seems a logical conclusion because the vascular flow is undoubtedly impeded during retraction with consequent damage and delay of the wound healing. However, the literature fails to disclose meaningful evidence which could be directly extrapolated to periradicular surgical procedures. Whether the retraction time is long or short, flaps should be irrigated frequently with saline solution during surgical procedures to prevent dehydration of the periosteal surface of the flap.[24]

Careful handling, undermining elevation and retraction using the groove technique are helpful to avoid unnecessary injuries to the reflected tissue. Keeping the flap moist at all times helps avoid shrinkage and dehydration.[27]

Closure of the Surgical Flap

Before suturing, is mandatory to take a postoperative radiograph. The flap is repositioned and a wet sterile gauze is positioned over the flap to keep it moist. After suturing, it is necessary to compress the repositioned flap with a saline-moistened gauze to create a thin fibrin layer between the flap and cortical bone.[24,26,28] The thin blood cloth with parallel fibrin fibers will be later replaced by new fibrous tissue, resulting in collagen adhesion.[28] Among other principles (incision, flap design, atraumatic and gentle tissue management), a passive and tension-free wound closure is fundamental for proper wound healing and for a successful functional and esthetic outcome.[3]

REFERENCES

1. Stropko J. *Micro-Surgical Endodontics*. In: Castellucci A, ed. *Endodontics*, vol. III. Florence, Italy: Il Tridente; 2005:342-411.
2. Gutmann JL, Harrison JW. *Surgical access: soft tissue management*. In: Gutmann JL, Harrison JW, eds. Surgical Endodontics. Oxford: Blackwell Scientific Publications; 1991:153-182.
3. Velvart P, Peters CI. *Soft tissue management in endodontic surgery*. J Endod. 2005;31(1):4-16.
4. Velvart P. *Surgical retreatment*. In: Bergenholtz G, Hørsted-Bindslev P, Reit C, eds. *Textbook of endodontology*. Oxford: Blackwell Munksgaard; 2003:312-26.
5. Vreeland DL, Tidwell E. *Flap design for surgical endodontics*. Oral Surg Oral Med Oral Pathol. 1982;54:461-5.
6. Lubow RM, Wayman BE, Cooley RL. *Endodontic flap design: analysis and recommendations for current usage*. Oral Surg Oral Med Oral Pathol. 1984;58:207-12.
7. Peters LB, Wesselink PR. *Soft tissue management in endodontic surgery*. Dent Clin North Am. 1997;41:513-28.
8. Luebke RG. *Surgical endodontics*. Dent Clin North Am. 1974;18:379-91.
9. Lang NP, Loe H. *The relationship between the width of keratinized gingiva and gingival health*. J Clin Periodontol. 1972;43:623-27.
10. Mormann, W, Meier C, Firestone A. *Gingival blood circulation after experimental wounds in man*. J Clin Periodontol. 1979;6:417-24.
11. Gutmann JL, Harrison WH. *Flap designs and incisions*. In: Gutmann JL, Harrison WH, eds. *Surgical endodontics*. St. Louis, Missouri: Ishijaku EuroAmerica, Inc; 1994:162-75.
12. Kim S, Pecora G, Rubinstein R. *Comparison of traditional and microsurgery in endodontics*. In: Kim S, Pecora G, Rubinstein R eds. *Color atlas of microsurgery in endodontics*. Philadelphia: W.B. Saunders; 2001:5-11.
13. Kim S, Kratchman S. *Modern endodontic surgery concepts and practice: a review*. J Endod. 2006; 32(7):601-623.
14. Kramper BJ, Kaminski EJ, Osetek EM, Heuer MA. *A comparative study of the wound healing of three types of flap design used in periapical surgery*. J Endod. 1984;10(1): 17-25.
15. Velvart P, Peters, OA. *Soft tissue management*. In: Torabinejad M, Rubinstein R eds. *The art and science of contemporary surgical endodontics*. Philadelphia: W.B. Saunders; 2001:5-11.
16. Lavagnoli G, Carnevale G. *Tecniche chirurgiche in endodonzia: note tecnico-cliniche sulla incisione della mucosa e sulla sutura*. Dental Cadmos. 1984:13 [In Italian].
17. Zimmermann U, Ebner J, Velvart P. *Papilla healing following sulcular full thickness flap in endodontic surgery*. J Endod. 2001;27:219.
18. Blatz MB, Hurzeler MB, Strub JR. *Reconstruction of the lost interdendal papilla - presentation of surgical and non surgical approaches*. Int J Periodont Restor Dent. 1999;19:395-406.
19. Velvart P. *Papilla base incision: a new approach to recession-free healing of the interdental papilla after endodontic surgery*. Int Endod J. 2002;35:453-60.
20. Tarnow DP, Magner AW, Fletcher P. *The effect of the distance from the contact point to the crest of bone on the presence or absence of the interproximal dental papilla*. J Periodont. 1992;63:995-96.
21. Michaelides PL, Wilson SG. *A comparison of papillary retention versus full-thickness flaps with internal mattress sutures in anterior periodontal surgery*. Int J Periodont Restor Dent. 1996;16:388-97.
22. Beer R, Baumann MA, Kim S. Endodontology. Stuttgart: Thieme Verlag. 2000;238-39.
23. Gutmann JL, Harrison JW. *Posterior endodontic surgery: anatomical considerations and clinical techniques*. Int Endod J. 1985;18:8-34.
24. Gutmann JL, Harrison JW. *Surgical access: soft tissue management*. In: Gutmann JL, Harrison JW, eds. *Surgical endodontics*. Boston: Blackwell Scientific Pubblications, Inc. 1991;153-202.
25. Carr G, Bentkover S. *Surgical Endodontics*. In: Cohen S, Burns R, eds. *Pathways of the pulp*. St. Louis, MO: Mosby Inc. 1998;608-56.
26. Harrison J, Jurosky K. *Wound healing in the tissues of the periodontium following periradicular surgery. 2. The dissectional wound*. J Endod. 1991;17:544-52.
27. Zuolo ML, Ferreira MO, Gutmann JL. *Prognosis in periradicular surgery: a clinical prospective study*. Int Endod J. 2000;33:91-8.
28. Selvig K, Torabinejad M. *Wound healing after mucoperiosteal surgery in the cat*. J Endod. 1996;22: 507-15.

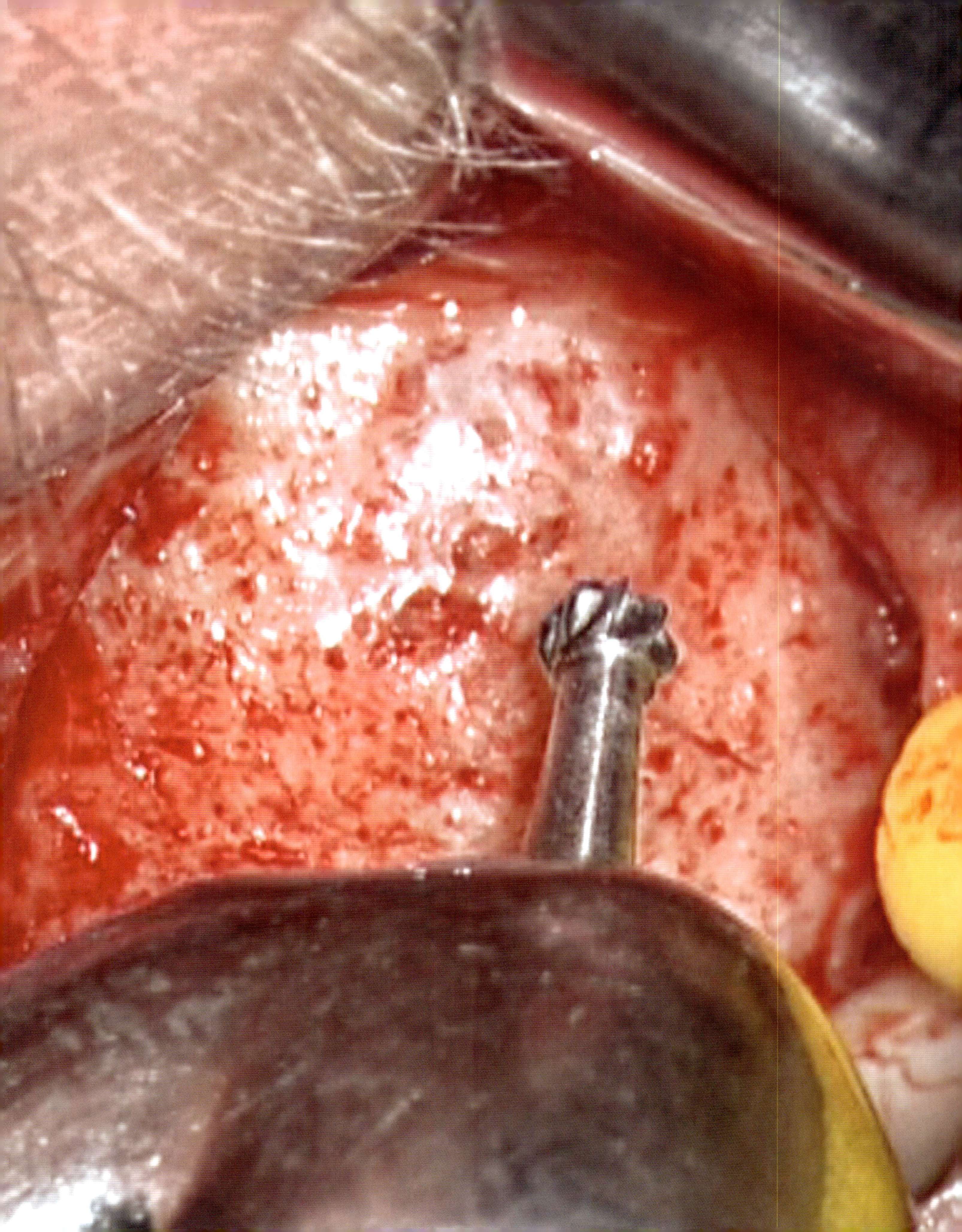

Hard Tissue Management

One of the primary objectives of microsurgical endodontics is to get surgical access through the cortical bone to the roots of the offending teeth. Once the surgical flap has been reflected and retracted, the root apex has to be located. In the event of a sinus tract or of a long-lasting resorptive pathosis that has perforated the cortical plate of bone and caused the total destruction of the facial bone covering the root tips of the teeth, then, once the granulation tissue has been removed, access to the apex can be achieved with little or no bone removal. On the other hand, as is the case most of the time, that, if the cortical bone is still partially or totally intact, then the apex can be exposed by removing the overlying bone with a high-speed surgical round bur. Before doing this, careful examination of the preoperative radiograph is advised to consider the approximate length of the root, the root anatomy and curvature, the distance between adjacent root tips and from surrounding structures. It can be very useful to superimpose a periodontal probe on the analogic radiograph to get an approxi-

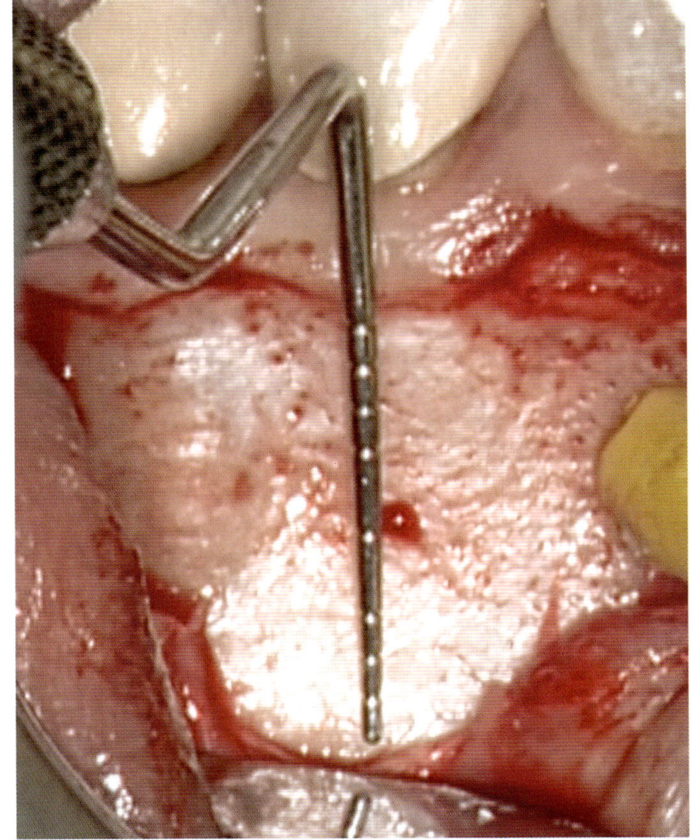

8.1 The periodontal probe is indicating the estimate location of the root apex, previously measured on the preoperative analogic radiograph.

mate idea of the location of the root apex and the length of the root and then to transfer that measurement to the healthy bone (8.1). The same measurement can be obtained by measuring the length on the screen of the digital radiograph (8.2). It is highly recommended to take a CBCT in order to obtain a precise knowledge of the anatomy of the roots and of the surrounding structures. The position of the root apex can be more accurately determined after a small amount of bone has been removed with a small round bur and then a small radiopaque marker placed in the shallow bony defect and a new radiograph exposed.[1,2] A convenient marker is a piece of sterilized lead sheet from a radiographic film packet (8.3) or a piece of sterilized gutta-percha. The radiopaque object will provide guidance both laterally and vertically for the position of the apex.[3]

Once an accurate location of the root apex has been determined, the bone is carefully removed in a shaving motion using a round surgical high-speed bur under copious irrigation with saline solution and very light pressure.

An osteotomy is done using a surgical length round #2 or #6 bur mounted on a specifically designed high-speed handpiece, such as the Impact Air 45 (Palisades Dental, NJ, USA) (8.4). This handpiece delivers only irrigating solution and no air exits from the working end, in order to avoid the risk of creating air emphysema or embolism in the surrounding soft tissue. The use of the bur is very gentle with a brushing motion, making sure that the bur is always cooled by the irrigating solution, using saline solution. A point 2-4 mm short of the estimated root length is selected and a bur hole is cut perpendicular to the anticipated long axis until the tooth structure is encountered (8.5).[1] The root surface can be easily distinguished from the surrounding bone tissue. The root structure is generally darker, yellowish and it does not bleed when probed and is surrounded by the periodontal ligament. On the other hand, the bone is white, soft and bleeds when scraped with a curette. In case of difficulty, methylene blue dye (8.6) can be used which will preferentially stain the periodontal ligament, allowing easier identification and orientation.[4] When the root becomes visible, more bone is gently removed in order to expose the root apex (8.7), creating enough space to provide adequate visibility, access for granulation tissue removal, resection of the apex and the establishment of an adequate apical retroseal. Of course, as much as is possible, the minimum amount of bone should be removed and the osteotomy should be as conservative as possible. The operator should always remember, however, that visibility is essential for a successful treatment and that during the healing process the bone will grow back.

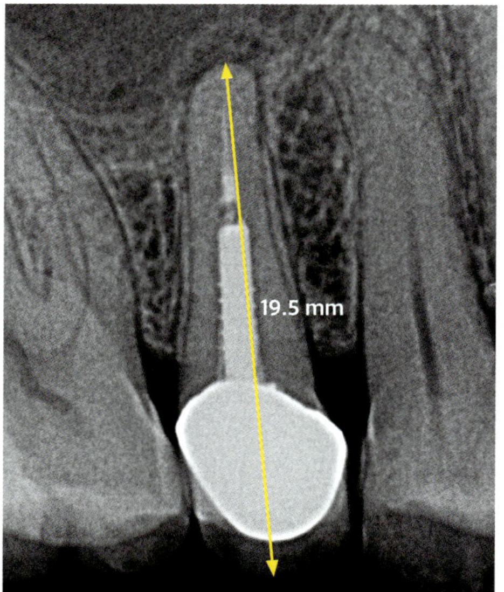

8.2 The same measurement can be done using digital radiology.

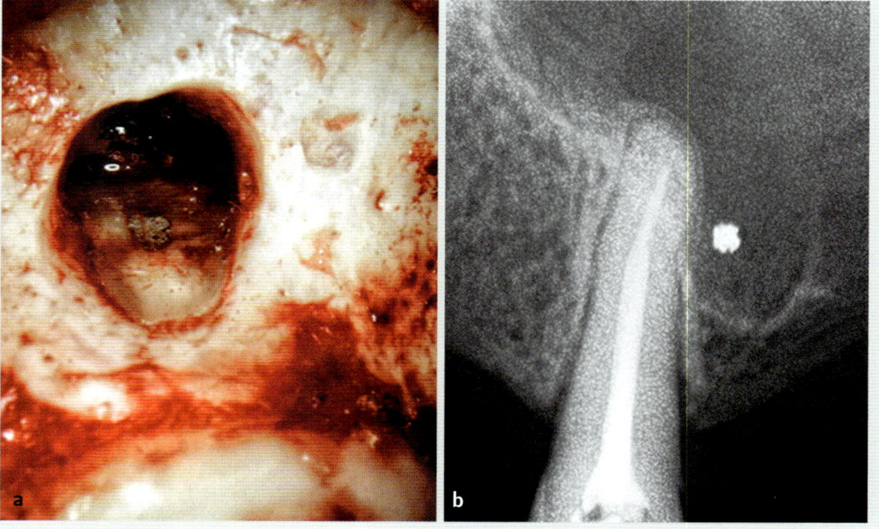

8.3 **a)** The convexity of the cortical bone could simulate the convexity of the root. For safety, a shallow cavity has been made on the cortical bone to lodge a small radiopaque marker before making the bony crypt. **b)** A radiograph has been taken. The convexity was due to the maxillary sinus and not to the root.

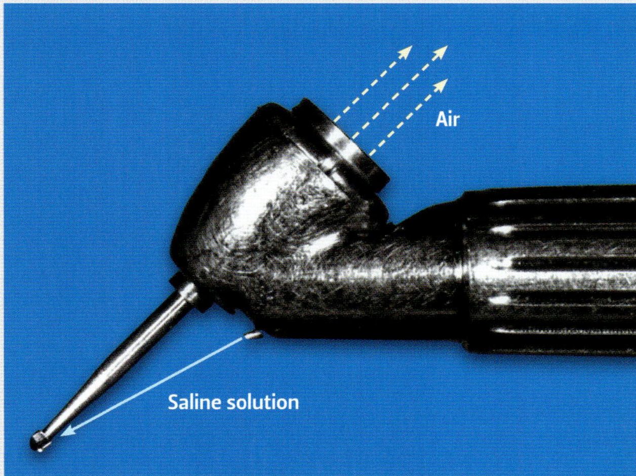

8.4 The Impact Air 45 (Palisades Dental, NJ, USA) is a 45° surgical high-speed handpiece, designed to irrigate the surgical field, while ejecting air from the back of the handpiece, to avoid pushing air in the soft tissue and causing air emphysema or embolism.

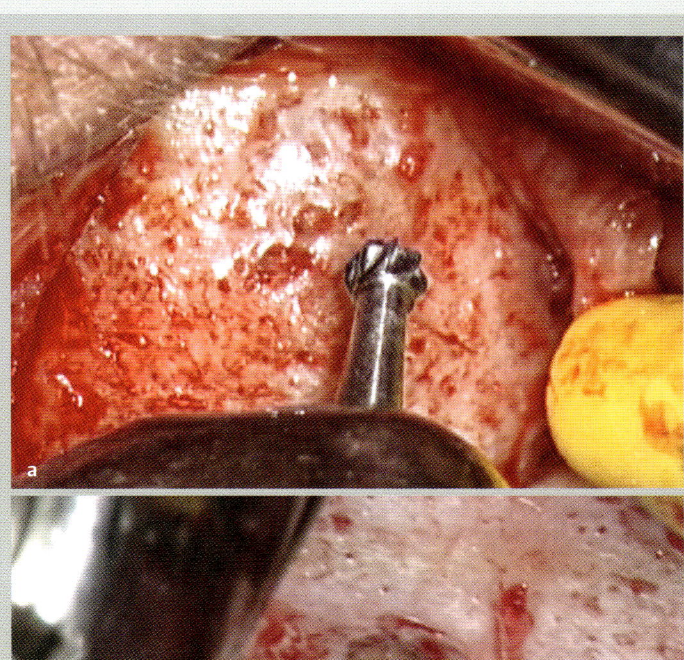

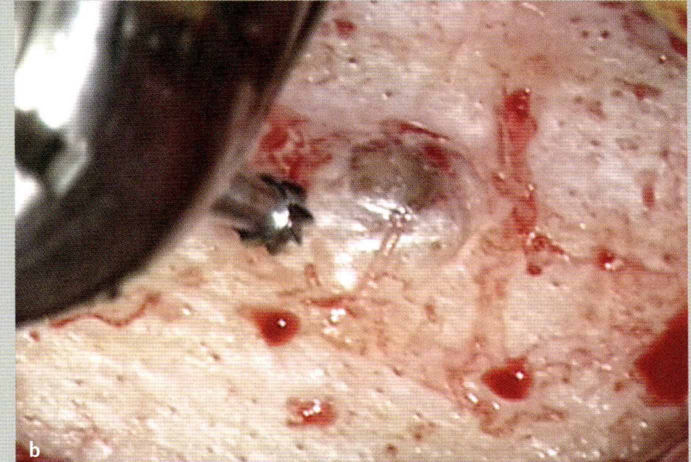

8.5 **a)** The bur is searching for the root structure. **b)** The root has been found and it can be easily recognized.

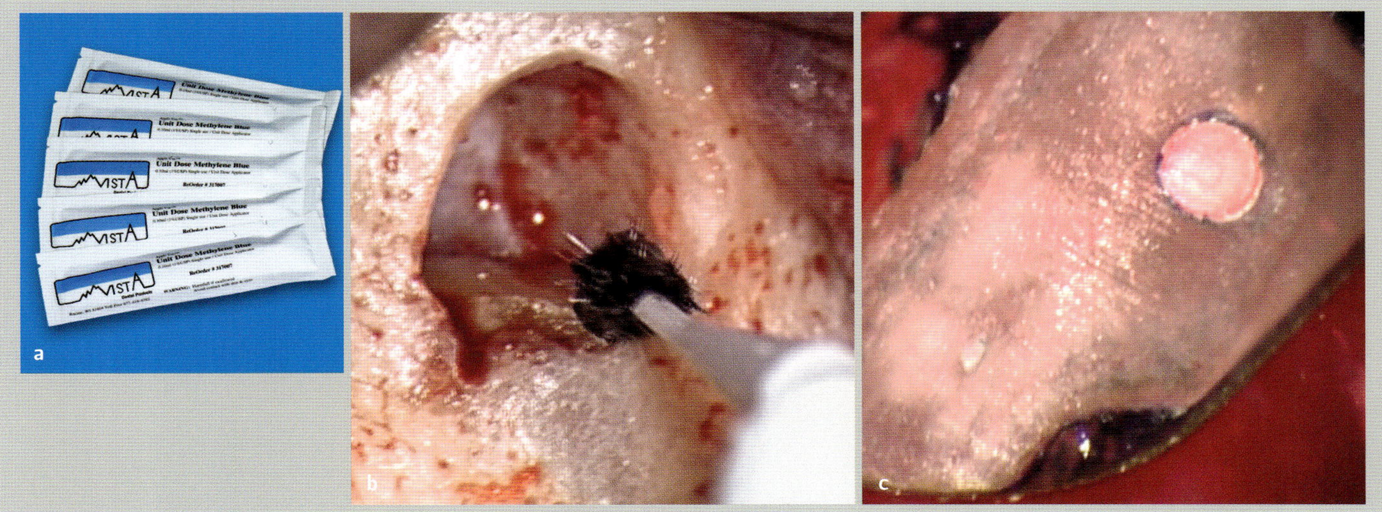

8.6 **a)** Unit dose Methylene Blue by Vista Dental, Racine, WI, USA. **b)** The Methylene Blue is carried with the specific micro-brush. **c)** Now the periodontal ligament is more visible.

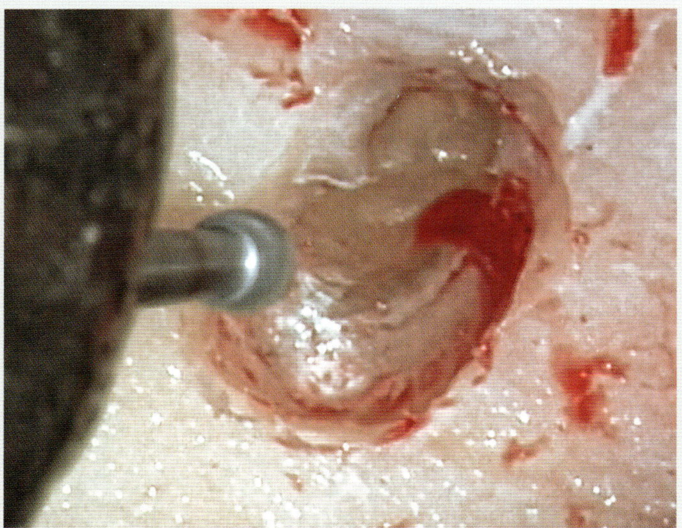

8.7 The high-speed bur is removing bone to have a better exposition of the root apex.

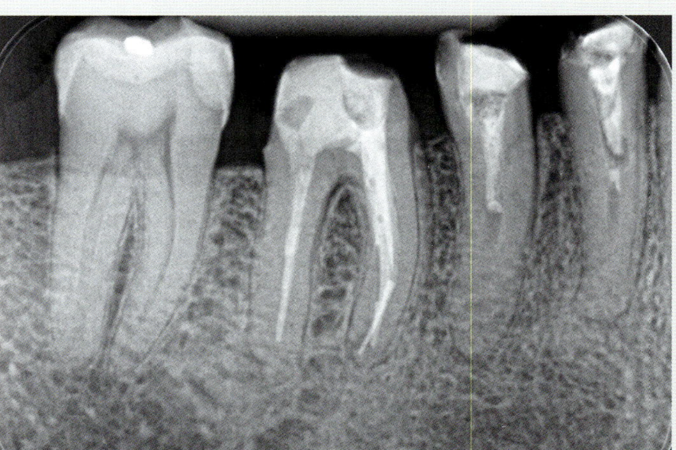

8.8 Preoperative radiograph of a lower right molar. A broken instrument is present in the mesial root. The patient has symptoms and there is no radiolucency.

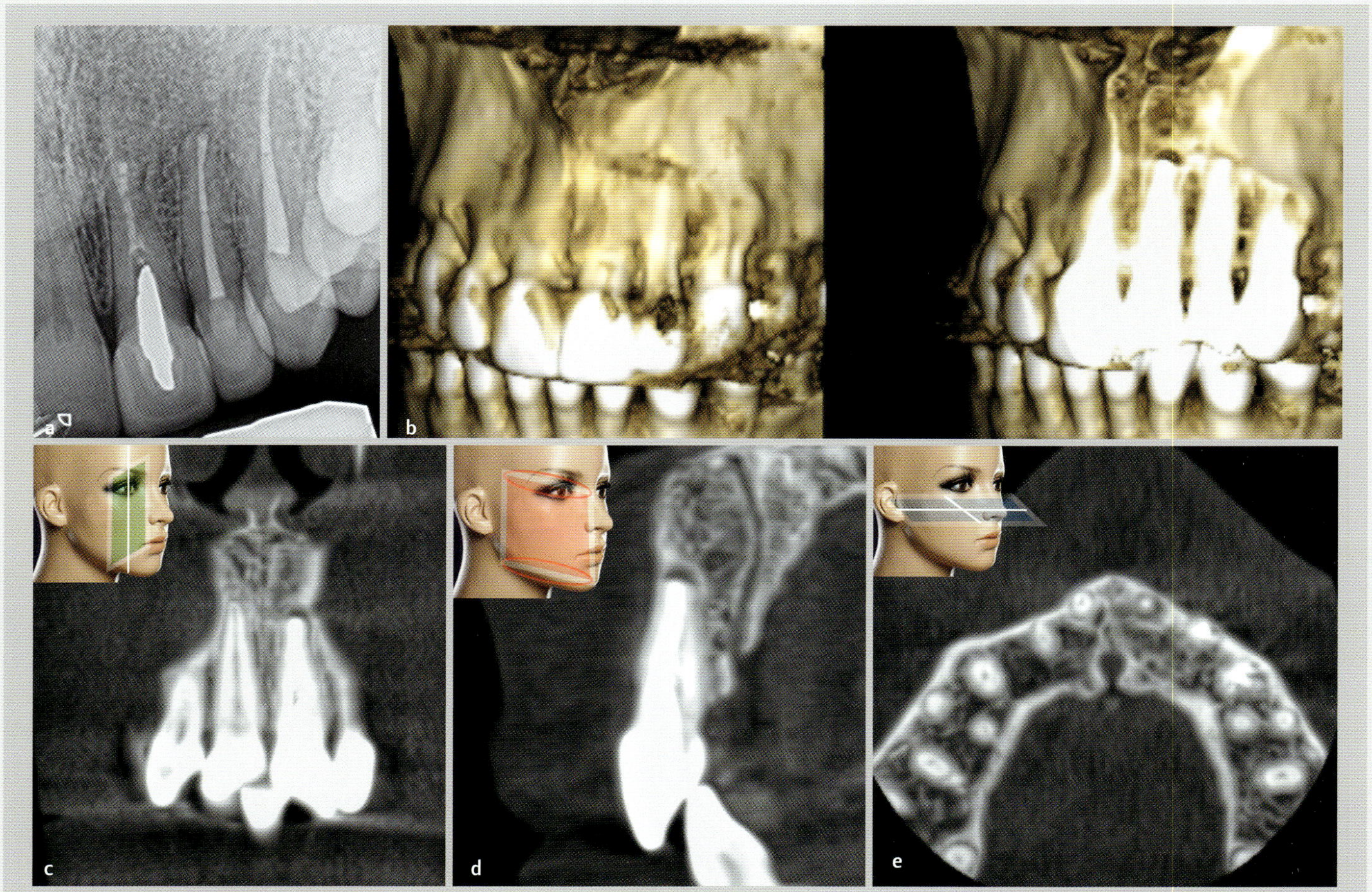

8.9 **a)** Preoperative radiograph of an upper left central incisor. The patient has symptoms and the radiograph shows no lesion. **b)** *Left*. The CBCT 3D rendering shows an intact cortical bone. *Right*. The CBCT 3D rendering shows a lesion at the apex of the central incisor. **c)** Coronal view showing the lesion. **d)** Sagittal view showing the lesion. **e)** Axial view showing the lesion.

After the elevation and retraction of the flap, the clinician may face three different situations:

1. the cortical bone is intact and radiographically there is no radiolucency evident
2. the cortical bone is intact and radiographically a lesion is present
3. the cortical bone has been fenestrated by the lesion.

No Periradicular Lesion and Intact Cortical Bone

In the author's opinion, this represents the most difficult situation in microsurgical endodontics. It typically occurs when a procedural error has been made and it cannot be corrected without surgery. Most often it is a broken instrument present in the root canal, the tooth is sensitive to percussion or palpation, the patient is experiencing discomfort and there is no radiolucency on the radiograph (8.8).

To be more precise, there may be a small lesion, but it is so small that it does not involve the internal wall at the junction of the cancellous and cortical bone. It is thus not visible on the radiograph and can only be detected on a CBCT, which with these cases is highly recommended to determine the root length and position of the apex in relation to the cusp tip and adjacent roots (8.9).

Periradicular Lesion and Intact Cortical Bone

This is the most common situation in microsurgical endodontics. Sometimes the cortical bone is so thin that it can be easily penetrated with a sharp endodontic

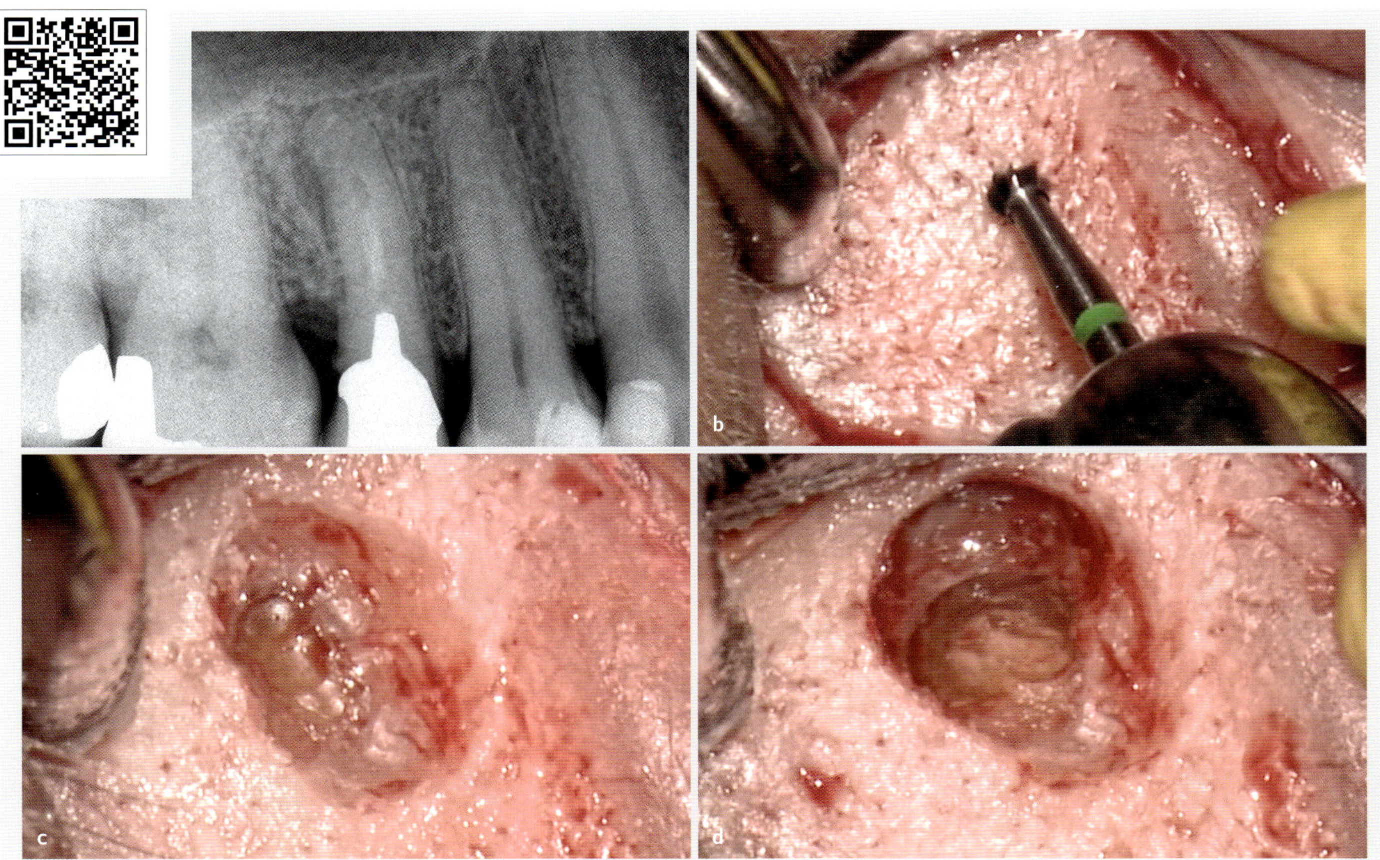

8.10 **a)** Preoperative radiograph of an upper right second premolar. **b)** The cortical bone is intact. **c)** After shaving the bone, the root apex is visible. **d)** After the removal of the granulation tissue, the root apex can now be prepared.

explorer or a curette and then peeled off, exposing the soft tissue of the lesion. The undermined bone can then be removed with the high-speed round bur as described before. When the intact cortical bone cannot be penetrated, the bone is shaved off until the granulation tissue or the root surface is exposed (8.10). The osteotomy should now be carefully enlarged and it should not be surprising that the final size of the bony crypt is larger than expected. It is a well-known fact that lesions are always larger than they appear on a radiograph. This is due to the fact that they begin in the cancellous bone and progress to the cortical bone, where the damage is of course smaller. Only the involvement of the cortical bone will make the lesion visible on the radiograph.[5]

Periradicular Lesion and Fenestrated Cortical Bone

This definitely represents the easiest situation in microsurgical endodontics. When the cortical bone is fenestrated because of the presence of a perforating lesion or a perforating sinus tract, the location of the root apex is immediate as soon as the granulation tissue is exposed (8.11). Just following the sinus tract and removing the granulation tissue will provide visibility, access to the root apex and good control of the bleeding inside the bony crypt. A shelf of bone apical to the soft tissue must be exposed to position the retractor during the

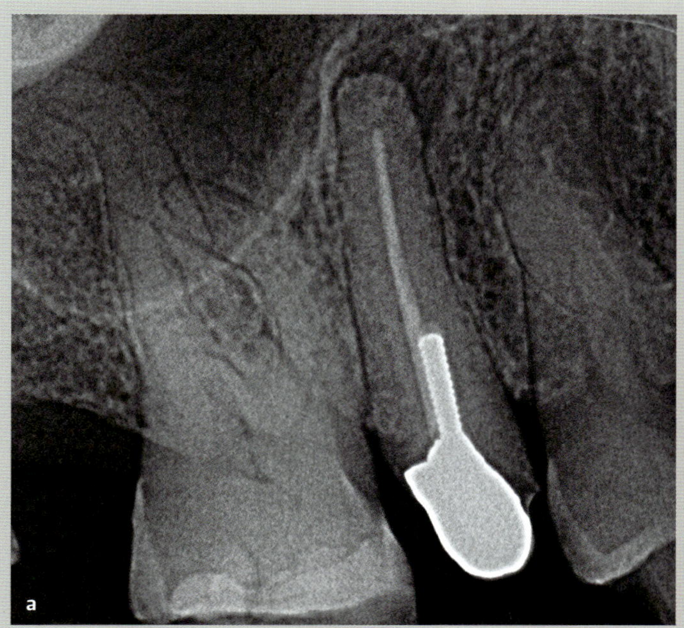

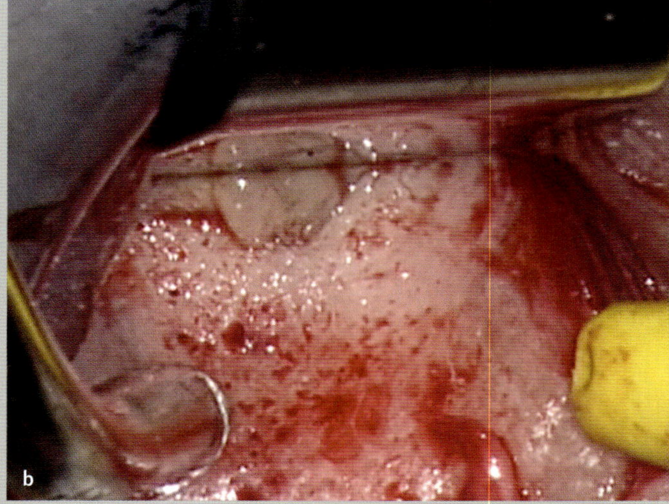

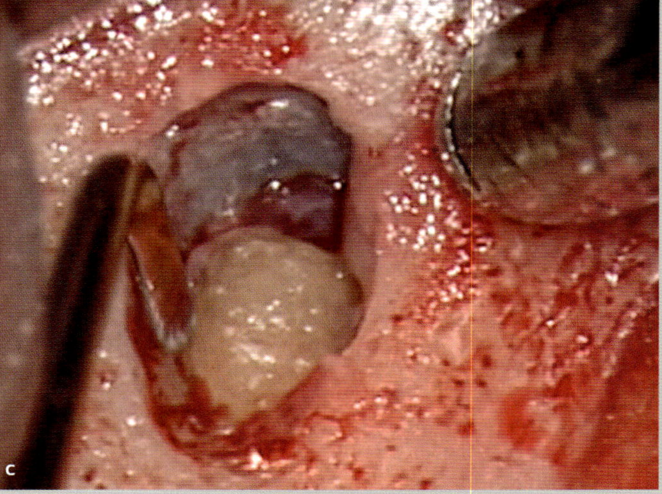

8.11 **a)** Preoperative radiograph of an upper right second premolar. **b)** The cortical bone is fenestrated. **c)** After the removal of the granulation tissue the root apex can now be prepared.

procedure. If necessary, the vertical releasing incisions should be extended and a greater amount of soft tissue should be reflected in order to avoid impingement of the soft tissue with the retractor and consequently to avoid tissue damage, delaying healing and postoperative discomfort.

Once the soft tissue of the lesion has been removed and good visibility of the root apex is obtained, the root-end resection and the establishment of an adequate apical seal can be accomplished.

Before the introduction of ultrasonic retrotips, an osteotomy was necessarily large to allow the use of large instruments and to reach the palatal or lingual canals (8.12). As we will discuss later, the root end resection was made with a steep bevel to allow direct visibility to the cut root surface and to allow a root end preparation using straight slow-speed handpieces and round surgical burs (8.13). The steep bevel required a large bony crypt, of at least 10 mm, a large amount of unnecessary removal of healthy buccal bone and had the risk of missing lingual or palatal root canal anatomy.

The osteotomy should be large enough to accommodate microsurgical instruments, first of all ultrasonic tips. The length of ultrasonic tips is 3 mm, therefore an osteotomy of about 4 mm is ideal, to give enough space to comfortably use the ultrasonic tips and other microinstruments, such

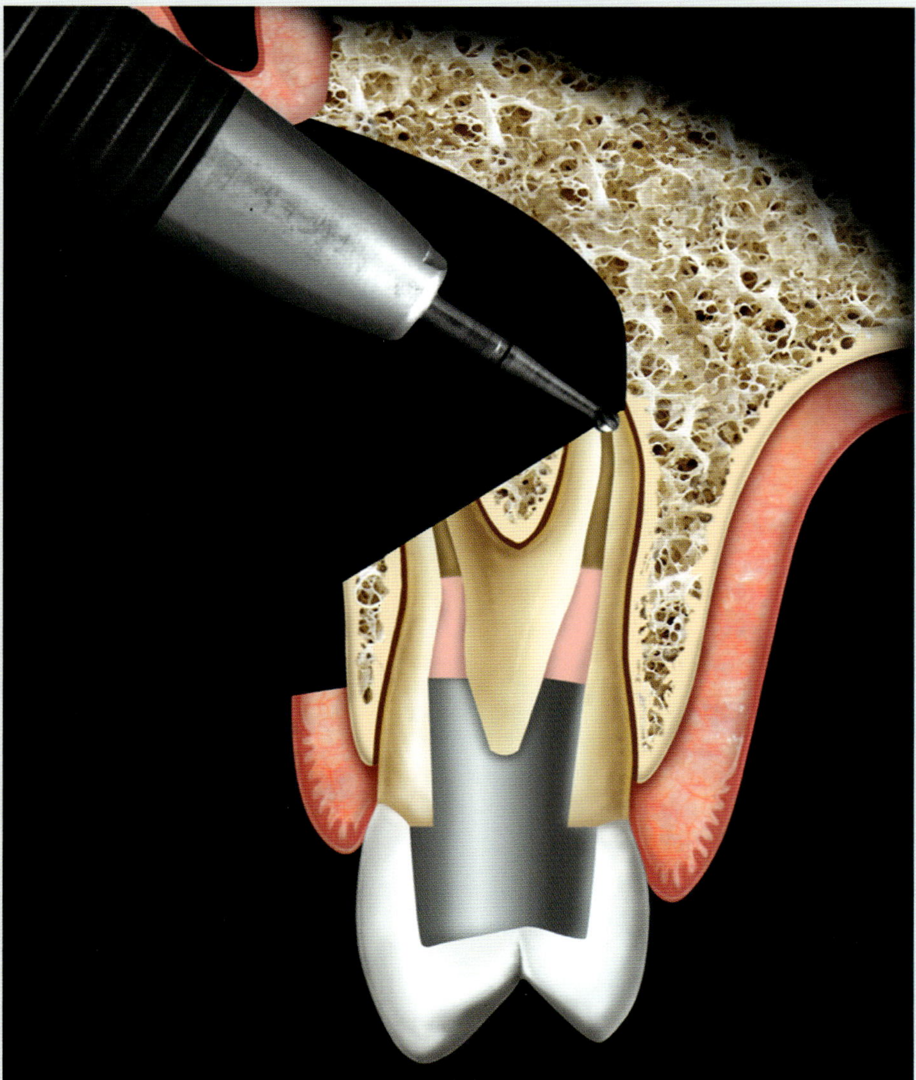

8.12 The long bevel obliges one to sacrifice more bone and tooth structure in order to reach the lingual or palatal anatomy.

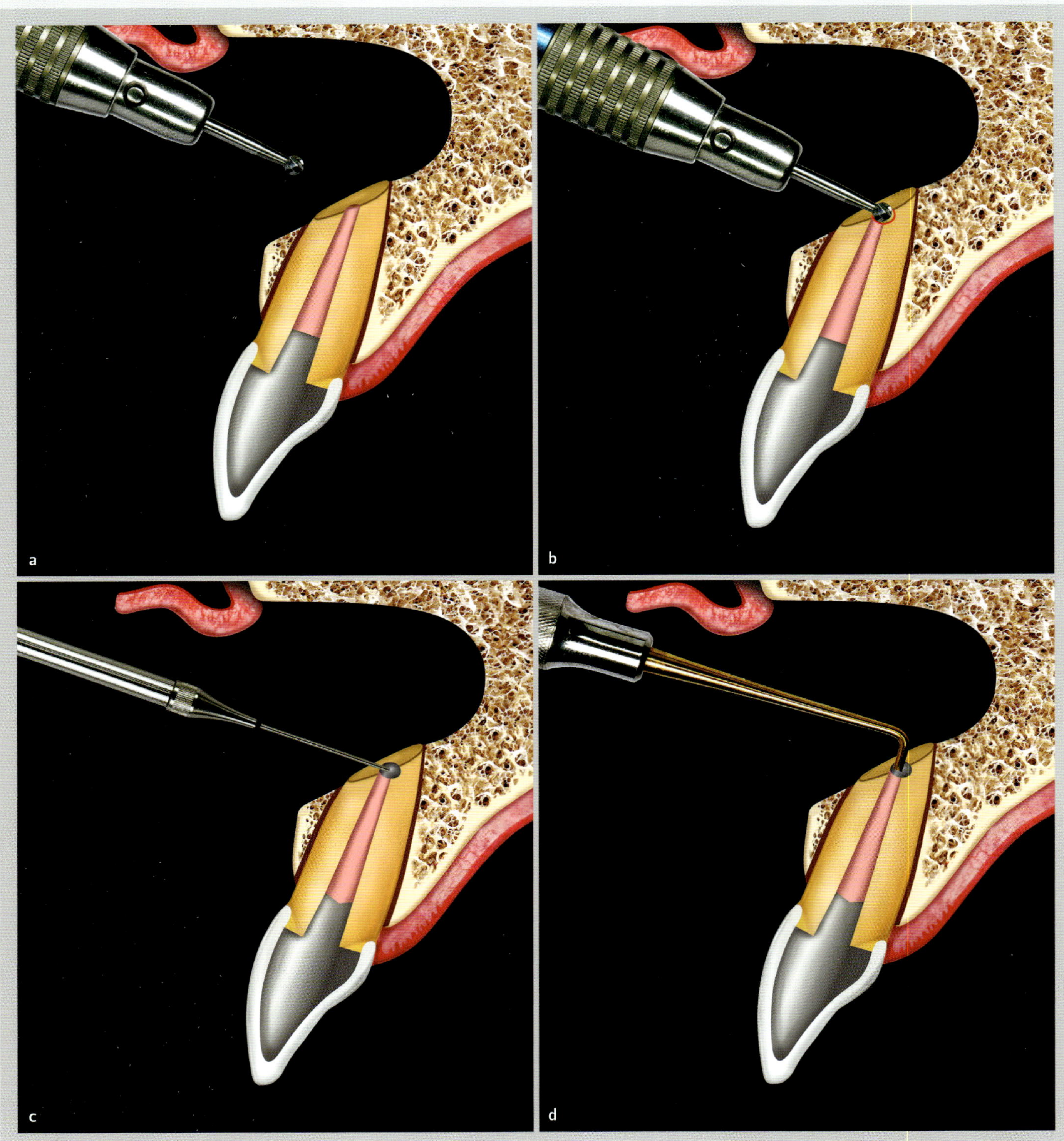

8.13 **a)** The steep bevel was necessary to reach the canal and prepare the root-end with a straight handpiece. **b)** The root-end cavity was made with a round bur mainly at the expenses of the palatal wall. **c)** The cavity was then filled with amalgam using the Messing Gun. **d)** The amalgam was then condensed using a plugger. It is evident that the retrofill was not along the main axis of the root canal.

as micromirrors, carriers, and micropluggers (📷 8.14). In some cases, a deeper retro-cavity is required; the typical situation is represented by an anterior tooth having a short postcemented in the root canal or a long portion of the root canal almost completely empty. In such cases, longer ultrasonic tips are required: 3 mm, 6 mm and 9 mm. These tips, as will be described later, must be used in sequence from the shortest to the longest and usually a larger osteotomy is not required. If needed, however, a small alteration to the previous osteotomy can be accomplished simply by creating a vertical extension in an apical direction,[6] keeping in mind that, as already stated, the bone will grow back during the healing process.

As far as the removal of the granulation tissue is concerned, as already stated, its complete removal is suggested to achieve a good hemostasis within the crypt, to have a better control of the bleeding and better visibility. On the other hand, in case of large cystic lesions, its complete removal can be performed only if this maneuver will not damage important anatomical structures, such as the blood supply of adjacent vital teeth, the floor of the nasal cavity and the maxillary sinus, the inferior alveolar nerve or the mental nerve (📷 2.13–2.15). The operator should always remember that we are dealing with lesions of endodontic origin that could heal with an adequate root canal therapy and without any surgery. Therefore, in such cases it is advisable to remove enough of the cystic wall that is sufficient to enable good access to the root apex for making the retroprep and positioning the retrofill.

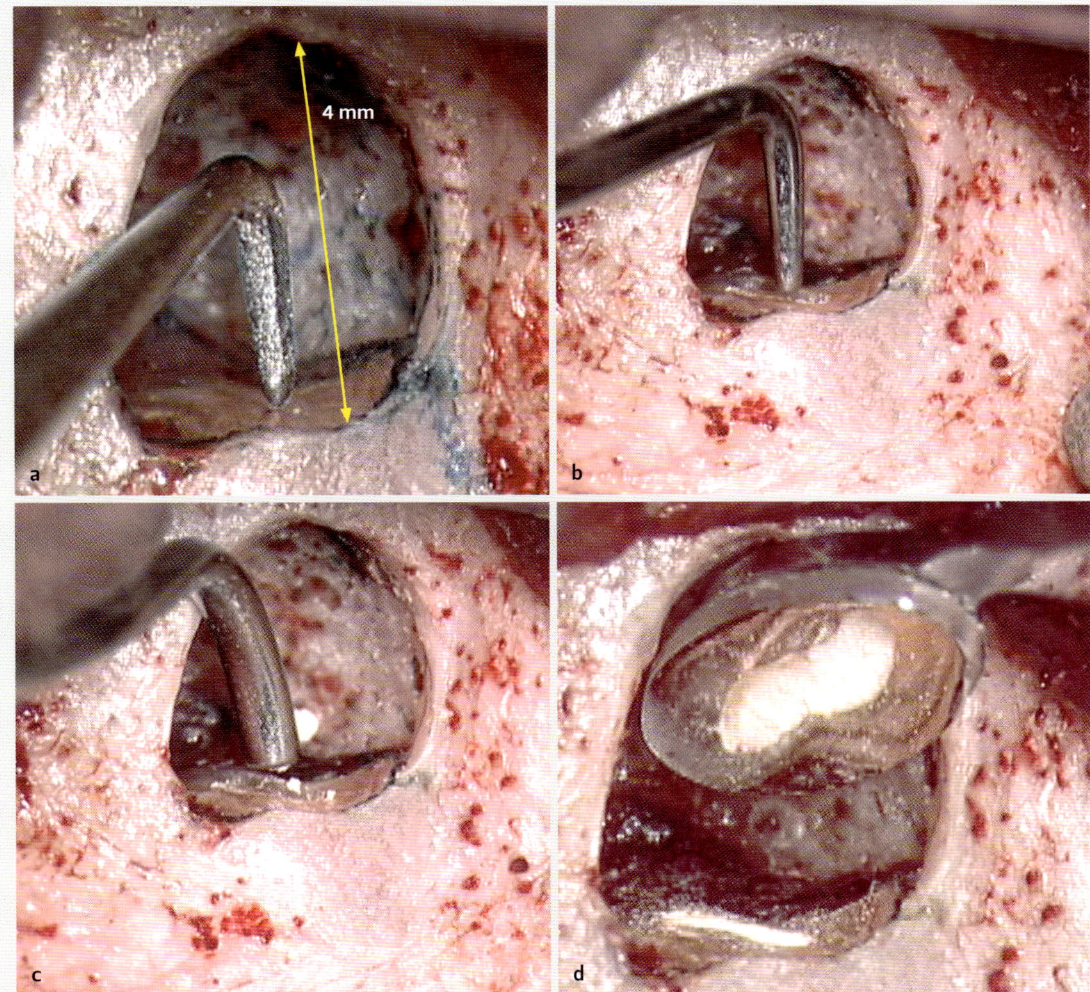

📷 **8.14** The bony crypt should be large enough to allow the introduction of ultrasonic tips **(a)**, micropluggers **(b)**, carriers **(c)**, micromirrors **(d)**.

Crypt Management

Sometimes, just the use of anesthesia the way it has been described is enough to have good hemostasis in the periapical surgical crypt. However, this is not the rule, and sometimes even after the complete removal of the granulation tissue there is still some bleeding that can compromise our visibility and then the entire procedure. In this situation, it is necessary to use other methods to guarantee hemostasis and to have a clean and relatively dry crypt. Among the several methods described in the literature, the most frequently used are ferric sulfate (*see* 5.8),[7,8] calcium sulfate,[9] and cotton pellets impregnated with epinephrine (*see* 5.9).[10] In the Author's experience, the epinephrine impregnated cotton pellets and the ferric sulfate are the most frequently used and the most efficient.

Before using the epinephrine impregnated cotton pellets, all the granulation tissue must be removed to ensure direct contact with the bone. After placing one epinephrine cotton pellet in the bony crypt, more cotton pellets are packed on top of it and pressure is applied over them for several minutes. The sterile cotton pellets are then removed one at the time, taking care not to dislodge the first epinephrine pellet (8.15). If bleeding still occurs, the procedure is repeated with a new epinephrine pellet until hemostasis is achieved. The com-

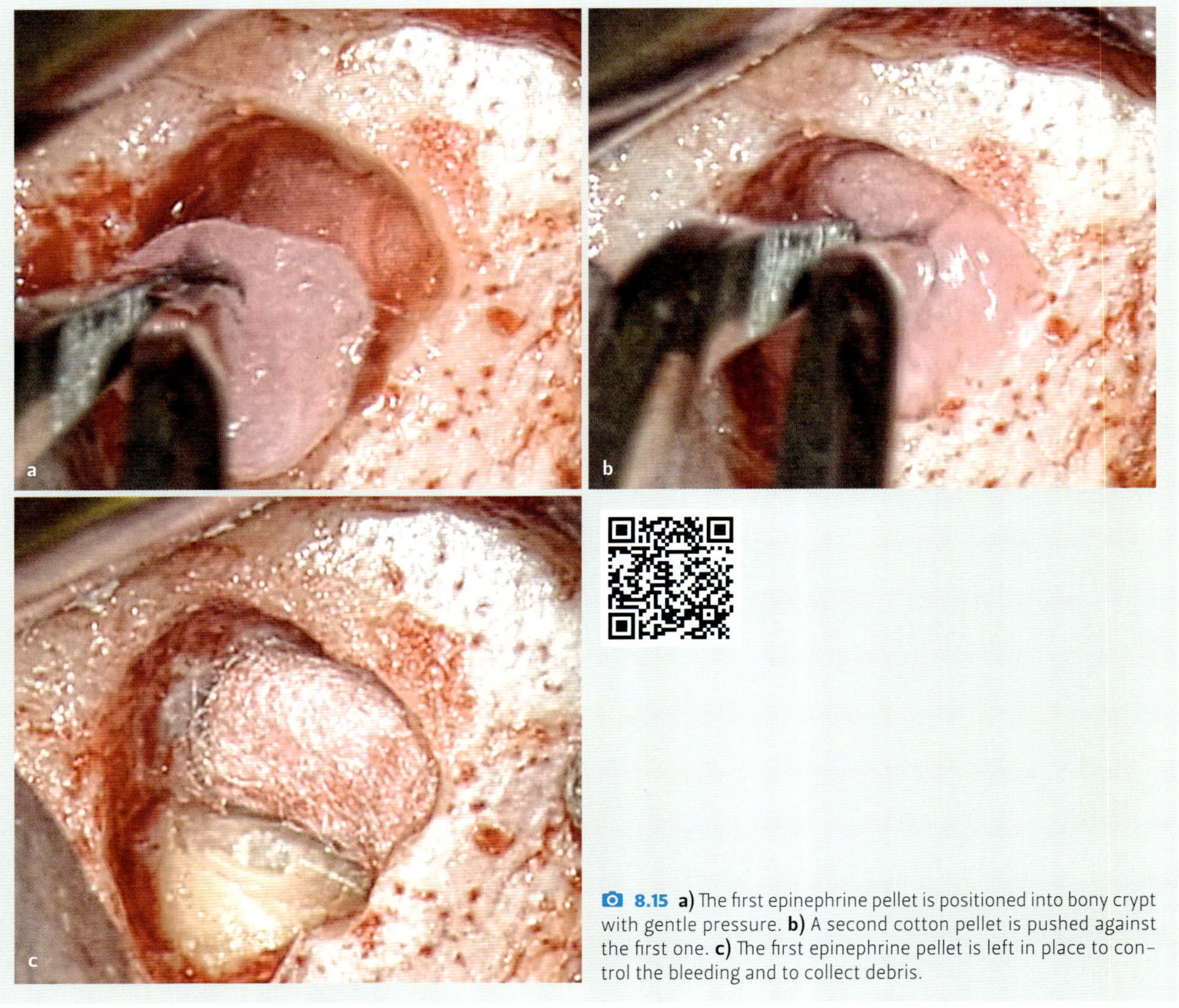

8.15 a) The first epinephrine pellet is positioned into bony crypt with gentle pressure. **b)** A second cotton pellet is pushed against the first one. **c)** The first epinephrine pellet is left in place to control the bleeding and to collect debris.

bination of both epinephrine and pressure has a synergistic effect that results in immediate and profound vasoconstriction.[10] Epinephrine causes local vasoconstriction by acting on the alpha receptors present in the wall of the blood vessels, and the pressure augments the hemostatic potential.[10] The cotton pellets are also used to collect the debris created during the retropreparation and the retrofill. They will be removed before the final irrigation and suturing (*see* chapter 5).

Ferric sulfate is available on the market in different forms and different concentrations. The most popular are Cut-Trol (Cut-Trol, Mobile, AL) and Astringedent (Ultradent Products, Inc. UT) (*see* 5.8). Ferric sulfate causes agglutination of blood proteins, and as soon as it comes in contact with bleeding vessels, a thick, brownish coagulum is formed and the bleeding stops almost immediately. As already stated, all granulation tissue should be removed prior to placement of the ferric sulfate to ensure direct contact with the bone. If some excess coagulum is present, it can be easily removed with gentle irrigation. The ferric sulfate is carried into the crypt using the specifically designed syringe and needle, which has a little brush at its extremity (*see* 5.8b). The brush should be just wet, not dripping, and the ferric sulfate is used by just brushing the crypt until the bleeding stops. To increase the efficacy, a cotton pellet impregnated with epinephrine is compressed into the crypt for a few seconds: if there is any bleeding, it will stop immediately. According to the literature,[7,8] there is no contraindication to the use of ferric sulfate, as long it is **only** used in the bony crypt and at the end of the procedure is removed with accurate curettage and irrigation, in order to stimulate new bleeding. If left *in situ*, it will cause a delay in the healing process. Furthermore, the operator must be very careful not to use the ferric sulfate on the cortical bone, the periosteum, the soft tissue and on the Schneiderian membrane. These structures must always be carefully avoided.

REFERENCES

1. ARENS DE, ADAMS WR, DECASTRO RA. *Endodontic Surgery*. Philadelphia: Harper & Row. 1981;124-125.
2. WEINE FS, GERSTEIN H. *Periapical surgery*. In: Weine FS, ed. *Endodontic therapy*. 4th edition. St. Louis: The CV Mosby Company. 1982;446-519.
3. GUTMANN, J.L., HARRISON, JW. *Surgical access: soft tissue management*. In: Gutmann JL, Harrison JW, eds. *Surgical endodontics*. Boston, MA: Blackwell Scientific Publications, Inc. 1991;153-202.
4. CAMBRUZZI JV, MARSHAL FJ. *Molar endodontic surgery*. J Can Dent Assoc. 1983;49:61-65.
5. BENDER IB. *Factors influencing the radiographic appearance of bony lesions*. J Endod. 1982;8:161-170.
6. MAGGIORE F, KIM S. *Osteotomy*. In: Kim S, Kratchman S, Eds. *Microsurgery in Endodontics*. Wiley Blackwell. 2018;57-65.
7. LEMON RR, STEELE PJ, JEANSONNE BG. *Ferric sulfate hemostasis: effect on osseous wound healing. I. Left in situ for maximum exposure*. J Endod. 1993;19:170-173.
8. LEMON RR, JEANSONNE BG, BOGGS WS. *Ferric sulfate hemostasis: effect on osseous wound healing. II. With curettage and irrigant*. J Endod. 1993;19:174-176.
9. PECORA G, ANDREANA S, MARGARONE JE, COVANI U, SOTTOSANTI JS. *Bone regeneration with a calcium sulfate barrier*. Oral Surg Oral Med Oral Path Radiol Endod. 1997;84:429-39.
10. KIM S, RETHNAM S. *Hemostasis in endodontic microsurgery*. Dent Clin North Am. 1997;41:499-511.

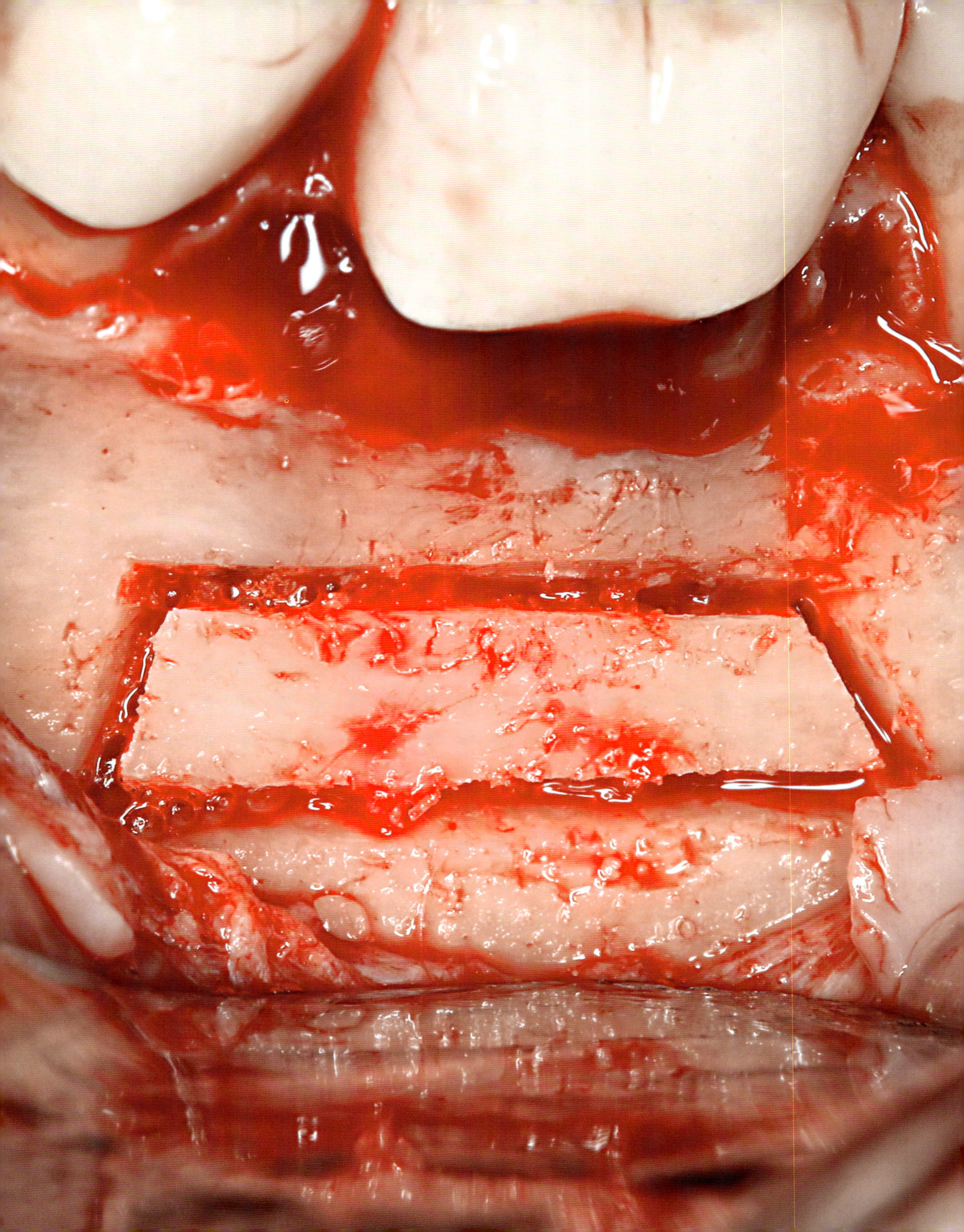

The Cortical Window

Yosi Nahmias, DDS, MSc, Ken Serota, DDS, MMSc,
Naheed Mohamed, DMD, MSD

Nonsurgical endodontic therapy requires access preparations that uncover entrances to the labyrinthine tunnels of the root canal system. The era of bio-minimalism has altered the traditional configuration of endodontic access cavities. These bio-minimalistic trends are also transforming endodontic surgery.[1] The use of surgical operating microscopes facilitates smaller crypt sizes and reduces the volume of bone removed. The wound architecture created by microsurgical scalpels is more precise resulting in minimal damage to the soft tissues.[2] Enhanced visibility facilitates perpendicular resection of the apical segment to the long axis of the root. Smaller resection angles reduce the number of tubuli exposed. Lateral canals, canal deltas, isthmus connections and microcracks can be identified prior to root resection, retropreparation and retrosealing.[3] Monofilament sutures minimize posttreatment inflammation. Soft and hard tissue augmentation corrects deficits in biotype and buttressing bone. These are but a few of the new adjuncts in endodontic microsurgical techniques.[2,4,5]

Studies of positive treatment outcomes for conventional endodontic surgical therapy show a diverse range of success dependent upon an array of predictors.[6,7] A study by Wang et. al reported an overall healed rate of 74% of assessed teeth; root filling length and size of preoperative lesions proved to be important predictors of treatment outcomes.[8] Positive treatment outcomes (94%) were demonstrated by microsurgical techniques.[2] Retreatment of failing endodontic procedures demonstrate statistically less positive treatment outcomes than those done by microsurgical techniques (86%); fewer failures ensue.[5] These conditions are more readily addressed with microsurgical techniques.[9]

Ultrasonic Osteotomy

Used in both periodontal and implant surgery, piezosurgery in microsurgical endodontics produces micrometric cuts which diminish cortical bone loss and retain root length. Saline pumped through irrigation lines cools the piezotome tip (NSK America Corp IL, Brasseler USA, Savannah GA) (9.1).

In deep spaces, ultrasonic vibrations break down the irrigation into very small particles readily suctioned from the surgical field. Reduction of heme in the crypt minimizes the use of hemostatic agents and interference with the setting of retroseal materials. The inclusion of piezo surgery in endodontic microsurgical protocols produces less morbidity during the healing phase. Ultrasound consists of mechanical waves of frequencies greater than 20 kHz. Generated by transducers (Lead Zirconate Titante), electrical energy is converted to ultrasonic waves with minimal heat production. The clinician controls the pressure applied, cutting frequency, pulse frequency, rate of delivery of coolant fluid and power (3-90 W). Minimal heat generation on cutting creates lower proinflammatory cytokine levels, an earlier increase in BMP4 and TGF2 and more active neo-osteogenesis.[10,11] Traditional osteotomies require large instruments to remove cortical bone in order to access the apical segment of the root. These instruments can lead to delayed healing, increased postoperative pain and/or complications. With microscopes and piezotome surgical tips, smaller osteotomies (less than 5 mm) are big enough to accommodate ultrasonic tips (tip length of 3 mm).

Cortical Window Technique

A cortical window (bone lid) access to the apical region is less invasive, minimizes bone loss and is less traumatic in comparison to alternative techniques. The perimeter of the window is determined from radiographs of the area. Radiographs are essential to all aspects of endodontics; however, flat films are two-dimensional images of three-dimensional structures. Historically, they were two-dimensional images of three-dimensional

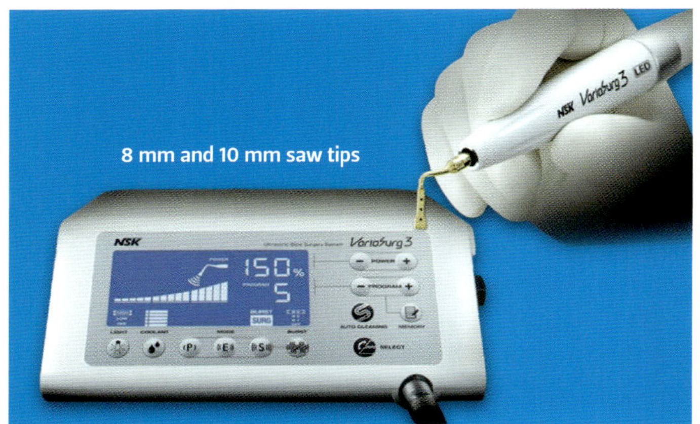

9.1 Piezotomes with fine-toothed saw tips of 8 and 10 mm length create smaller osteotomies and minimal osseous trauma (*NSK America Corp IL, Brasseler USA, Savannah GA*).

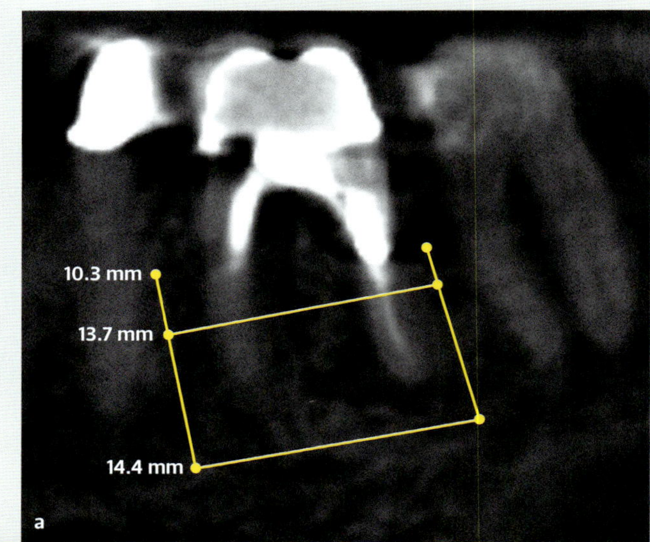

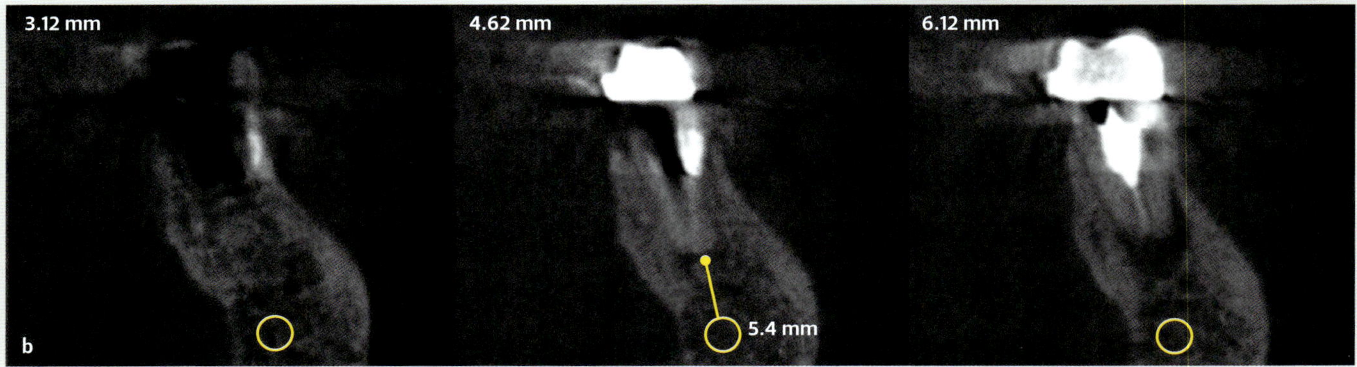

9.2 **a)** Cone beam tomography facilitates measurements of crypt dimension in sagittal, axial and coronal views (x, y, z axes). **b)** Proximity to the inferior alveolar nerve can be calculated. This is a crucial measurement in all microsurgical procedures.

structures; as such, data interpretation was subjective. The introduction of cone beam computed tomography (CBCT) and digital volume technology (DVT) provides images in sagittal, axial and coronal planes showing previously indeterminable views.[12,13]

Three-dimensional imaging provides more substantial data for diagnosis, pretreatment planning, post-treatment assessment and reassessment evaluations.[12,14] Data gathered from the CBCT scan allows a preplanned window to be made to access the apical portion of the roots (📷 9.2). A printed stereolithographic surgical template can guide the osteotomies during the surgery minimizing deviation from the digital surgical plan. Surgical templates printed from three-dimensional imaging optimize site preparation, the perimeter of the osteotomy, depth of cortical bone, extent of pathology and volume of bone graft required.[15–18]

The use of CBCT imaging in conjunction with piezosurgery provides a precise and less traumatic outline for the cortical bone window in contrast to traditional freehand guided crypt creation. The cortical bone window is sectioned so that the facial or palatal wall converges from the external surface to the internal surface. This ensures the accuracy of removal of the cortical bone plate and reseating when the window is replaced.

Piezotome Osteotomy

Traditional osteotomies use large round burs which remove significant cortical bone. Delayed healing increased postoperative pain and other complications may ensue. With microscopes, piezotomes and ultrasonic tips, a smaller osteotomy is created thus minimizing the aforementioned sequelae. Piezosurgery enables micrometric saw cuts which preserve cortical bone loss and facilitates preservation of root length by lower resection angles and enhanced visibility. In deep spaces, ultrasonic vibrations break down irrigant into small particles readily washed from the crypt. Less vascular presence in the crypt minimizes the use of hemostatic agents (Viscostat® Clear UPI, South Jordan, UT) and interference with retroseal setting time. The use of a piezosurgical devices enables accurate shaping of the cortical window and diminished osseous removal.[11] This is in contrast to traditional crypt creation which is free hand guided (📷 9.3–9.14).

Conclusion

The basic framework of endodontic surgery by incorporation of interdisciplinary precepts has evolved into microsurgical endodontics. The benefits of this cortical window approach include greater access to the roots for better visibility without greater risk for bone loss. The minimally invasive approach to access the roots by way of removal of a cortical bone plate has its greatest advantage simply because the bone plate is conserved and then replaced, allowing maximum regenerative potential. Advances in the surgical armamentarium, based on biological concepts has enabled a microsurgical approach which ensures enhanced positive treatment outcomes. The past is not being rejected; the future is being embraced. It is the natural progression of all things.

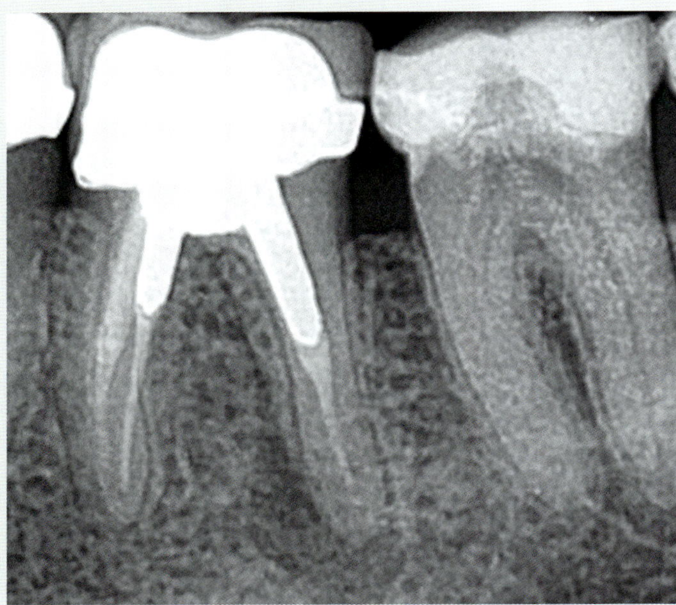

9.3 Preoperative radiograph of the lower left first molar. All canals are underinstrumented and demonstrate obturation density deficit. Retreatment of the tooth would necessitate removal of the cast post core which could lead to fracture of the mesial and distal roots.

9.4 The CBCT demonstrates a more definitive extent of the pathology. A sagittal view (CBCT) was used to determine the width and height of the cortical window required. The window cut is angled convergent from the external to the internal cortical plate, the base larger apically than coronally, thus preventing the bone segment from collapsing into the crypt when replaced.

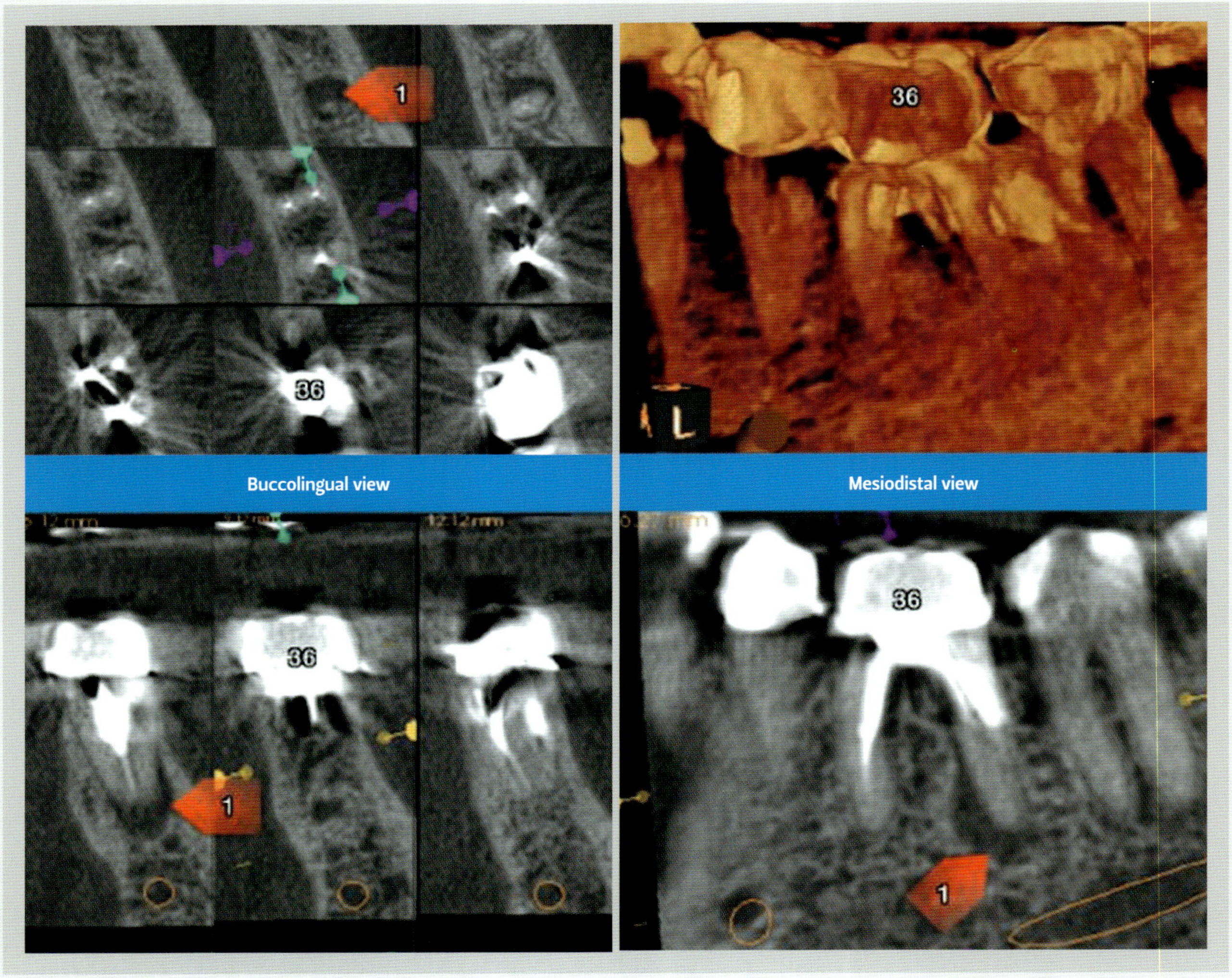

Buccolingual view

Mesiodistal view

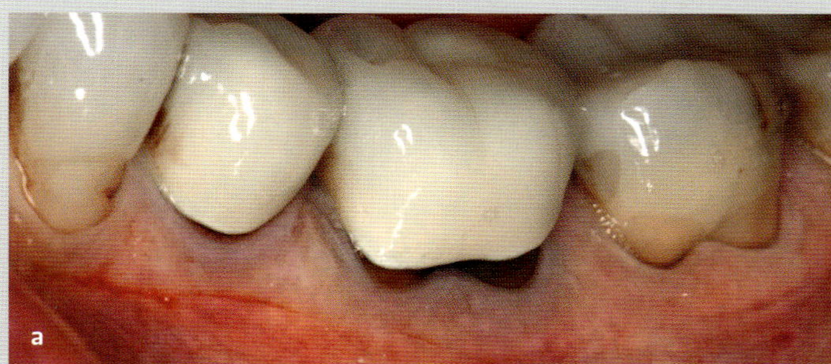

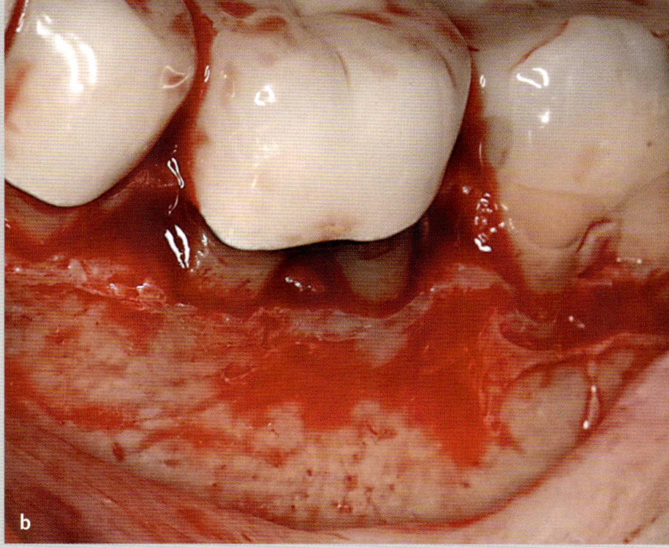

9.5 **a, b)** The flap is designed to correct the areas of recession. Vertical and horizontal incisions present pressure of the flap on retraction; the roots were planed to ensure a clean surface enhancing improved adherence of flap to the root.

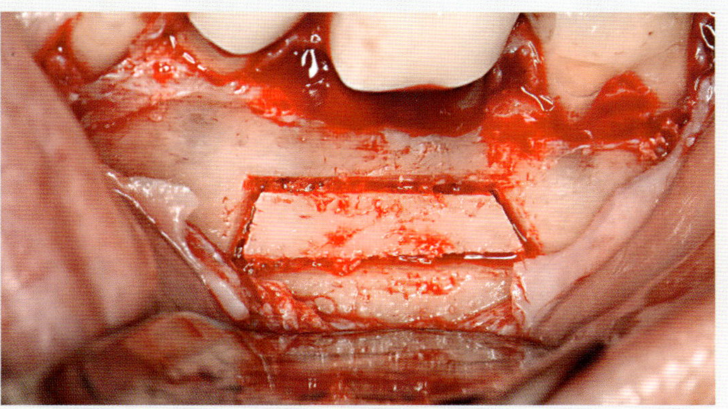

9.6 The piezotome (NSK VarioSurg 3 1800 Global Parkway Hoffman Estates, IL 60192, USA) creates an osseous window that will be replaced after completion of the root-end surgery.

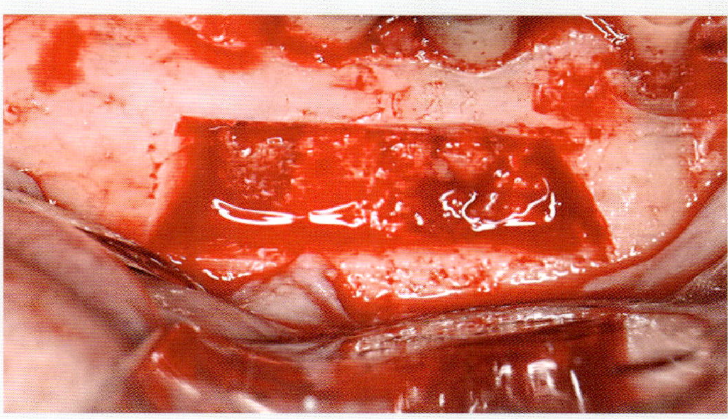

9.7 The cortical window was removed with a fine chisel.

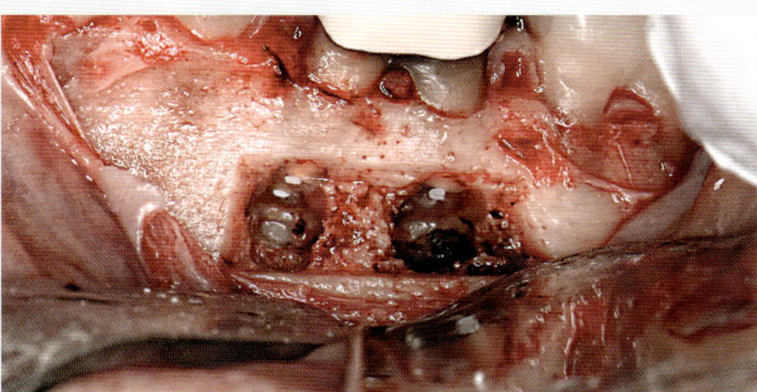

9.8 A truss is retained between the two roots to expedite osseous regeneration. The retroseals (SuperEBA) are burnished and the root face polished with a multi-fluted carbide bur.

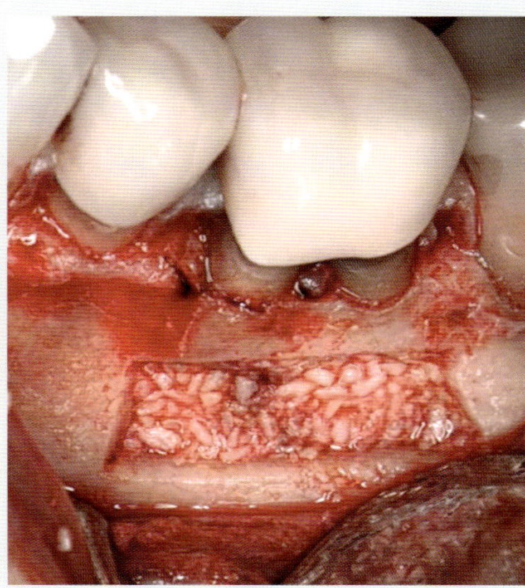

9.9 Allograft is placed in the crypt.

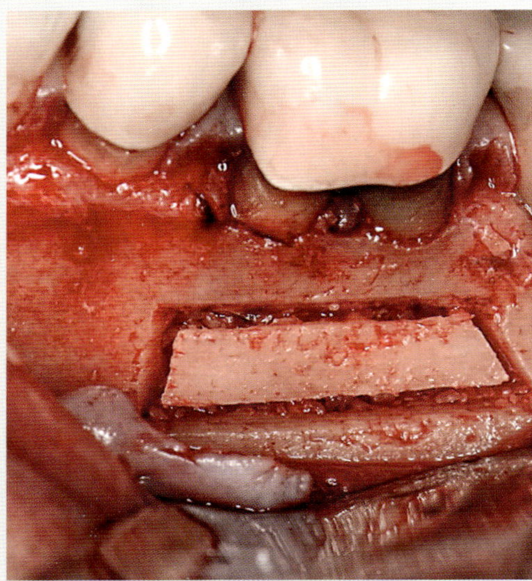

9.10 The cortical bone plate is replaced over the access window.

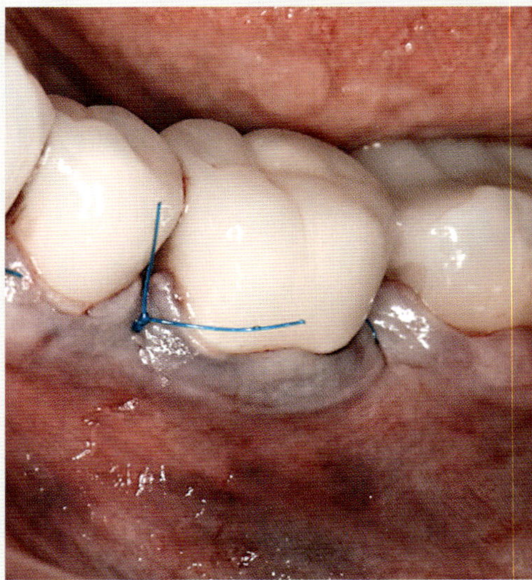

9.11 The flap is coapted and sutured to place. Note that the areas of recession are covered with tissue.

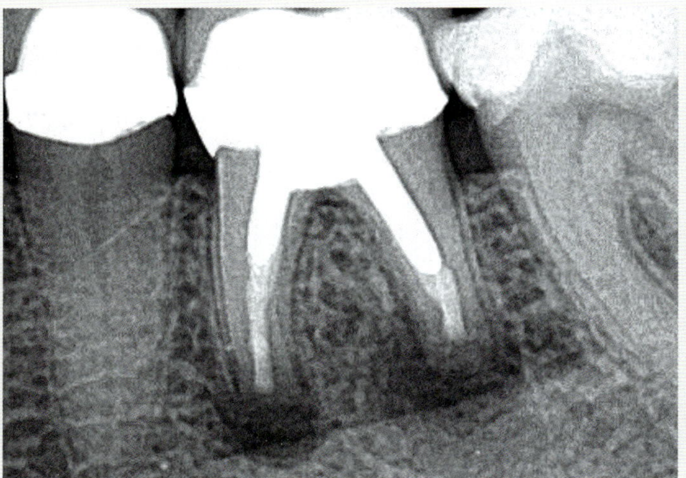

9.12 Posttreatment radiograph.

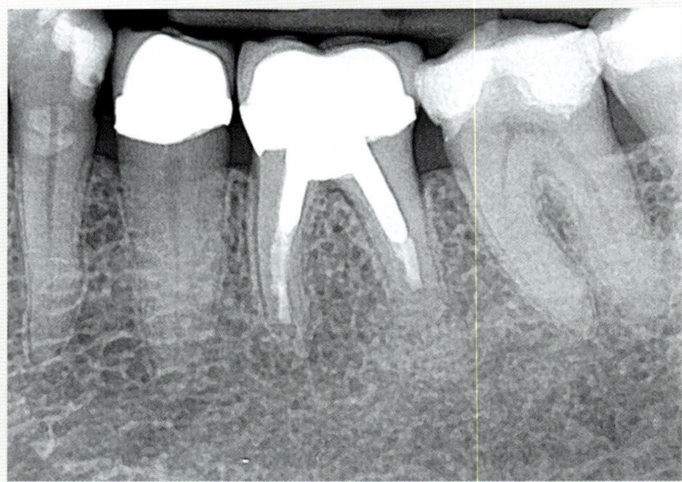

9.13 Six-month recall appointment shows healing to be almost complete.

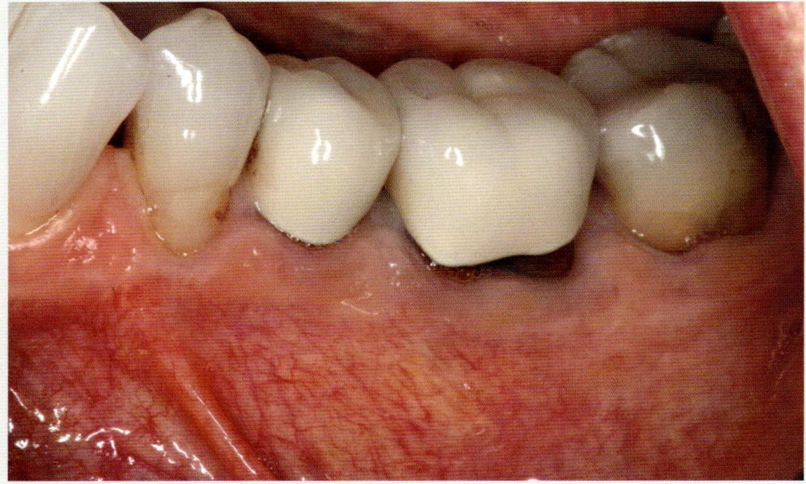

9.14 Six-month follow up showing clinical healing and healthy tissue response.

REFERENCES

1. Wang N, Knight K, Dao T, Friedman S. *Treatment outcome in endodontics: the Toronto Study. Phases I and II: apical surgery.* J Endod. 2004;30(11):751-61.
2. Tsesis I, Rosen E, Taschieri S, et al. *Outcomes of surgical endodontic treatment performed by a modern technique: an updated meta-analysis of the literature.* J Endod. 2013;39(3):332-9.
3. Weller RN, Niemczyk SP, Kim S. *Incidence and position of the canal isthmus. Part 1. Mesiobuccal root of the maxillary first molar.* J Endod. 1995;21(7):380-383.
4. Kim S, Kratchman S. *Modern endodontic surgery concepts and practice: a review.* J Endod. 2006; 32(7):601-23.
5. Setzer FC, Kohli MR, Shah SB, Karabucak B, Kim S. *Outcome of endodontic surgery: a meta-analysis of the literature - Part 2: Comparison of endodontic microsurgical techniques with and without the use of higher magnification.* J Endod. 2012;38(1):1-10.
6. Guerreo CG, Quijano Guaugue S, et al. *Predictors of clinical outcomes in endodontic microsurgery: a systematic review and meta-analysis.* Giornale Italiano di Endondonzia. 2017:31(1):2-13.
7. De Chevigny Dao TT, Basrani B, et al. *Treatment Outcomes in Endodontics: The Toronto Study-Phase 4: Initial treatment.* J Endod. 2008;34(3);258-263.
8. Wang N, Knight K, Dao T, Friedman S. *Treatment outcome in endodontics: the Toronto Study. Phases I and II: apical surgery.* J Endod. 2004;30(11):751- 61.
9. Floratos S, Syngcuk K. *Modern Microsurgical Concepts.* Dent Clin North Am. 2017;61(1):81-91.
10. Vercellotti T. A. *Essentials in piezosurgery: Clinical advantages in dentistry.* 1st ed. Surry, UK: Quintessence Publishing Co; 2009.
11. Abella F, de Ribot J, Doria G, et al. *Applications of piezoelectric surgery in endodontic surgery: a literature review.* J Endod. 2014;40(3):325-326.
12. Venskutonis T, Plotino G, Juodzbalys G, et al. *The importance of cone-beam computed tomography in the management of endodontic problems: a review of the literature.* J Endod. 2014;40(12):1895-1901.
13. Leonardi Dutra K, Haas L, Porporatti AL, et al. *Diagnostic accuracy of cone-beam computed tomography and conventional radiography on apical periodontitis: a systematic review and meta-analysis.* J Endod. 2016;42(3):356-64.
14. Ahlowalia MS, Patel S, Anwar HM, et al. *Accuracy of CBCT for volumetric measurement of simulated periapical lesions.* Int Endod J. 2013;46(6):538-46.
15. Kuhl S, Payer M, Zitzmann NU, et al. *Technical accuracy of printed surgical templates for guided implant surgery with the coDiagnostiX software.* Clin Implant Dent Relat Res. 2015;17(Suppl 1):e177-82.
16. D'Haese J, Van De Velde T, Komiyama A, et al. *Accuracy and complications using computer-designed stereolithographic surgical guides for oral rehabilitation by means of dental implants: a review of the literature.* Clin Implant Dent Relat Res. 2012;14(3):321-35.
17. Pinsky HM, Champleboux G, Sarment DP. *Periapical surgery using CAD/CAM guidance: preclinical results.* J Endod. 2007;33(2):148-51.
18. Strbac GD, Schnappauf A, Giannis K, Moritz A, Ulm C. *Guided Modern Endodontic Surgery: A Novel Approach for Guided Osteotomy and Root Resection.* J Endod. 2014;43(3):496-501.

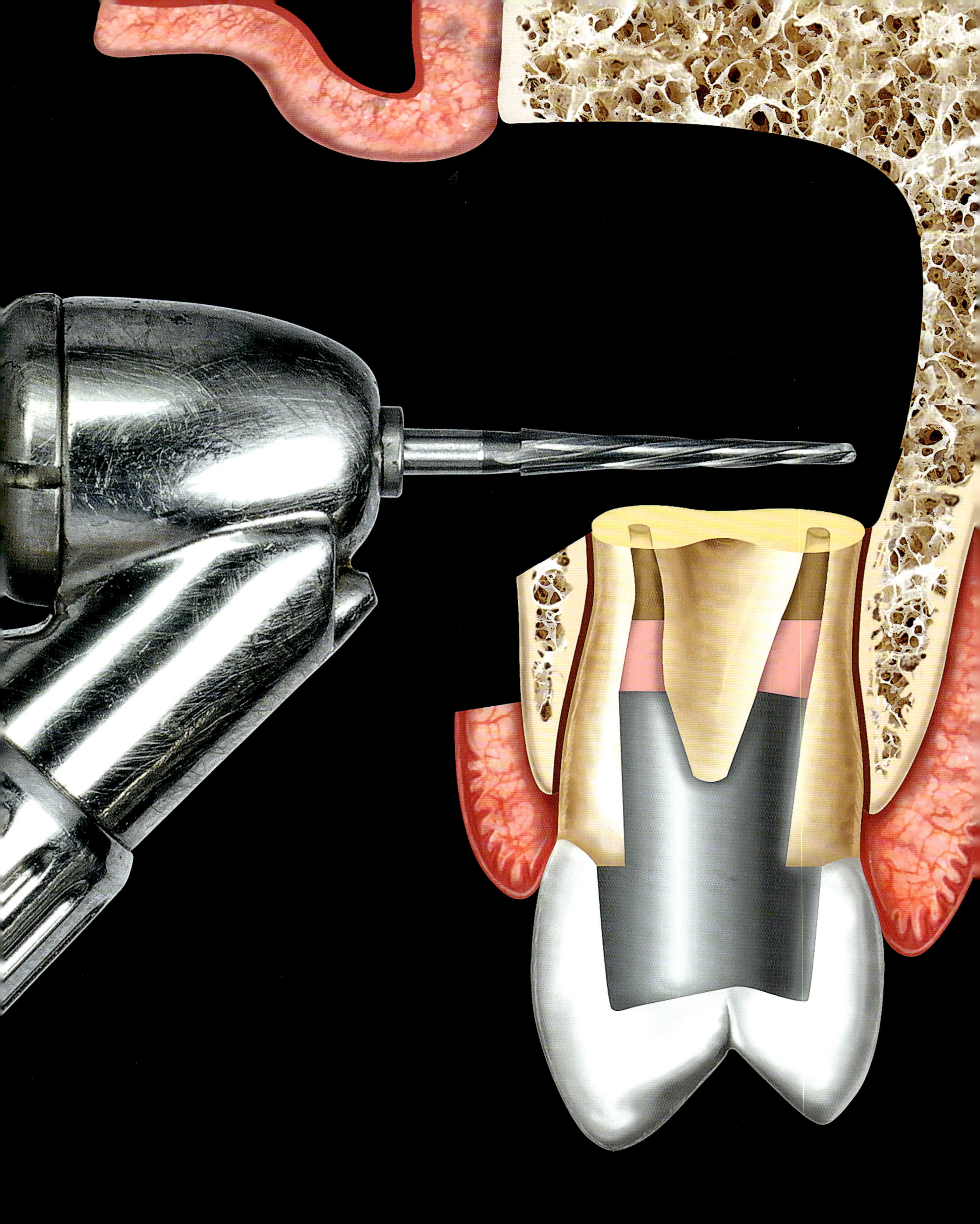

Root-end Resection

Root Resection versus Periapical Curettage

Over the years several authors have advocated periradicular curettage as definitive treatment for endodontic lesions, without subsequent root-end resection and retroseal.[1-7] This approach was advocated mainly to maintain root length for stability. However, no studies are available which address loss of tooth stability due to root-end resection, especially considering that usually root-end resection means removal of only 3 mm. While it is true that some cases demonstrate repair following curettage only,[7-9] on the other hand many of these are one-visit treatment cases or open system cases where the canal has been cleaned and obturated during the surgical procedure,[10] similar to the one described in Fig. 1.2. This generally enables the surgeon to eliminate the etiologic factors in the root canal system during the surgical procedure without root-end resection.[11] In other words, these cases were treated surgically and if the canal could have been negotiated nonsurgically, they could have been healed without any surgery. In conclusion, in the large majority of cases, if not always, the surgical approach is indicated to improve the apical seal in cases that could not be treated nonsurgically; therefore, the curettage by itself makes no sense and the apical resection and the retroseal are mandatory for success. As already stated, the apical curettage is done to control the bleeding, to improve visibility, to gain access to the root apex and finally to procure a specimen for histologic examination. It is *not enough* if we want healing to take place and to have a successful outcome.

Sometimes the removal of the granulation tissue is painful for the patient, and in such cases the soft tissue is injected with an anesthetic solution containing a vasoconstrictor 1:50,000. This will ensure comfort during the curettage and control hemorrhage in the surgical site.[12,13] The bone curettes are initially used to peel the soft tissue from the lateral borders of the bony crypt using the convex surface of the curette facing the bony wall. Once the tissue is freed along the lateral margins, the bone curette can be turned and used scraping the root surface. This is done because the lesion is initially formed at the expenses of the periodontal ligament and maintains its attachment to the root surface while it has no connection to the surrounding bone.

Root-end Resection. Indications and Rational

An old theory about the root-end resection was that the amount of root removed could greatly influence the outcome, so that often the patients were left with less than a one-to-one crown-root ratio.[14] Another theory often suggested by oral surgeons and maxillofacial surgeons advocated the removal of the entire root length that is surrounded by the lesion, up to the depth of the bony cavity. According to this theory, the portion of the root which penetrated into the diseased tissue has to be removed to a point flush with the base of the bony cavity or slightly below the cavity.[14] This theory was based on the assumption that the hard dental tissue and especially the cementum surrounded by the granulation tissue or by the cyst, is necrotic.[15] However, this concept has never been demonstrated[16] and we can conclude that this approach is completely wrong and certainly can compromise the stability of the tooth itself.

Once the granulation tissue has been removed and the root apex has been isolated, the root can be resected using the Lindemann bur on the high-speed handpiece Impact Air 45 (10.1), perpendicular to the long axis of the root.

Before the use of ultrasonic tips, with the traditional rotary bur, the cut was made at an angle of about 45° with a lingual to buccal steep bevel (10.2a). This was primarily designed for surgical access and direct visibility to the cut root surface, in order to orient the canal orifice towards the clinician who then used a straight slow-speed handpiece to prepare the cavity for the retroseal (10.2b). However, there is no biological justi-

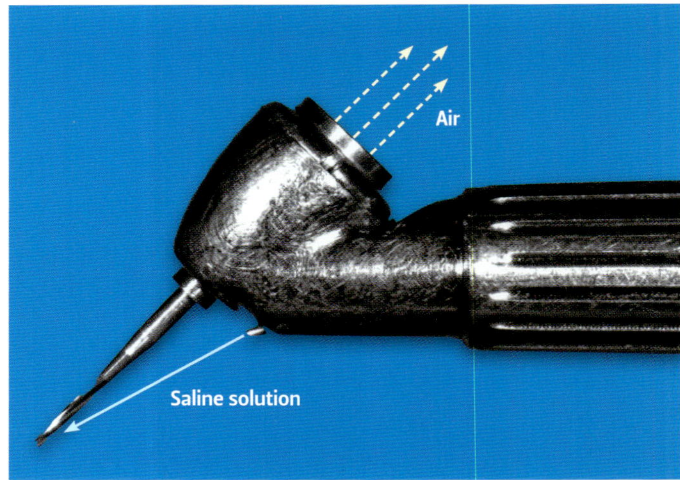

10.1. The Impact Air 45 (Palisades Dental, NJ, USA) is a 45° surgical high-speed handpiece, with the Lindemann bur.

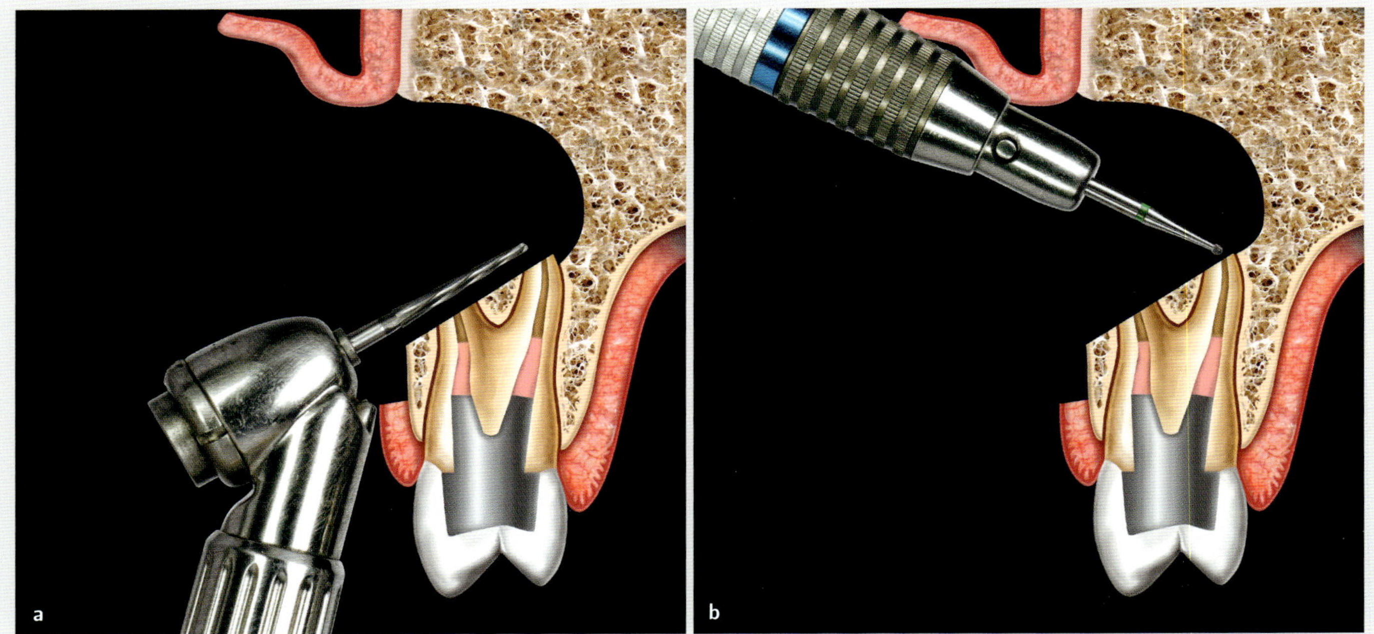

10.2 a, b) The 45° steep bevel involves an excessive and unnecessary removal of buccal supporting bone and tooth structure.

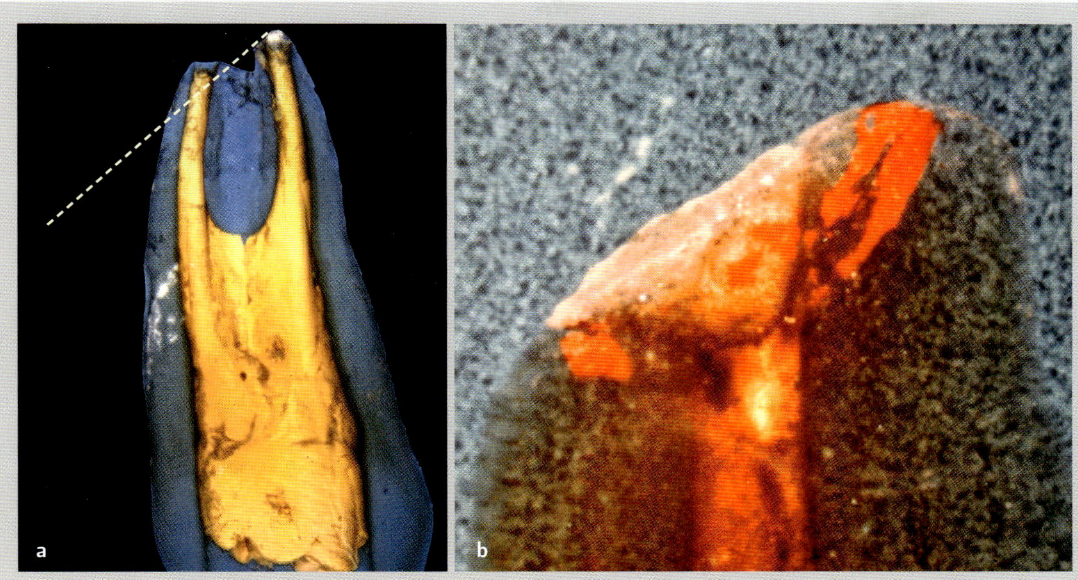

10.3 **a)** The 45° steep bevel involves the risk of missing palatal or lingual anatomy. **b)** The retrofill has been positioned without completely resecting through the root: the apical delta remained untouched, leaving three portals of exit unsealed (*Courtesy of Dr. John West*).

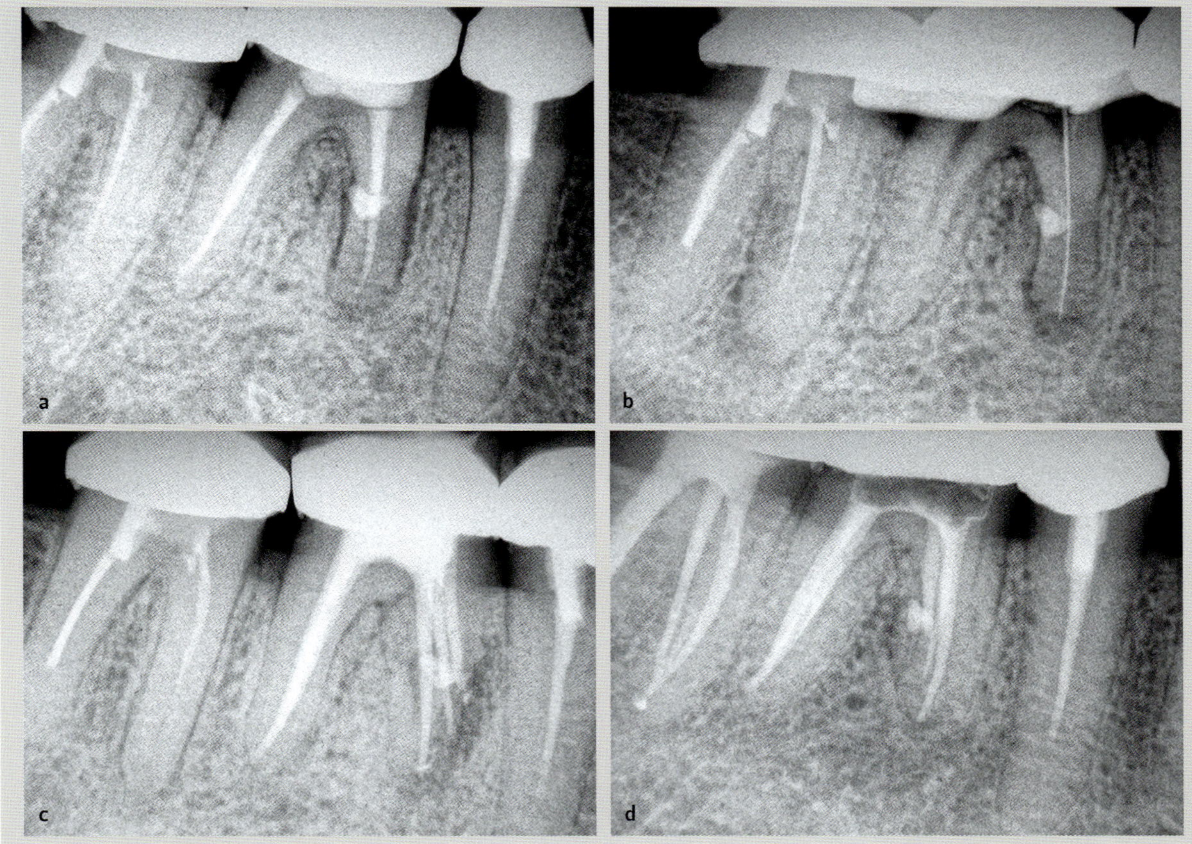

10.4 **a)** Preoperative radiograph of the lower right first molar. The oral surgeon was trying to be conservative with a very long bevel and positioned a retroseal in a very coronal portion of the root. **b)** During the nonsurgical retreatment, the mesiolingual canal appeared to be intact. **c)** The long bevel and two canals that were completely missed is evident. **d)** Two-year recall.

fication for creating a steep bevel angle on the resected root-end.[17] A steep bevel will cause:

- an excessive and unnecessary removal of buccal supporting bone and tooth structure (10.2b)
- an incomplete root resection which can lead to missing lingual or palatal root canals (10.3, 10.4)
- impossibility to seal the dentinal tubules present on the palatal aspect of the bevel (10.5).

It is a frequent occurrence in failed surgical cases, that only the buccal aspect of the root was resected, leaving the lingual aspect *in situ* (10.4). The result is a continuous infection from the lingual apex.[18]

Since the advent of the ultrasonic tips, the resection is made with a 0° bevel, working at 90° to the long axis of the tooth, to prepare a Class I cavity along the main axis of the tooth (10.6).

A 0° bevel has the following advantages:

- preservation of root length
- smaller osteotomy
- less chances of missing lingual canals
- less exposed dentinal tubules
- easier preparation of a Class I cavity along the main axis of the root canal
- less risk of palatal or lingual perforations.

Usually, the amount of root removed is about 3 mm,[19] however the amount of the apex to be resected is never established in advance but is dictated by the amount of the remaining tooth structure which must be the same on the buccal and on the lingual or palatal aspects of the resected root. What indicates that the removal is completed is the fact that the canal orifice is in the center of the root surface, surrounded by the same amount of dentine both buccally and lingually. In the case of two canals in the same root, as happens in the mesiobuccal root of the upper molars, in the mesial root of the lower molars, and every time there are two canals in the same root, the amount of dentine buccal to the buccal canal and the amount of dentine lingual to the lingual canal must be the same. This is important in order to have enough tooth structure to make an adequate root-end preparation.

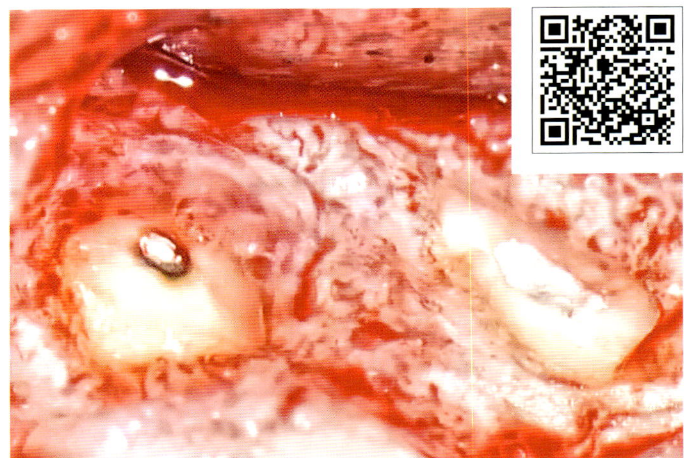

10.5 Intraoperative images of upper right central and lateral incisors treated by a maxillofacial surgeon one month before. Note the acute bevel and the absence of a retrofilling. The 45° steep bevel makes it impossible to seal the dentinal tubules present on the palatal aspect of the bevel, and the exposed dentinal tubules can be responsible for bacterial microleakage postoperatively. It is obvious why one month after surgery the patient presented a sinus tract originating from the central incisor, whose dentinal tubules are completely infiltrated by bacteria.

Once the granulation tissue has been removed and the root apex has been exposed, the root-end can be resected positioning the bur at 90° angle to the long axis and the root is shaved, cutting in a mesiodistal and apical/coronal direction (10.7). The bur is moved from mesial to distal, shaving the root smooth and flat, and exposing the entire root canal system and root outline.[11] As already stated, the removal is completed when the canal or canals are surrounded by the same amount of dentin buccally and lingually, visibility and access to the resected surface is obtained and the root outline is visible.

Sometimes in cases when a biopsy is desired, instead of shaving the root-end, the root apex is resected by a predetermined amount, cutting with a thin fissure bur through the root from mesial to distal. The same technique must be used when a fragment of a broken instrument is present at the apex or through the foramen (10.8). Shaving the root-end in this situation could cause the production of metal fragments that will easily enter in the surrounding soft tissue, causing a later tattoo.

The removal of about 3 mm of the root apex will allow the operator to remove 98% of apical ramifications and 93% of lateral canals (10.9).[19] A root-end amputation

Cont'd on page 189

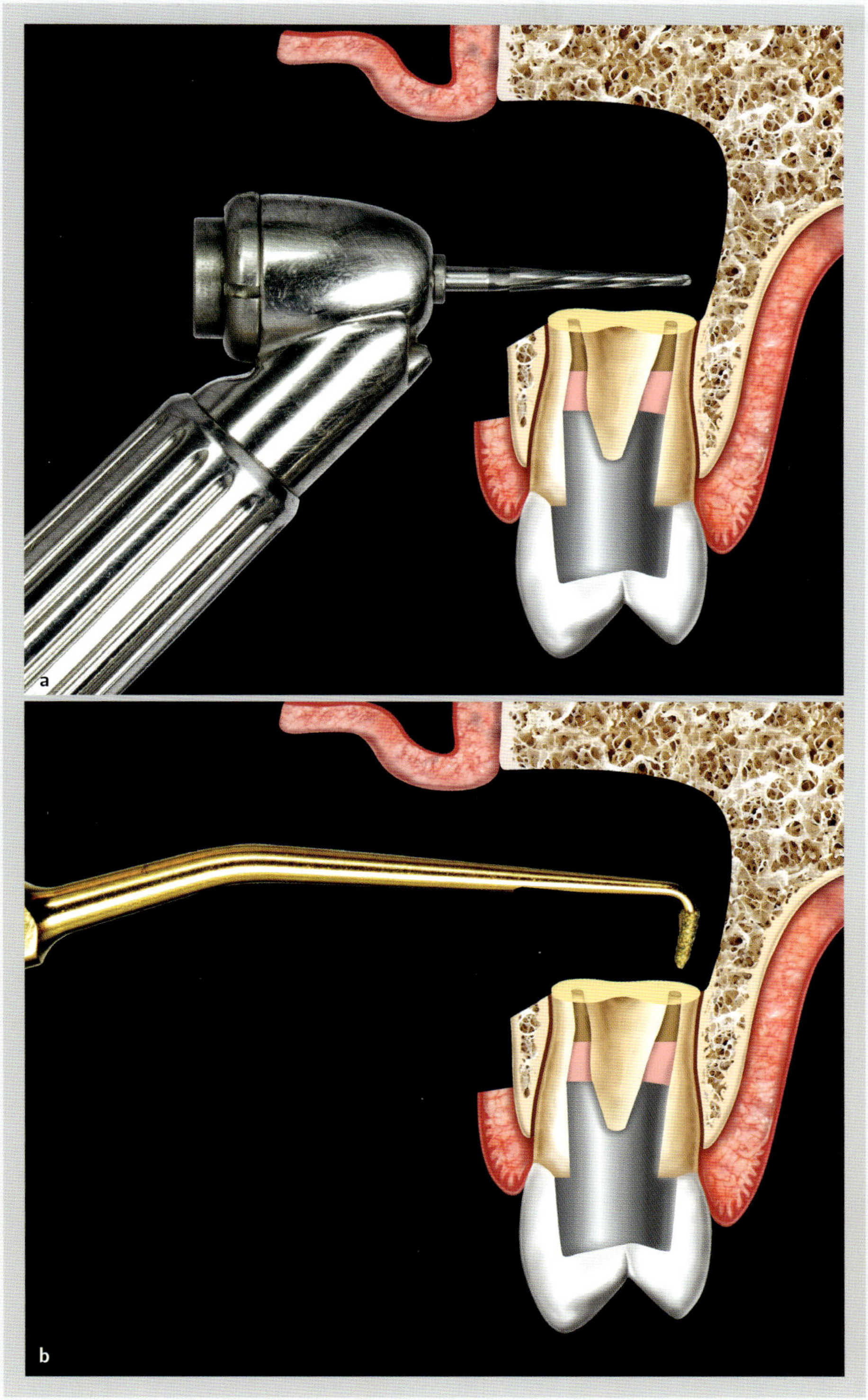

10.6 **a)** The root-end resection is currently made with a 0° bevel, perpendicular to the long axis of the tooth. **b)** The root-end preparation makes a class-one cavity along the main axis of the tooth.

10.7 The exposed root apex is shaved moving the Lindemann bur in a mesiodistal (M–D) and apical/coronal (A–C) direction.

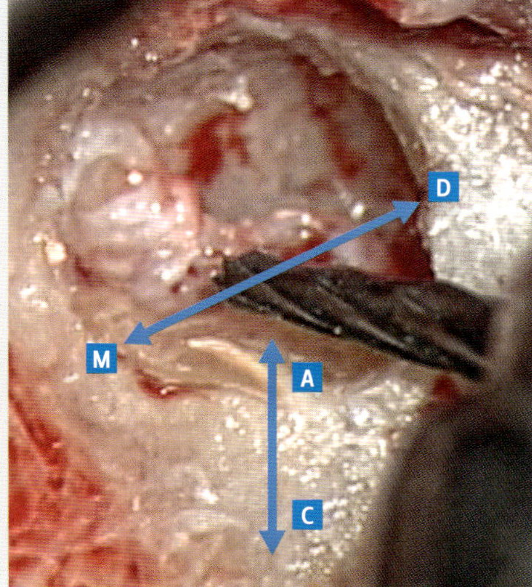

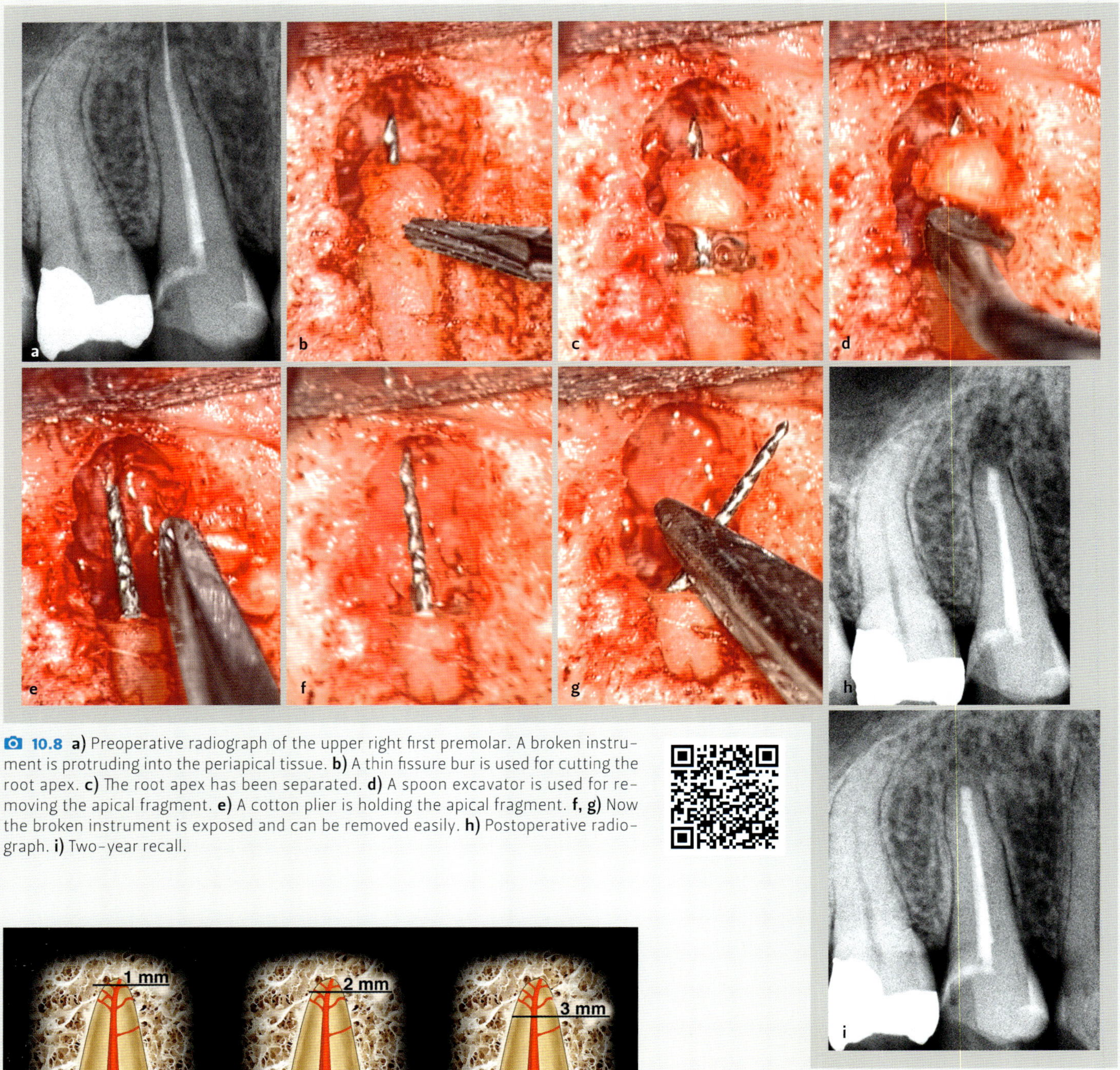

10.8 a) Preoperative radiograph of the upper right first premolar. A broken instrument is protruding into the periapical tissue. **b)** A thin fissure bur is used for cutting the root apex. **c)** The root apex has been separated. **d)** A spoon excavator is used for removing the apical fragment. **e)** A cotton plier is holding the apical fragment. **f, g)** Now the broken instrument is exposed and can be removed easily. **h)** Postoperative radiograph. **i)** Two-year recall.

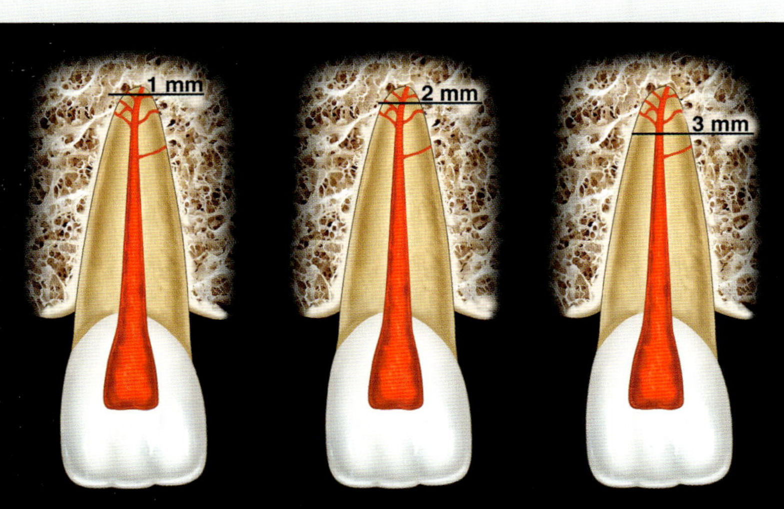

10.9. Removing the apical 3 mm: 98% of the apical ramifications and 93% of lateral canals can be eliminated.

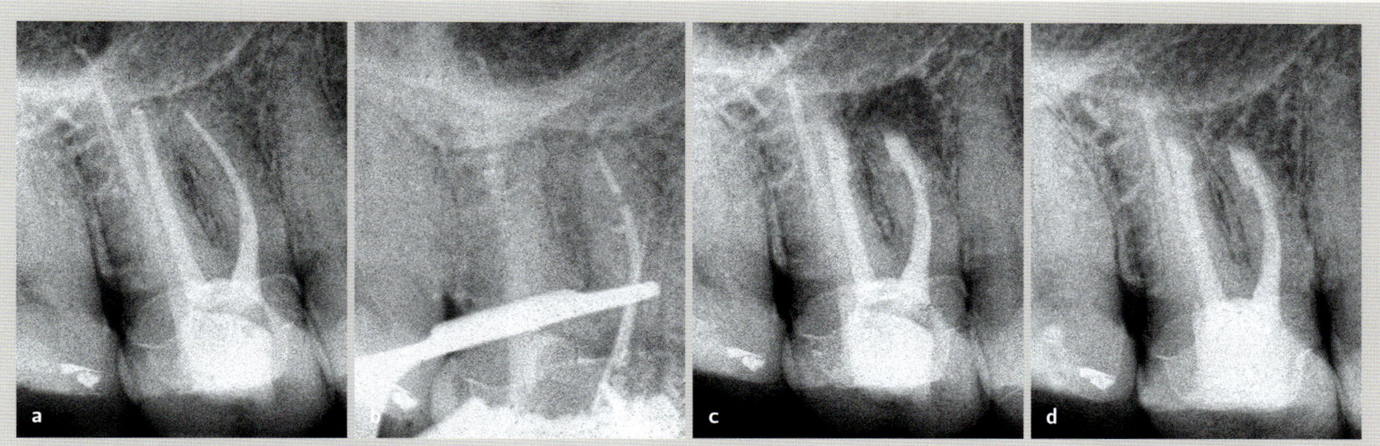

10.10 **a)** Preoperative radiograph of the upper right first molar. The patient has symptoms and is scheduled for nonsurgical retreatment. **b)** In the attempt to bypass the plastic carrier of the Thermafil® a perforation was made. **c)** Postoperative radiograph. During the surgical procedure, the root was resected coronal to the level of the perforation. **d)** Two-year recall.

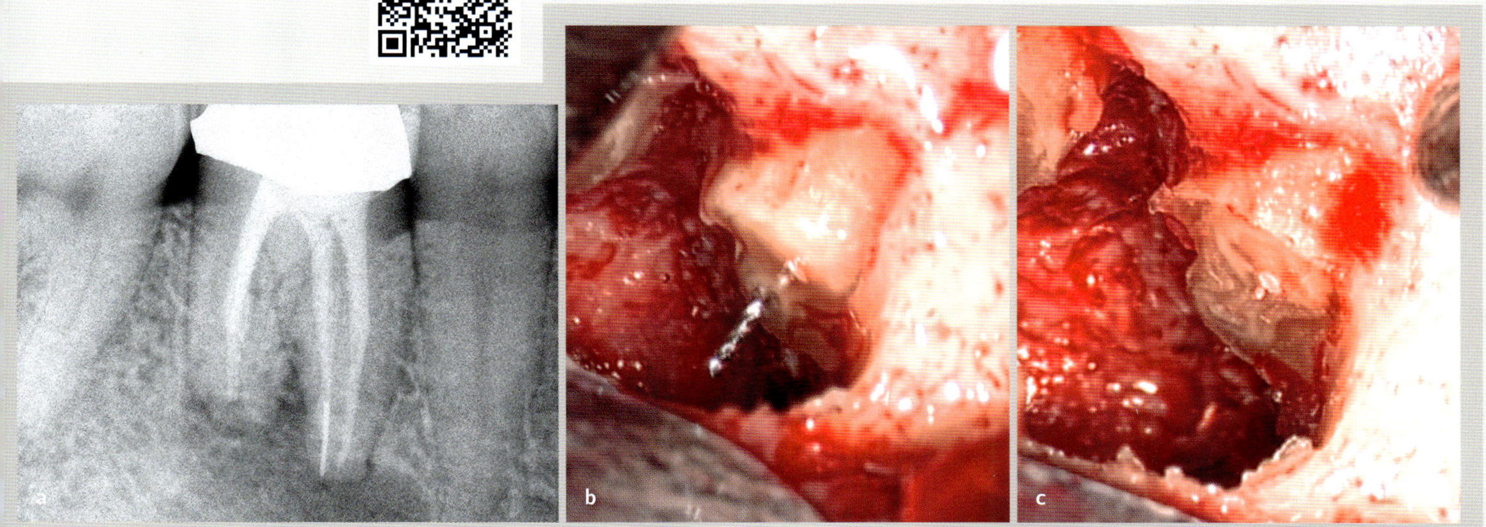

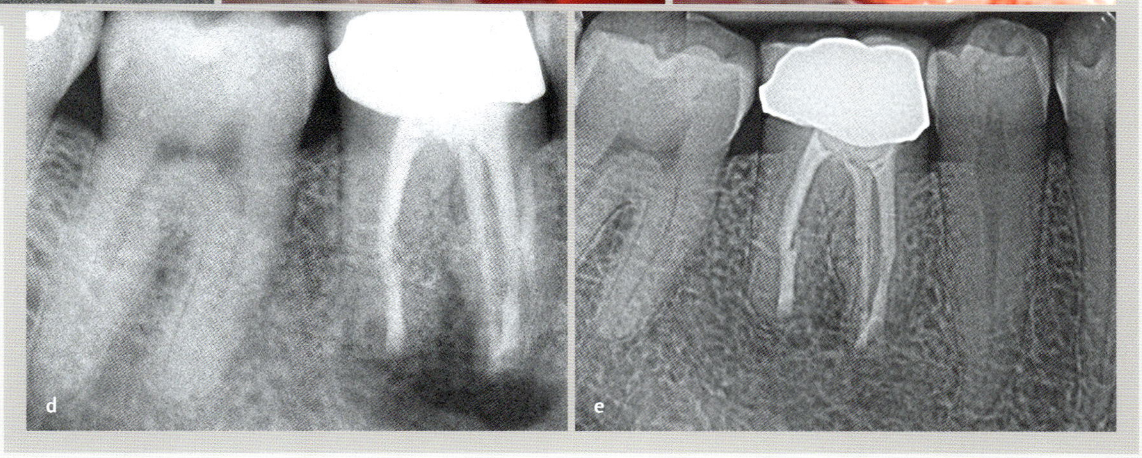

10.11 **a)** Preoperative radiograph of the lower right first molar. A broken instrument is present in the mesial root. **b)** The mesial root was resected sufficiently to expose the fragment. **c)** The broken instrument has been removed. **d)** Postoperative radiograph. **e)** Two-year recall.

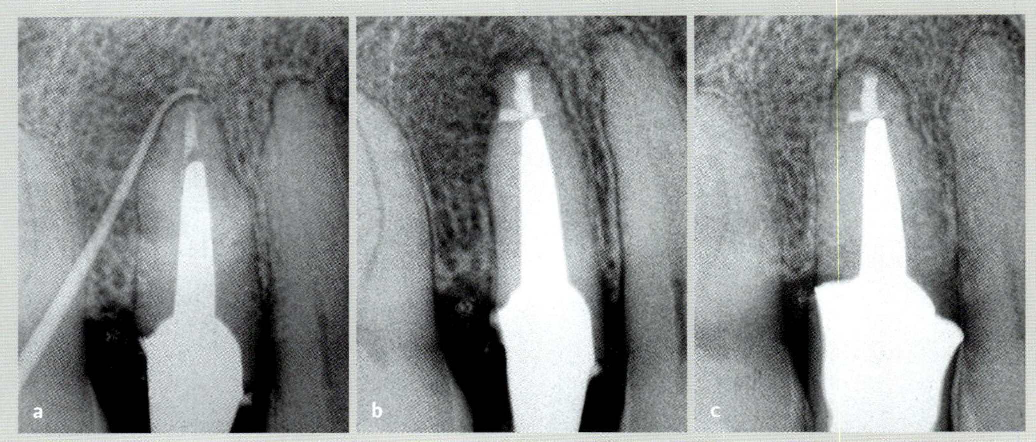

10.12 **a)** Preoperative radiograph of the upper right second premolar. The root has a big cast post, a lateral lesion, and a sinus tract. **b)** Instead of removing 3 mm of the root apex, the main canal and the lateral canals were prepared and sealed, in order to avoid exposing the cast post. **c)** Two-year recall.

10.13 **a)** Preoperative radiograph of the upper right central incisor. **b)** A vertical root fracture is present. **c)** After shaving a few millimeters of root structure, the fracture line is no longer evident. **d)** A retrofill was positioned in the root-end preparation. **e)** Postoperative radiograph. **f)** Seventeen-year recall.

Cont'd from page 184
of less than 3 mm, most likely, does not remove all of the lateral canals and apical ramifications, therefore posing a risk of reinfection and eventual failure.[20]

However, the 3 mm rule does not apply to every situation and depends on several factors, namely presence and location of a perforation (10.10), ledge or broken instrument (10.11), apical extent of a metal post (10.12), presence of an incomplete vertical root fracture (10.13).

The resected root can be precisely examined directly or via a microsurgical mirror (under a medium/maximum magnification of the operating microscope) after staining the periodontal ligament with Methylene blue (Vista Dental, Racine, WI, USA) (10.14a).[21] The stain-

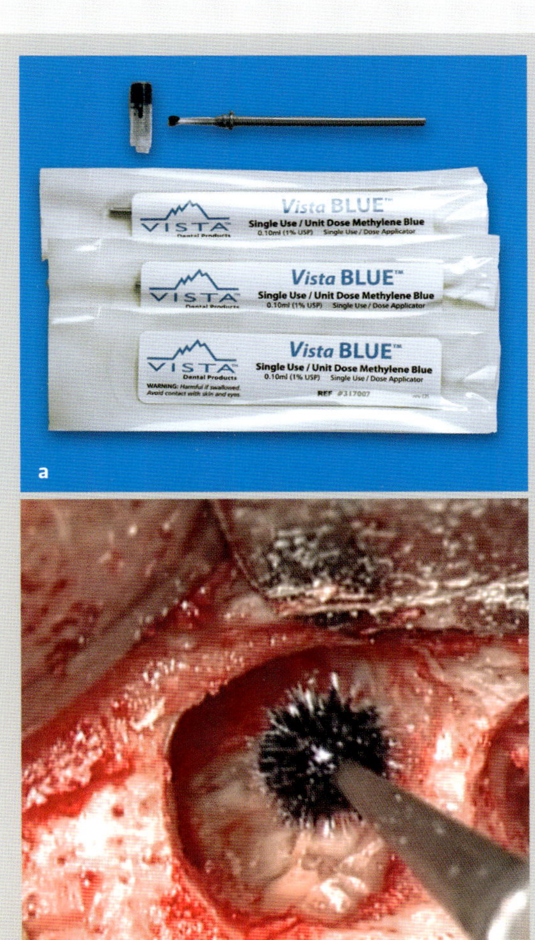

10.14 **a)** The single dose Methylene Blue by Vista Dental (Vista Dental, Racine, WI, USA). **b)** The microsurgical brush is carrying the methylene blue.

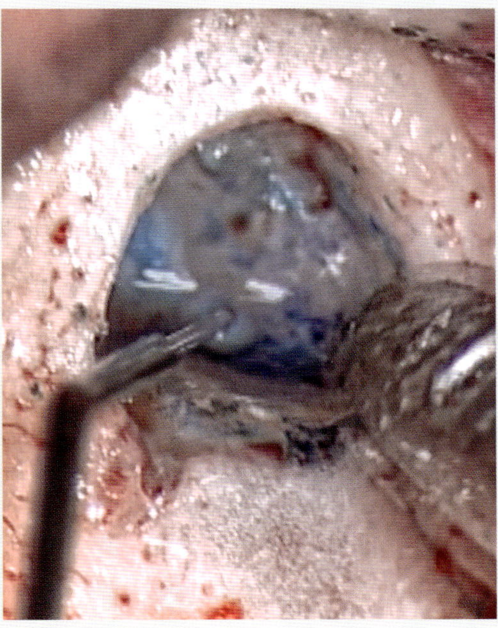

10.15 The excess of the dye is removed with irrigation with saline solution.

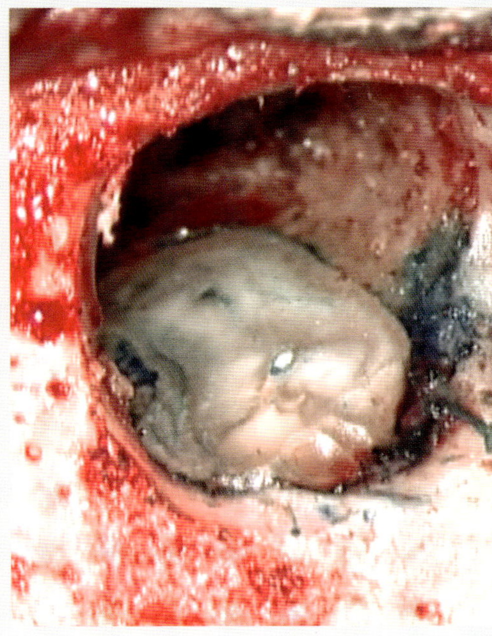

10.16 Now the PDL and the root canals are quite visible.

ing solution is gently applied with specific microsurgical applicators (10.14b) and after a short period of time is flushed with sterile water or saline solution using the Stropko irrigator (10.15).

The PDL will appear uninterrupted all around the root surface and the blue dye will show the periodontal ligament 360° around the bevel, to confirm that the resection has completely involved the root structure in a buccal to lingual direction (10.16). This will allow the operator to easily visualize any anatomical variations, fracture lines, isthmus (roots with two canals have an isthmus 100% of the time! [22]), accessory canals and to confirm that the root has been completely resected. If the periodontal ligament is not visible on the palatal side, it means that the resection did not involve the entire root surface (10.13c).

The indications for root resection are the following:

1. It allows the removal of pathologic processes, like fractured root-tips and resorptive processes.[14,23,24] However, the presence of an apical root resorption is not an indication for surgery and root resection. The apical external root resorption is the common consequence of the inflammation due to the presence of bacteria in the necrotic root canal and usually is a self-limiting process if the root canal therapy is performed correctly: root canal debridement, disinfection and obturation will arrest the process. This kind of external root resorption can involve every apex of every necrotic tooth as well as the apex of the adjacent vital tooth. In a case like this, the resorption will involve the hard tissue, bone, cementum and dentine, but will never involve the soft tissue, therefore the vitality of the adjacent tooth is never compromised (10.17).[24] Only in cases where the nonsurgical therapy failed, that the surgical approach is indicated, and in this situation the resorbed portion of the root apex will be removed and the apical seal will be surgically improved. The same is valid in the case of an apical root fracture (10.18). Only in the presence of signs or symptoms of pathosis is the surgical approach indicated (10.19).
2. It facilitates the removal of the granulation tissue, especially if it is deeply placed behind the root apex and it also makes a biopsy possible.[25]
3. It allows the removal of iatrogenic mishaps, like transported foramina, broken instruments, blocked root canals, ledges that are not negotiable nonsurgically.[14] When these operator errors are present, the clinician should always evaluate the difficulties of their elimination nonsurgically as well as his/her skill and expertise. However, as suggested by Nygaard-Ostby and Schilder,[26] when these situations occur, it is usually recommended filling as much of the root canal by conventional method as possible.
4. It allows the removal of the great majority of canal

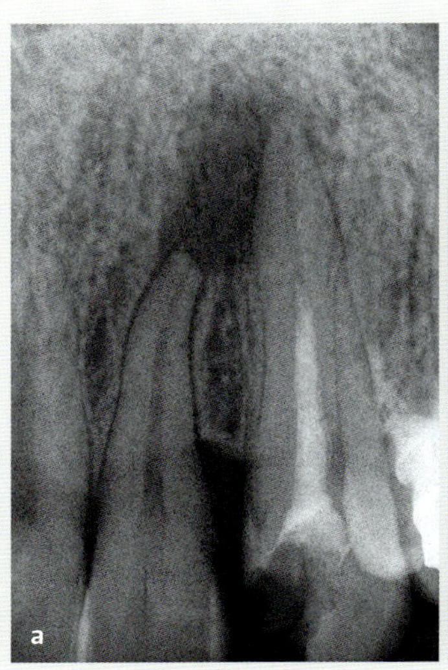

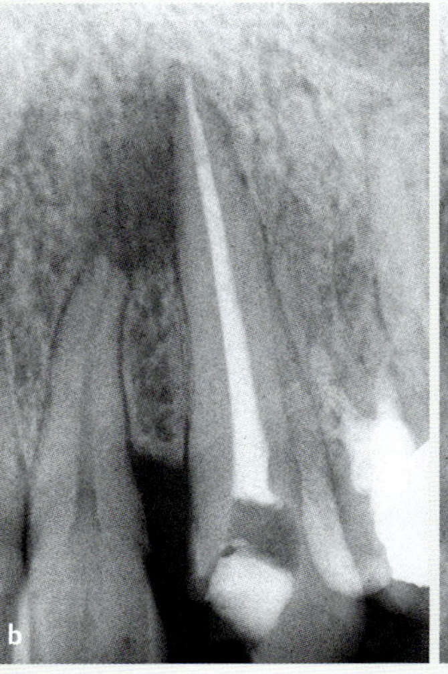

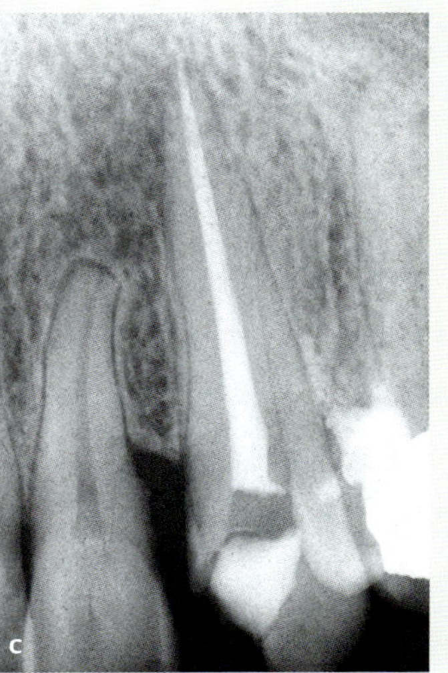

10.17 External resorption (progressive inflammatory resorption secondary to infection) of the apex of an upper left lateral incisor, caused by pulp necrosis of the adjacent canine, treated inadequately. The lateral incisor responds positively to the pulp tests. **a)** Preoperative radiograph. **b)** Postoperative radiograph. **c)** Recall radiograph 12 months later: the resorption has been arrested, the lesion has healed, and one can identify the lamina dura around the apex of the lateral incisor. The pulp has obviously preserved its vitality.

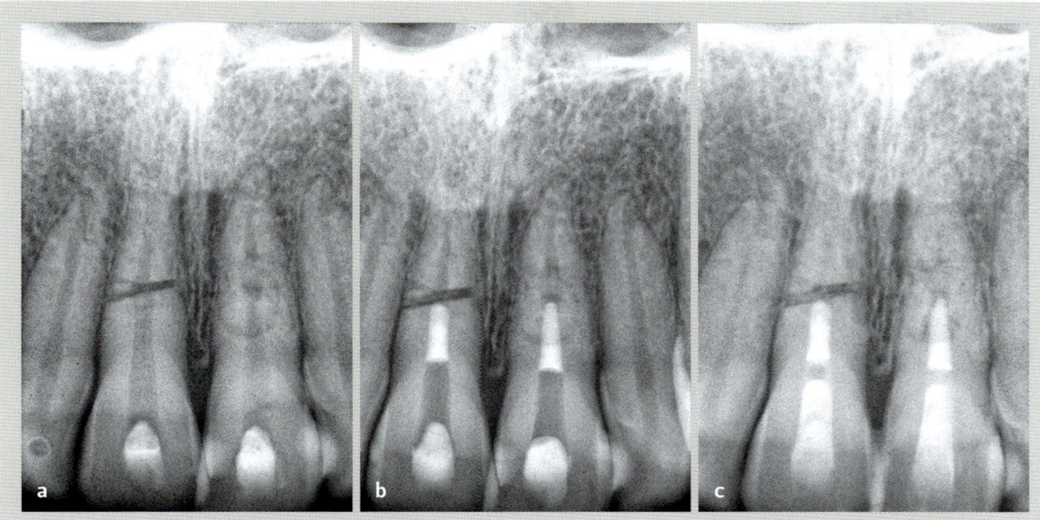

10.18 a) Both central incisors have a horizontal fracture consequent to a trauma. Both pulps were necrotic and the referring dentist had already opened the access cavity. **b)** The coronal portions of the root canals have been treated with white MTA at the level of the fracture and warm gutta-percha. **c)** At the two-year recall, the apical fragments maintained their vitality; there is no sign of inflammation around the horizontal fractures. Therefore, there is no reason to surgically remove the apical fragments.

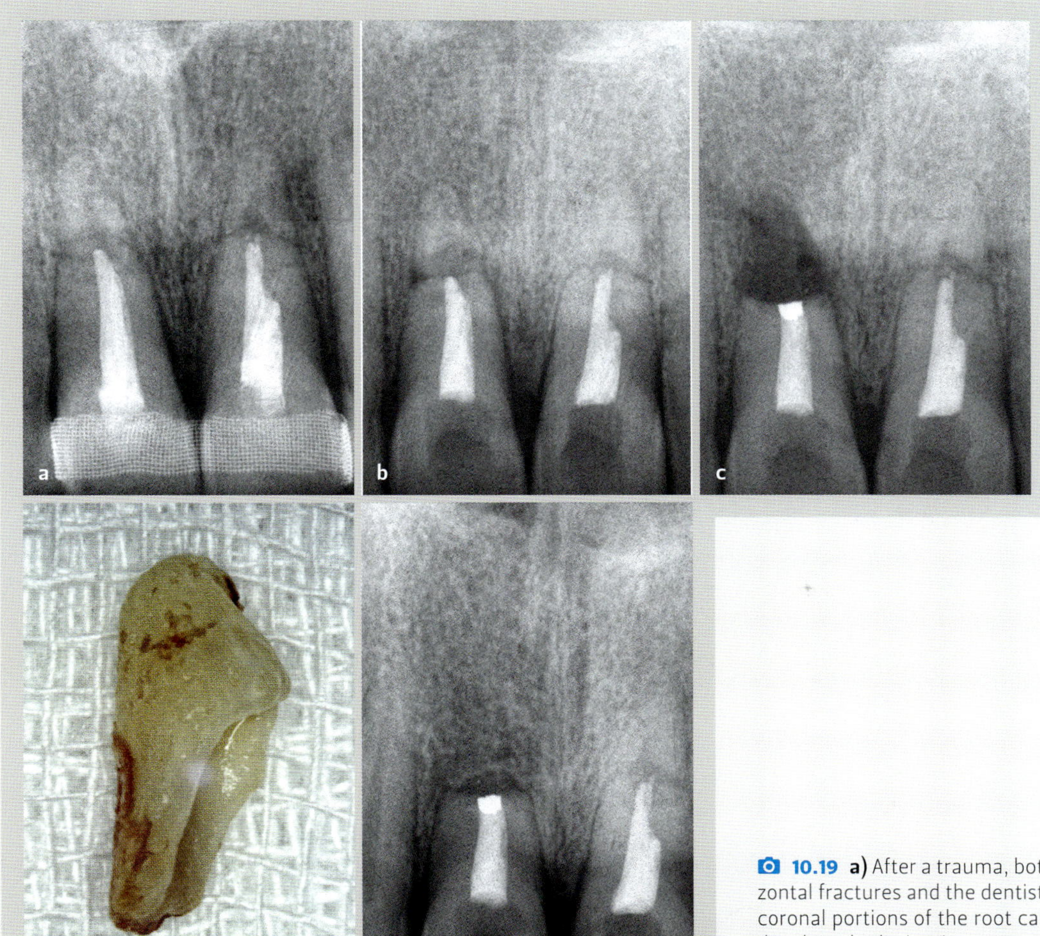

10.19 a) After a trauma, both central incisors presented with horizontal fractures and the dentist performed root canal therapy on both coronal portions of the root canals. **b)** A few months later the patient developed a lesion in correspondence with the fracture line of the right incisor. **c)** The necrotic fragment was removed and a retroseal with amalgam positioned. **d)** The apical fragment. **e)** Two-year recall.

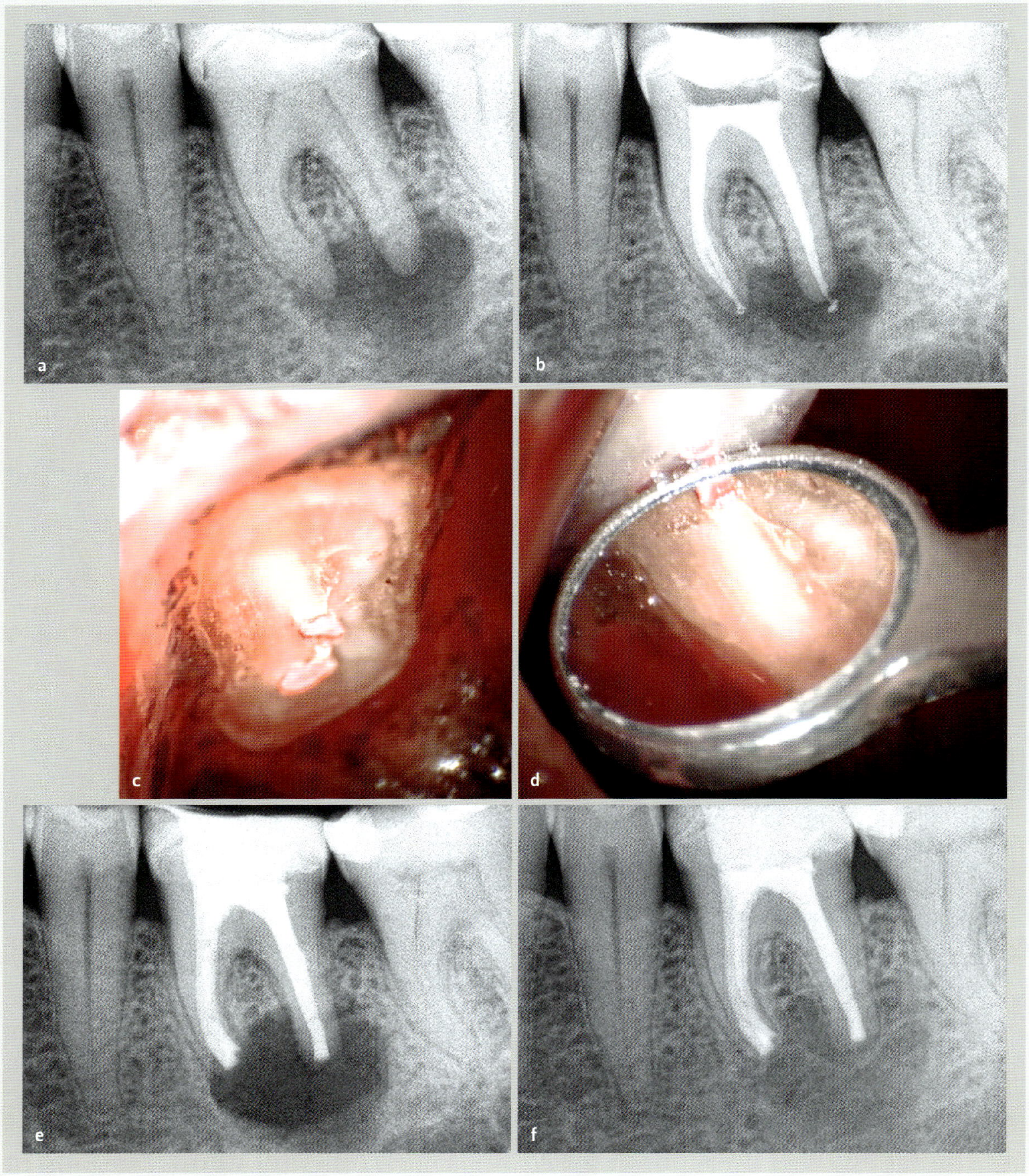

10.20 **a)** Preoperative radiograph of the lower left first molar. **b)** Several months after the root canal therapy there is no sign of healing and the patient has symptoms. **c)** The mesial root is showing the presence of a third canal full of debris. **d)** The untreated canal is now more evident in the microsurgical mirror. **e)** Postoperative radiograph. Both roots have been sealed with white MTA. **f)** Two-year recall.

ramifications, apical deltas, lateral and accessory canals (10.9) and severe curves.[14,27,28] It is possible that these aberrant anatomic variations contain bacteria or necrotic debris impossible to be removed nonsurgically and responsible for the failure of what apparently was a well performed nonsurgical treatment (10.20). Surgical removal of these aberrant anatomic entities will transform the failure into a success.

5. It allows the creation of an adequate apical seal, impossible to be obtained nonsurgically.[29] This is the most common indication for root-end resection. When the root canal system cannot be negotiated in its entire length for whatever reason, e.g. a post and core is present, and the apical portion had not been properly cleaned, shaped and obturated, or the apical portion is blocked by calcifications or debris (10.21) the root-end resection will allow one to manage the apical portion of the root canal and to obtain and adequate apical seal.

6. It will allow the reduction of fenestrated root apices.[29,30,35] This situation is common mainly in maxillary premolars and molars but can also be present in anterior maxillary teeth (2.47, 2.48). By definition, the "fenestrated apex" is surrounded by inflamed periosteum and is associated with symptoms on palpation of the apical area. The root resection is indicated in order to remove the root apex to the level of the bone, to place the remainder of the root within its bony housing. This way the root will be completely surrounded by bone and the symptoms will be eliminated.

Of course, as it will be discussed later, in all the above mentioned indications after the root resection a retroprep and a retroseal should always be performed.

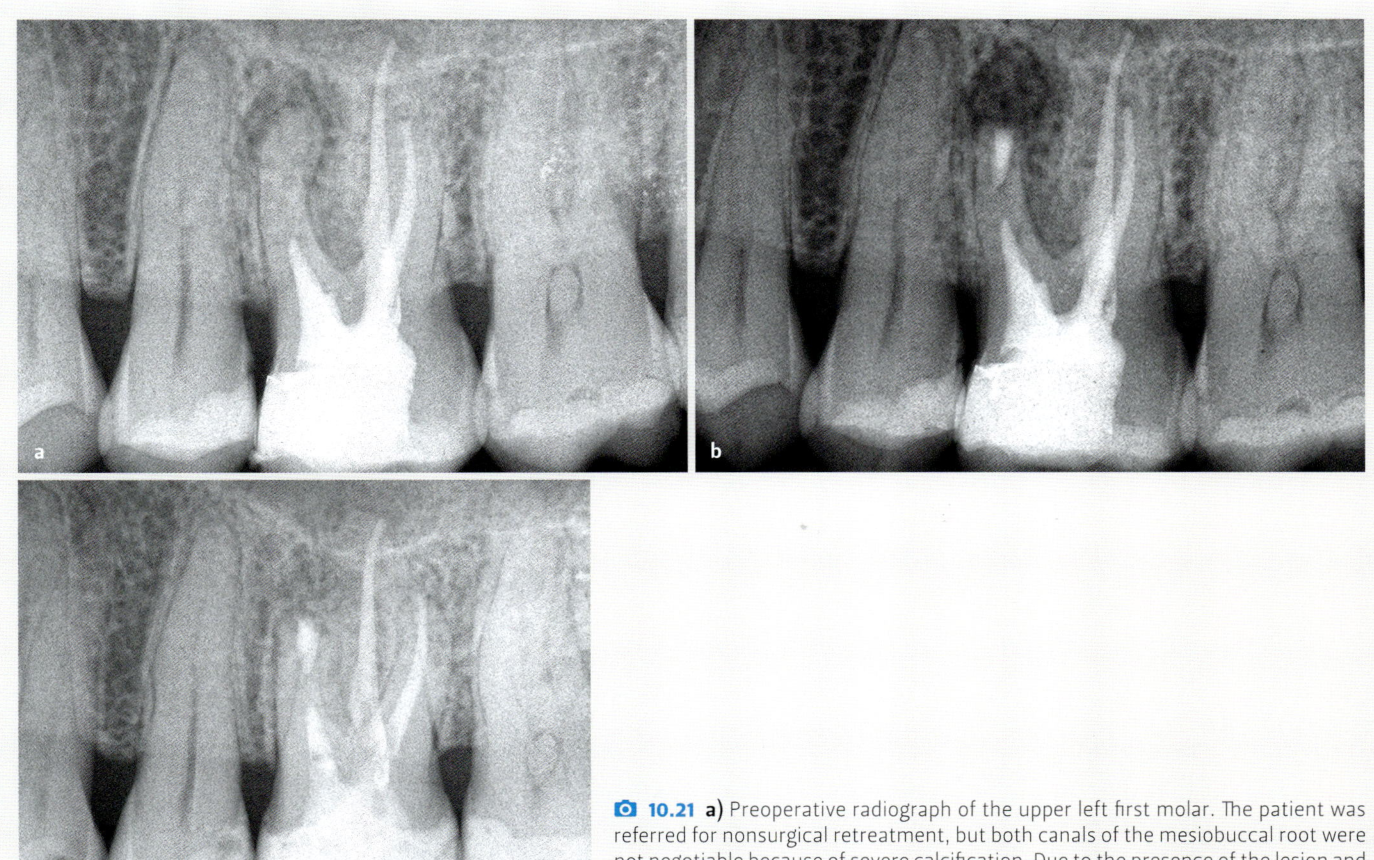

10.21 a) Preoperative radiograph of the upper left first molar. The patient was referred for nonsurgical retreatment, but both canals of the mesiobuccal root were not negotiable because of severe calcification. Due to the presence of the lesion and symptoms, the patient was scheduled for surgery. **b)** Both canals and the isthmus were sealed with white MTA. **c)** Two-year recall.

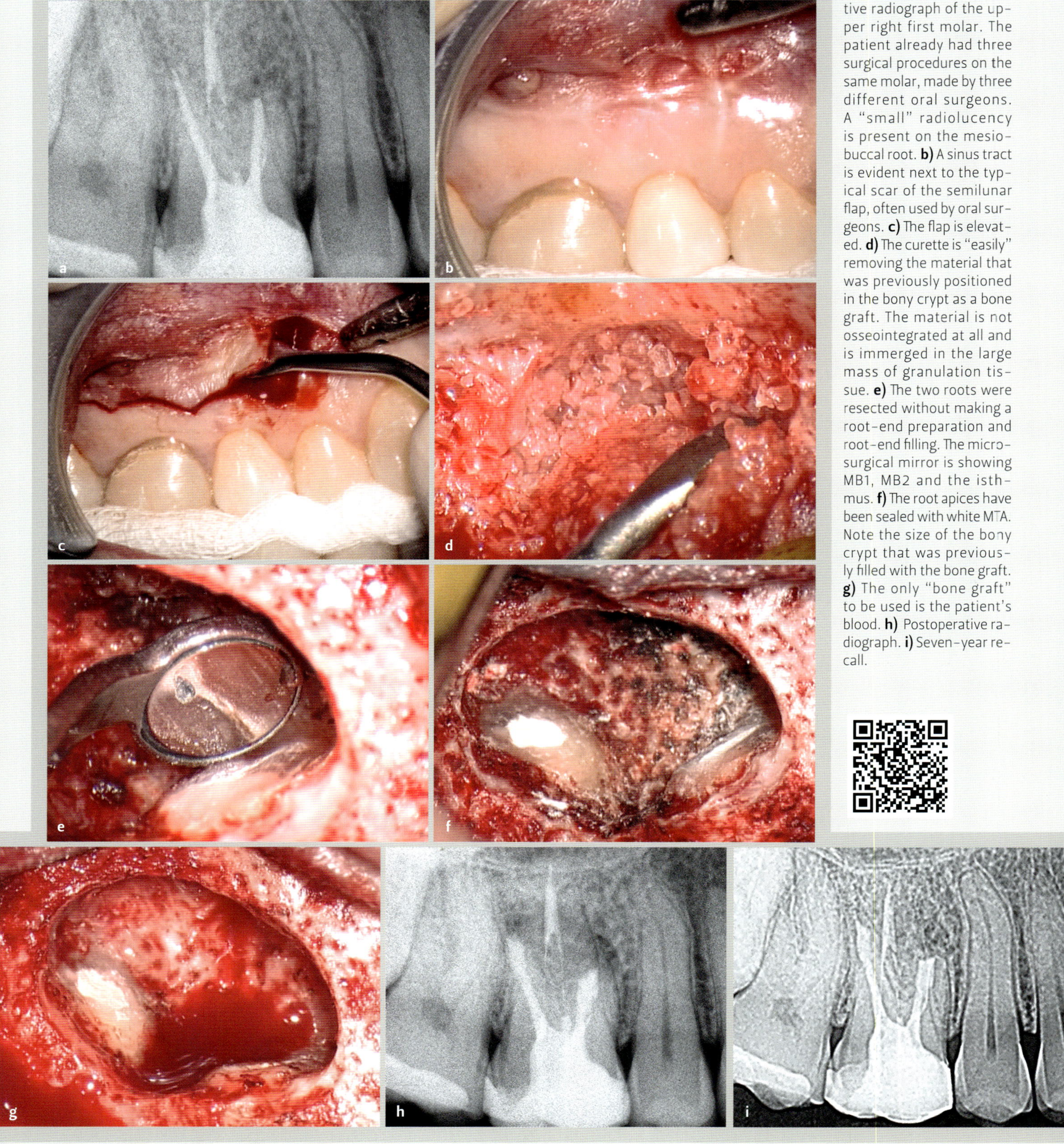

10.22 **a)** Preoperative radiograph of the upper right first molar. The patient already had three surgical procedures on the same molar, made by three different oral surgeons. A "small" radiolucency is present on the mesiobuccal root. **b)** A sinus tract is evident next to the typical scar of the semilunar flap, often used by oral surgeons. **c)** The flap is elevated. **d)** The curette is "easily" removing the material that was previously positioned in the bony crypt as a bone graft. The material is not osseointegrated at all and is immerged in the large mass of granulation tissue. **e)** The two roots were resected without making a root-end preparation and root-end filling. The microsurgical mirror is showing MB1, MB2 and the isthmus. **f)** The root apices have been sealed with white MTA. Note the size of the bony crypt that was previously filled with the bone graft. **g)** The only "bone graft" to be used is the patient's blood. **h)** Postoperative radiograph. **i)** Seven-year recall.

Inspection of the Resected Root Surface

Once the root-end has been resected, it should be carefully examined using a microsurgical mirror under the operating microscope, to make sure that the resection has involved the entire surface bucco-lingually.[18,19,31–34] For this reason it is highly recommended to use methylene blue dye on the root surface as it stains the periodontal ligament and pulp tissue selectively.[18,32] The excess of dye is then removed by irrigating with saline solution and through the microsurgical mirror the uninterrupted PDL should be visible. Furthermore, the blue dye will make additional foramina, fracture lines and the quality of the apical seal visible.

Evaluation of the Apical Seal

According to Harrison and Todd,[36] resection of roots obturated using the lateral condensation technique does not adversely affect the apical seal or adaptation of the material against the prepared canal walls. However, SEM study by Cunningham [37] and Tanzilli et al.[38] could not support the good adaptation of the gutta-percha to the canal walls subsequent to resection alone. Therefore, regardless of the technique used to obturate the root canal system, the root resection should *always* be followed by the root-end preparation and root-end fill. This is due to the fact that even a well compacted gutta-percha, after the resection, will be dislodged by the cutting bur, overlapping the root surface on one side and leaving a gap on the other side. Cold burnishing of the gutta-percha has been suggested, but according to Minnich et al.[39] cold burnishing the gutta-percha exposed after apical root resection of a well-obturated canal results in a poorer apical seal than did without burnishing, therefore the root-end preparation and fill should always be performed after apical root resection (📷 2.1).

According to Shaw et al.[40] cold burnishing of gutta-percha after apicoectomy does not produce a hermetic seal, therefore a reverse filling should be inserted into the resected root-ends of teeth if the operator is of opinion that clinical success may be dependent on creating a seal which will permit the least amount of leakage. Since this is exactly the goal, one can conclude that the reverse filling must be always performed. The removal of the diseased periapical tissue alone eliminates only the effect of the leakage, not the cause. Exactly the same is obtained if the root apex is resected and the endodontic seal has not been improved by a root-end obturation. Apical surgery entails not just the removal of the diseased tissue or the root-tip, but most importantly resealing of the root canal system.[20] Unfortunately, some oral surgeons and maxillofacial surgeons put all their efforts in the periapical curettage, in the resection of the root apex, sometimes put some bone graft in the bony lesion and they don't do anything to improve the apical seal of the resected root (📷 10.22)!

The Isthmus

As already stated before, one of the key steps in microsurgery is the careful inspection of the resected root surface, that can reveal all the details and complexity of the root canal anatomy, like the presence of an isthmus. First of all, one must understand and remember that two canals of the same root are *always* connected by a thin communication that in vital teeth contains pulp tissue, while in necrotic teeth contains bacteria. An isthmus is a part of the canal system and not a sep-

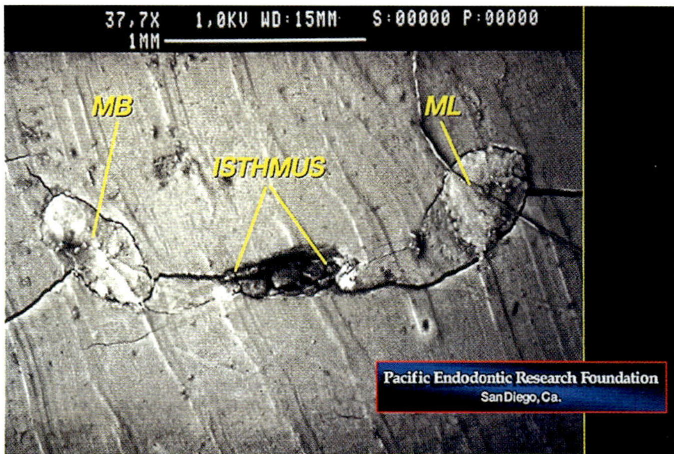

📷 **10.23** The SEM picture shows the presence of an isthmus between a mesiobuccal and a mesiolingual canal (*Courtesy of Dr. Gary Carr*).

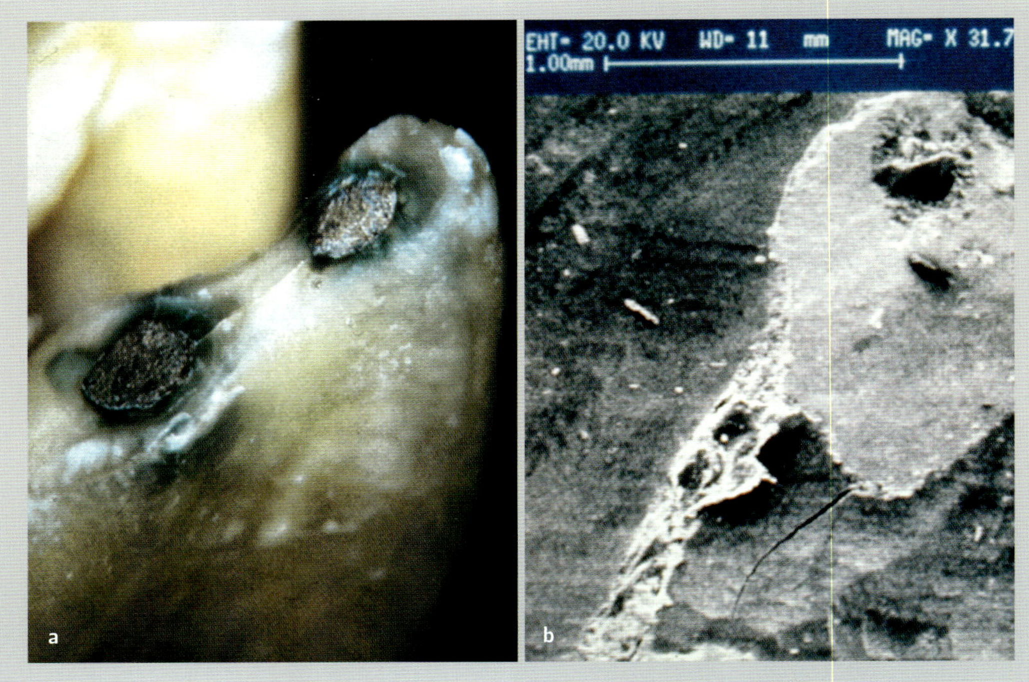

10.24 a, b) Examples of missed isthmuses (*Courtesy of Dr. Gary Carr*).

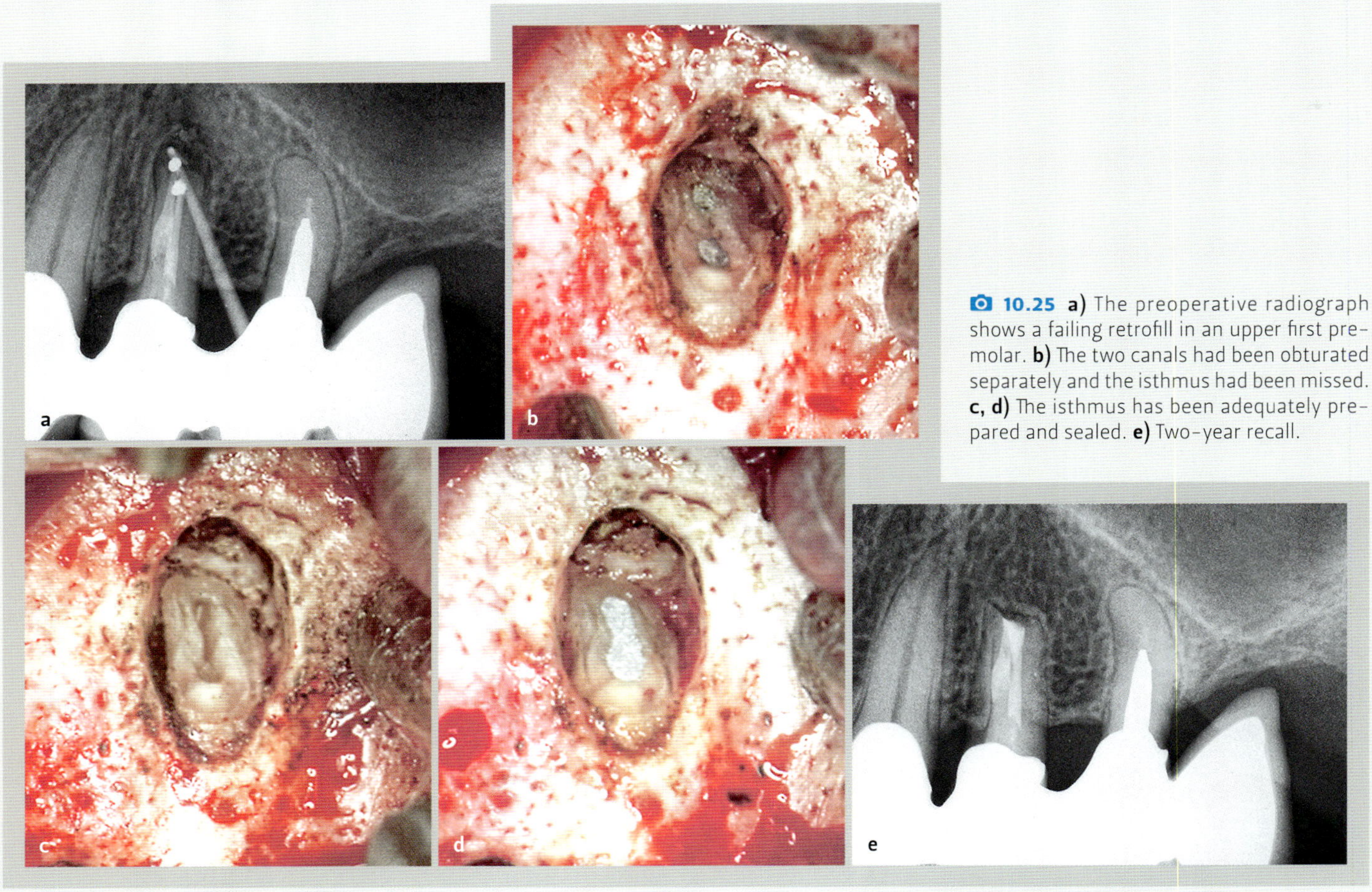

10.25 a) The preoperative radiograph shows a failing retrofill in an upper first premolar. **b)** The two canals had been obturated separately and the isthmus had been missed. **c, d)** The isthmus has been adequately prepared and sealed. **e)** Two-year recall.

arate entity, therefore it must be cleaned, shaped and filled as thoroughly as any other canal spaces (10.23, 10.24).[20] This is true even though the isthmus is not visible under the operating microscope. When making the root-end preparation of two canals of the same root, the preparation must always include the isthmus, so that the final shape of the cavity will be ribbon-shaped. Missing the preparation and the obturation of the isthmus can be the cause of the surgical failure. The case presented in Fig. 10.25 is a typical case that failed because of not treating the isthmus and healed subsequent to surgical retreatment. The main cause of failure in mesial roots of mandibular molars done with the bur and amalgam is the inability to treat the isthmus (10.26).

Regarding its incidence, the isthmus must always be considered present between two canals within one root. Considering the fact that the mesiobuccal root of upper first molars has two canals (MB1 and MB2) in about 93% of the cases,[41] it is obvious that the isthmus in present exactly in the same percentage. The same is valid for the mesial root of mandibular first molar and upper premolars. This is one of the reasons why apicoectomy alone, without root-end preparation and root-end filling on the mentioned teeth, usually fails.[20] As far as the management is concerned, the isthmus requires a careful approach with thin ultrasonic tips troughing along the entire isthmus and preparing it to a depth of 3 mm.[42]

Evaluation of Fracture Lines

The presence of a fracture can explain cases where the root canal obturation is judged satisfactory radiographically but there is the persistence of clinical symptoms (2.59).[17]

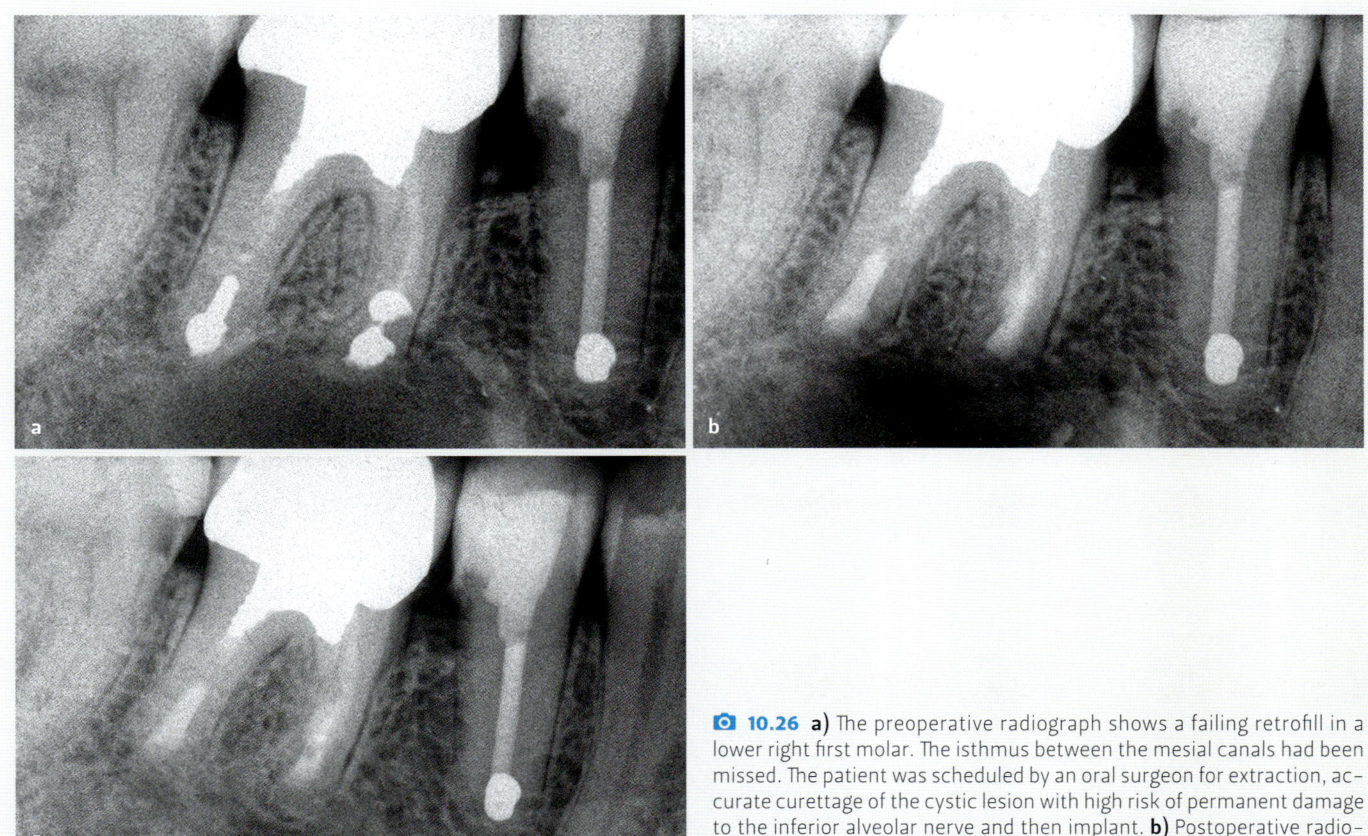

10.26 a) The preoperative radiograph shows a failing retrofill in a lower right first molar. The isthmus between the mesial canals had been missed. The patient was scheduled by an oral surgeon for extraction, accurate curettage of the cystic lesion with high risk of permanent damage to the inferior alveolar nerve and then implant. **b)** Postoperative radiograph. The canals have been sealed with white MTA. **c)** Four-year recall.

In the presence of a fracture line, the operator must take a decision as to whether to extract the tooth or try to reduce the fractured apex, shaving the root structure up to within a sound bony housing and make sure that the fracture line completely disappears. If this happens, the prognosis remains excellent (📷 10.13). If the fracture line continues to be visible in a coronal direction on the internal wall of the root-end preparation, the prognosis is poor and the patient must be informed that soon the tooth will have to be extracted. One is of course referring to apical root fractures, with no periodontal probing on the coronal aspect of the tooth. They could be the consequence of a "well performed" cold lateral condensation.[43]

REFERENCES

1. BARRON SL, GOTTLIEB B, CROOK JH. *Periapical curettage or apicectomy.* Texas Dent J. 1947;65:37-41.
2. PEARSON HH. *Curette or resect?* J Can Dent Assoc. 1949;14:508-509.
3. WAKELY JW, SIMON WJ. *Apical curettage or apicoectomy?* Dent Assist. 1977;46:29-32.
4. CURSON J. *Endodontics techniques - apical surgery.* Br Dent J. 1966;121:470-474.
5. KUTTLER Y. *Fundamentos de endometaendodoncia practica.* 2nd ed. Mexico City: Institute De Endo-Metaendodoncia; 1980:241-252 [In Spanish].
6. WEAVER SM. *Root canal treatment with visual evidence of histologic repair.* J Am Dent Assoc. 1947;35:483-497.
7. RUD J, ANDREASEN JO. *Operative procedures in Periapical surgery with contemporaneous root filling.* Int J Oral Surg. 1972;1:297-310.
8. WEINE FS, GERSTEIN H. *Periapical Surgery.* In: Weine FS. *Endodontic Therapy.* 4th ed. St. Louis: The CV Mosby Company; 1989:446-519.
9. RUD J, ANDREASEN JO, JENSEN JEM. *A follow-up study of 1,000 cases treated by endodontic surgery.* Int J Oral Surg. 1972;1:215-228.
10. CARTIN S. *Root canal curettage - a review of 1,000 cases.* Dent Dig. 1955;61:8-15.
11. GUTMANN JL, HARRISON JW. *Surgical Endodontics.* Boston: Blackwell Scientific Publications; 1991:203-277.
12. CUMMINGS RR, INGLE JI, FRANK AL, GLICK DH, ANTRIM D. *Endodontic surgery.* In: Ingle JI, Taintor JF, eds. Endodontics. 3rd ed. Philadelphia: Lea & Febiger; 1982:619-701.
13. JASTAK JT, YAGIELA JA. *Vasoconstrictors and local anesthesia: a review and rational for use.* J Am Dent Assoc. 1983;107:623-630.
14. ARENS DA, ADAMS WR, DECASTRO RA. *Endodontic surgery.* Philadelphia: Harper & Row Publishers; 1981:109-141.
15. EULER E. *Anatomische und pathologische Grundlagen fur das Misslingender Wurzelbehandlung.* DZW. 1934;37:100 [In German].
16. ANDREASEN JO, RUD J. *A histobacteriologic study of dental and periapical structures after endodontic surgery.* Int J Oral Surg. 1972;1:272-281.
17. FLORATOS S, AL-MALKI F, KIM S. *Root end resection.* In: Kim S, Kratchman S, eds. *Microsurgery in Endodontics.* New Jersey: Wiley Blackwell; 2018:67-72.
18. CARR GB. *Microscope in endodontics.* J Calf Dent Assoc. 1992;20:55-61.
19. KIM S, PECORA G, RUBINSTEIN R. *Comparison of traditional and microsurgery in endodontics.* In: Kim S, Pecora G, Rubinstein R, eds. *Color atlas of microsurgery in endodontics.* Philadelphia: W.B. Saunders; 2001:5-11.
20. KIM S, KRATCHMAN S. *Modern endodontic surgery concepts and practice: a review.* J Endod. 2006; 32(7):601-623.
21. CAMBRUZZI JV, MARSHAL FJ. *Molar endodontic surgery.* J Can Dent Assoc. 1983;49:61-65.
22. WELLER RN, NIEMCZYK SP, KIM S. *Incidence and position of canal isthmus. Part 1. Mesiobuccal root of the maxillary first molar.* J Endod. 1995;21:380-3.
23. LUEBKE RG, GLICK DH, INGLE JI. *Indications and contraindications for endodontic surgery.* Oral Surg. 1964; 18:907-113.
24. FRANK AL. *Inflammatory resorption caused by an adjacent necrotic tooth.* J Endod. 1990;16:339-341.
25. GUTMANN JL, HARRISON JW. *Posterior endodontic surgery: anatomical considerations and clinical techniques.* Int Endod J. 1985;18:8-34.
26. NYGAARD-OSTBY B, SCHILDER H. *Inflammation and infection of the pulp and periapical tissues: a synthesis.* Oral Surg. 1972;34:498.
27. NICHOLS E. *The role of surgery in endodontics.* Br Dental J. 1965;118:59-71.
28. BARNES IE. *Surgical endodontics. A color manual.* Littleton, MA: PSG Publishing Co Inc; 1984:15-16.

29. **Gerstein H.** *Surgical endodontics.* In: Laskin DN, ed. *Oral and maxillofacial surgery.* Vol. II. St. Louis: The CV Mosby Co; 1985:143-171.

30. **Gutmann JL.** *Principles of endodontic surgery for the general practitioner.* Dent Clin North Am. 1984;28:895-908.

31. **Rubinstein RA, Kim S.** *Short-term observation of the results of endodontic surgery with the use of a surgical operation microscope and Super-EBA as root-end filling material.* J Endod. 1999;25:43-8.

32. **Carr GB.** *Microscope in endodontics.* J Calif Dent Assoc 1992;20:55- 61.

33. **Lubow RM, Wayman BE, Cooley RL.** *Endodontic flap design: analysis and recommendations for current usage.* Oral Surg. 1984;58:207-12.

34. **Kim S.** *Endodontic microsurgery.* In: Cohen S, Burns R, eds. *Pathways of the pulp,* 8th ed. St Louis: Mosby; 2002:683-721.

35. **Frank AL, Simon JHS, Abou-Rass M, Glick DH.** *Clinical and surgical endodontics - concepts in practice.* Philadelphia: JB Lippincot; 1983:85-123.

36. **Harrison JW, Todd MJ.** *The effect of root resection on the sealing property of root canal obturations.* Oral Surg. 1980; 50:264-272.

37. **Cunningham J.** *The seal of root fillings at apicectomy. Br* Dent J. 1975;139:430-435.

38. **Tanzilli JP, Raphael D, Moodnik RM.** *A comparison of the marginal adaptation of retrograde techniques: a scanning electron microscopic study.* Oral Surg. 1980;50:74-80.

39. **Minnich SG, Harwell GR, Portell FR.** *Does cold burnishing gutta-percha create a better apical seal?* J Endod. 1989;15(5):204-209.

40. **Shaw CS, BeGole EA, Jacobsen EL.** *The apical sealing efficacy of two reverse filling techniques versus cold-burnished gutta-percha.* J Endod. 1898;15(8):350-354.

41. **Stropko J.** *Canal morphology of maxillary molars: clinical observations of canal configurations.* J Endod. 1999;25(6):446-450.

42. **Carr GB.** *Ultrasonic root-end preparation.* Dent Clin North Am. 1997;41:541-4.

43. **Gimlin DR, Parr CH, Aguirre-Ramirez G.** *A comparison of stresses produced during lateral and vertical condensation using engineering models.* J Endod. 1986;12:235.

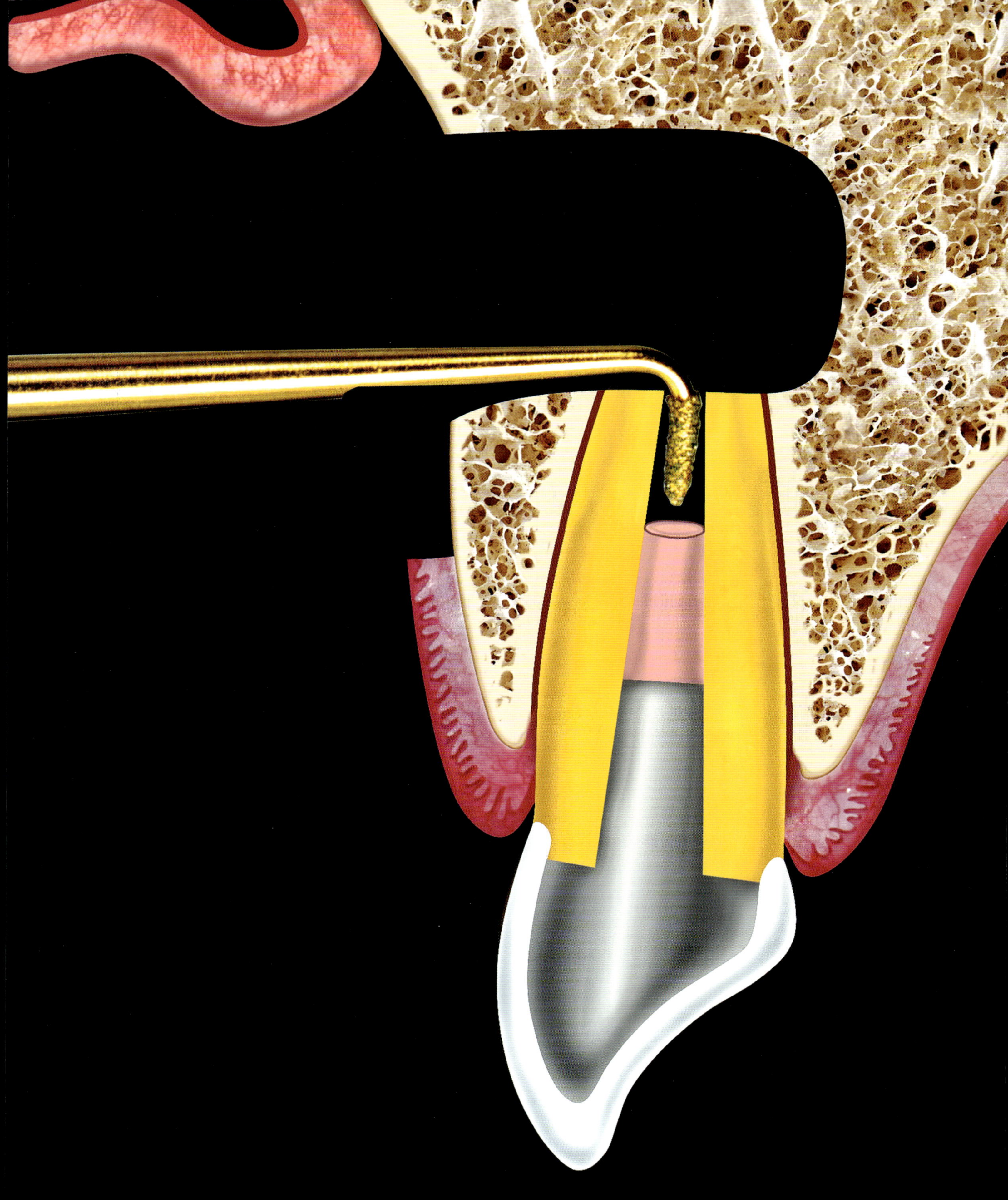

Ultrasonic Root-end Preparation

At the end of the '80s Gary Carr made a big revolution in the field of the periapical surgery: he introduced the ultrasonic retrotips specifically designed for the root-end cavity preparation during surgical endodontics and since then the use of slow speed handpieces and burs are no longer accepted as the standard of care for apical surgery.[1,2]

These tips are driven by a variety of ultrasonic units, where a piezoelectric crystal made of quartz or ceramic located in the handpiece is vibrated at 28,000 to 40,000 cycles per second, and the energy is transferred to the ultrasonic tip, which then moves forward and backward in a single plane, brushing away the dentin with gentle strokes.[3]

Advantages and Disadvantages of Ultrasonic Tips

There are many more **advantages** of using the ultrasonic root-end preparation compared to using rotary handpieces and burs:

- the preparation is a Class I cavity at least 3 mm deep, made along the main axis of the root canal, with walls parallel to the anatomic outline of the root canal space (11.1)
- it is now possible to clean the apical root canal at 360°, including the buccal aspect of the preparation (11.2)
- the retroprep is smaller and consequently is easier to seal
- the bony crypt is smaller and less dentin is removed using a short bevel
- it is much easier to follow the root canal anatomy and to prepare isthmuses (11.3)
- the access is comfortable even in canals difficult to be reached, like the palatal canal of a first premolar, the MB2 of upper molars and the ML of lower molars
- there is no need to make undercuts to give retention to the cavity and this means less risk of causing perforations on the palatal aspect of the retroprep (11.4)
- it is much easier to retreat a surgical failure and to remove the old amalgam retrofill, which most of the times can be removed in one single piece (11.5), while using a bur a lot of amalgam dust is made with consequent high risk of tattoo in the soft tissue (11.6).

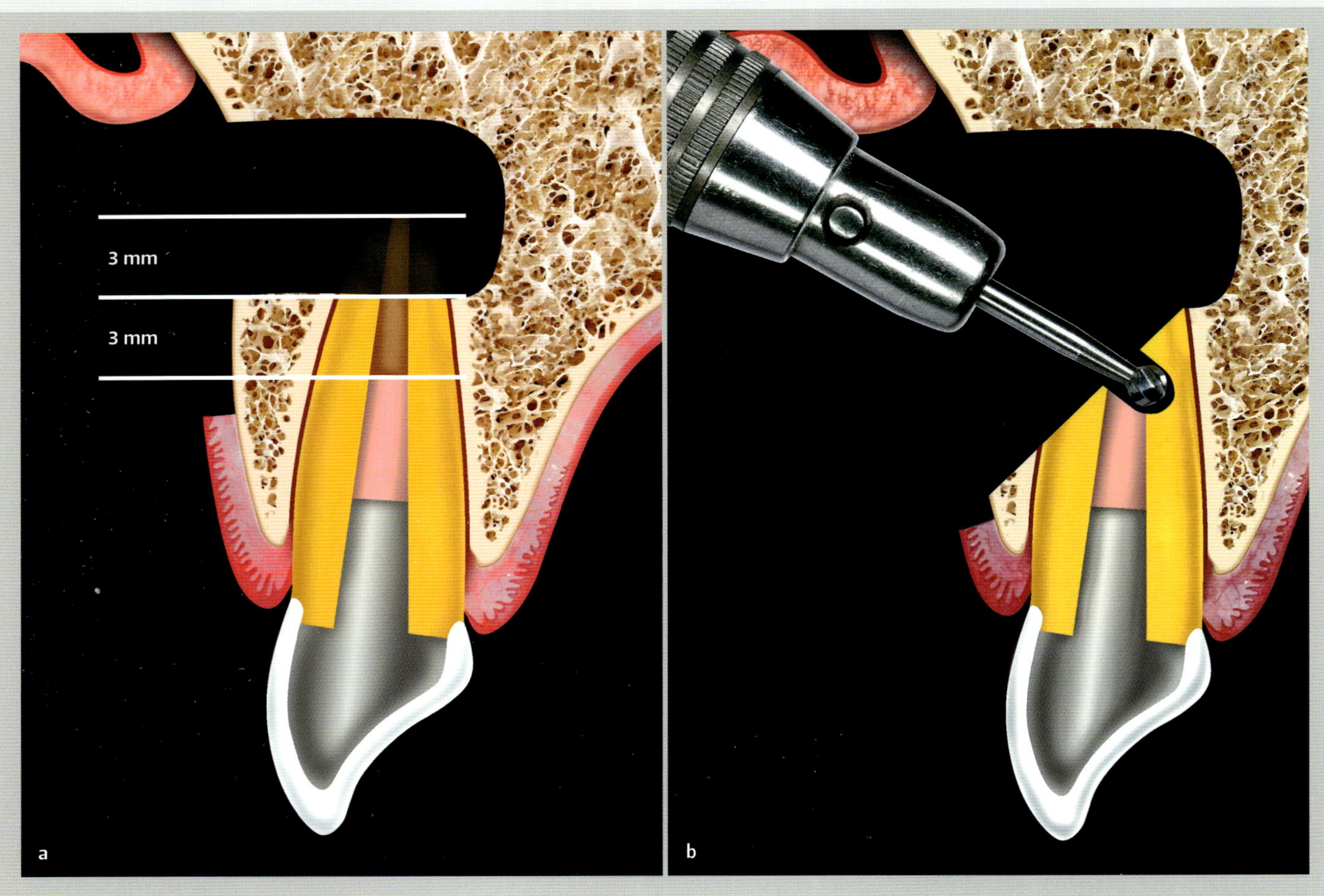

11.1 **a)** The drawing shows the ideal root-end preparation accomplished with an ultrasonic tip. **b)** Preparation with a slow speed handpiece and a bur ends up in a dome-shaped preparation, having compromised retention of the root-end filling material and a high risk of palatal perforation.

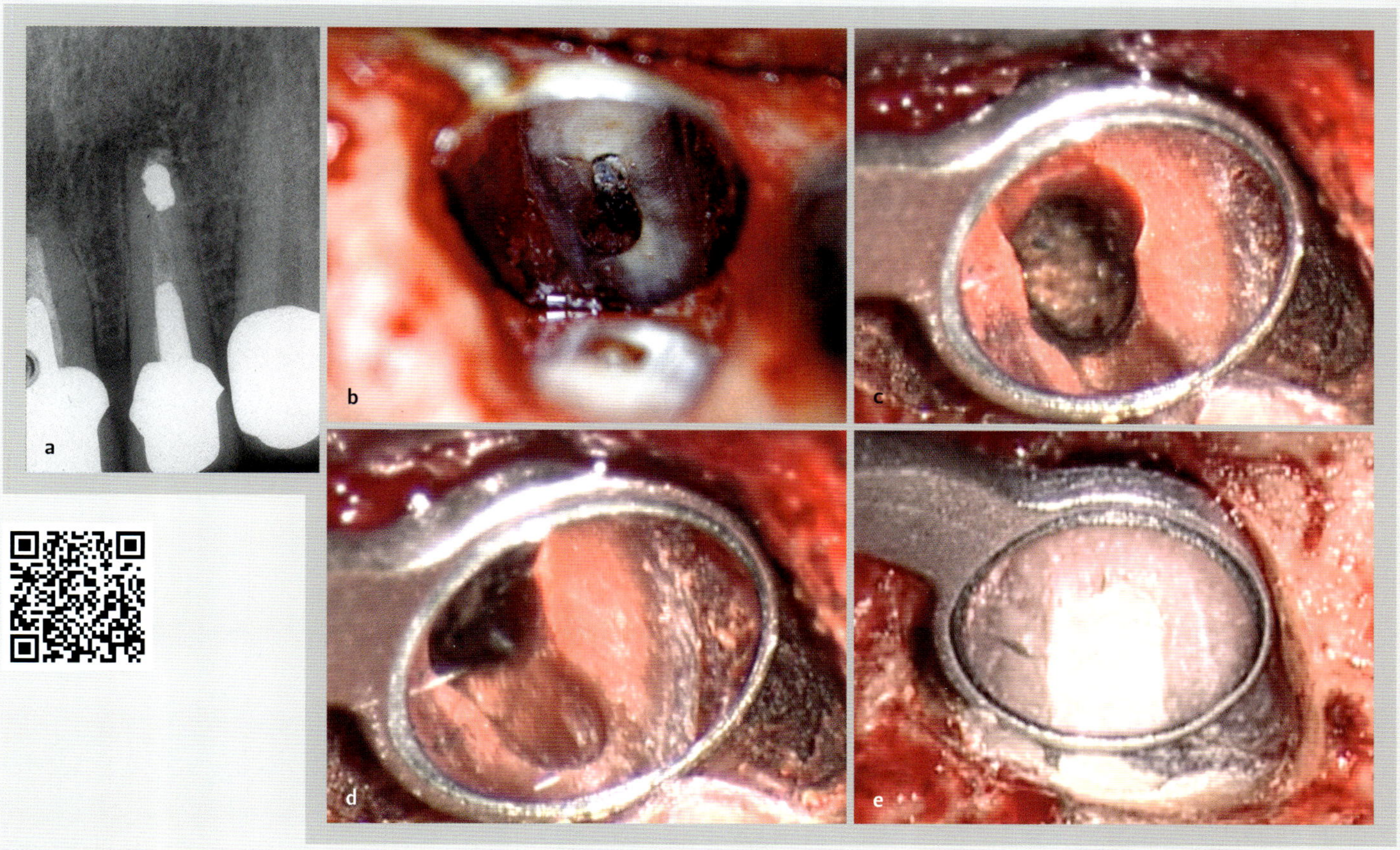

11.2 **a)** Preoperative radiograph of the upper left lateral incisor. **b)** After the removal of the amalgam retrofilling, it is evident that the root-end preparation was made mainly if not only at the expenses of the palatal wall, with the original canal remaining completely untouched. **c)** The Class I cavity has been prepared in the main canal. **d)** To save tooth structure, the previous dome-shaped cavity has not been removed. **e)** Root-end obturation with white MTA.

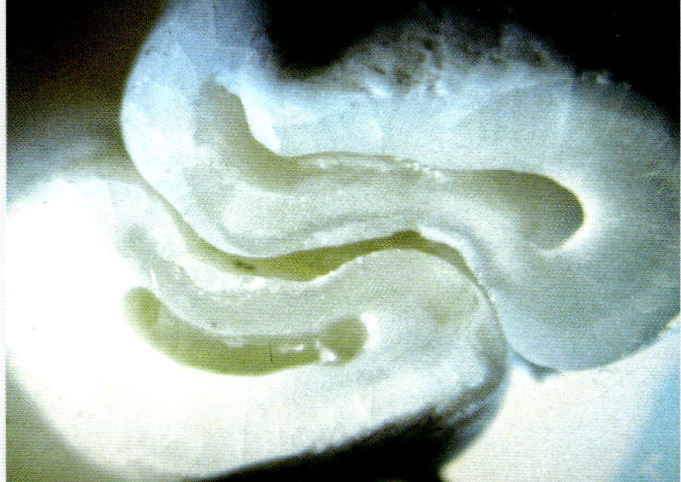

11.3 The root-end preparations and the isthmuses of this extracted third molar have been easily accomplished with ultrasonic tips.

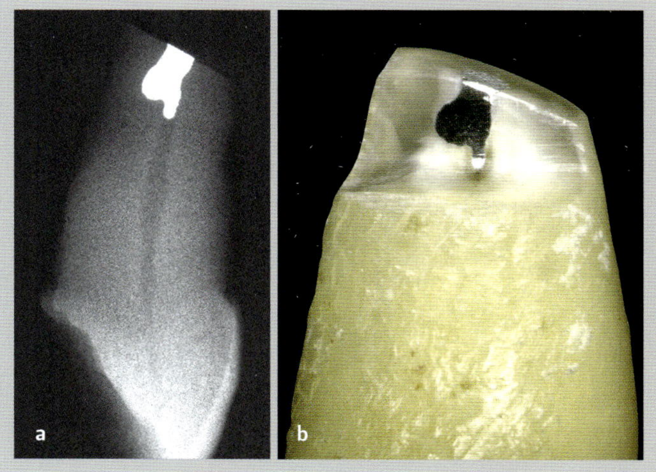

11.4 **a)** The root-end preparation of this extracted tooth has been accomplished with a bur. Notice the "dome-shaped" preparation on the palatal wall, made to give retention to the filling material. **b)** The same tooth after sectioning the apex.

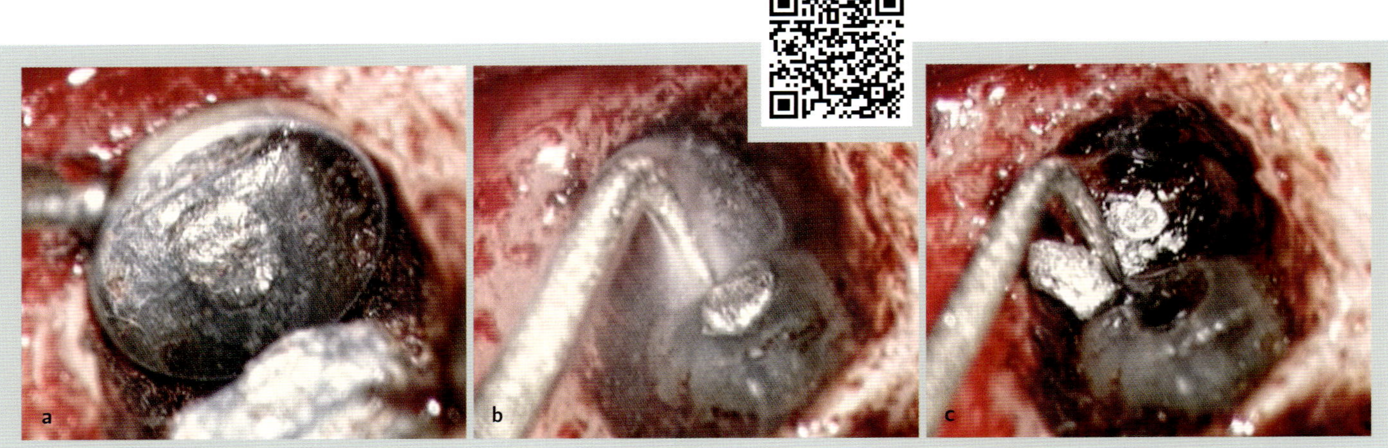

11.5 **a)** Retreatment of a surgical failure. The amalgam needs to be removed. **b)** The ultrasonic tip working all around the amalgam. **c)** The old amalgam was removed in large fragments.

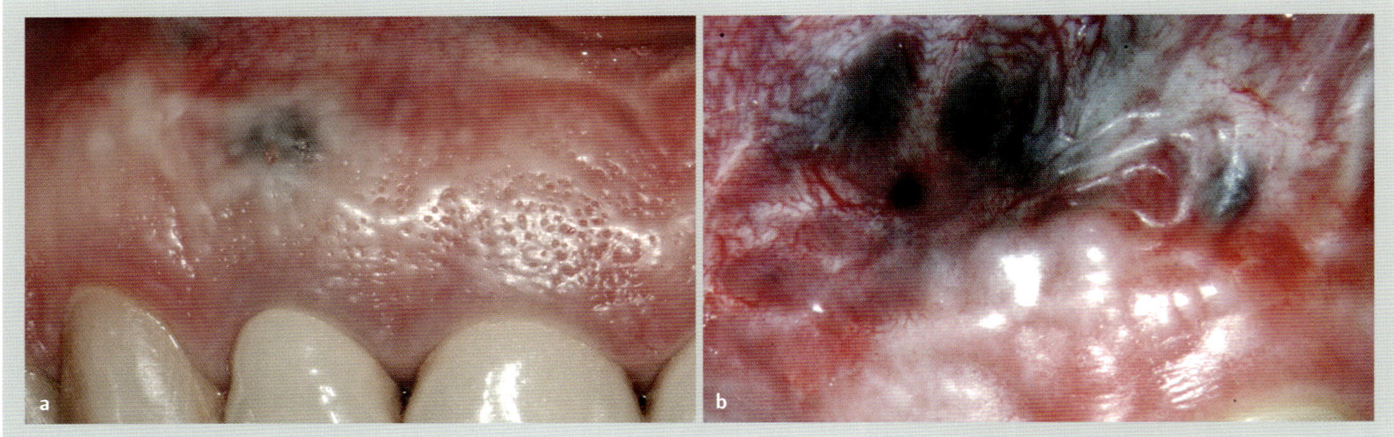

11.6 **a, b)** Two examples of a tattoo on the buccal mucosa.

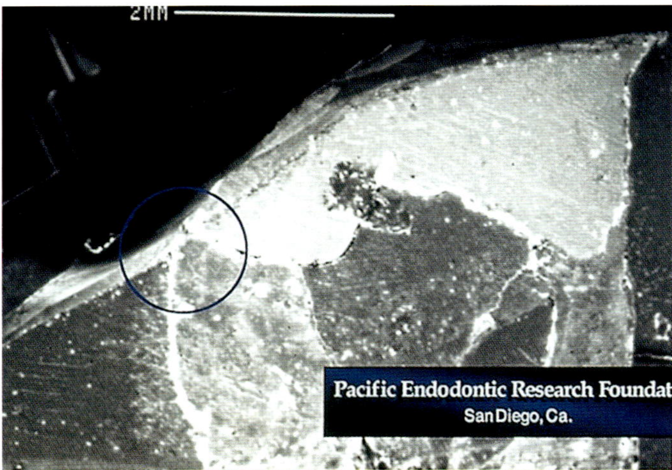

11.7 The preparation is not within the long axis of the root (*Courtesy of Dr. Gary Carr*).

The only "**disadvantages**" of the use of ultrasonic tips are:

- the tips are fragile and for certain they don't last as long as the burs
- more instruments are needed, like tips, ultrasonic units, and many microinstruments, like mirrors, pluggers, carriers etc.
- the cost is therefore higher
- the technique is not familiar for the operator who is advised to practice with the instruments first on extracted teeth.

The common **mistakes** made when using rotary handpieces are the following:

- the root apex has not been resected completely (10.3)
- the preparation is not made along the main axis of the root canal (11.7, 11.8)
- the isthmus has not been involved in the retroprep (10.25)
- anatomical variations or complexities have not been recognized (*see* 1.1).

The **disadvantages** of the use of rotary bur are:

- the access to the root apex is limited
- the bony crypt is too large
- high risk of perforation on the palatal/lingual aspect of the root-end preparation
- impossible to adequately clean the buccal aspect of the root-end preparation
- very limited retention for the obturating material (11.9)
- using a steep bevel, many dentinal tubules remain unsealed
- the isthmus cannot be prepared without high risk of perforating the root wall.

In conclusion, the use of rotary burs in microsurgical handpieces (11.10) or in straight handpieces (11.11), commonly used in the traditional surgical techniques, can no longer be recommended.

The combination of the operating microscope and ultrasonic tips make previously challenging cases routine and the root-end preparation can be visualized and executed with a high level of confidence that was previously unattainable.[3]

Many recent articles agree that the use of microsurgical techniques is superior in achieving predictably high success rates for root-end surgery (93.52%) when compared with traditional techniques (59%).[4–12]

Dentinal Cracks

Despite the many advantages of using ultrasonics, Saunders et al.[13] while using smooth stainless steel tips on extracted teeth reported crack formation in the walls of the cavity. Two years later Layton et al.[14] in another article suggested that the cracks might be a result of the fact that the previous study used demineralized and dehydrated teeth, which may have been predisposed towards crack formation. However, using smooth stainless steel tips on extracted teeth Layton concluded that

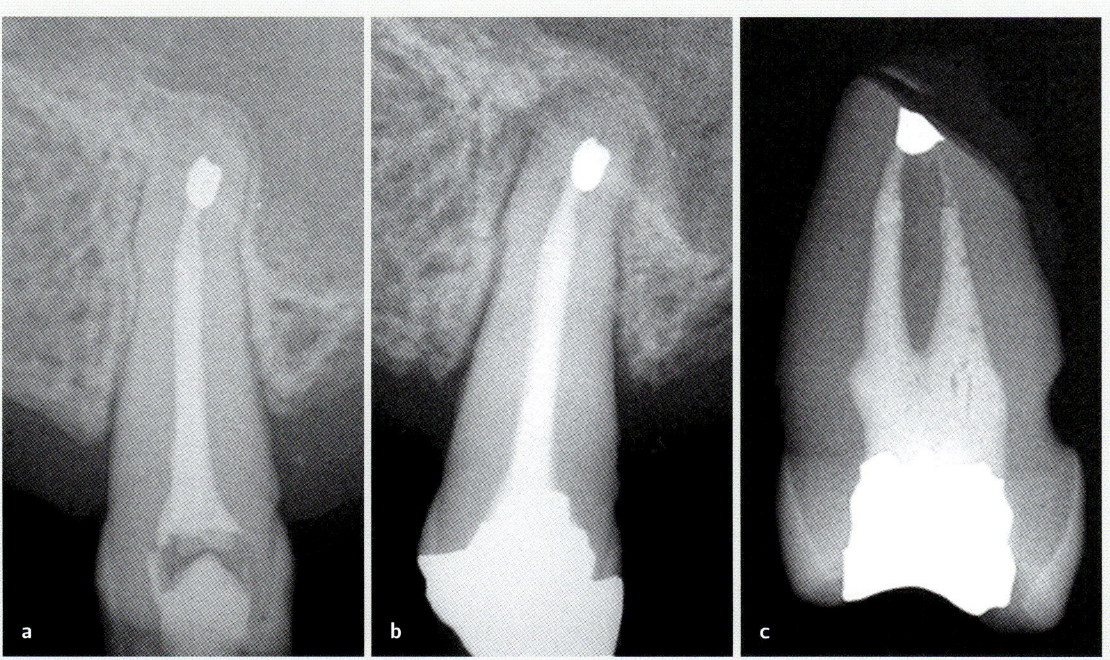

11.8 **a)** Postoperative radiograph of an upper left second premolar. The tooth was treated in the 80's with a steep bevel, rotary bur and amalgam. **b)** Fifteen years later the tooth has a vertical root fracture and needs to be extracted. **c)** The extracted tooth shows the steep bevel and the preparation that was not within the long axis of the root. The buccal canal was "almost" missed.

ultrasonic preparations do lead to increased number of cracks in the wall of the preparation and that a higher prevalence of microfractures was observed when the tips were used at a higher power setting. Walpington et al.[15] later suggested using low to moderate intensity for 2 minutes to minimize the risk of dentine microfractures. Because both the Saunders and Layton studies were performed on extracted teeth (more brittle, desiccated and without periradicular tissue), Min et al.[16] suggested the use of cadavers to get more clinically relevant results. In agreement with Min's study, Grey et al.[17] also using cadavers, reported that the ultrasonic tips did not cause a greater than average number of cracks and they seemed to be insignificant. However, most ultrasonic instruments used in the prior study were smooth, stainless steel tips. In recent years diamond coated ultrasonic tips have been introduced to minimize dentinal fractures through their ability to abrade dentine more quickly, minimizing the time that the instrument is in contact with the dentinal walls.[18]

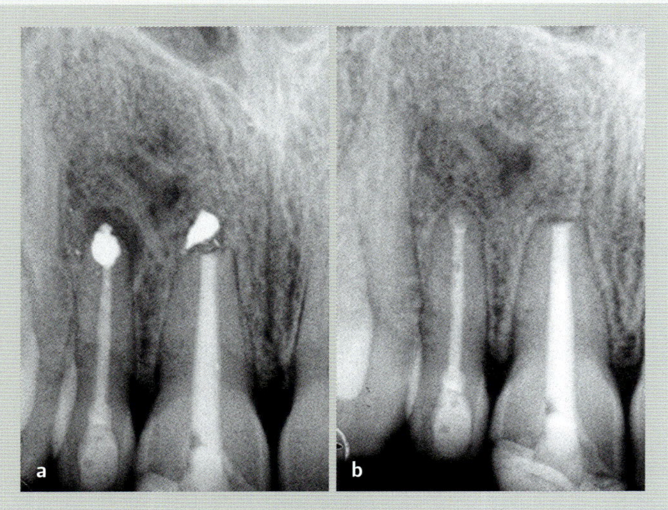

11.9 a) Retreatment of a surgical failure. The preparation was not retentive and the amalgam is floating in the granulation tissue. **b)** Two-year recall.

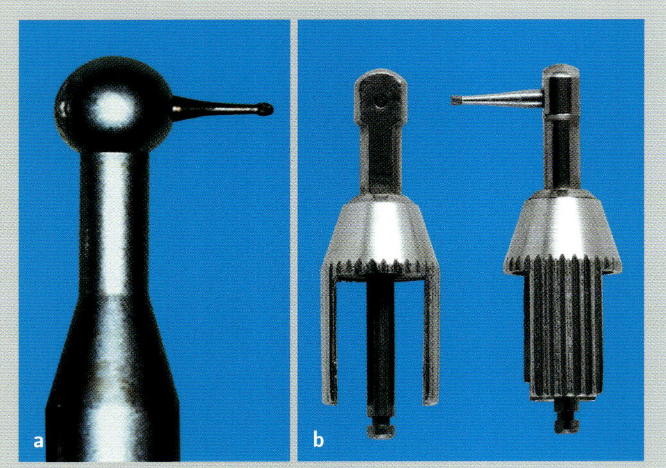

11.10 Two examples of mini-handpieces specifically designed for periapical surgery, to make preparations within the long axis of the root. **a)** The Miniature handpiece by Kavo. **b)** The Reproxidrill. They needed a bony crypt of at least 12 mm!

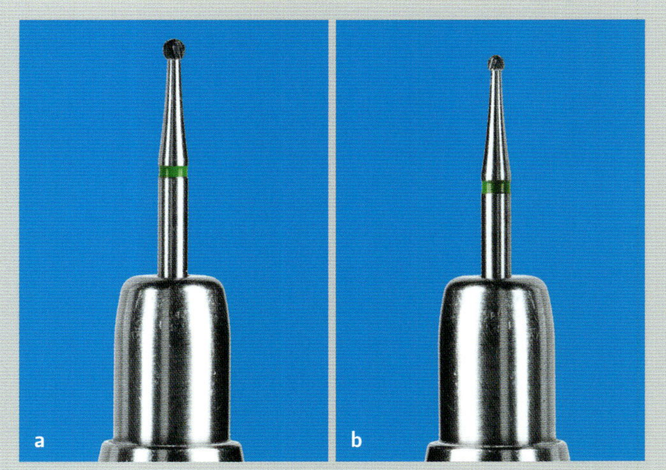

11.11 The straight handpiece was used both for the bony crypt **(a)** and for the root-end preparation **(b)** especially in posterior teeth.

Several piezoelectric units are available in the market, like Obtura/Spartan (11.12a), Acteon (11.12b), Amadent, EMS (11.12c), and they are all very efficient. Also, several different kinds of ultrasonic tips are available and the operator can choose depending on the requested efficiency. Most of them are 0.25 mm in diameter and approximately 3 mm in length. The tips in stainless steel with no coating are the less effective, the tips chemically coated (zirconium or titanium nitride) (11.13) are more efficient, however the diamond coated are definitely the most efficient.[19] Recently new tips were introduced by B&L Biotech: the Jet Tips. What makes these tips very special are the microprojections of the cutting surface (11.14), allowing quick and complete removal of gutta-percha or broken instruments from the root canal. Some of these ultrasonic tips are bendable, so that the operator can bend them in any direction for better access (11.14d–h).

All of them have a water port for the irrigation (11.15), since they must never work dry. The amount of irrigat-

Cont'd on page 211

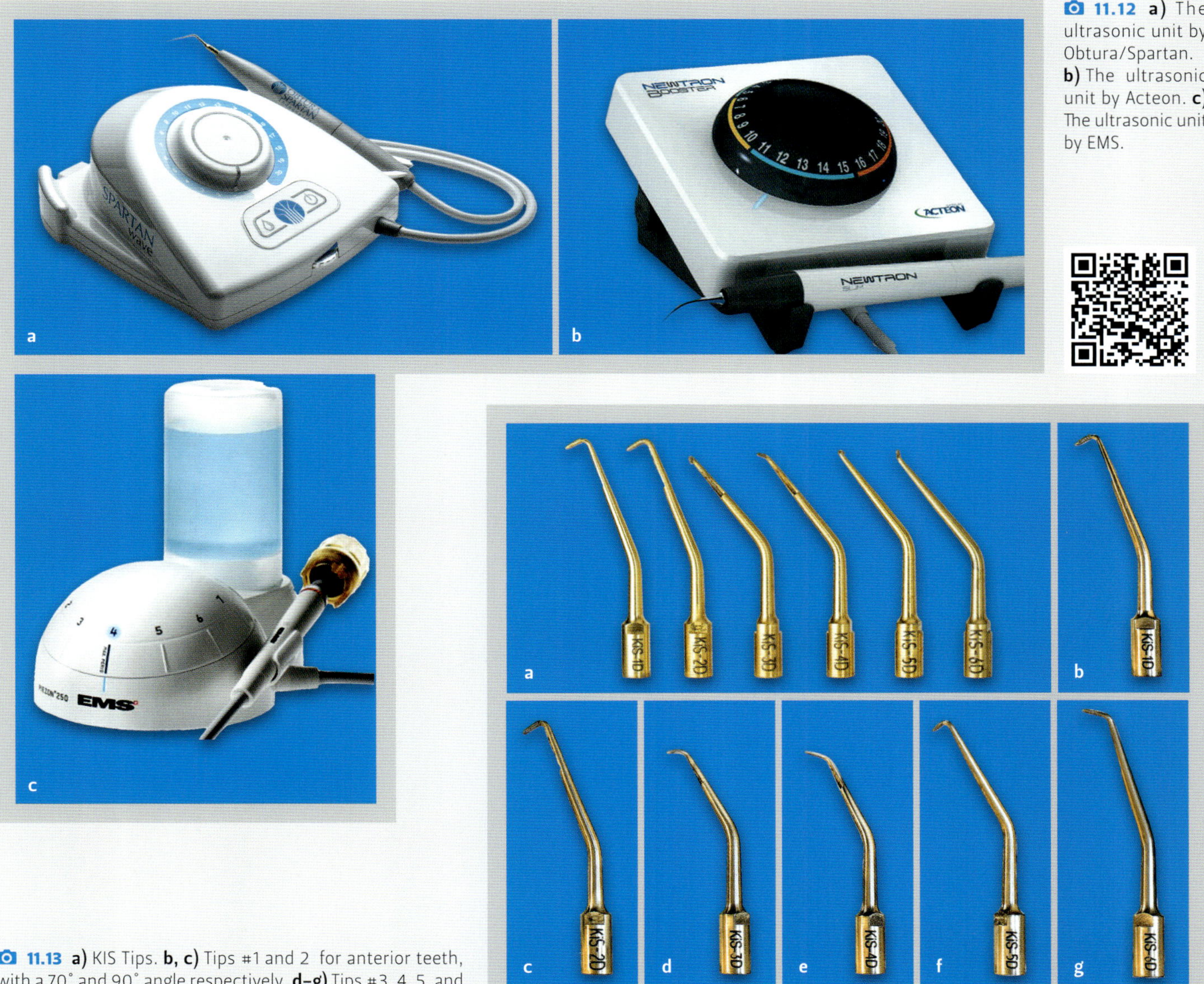

11.12 a) The ultrasonic unit by Obtura/Spartan. **b)** The ultrasonic unit by Acteon. **c)** The ultrasonic unit by EMS.

11.13 a) KIS Tips. **b, c)** Tips #1 and 2 for anterior teeth, with a 70° and 90° angle respectively. **d–g)** Tips #3, 4, 5, and 6 for posterior teeth.

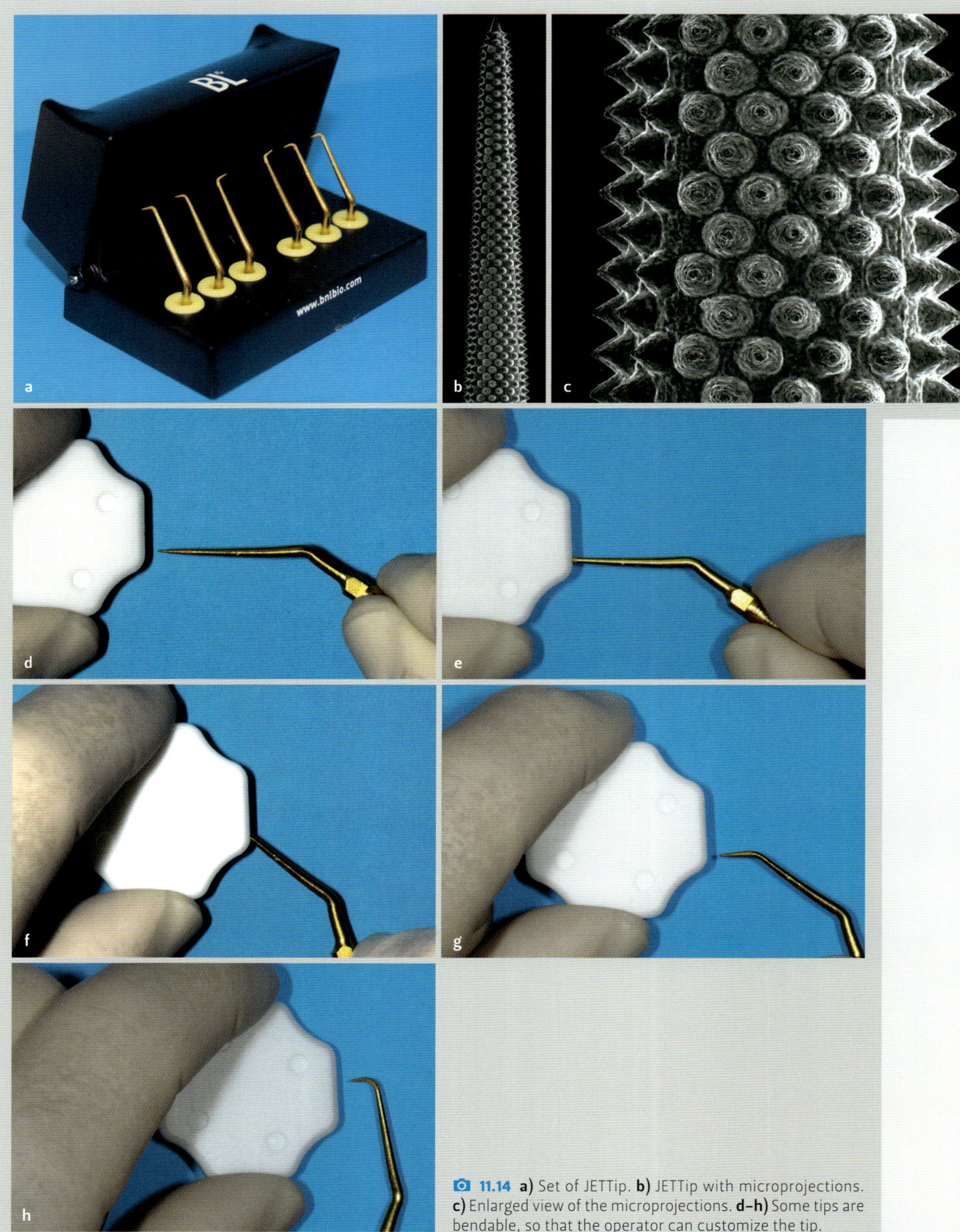

11.14 **a)** Set of JETTip. **b)** JETTip with microprojections. **c)** Enlarged view of the microprojections. **d–h)** Some tips are bendable, so that the operator can customize the tip.

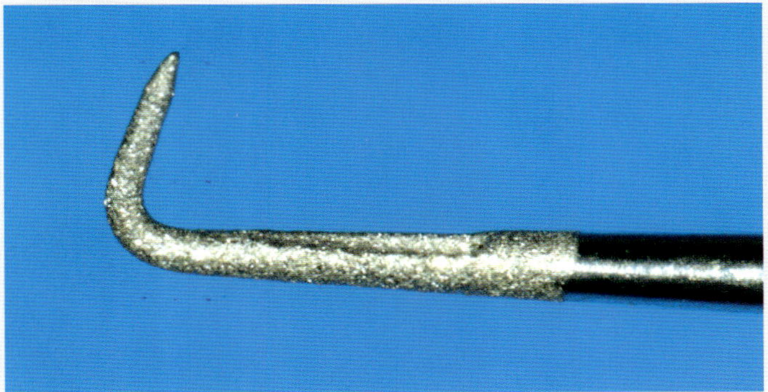

11.15 The water port for the irrigation is very close to the working portion.

11.16 **a)** The drawings show an off-angle preparation consequent to a wrong angulation of the ultrasonic tip, which was not aligned with the long axis of the root. **b)** Preoperative radiograph of the upper left first and second premolars. **c)** Postoperative radiograph. The second premolar was treated keeping the ultrasonic tip at the same angulation used for the first premolar, not taking into account that the teeth were not parallel. **d)** Two-year recall. The off-angle preparation is evident.

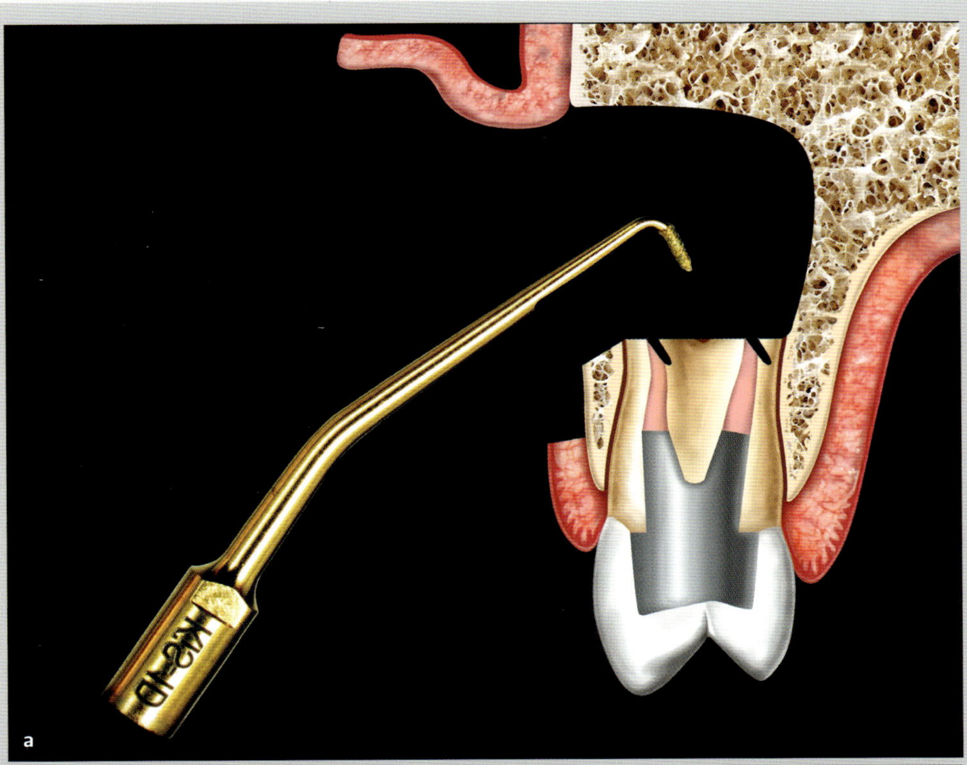

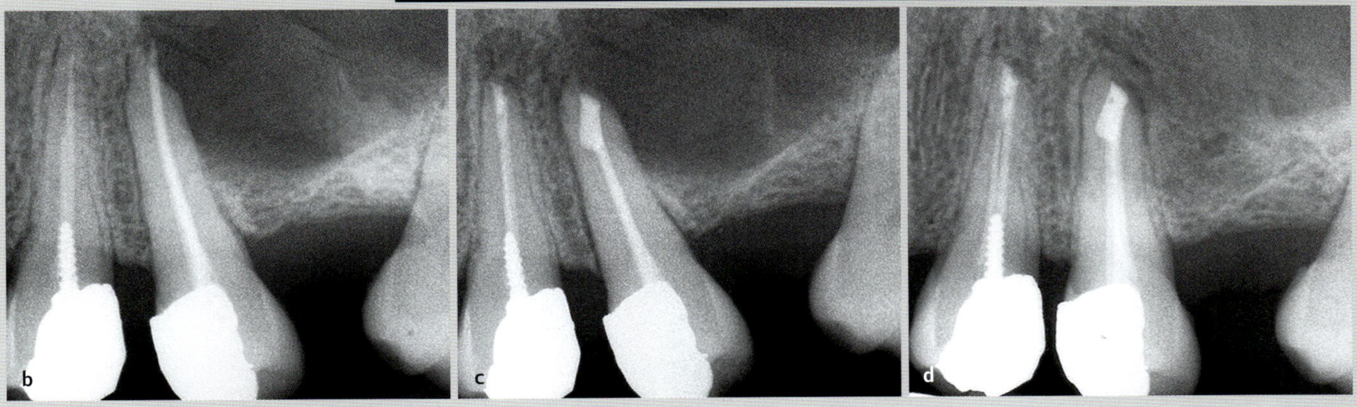

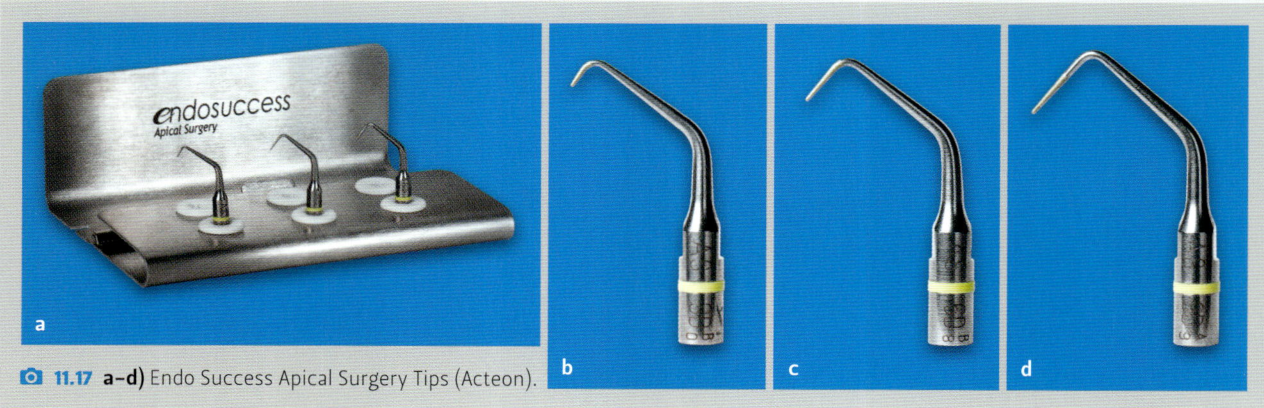

11.17 **a–d)** Endo Success Apical Surgery Tips (Acteon).

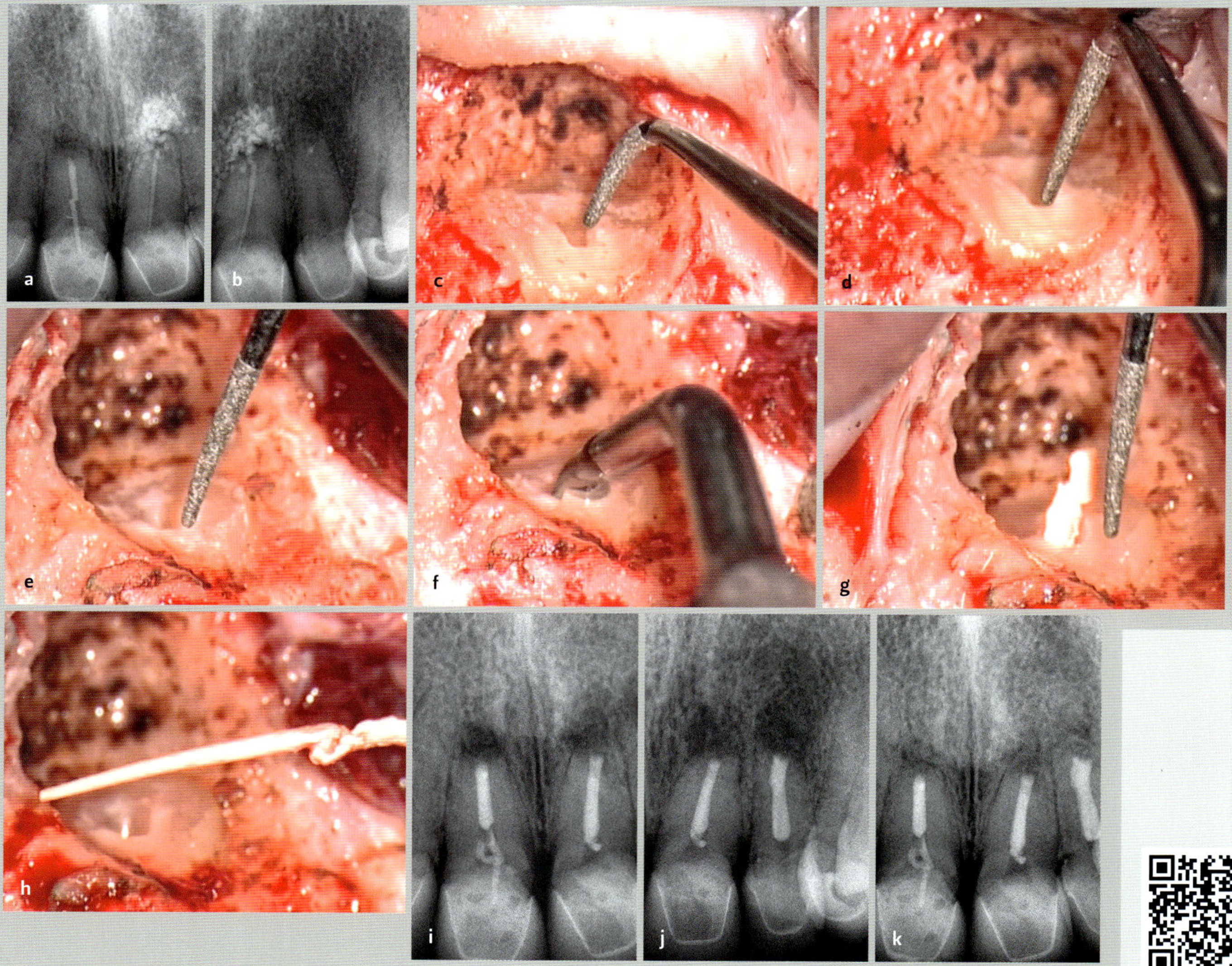

11.18 **a)** Retreatment of a surgical failure. Preoperative radiograph of the upper central incisors. Both teeth were treated by an oral surgeon who placed gutta-percha points from the apex and a bone graft at the apex of the left incisor. **b)** The lateral left incisor was left completely empty. **c)** The Endo Success Apical Surgery Tip of 3 mm of length. **d)** The tip of 6 mm of length. **e, f)** The tip of 9 mm of length. **g)** The tip of 9 mm removing the gutta-percha point from the canal of the upper left central incisor. **h)** The gutta-percha point has been removed. **i, j)** Postoperative radiograph. **k)** Two-year recall.

Cont'd from page 207

ing solution is also very important: too much irrigation will decrease the visibility, too little will overheat the dentin and can cause the fracture of the tips. They have to be used at the minimum power, very gently, without finding any resistance while preparing the retrocavity. If needed, the setting of the ultrasonic unit can be increased incrementally until an adequate efficiency is achieved. If the power setting initially is too high, the tip may fracture. During the preparation of the retrocavity it is suggested to work with the microscope al lower magnification, in order to take into consideration the long axis of the root and consequently to orient the retrotip parallel to the root canal. If this step is not taken, then transportation or a perforation of the root may occur either on the lingual (📷 11.16a) or mesial/distal dentinal wall (📷 11.16b-d).

Recently Dr. Khayat designed new longer ultrasonic tips diamond coated of 3, 6, and 9 mm of length (📷 11.17). They are particularly useful in the case when the surgical procedure is performed in root canals partially empty and therefore the retroprep has to be particularly long. The typical situation is when a post has been placed without orthograde treatment and therefore the canal space is full of pulpal remnants, debris

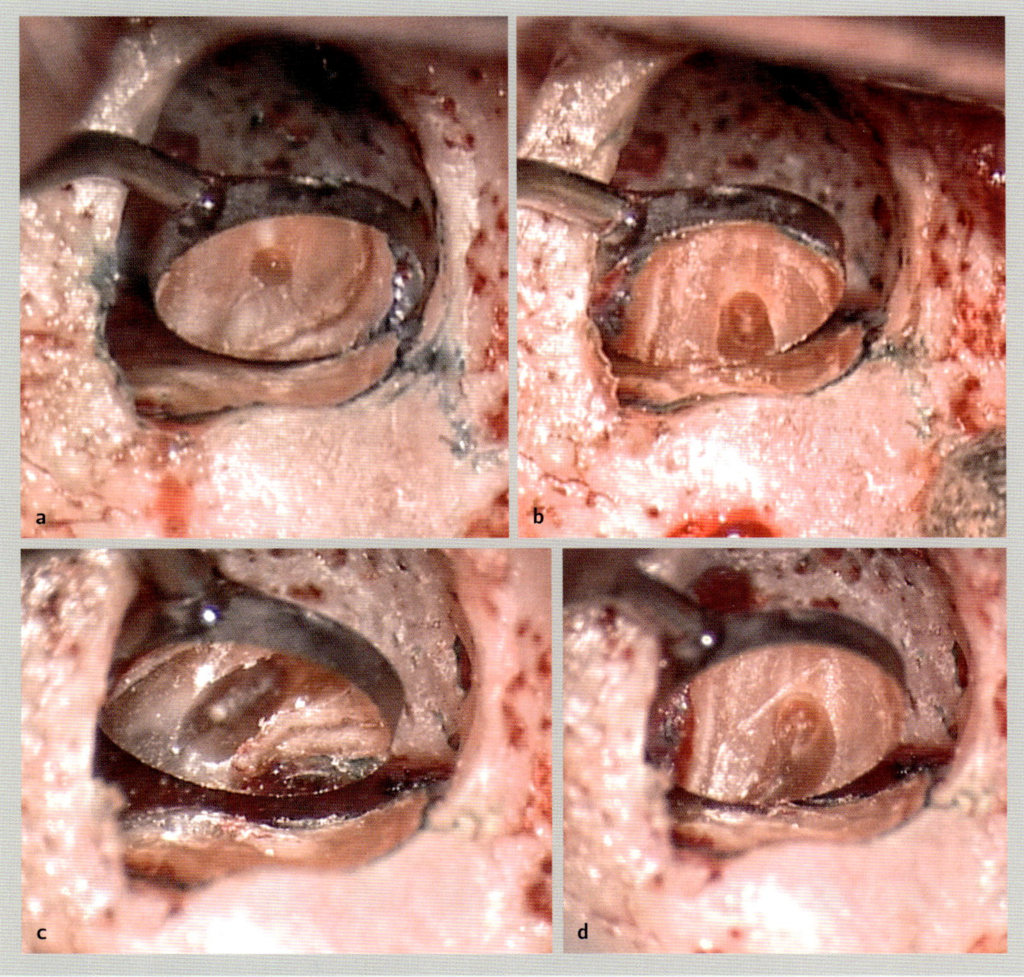

📷 **11.19** Preparation of the root-end cavity in a completely calcified mesiobuccal root of un upper molar. **a)** The little white spot in the center of the preparation is the calcified MB1 canal. **b)** The preparation is deeper and the calcified canal is still in the center of the cavity. **c)** The little white spot in the center of the preparation is the calcified MB2 canal. **d)** MB1 and the isthmus have been prepared.

and bacteria. Endo Success Apical Surgery Tips by Acteon address this problem. Of course these cases must still have the real indication for the surgical endodontic treatment in that they cannot be treated nonsurgically. The three tips of different length have to be used in sequence, always starting with the small one of 3 mm and then if there is room enough for the others, proceed with the one of 6 and then 9 mm of length (11.18).

Usually the surgery is made to retreat non-surgical failures and the root canal contains at least sealer or possibly sealer and gutta-percha. Therefore, the tip should not meet resistance while it is cleaning the root canal from the previous material. If the operator feels resistance, it means that the tip is working against the dentinal wall instead of just removing material from the root canal. The only time when the operator will feel resistance is when the canal is completely calcified, has not been negotiated previously and doesn't contain any obturating material. In such a case, the risk of transportation is very high, therefore it is suggested to work under low magnification, progress coronally very slowly, checking every few seconds that the tip is going in the right direction and constantly confirming that the ultrasonic tip is coaxial to the root. The operator should stop, dry the operative field with the Stropko and check with the micromirror that the calcified canal is always in the center of the retroprep (11.19).

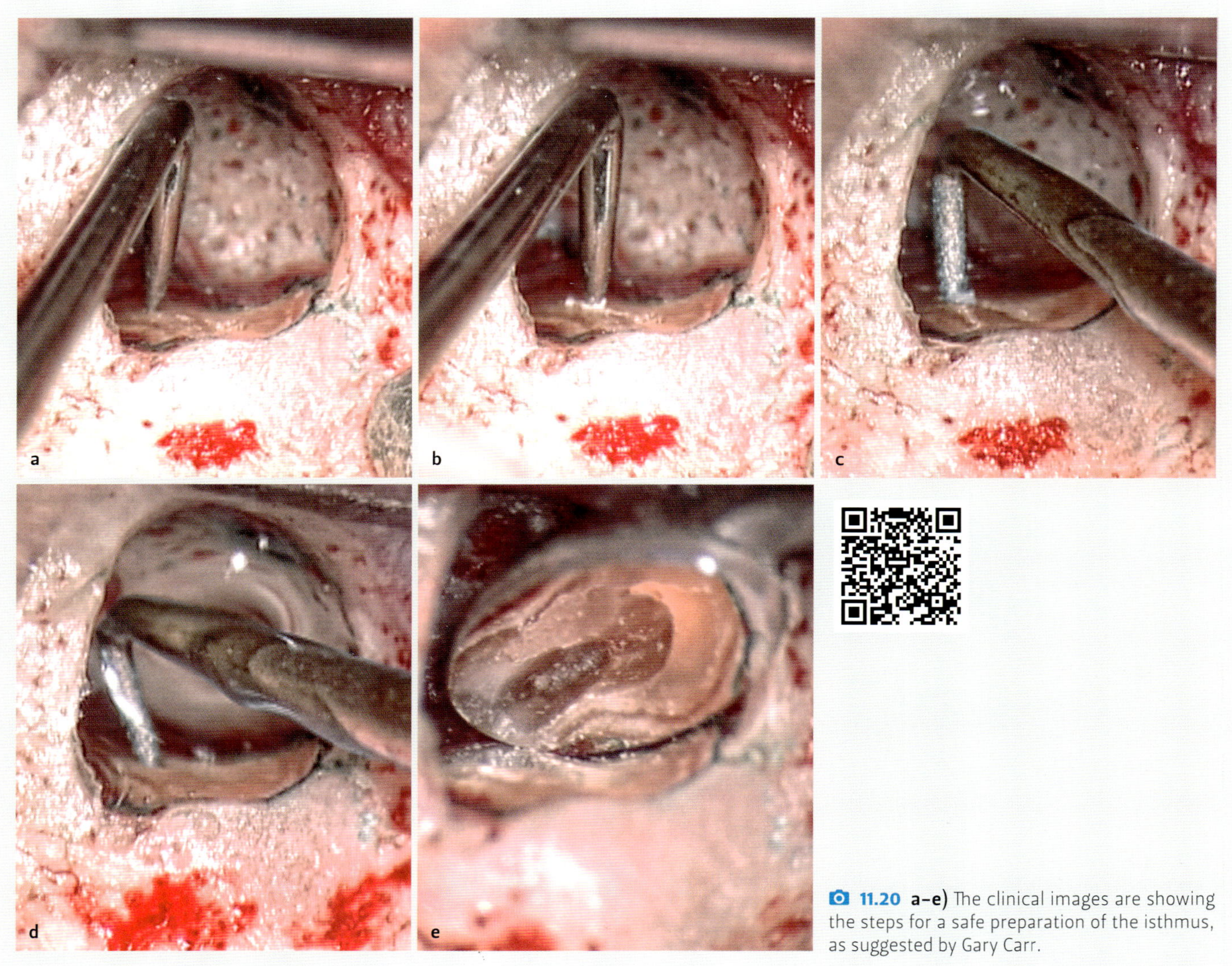

11.20 a–e) The clinical images are showing the steps for a safe preparation of the isthmus, as suggested by Gary Carr.

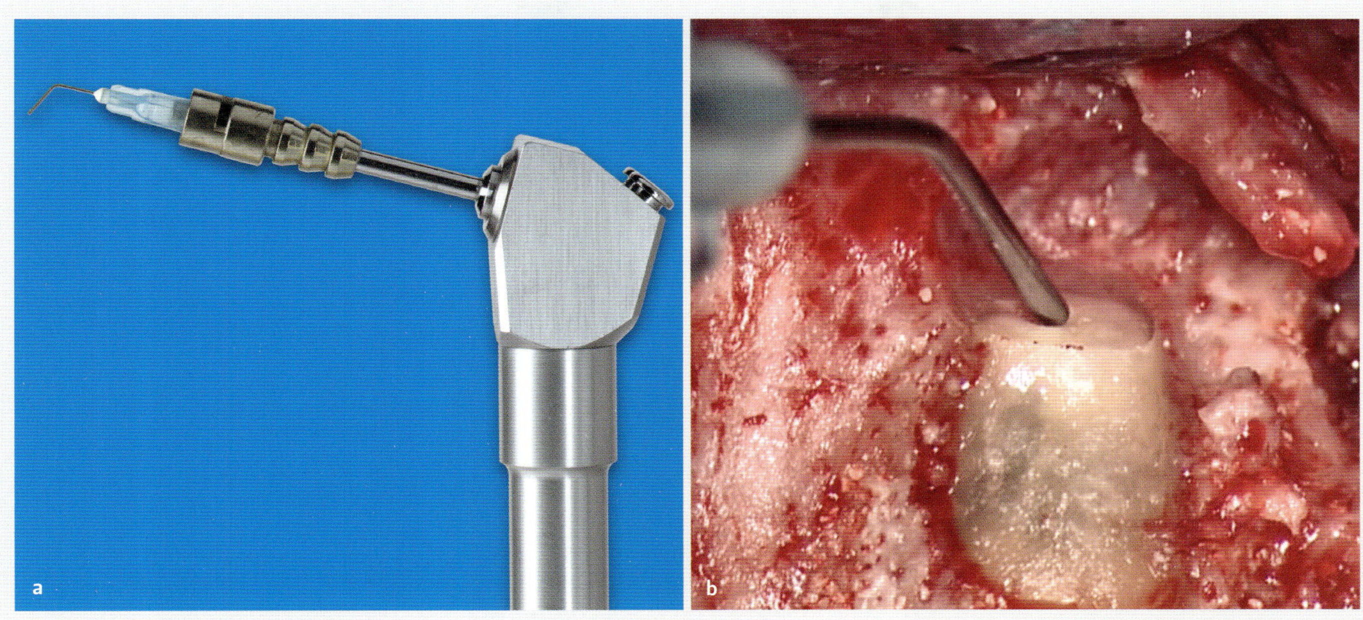

11.21 **a)** Adec syringe with the Stropko irrigator. **b)** The Stropko is gently blowing air to dry the root-end cavity.

As already stated, the retrotips always work at the minimum power. If this is not enough to clean the root canal from the previous obturating material, then the operator can increase the power little by little until the desired efficiency is reached. This is because sometimes the old gutta-percha is not so easy to be removed during the surgical procedure, especially if it had been well compacted.

The selection of the tip depends also on the anatomy and the quadrant of the operative field. The tips for anterior teeth have an angle of 90° and 70° (back action tip, particularly useful for upper lateral incisors); the tips for posterior teeth have a double or triple angle to guarantee a better access in distal quadrants.

In case of a root with two canals the operator should always remember that there is an isthmus, even though it is not visible with the microscope. The isthmus used to contain vital pulp tissue, now it contains bacteria, therefore it must always be included in the retropreparation and must be cleaned and filled with the obturating material. We know from the recent literature that the mesiobuccal root of upper first molars has two canals 93% of the time.[20] This means that the isthmus is present in the same percentage. The same is valid for

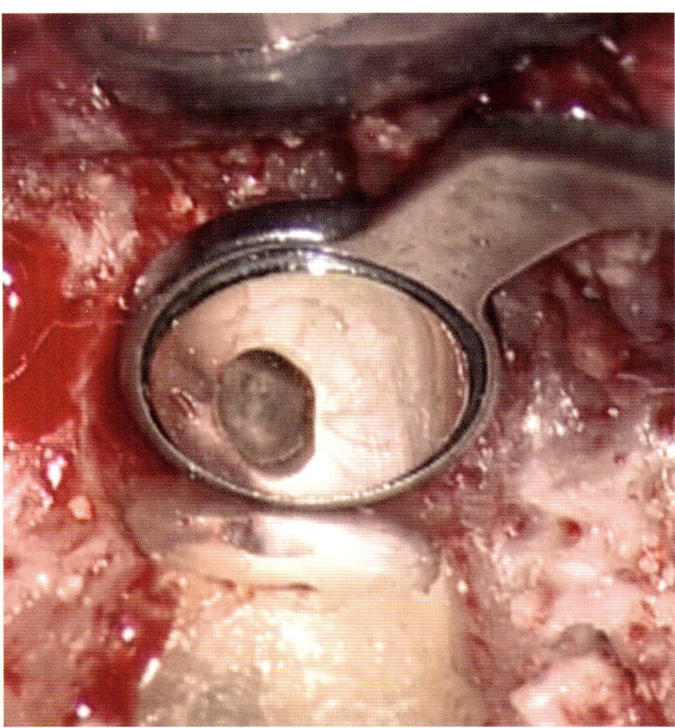

11.22 The micromirror is showing the root-end cavity ready to be obturated.

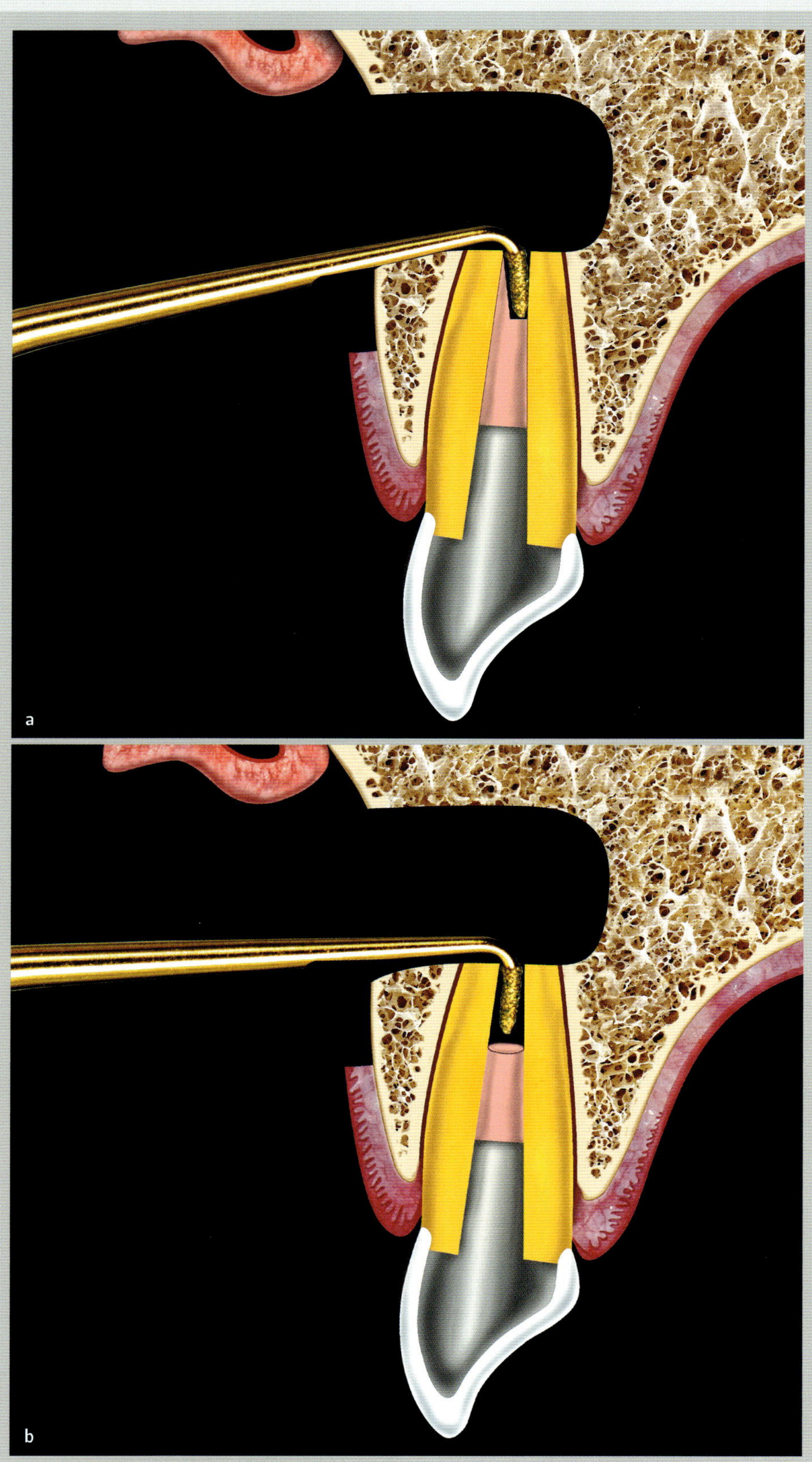

11.23 Inspection of the root-end preparation. **a)** A part of the gutta-percha is still visible on the buccal aspect of the preparation. **b)** In order to remove the remaining gutta-percha, the ultrasonic tip can be tilted so that the tip can vibrate against the buccal wall and loosen the remaining material.

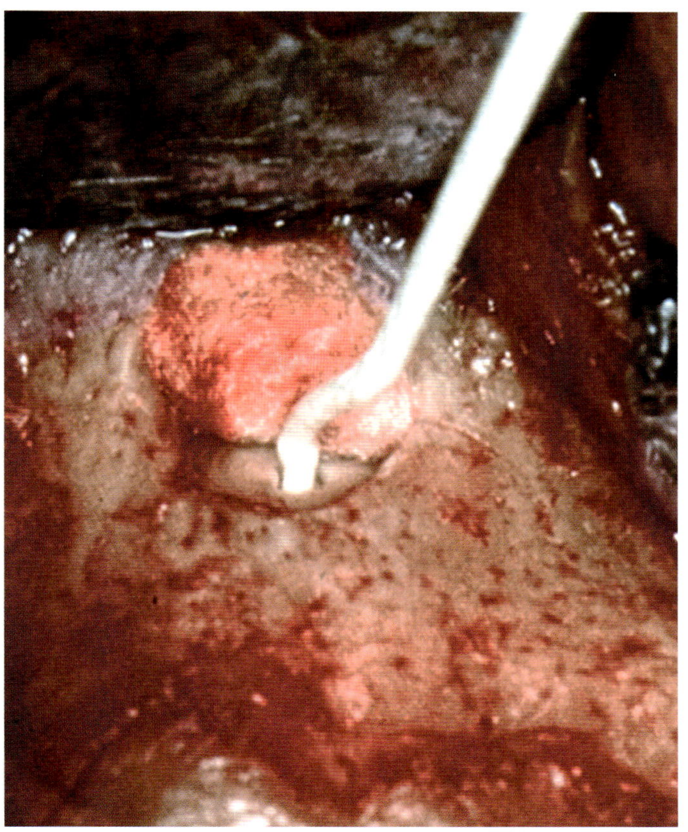

11.24 Traditionally the root-end cavity was dried with paper points, but this is not recommended anymore.

upper second molars (59%) and for the mesial roots (80%) and distal roots (20%) of lower molars.[21]

For the preparation of the isthmus, these are the steps:[1,2]

- using the Carr Explorer CTX make a "tracking groove" over the isthmus (11.20a, b)
- with the irrigation turned off, use a sharp ultrasonic tip following the previous "scratch" and make it a little bit deeper (11.20c)
- now with the irrigation turned on, make it even deeper until it has the desired depth (11.20d, e).

The tracking groove works as a guide for the ultrasonic tip, which will be used at first without any irrigation just to have a perfect visibility and then with irrigation to make it deeper about 2-3 mm. Now a larger tip can be used to flatten out the floor of the root-end preparation.

From time to time it is suggested to stop the use of the tip and the irrigation, to dry the area with the Stropko (11.21) and to check the preparation with a micromirror (11.22). If some gutta-percha is still remaining along the buccal wall, instead of insisting with the retrotip it is easier and better to capture the maximum cushion of thermoplasticized gutta-percha with a small plugger and condense it coronally, until the wall is clean and free of debris. As an alternative, facial wall debris can be removed using a back-action ultrasonic tip, having an angle of about 70° or tilting the tip buccally (11.23), so that the end of the tip can vibrate against the facial wall and gradually loosen the remaining filling material. If this part of gutta-percha is not removed before placing the retrofilling material, it may potentially cause leakage and then failure of the surgery.

Once the retropreparation is completed, it is rinsed with the retrotip irrigation and dried with the Stropko irrigator and inspected with a micromirror of adequate size, checking the cleanliness at various magnifications. Historically, apical preparations were dried with paper points before placing retrofilling materials (11.24). This technique is incorrect as particles of paper may be left in the preparation, remaining debris will be compacted in the preparation and a thorough drying of the cavity may not be obtained. Today better results are accomplished with a controlled blast of air, using a small blunt microtip irrigating needle (Vista Dental) mounted on a Stropko Irrigator, where water is not connect and the air is delivered at a minimum pressure.

Upon inspection of the root-end preparation, the cavity should be a Class I cavity, dry and clean, coaxial to the root, with no debris of previous filling material on any wall (11.25).

Now the cavity is ready to be filled.

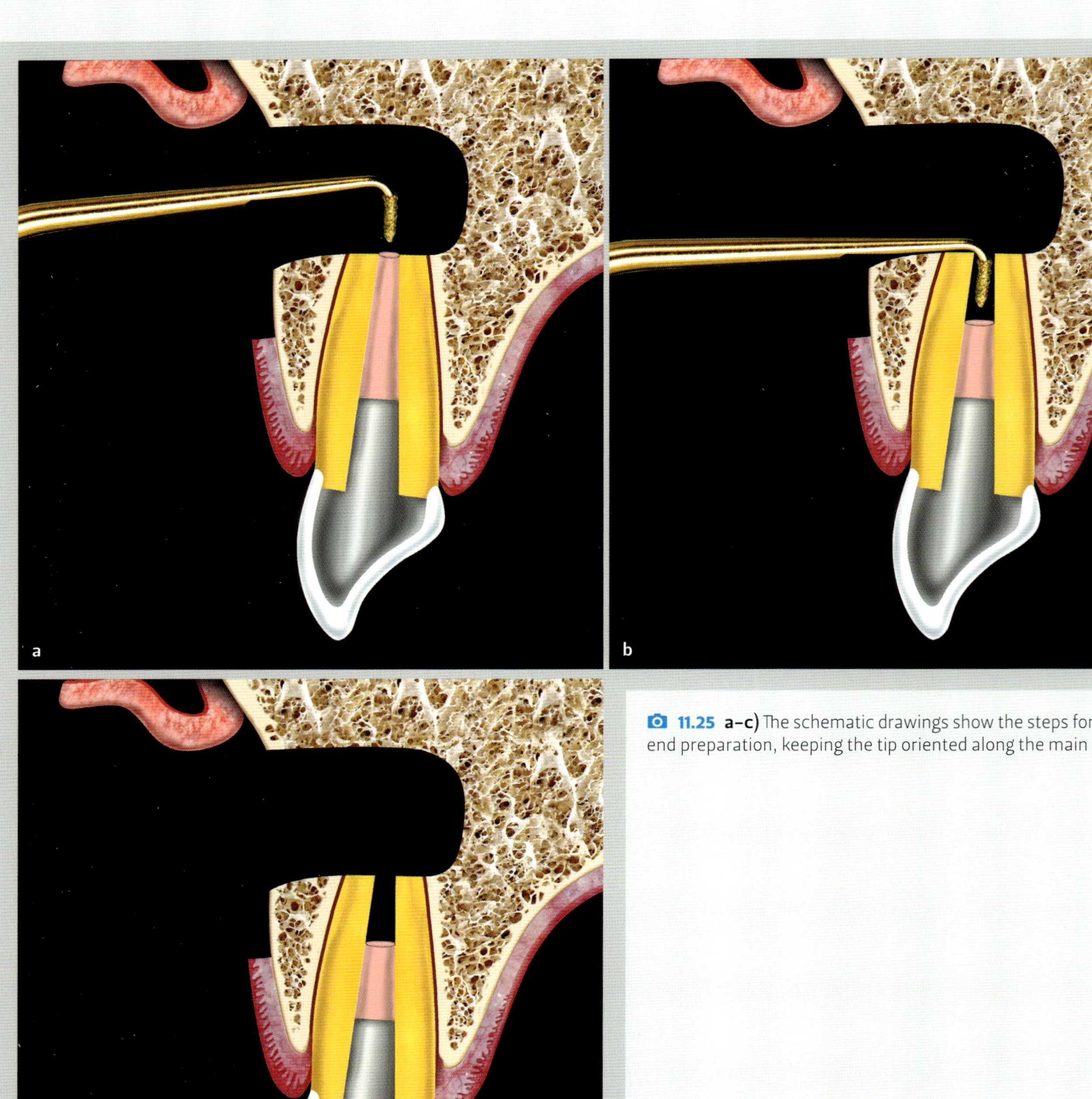

11.25 a–c) The schematic drawings show the steps for a correct root-end preparation, keeping the tip oriented along the main axis of the root.

REFERENCES

1. Carr GB. *Surgical Endodontics*. In: *Pathways of The Pulp*, 6th ed. St. Louis: Mosby. 1994;544-52.
2. Carr GB. *Ultrasonic root end preparation*. Dent Clin North Am. 1997;41:541-544.
3. Rubinstein R, Fayad MI. *Apical microsurgery: application of armamentaria, materials, and methods*. In: Torabinejad M, Rubinstein R. eds. *The art and science of contemporary surgical endodontics*. Quintessence Publishing Co, Inc. 2017;155-178.
4. Friedman S, Stabholz, A. *Endodontic retreatment—case selection and technique. Part 1: criteria for case selection*. J Endod. 1986;12:28-33.
5. Lin CP, Chou HG, Cuo JC, Lan WH. *The quality of ultrasonic root-end preparation: a quantitative study*. J Endod. 1998;24:666-70.
6. Setzer FC, Kohli MR, Shah SB, Karabucak B, Kim S. *Outcome of endodontic surgery: a meta-analysis of the literature-Part 2: Comparison of endodontic microsurgical techniques with and without the use of higher magnification*. J Endod. 2012;38(1):1-10.
7. Setzer FC, Shah SB, Kohli MR, Karabucak B, Kim S. *Outcome of endodontic surgery: a meta-analysis of the literature-Part 1: Comparison of traditional root-end surgery and endodontic microsurgery*. J Endod. 2010;36:1757-1765.
8. Song M, Shin S-J, Kim E. *Outcomes of endodontic micro-resurgery: a prospective clinical study*. J Endod. 2011;37:316-320.
9. Song M, Jung I, Lee SJ, Lee CY, Kim E. *Prognostic factors for clinical outcomes in endodontic microsurgery: a retrospective study*. J Endod. 2011;37(7):927-933.
10. Tsesis I, Rosen E, Schwartz-Arad D, et al. *Retrospective evaluation of surgical endodontic treatment: traditional versus modern technique*. J Endod. 2006;32: 412-416.
11. Tsesis I, Faivishevsky V, Kfir A, Rosen E. *Outcome of surgical endodontic treatment performed by a modern technique: a meta-analysis of literature*. J Endod. 2009;35:1505-1511.
12. Tsesis I, Rosen E, Taschieri S, Strauss YT, Ceresoli V, Del Fabbro M. *Outcomes of surgical endodontic treatment performed by a modern technique: an updated meta-analysis of the literature*. J Endod. 2013;39(3):332-339.
13. Saunders WP, Saunders M, Gutmann JL. *Ultrasonic root end preparation: part 2-microleakage of EBA root end fillings*. Int Endod J. 1994;27:325-329.
14. Layton CA, Marshall G, Morgan L, Baumgartner C. *Evaluation of cracks associated with ultrasonic root end preparations*. J Endod. 1996;22:157-160.
15. Waplington M, Lumley PJ, Walmsley AD, Blunt L. *Cutting ability of an ultrasonic retrograde cavity preparation instrument*. Endod Dent Traumatol. 1995;11:177-180.
16. Min MM, Brown CE Jr, Legan JJ, Kafrawy AH. *In vitro evaluation of effects of ultrasonic root end preparation on resected root surfaces*. J Endod. 1997;23:624-628.
17. Gray JG, Hatton J, Holtzmann DJ, Jenkins DB, Neilsen CJ. *Quality of root end preparations using ultrasonic and rotary instrumentations in cadavers*. J Endod. 2000;26:281-283.
18. Navarre SW, Steiman R. *Root-end fracture during retropreparation: a comparison between zirconium nitride-coated and stainless steel microsurgical ultrasonic instruments*. J Endod. 2002;28:330-332.
19. Brent PD, Morgan LA, Marshall JG, Baumgartner JC. *Evaluation of diamond-coated ultrasonic instruments for root-end preparation*. J Endod. 1999;25:672-675.
20. Stropko JJ. *Canal morphology of maxillary molars: clinical observation of canal configurations*. J Endod. 1999;25:446-50.
21. Hsu YY, Kim S. *The resected root surface. The issue of canal isthmuses*. Dent Clin North Am. 1997;41:529-540.

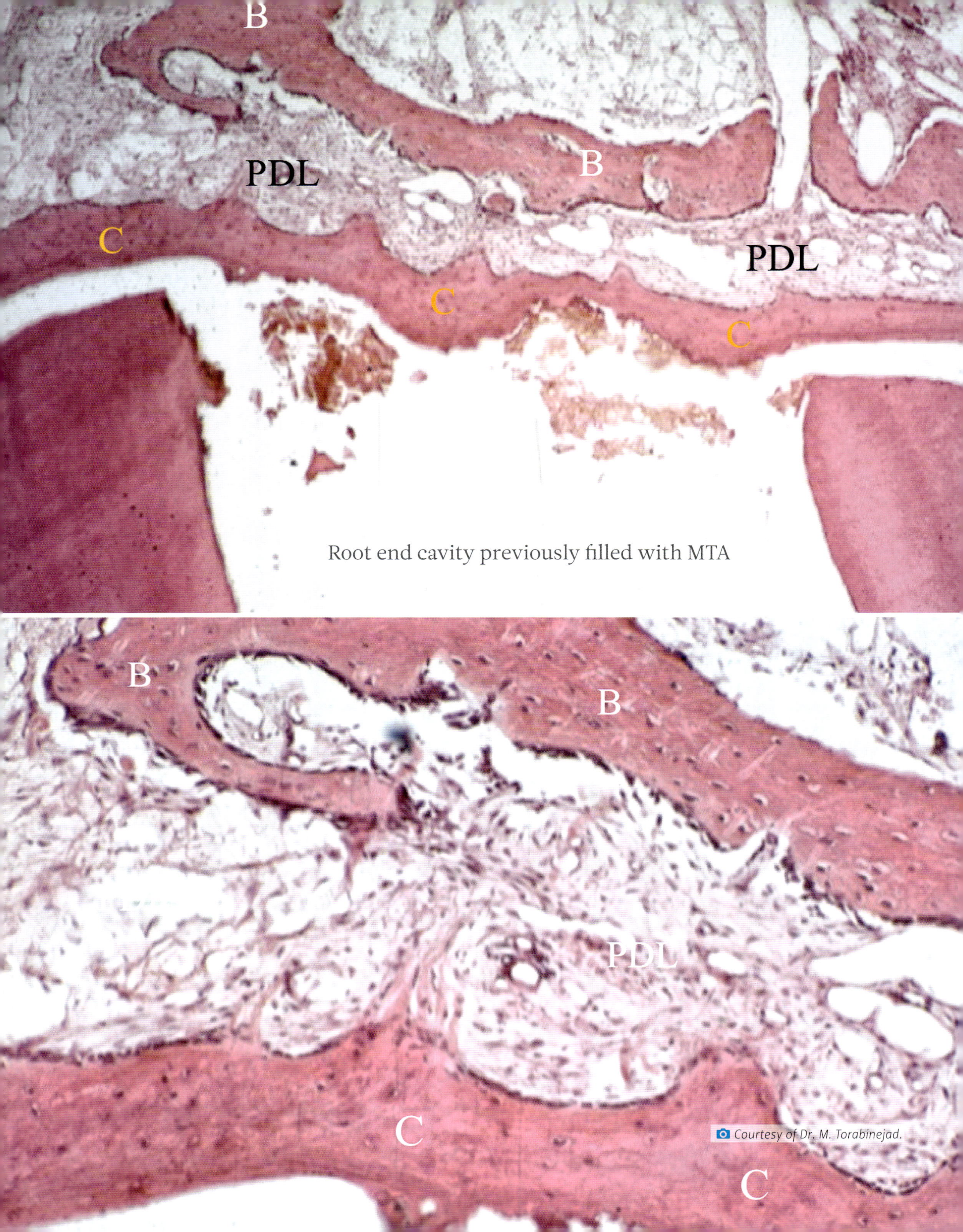
B
PDL
B
C
PDL
C
C
Root end cavity previously filled with MTA
B
B
PDL
C
C
Courtesy of Dr. M. Torabinejad.

Root-End Filling Materials

The ideal retrofilling material should have the following characteristics:

- capable of guaranteeing a perfect cavity seal
- easy to carry and to manipulate
- relatively fast setting time
- dimensionally stable and nonresorbable
- biocompatible
- osseo and cementogenic
- nontoxic
- insoluble in tissue fluids
- bactericidal or bacteriostatic
- does not stain the root and the surrounding tissues
- sterile or easily sterilizable before use
- radiopaque
- easy to remove if necessary

Many retrofilling materials have been used through the years: amalgam, gold foil, zinc oxide eugenol cements, glass ionomer cements, IRM (Caulk, Dentsply, Milford, DE, USA), SuperEBA (Keystone Industries, Gibbstown, NJ), Optibond, Gerestore and more recently Mineral Trioxide Aggregate (ProRoot MTA, Dentsply International, Dentsply Tulsa Dental, Tulsa OK, USA) and EndoSequence Root Repair Material (Brasseler, USA).

Amalgam

Amalgam has been the most commonly used root-end filling material since it was first recommended in the literature by Farrar in 1884.[1] Amalgam remained the standard until 1959, when Omnell demonstrated the presence of a cytotoxic precipitate of zinc carbonate, then the "zinc-free amalgam" became the material of choice for root-end filling.[2]

However, amalgam has been abandoned for many reasons, like toxicity, leakage,[3] corrosion,[4] blood mercury level,[5] tattoos on soft tissue,[6] microcracks in the root (📷 10.13b), and more so that it can be concluded that there is no valid reason today to continue its use. Nevertheless, many oral surgeons and maxillofacial surgeons still use amalgam[7,8] (📷 1.2). The only advantage of amalgam was its radiopacity (📷 12.1).

Intermediate Restorative Material (IRM)

Intermediate Restorative Material (IRM) is a zinc oxide eugenol material reinforced with polymethacrylate. It became an alternative to amalgam and it has been recommended as a root-end filling material because of its biocompatibility,[9,10] marginal integrity,[11,12] and reported success in a retrospective clinical study.[6] This material has the added advantages of being readily available, inexpensive, and easy to manipulate (good working properties).

SuperEBA

SuperEBA (12.2) is a zinc oxide eugenol cement reinforced with ethoxy benzoic acid. It has been proposed as a root-end filling as a result of its good sealing properties as stated in *in vitro* dye leakage and fluid filtration studies [13] as well as the good tissue response to SuperEBA cement.[14] It has been used for many years, especially after the advent of the ultrasonics preparation.[15] In the Author's experience SuperEBA demonstrated to be an excellent material, showing a long term success rate of more than 91,5%.[16] According to Song et al. there is no significant difference in the clinical outcomes of microsurgical endodontics when SuperEBA and ProRoot MTA are used as root-end filling materials.[17]

On the other hand, as it will be discussed later, MTA is more biocompatible, hydrophilic and has so many characteristics that in this Author's opinion can be considered a lot superior to SuperEBA, which also has few drawbacks. First of all, it is technique sensitive, it requires three and half minutes of mixing, until it is thick, putty consistency. Then the dental assistant has about three minutes to prepare small truncated cones 1 to 2 mm in size that remain attached to a small spatula to hand to the doctor (12.3). Now the material is condensed with slight excess into the cavity with small pluggers and a ball burnisher (12.4, 12.5), then it will take several minutes for setting and finally it can be finished with a high speed finishing bur (12.6, 12.7). If

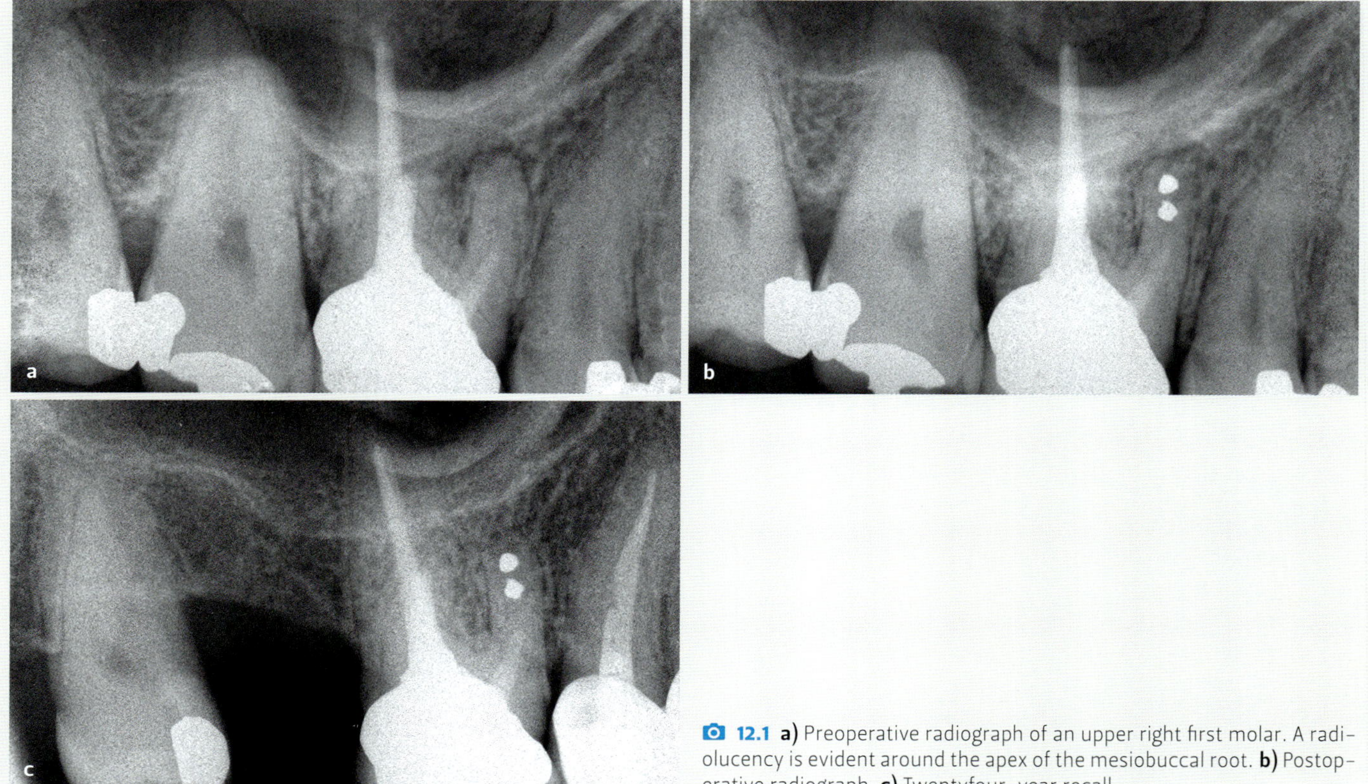

12.1 a) Preoperative radiograph of an upper right first molar. A radiolucency is evident around the apex of the mesiobuccal root. **b)** Postoperative radiograph. **c)** Twentyfour-year recall.

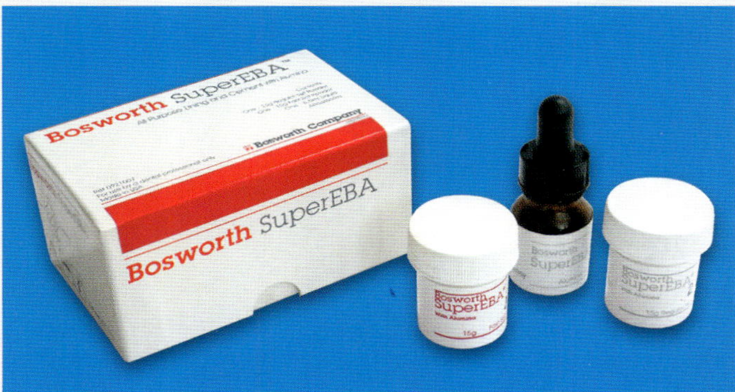

12.2 SuperEBA with the regular and fast setting powders.

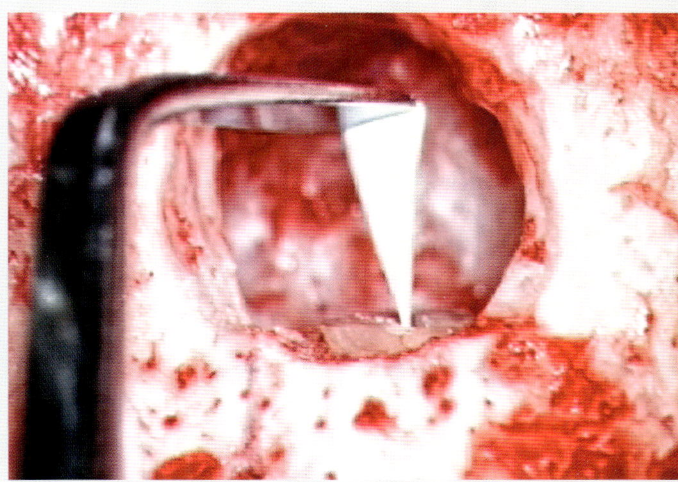

12.3 A cone of SuperEBA is ready to be introduced into the root-end cavity.

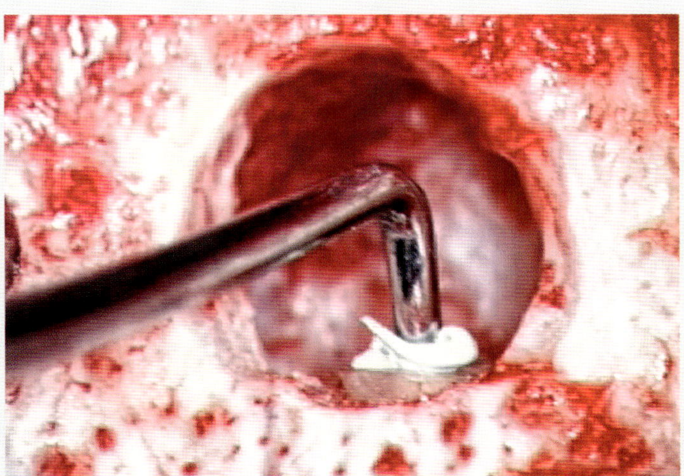

12.4 A microsurgical plugger condenses the retrofilling material.

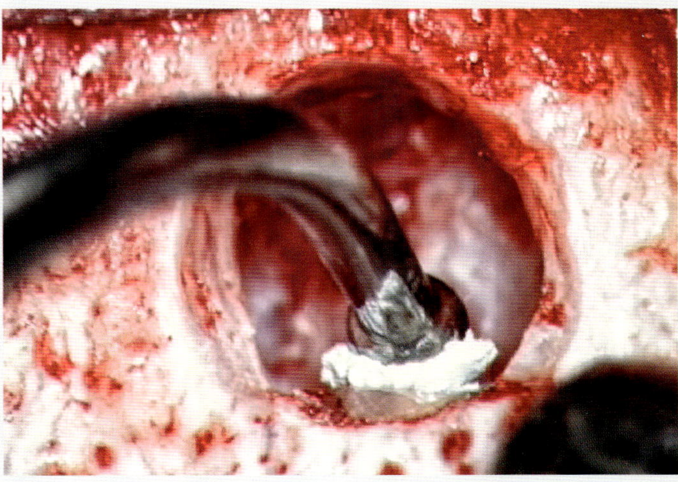

12.5 A ball burnisher condenses the excess material.

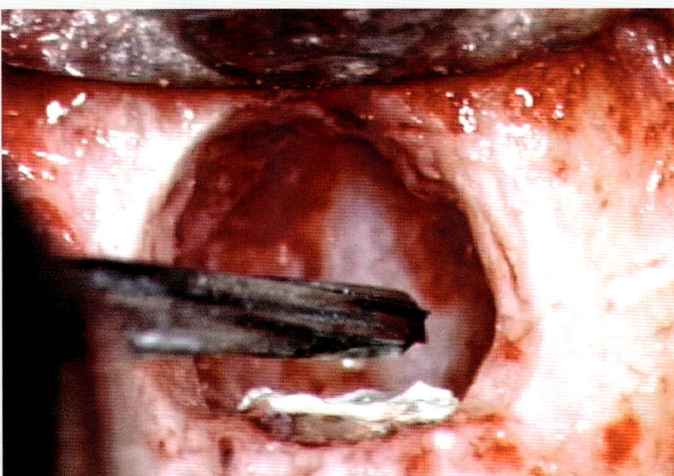

12.6 After setting, the Lindemann bur removes the excess material.

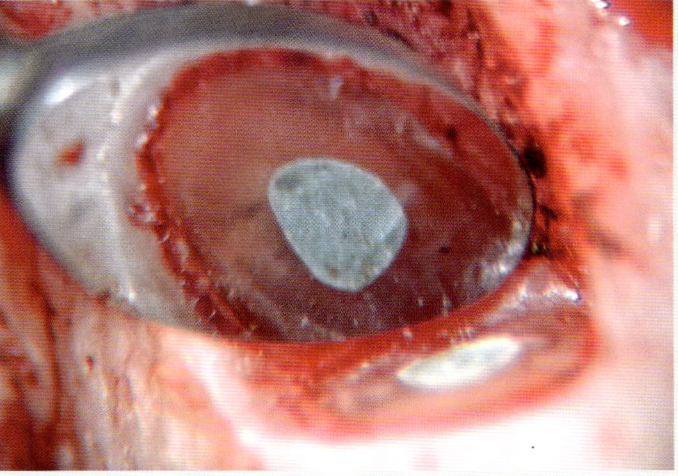

12.7 The retrofill made of SuperEBA has been finished.

we count the total time, we can realize that it is a way too much and the most difficult thing to do is to be synchronized with the dental assistant. Since it takes about 5 minutes of manipulation before being condensed into the cavity, it means that the dental assistant has to start the mixing about 5 minutes before the doctor is ready.

The material comes with two different kinds of powder, fast and slow setting time. It is not always easy to make the right choice, so that sometimes the setting time is too fast and the material starts to set during the compaction, while other times the setting takes forever... During the compaction the bleeding control must be perfect because the material cannot be contaminated by blood. If this happens, the damaged material needs to be removed and the filling had to start all over again. A disadvantage that appeared immediately evident after replacing the old amalgam is that it is less radiopaque as it has the same radiopacity of gutta-percha, so that it can be difficult to recognize (📷 12.8). Another drawback is the long term dimensional stability and the resorbability.[18] In two cases the Author had to retreat his surgical failures and he found that the SuperEBA that he had positioned several years before was completely washed out (📷 12.9).

In conclusion, SuperEBA is well tolerated by tissues, is fast setting, polishable, and provides excellent apical seals. However, it is difficult to manipulate, sensitive to temperature and humidity, only moderately radiopaque, and its long term dimensional stability is questionable.

Composite Materials

Composite materials like OptiBond™ (SybronEndo) and Geristore® (DenMat, USA) can be used today thanks to the perfect crypt control and the absolutely dry operative field. [19] Just as in restorative dentistry, the material must not be contaminated by any moisture and being positioned under the microscope, it is important to reduce the intensity of the illumination as much as possible and use a filter to prevent a significant reduction of the setting time.[19] In summary, the major disadvantage of these resin-type materials is difficulty in avoiding blood/moisture contamination. If contaminated, these root-end filling materials will not provide an adequate seal. For these reasons, the materials are not as popular as hydrophilic substances such as MTA and bioceramics.[20]

Mineral Trioxide Aggregate

Mineral Trioxide Aggregate (MTA; ProRoot® MTA, Dentsply Tulsa Dental) became recently available and today there are many articles in the literature showing that MTA can be considered the material of choice.[21–24] MTA was originally developed from Portland cement as a grey powder by Dr. Torabinejad (Loma Linda University, CA, USA) and sold as ProRoot® MTA, manufactured by Dentsply Tulsa Dental, Tulsa, OK. More recently, due to esthetic concerns, a tooth-colored formula was introduced as White MTA, which differs from the original Grey MTA in the absence of iron. Holland et al.[25] made an *in vivo* research study, implanting dentin tubes filled with MTA inside rat connective tissue and demonstrated that Grey and White MTA are identical as to their mechanisms of action and biocompatibility. Several studies later confirmed that there is no statistically significant difference between the two materials, indicating that their mechanism of action is similar.[26–29]

However, White MTA has smaller particle sizes and for this reason it is preferable to the Grey during surgery, because the carrier doesn't remain plugged so easily. MTA is an endodontic cement that is extremely biocompatible, capable of stimulating healing and osteogenesis, and is hydrophilic. MTA is a powder that consists of fine trioxides (tricalcium oxide, silicate oxide, bismuth oxide) and other hydrophilic particles (tricalcium silicate, tricalcium aluminate, responsible for the chemical and physical properties of this aggregate), that set in the presence of moisture. Hydration of the powder results in formation of a colloidal gel with a pH of 12.5, that solidifies to a hard-solid structure in approximately three to four hours.[30] This cement is different from other materials currently in use because of its biocompatibility, antibacterial properties, marginal adaptation and sealing properties, and its hydrophilic nature.[30]

In the Author's experience, MTA has replaced all the previously mentioned materials for many reasons, first of all its biocompatibility,[31–33] its hydrophilic nature,[30]

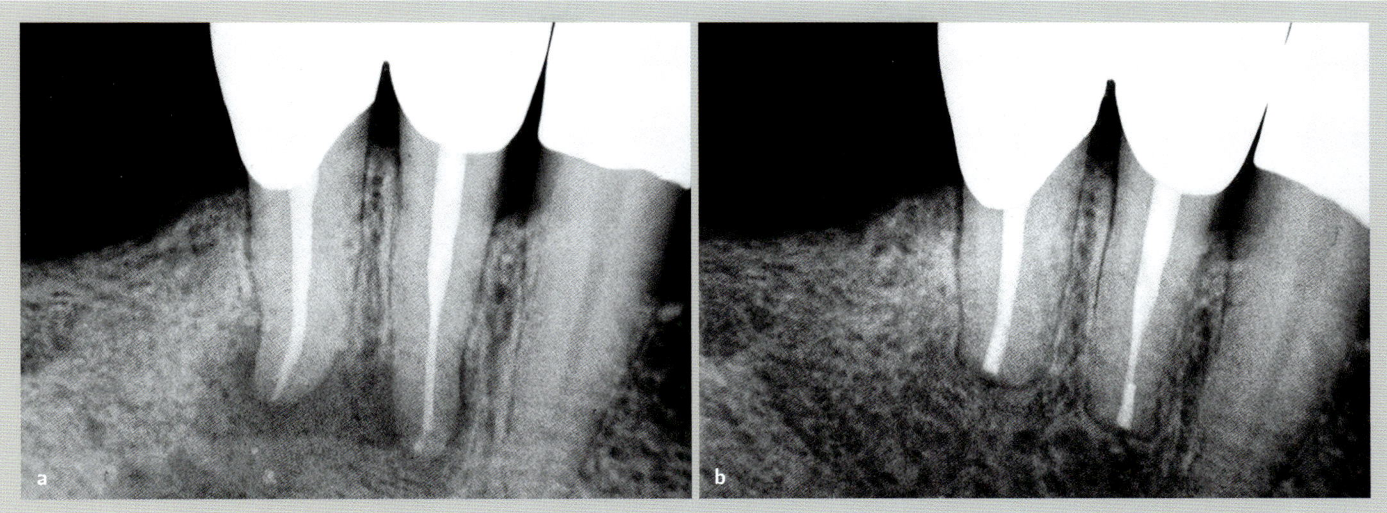

12.8 **a)** Preoperative radiograph of lower right first and second premolars. **b)** Two-year recall. The retrofill made of SuperEBA has almost the same radiopacity as gutta-percha.

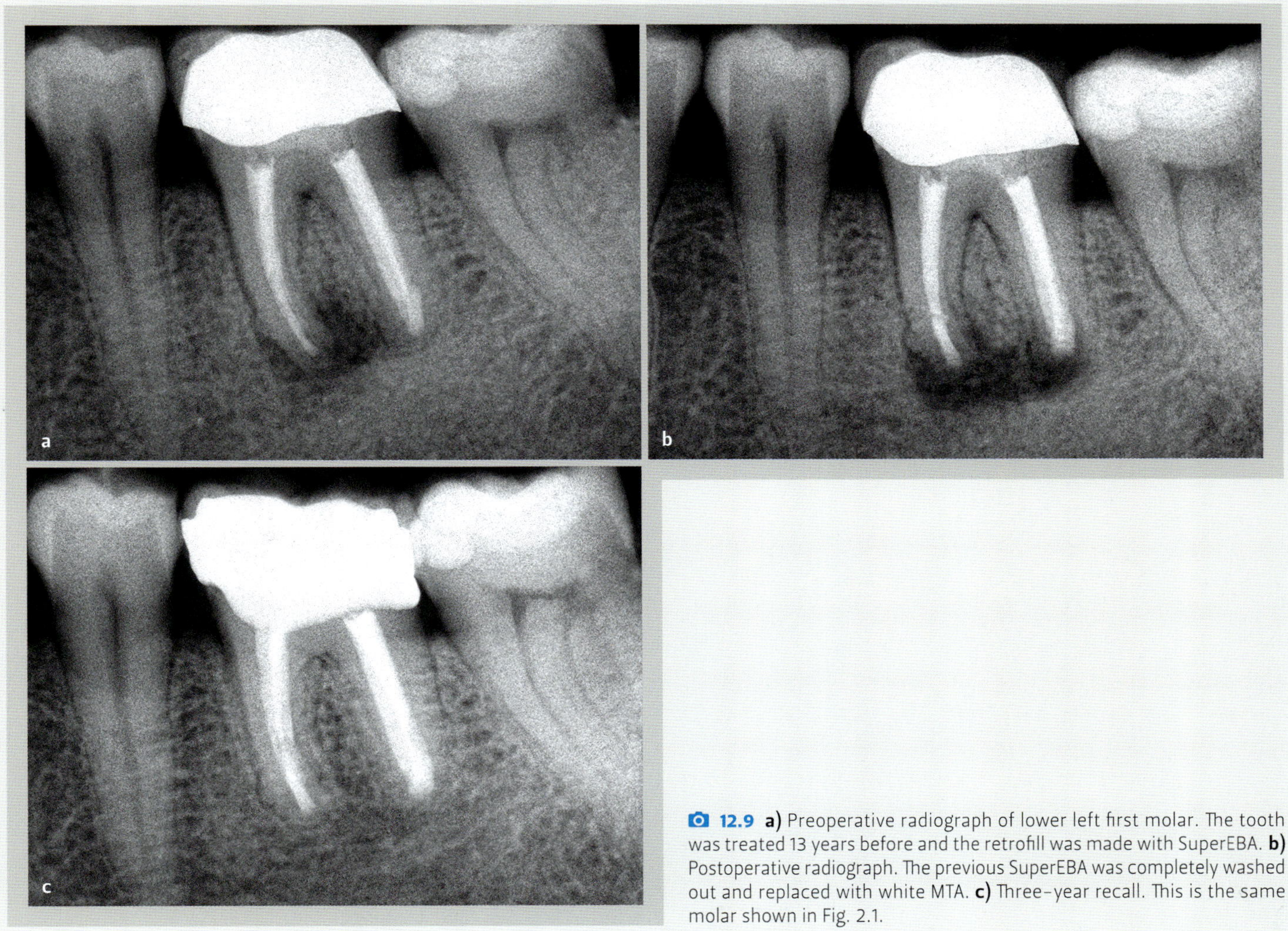

12.9 **a)** Preoperative radiograph of lower left first molar. The tooth was treated 13 years before and the retrofill was made with SuperEBA. **b)** Postoperative radiograph. The previous SuperEBA was completely washed out and replaced with white MTA. **c)** Three-year recall. This is the same molar shown in Fig. 2.1.

also because it has superior sealing quality,[34-39] is not affected by moisture or blood contamination,[38] it is relatively easy to manipulate and currently has an excellent carrier available. MTA has several advantages:

1. easy to mix and place into the cavity with a small carrier
2. since it sets in the presence of moisture, it is not moisture sensitive and is not affected by blood contamination
3. seals better than amalgam, SuperEBA or IRM
4. has a better adaptation to the surrounding dentin
5. has excellent biocompatibility
6. activates regeneration of periapical tissues including periodontal ligament and cementum (12.10, 12.11).[40]

The only disadvantage that existed years ago when the material was first introduced into the market was the difficulty of handling it because there was no adequate carrier available. The first carrier that became available was the Dovgan Carrier (Quality Aspirators, Duncanville, TX, USA) (12.12), but even though the needles were bendable, its use was not comfortable during surgery, especially in posterior teeth. Its diameters were too large, they didn't fit into the apical preparations and they got blocked up easily.

In the year 2000 another carrier was proposed by Edward Lee,[41,42] the MTA Pellet Forming Block (12.13). This carrier was designed by cutting grooves into a

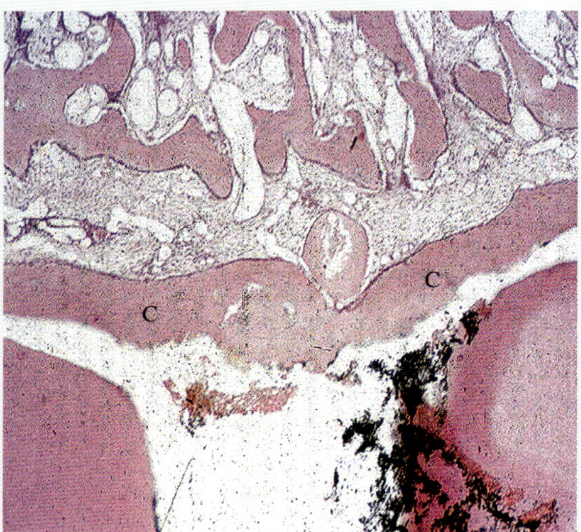

12.10 A histological section of a maxillary central incisor of a monkey after periapical surgery and use of MTA as root-end filling material showing formation of cementum (C) over resected root-end surface and MTA. Note the presence of normal periodontal ligament and bone adjacent to the newly formed cementum (*Courtesy of Dr. M. Torabinejad*).

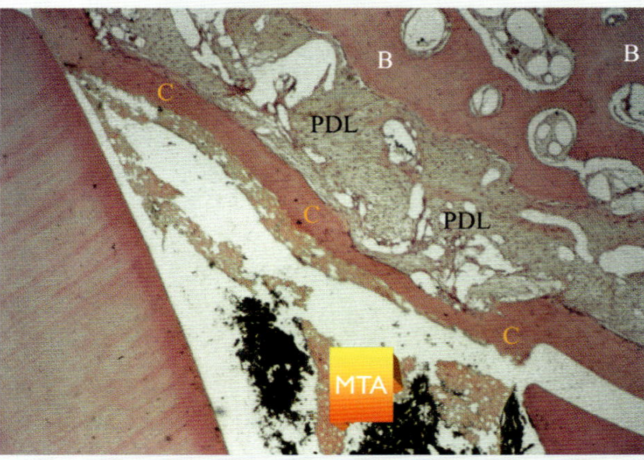

12.11 Tissue response to an MTA root-end filling. New cementum has grown over the cut root-end dentin and over the root-end filling; there is no inflammation in the adjacent connective tissue (*Courtesy of Dr. M. Torabinejad*).

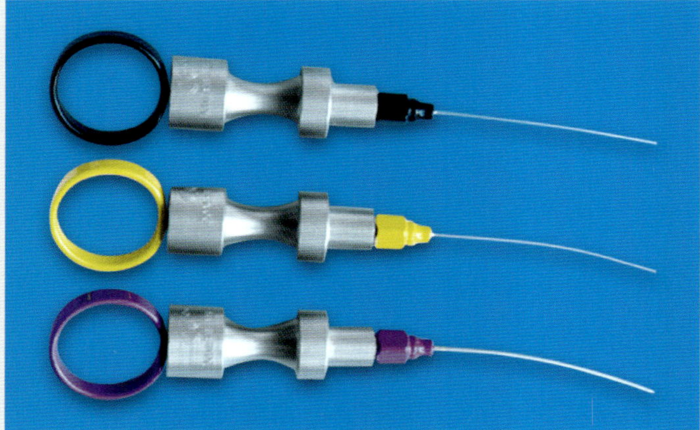

12.12 The Dovgan Carriers in three different sizes (Quality Aspirators, Duncanville, TX, USA).

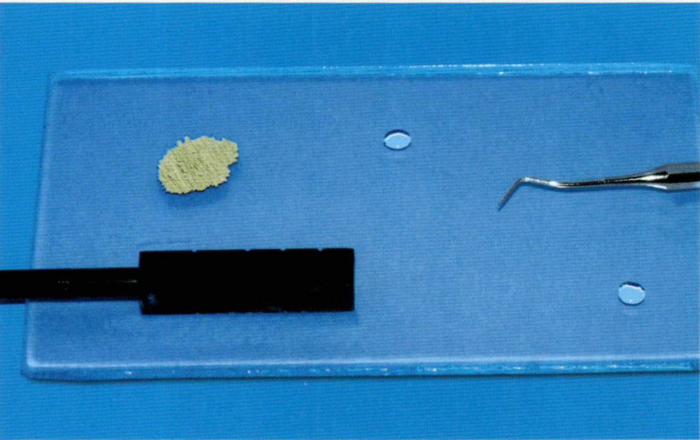

12.13 The MTA Block (G. Hartzell & Sons, Concord, CA, USA).

1.2 cm × 1.2 cm × 5 cm plastic block. After being properly mixed to a putty-like consistency (not too dry and not too wet), the MTA is just pressed into the previously selected groove of the Lee block, then a small spatula slides into the groove to take the selected length of material, this adheres to the tip of the spatula and it is ready to be easily placed into the retroprep (12.14).

Recently, another carrier has been designed and manufactured by Produits Dentaires SA (Vevey, Switzerland) in cooperation with Dr. Bernd Ilgenstein, called The MAP (Micro Apical Placement) System (12.15) and this can be considered a "universal" carrier, since it has special needles that can be used both in clinical and in surgical endodontics and that during surgery allows an easy positioning of MTA also in posterior teeth and in lateral canals.[43] The needles are available in NiTi or as stainless steel triple-bent and single bent needles.

The surgical triple-bent needles are available in two variants, right-angled and left-angled, each with two external diameters, 0.9 mm (yellow) and 1.1 mm (red). The internal diameter of the cannulas is 0.6 mm (yellow) and 0.8 mm (red), which allows for sufficient portions of the retrofilling material to be applied successively. The NiTi needle is available also in 1.3 mm to be used in large preparations, resorbed roots and immature roots.

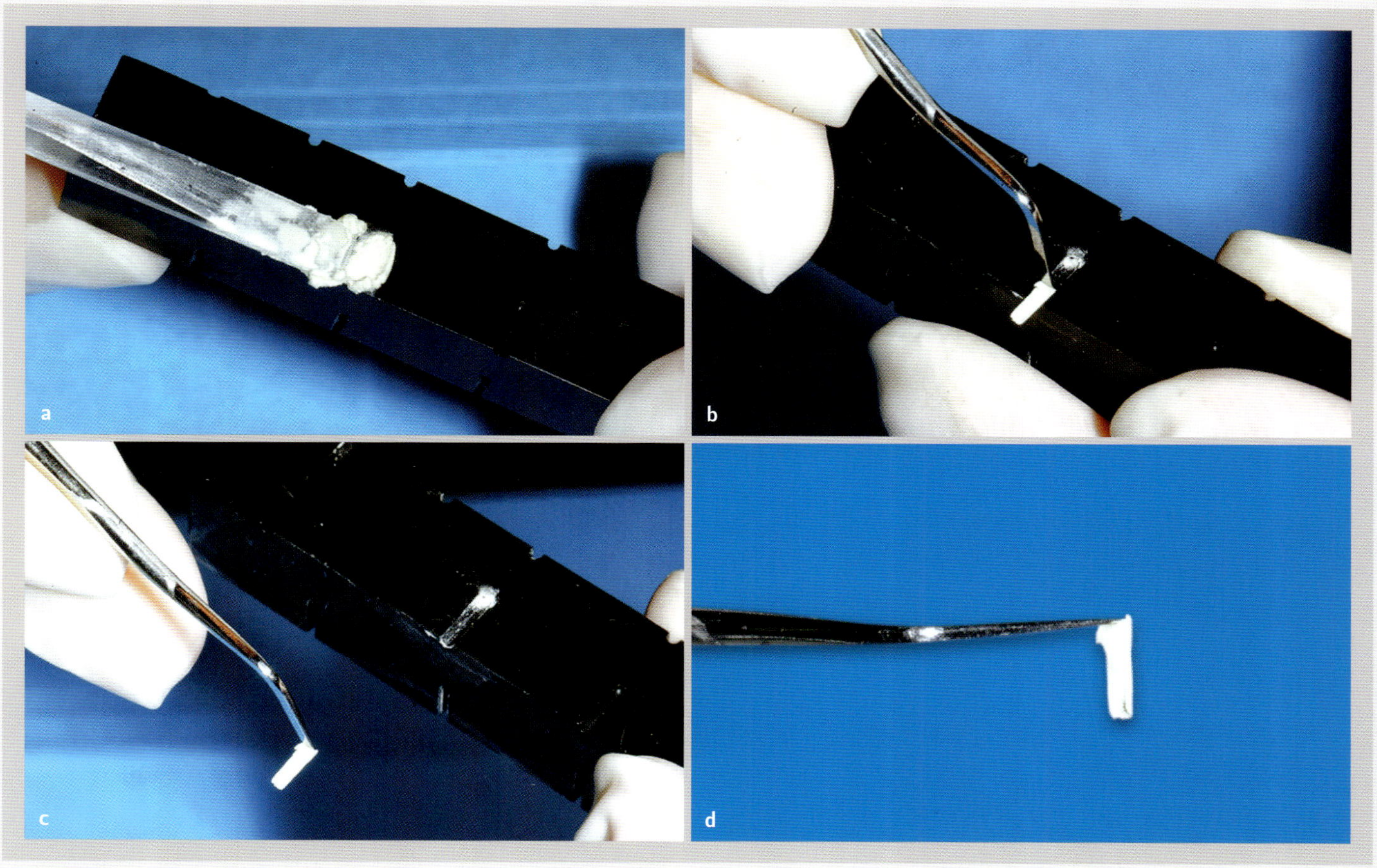

12.14 **a)** The mixed MTA is filled into a groove of the MTA block. **b)** Using a small spatula, a small amount of MTA pellet is scooped out of the groove. **c, d)** The little cylinder of MTA is now ready to be easily placed into the retroprep.

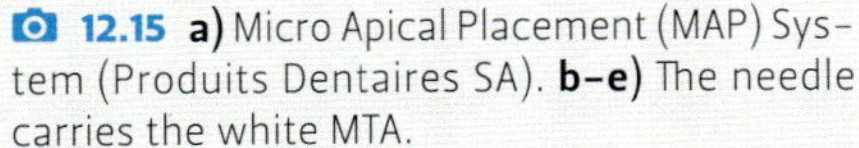

12.15 **a)** Micro Apical Placement (MAP) System (Produits Dentaires SA). **b–e)** The needle carries the white MTA.

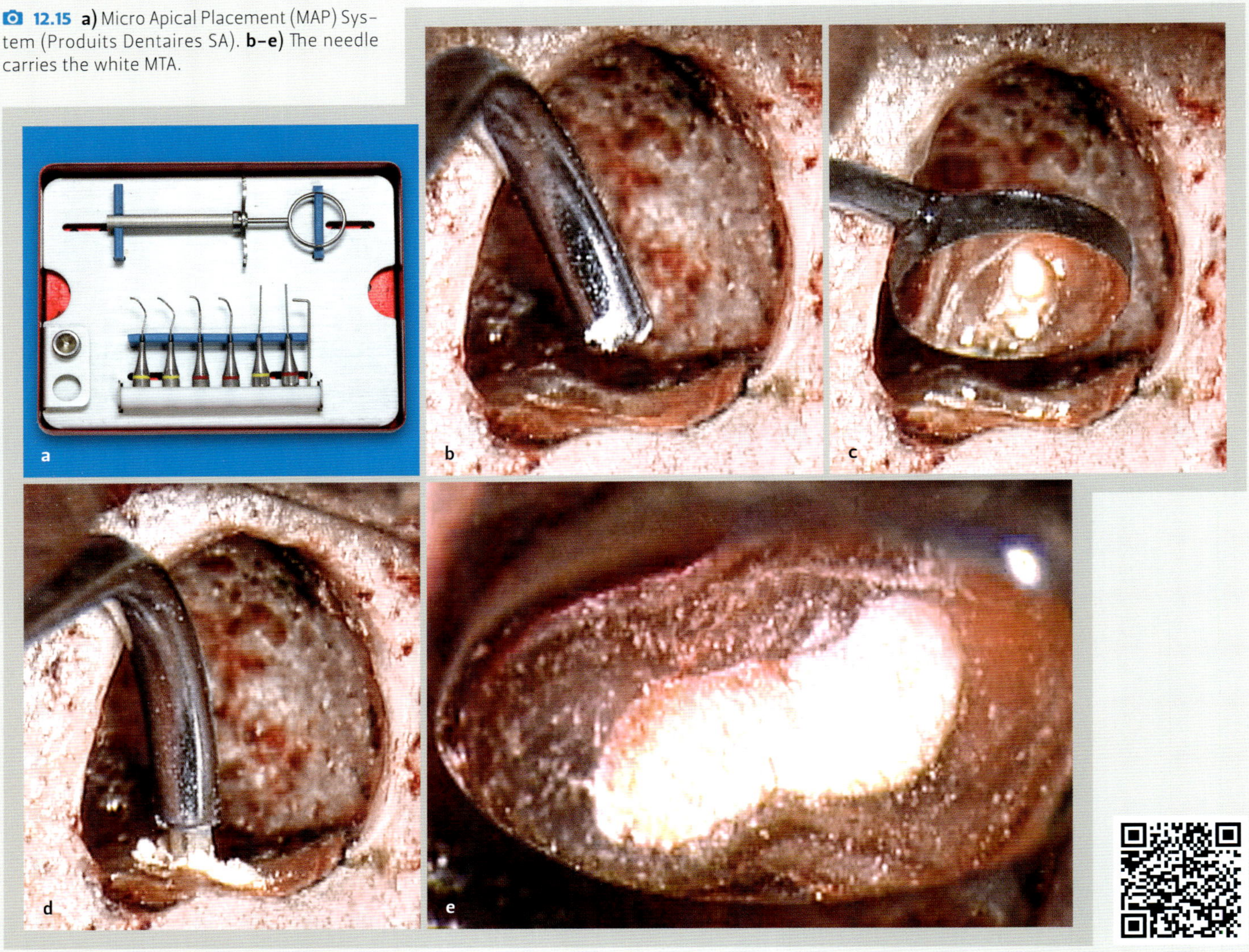

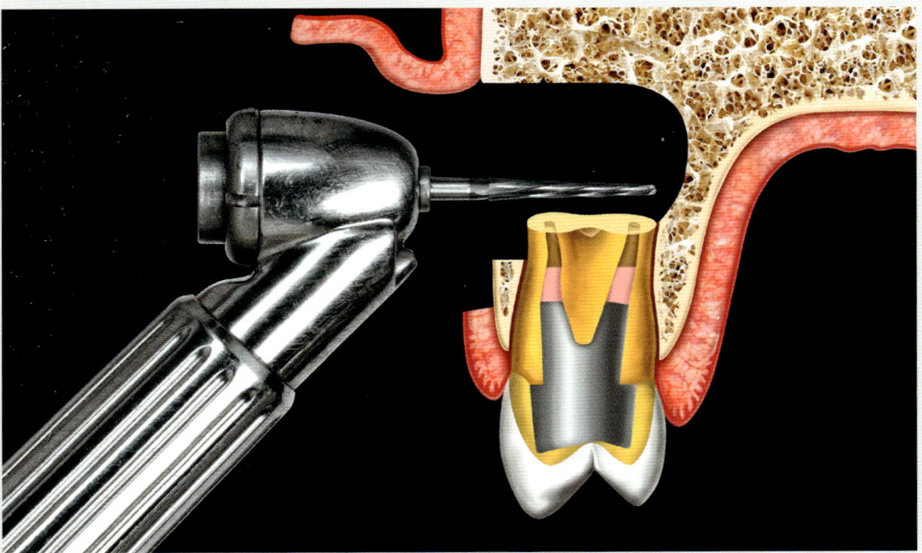

12.16 The apical root tip is resected perpendicular to the long axis of the tooth.

It is well known that since the ultrasonic tips have been introduced onto the market, the root surface is no longer cut with a bevel at 45°, but rather with an almost 90° angle (12.16). This involves the need for a specific carrier in order to deliver the retrofilling material at a 90° angle (12.17). The MAP System is the perfect carrier for this purpose, having several needles in different sizes and with different angulations (12.18).

The triple angle needles are best indicated for posterior teeth. They are available in two variants, right-angled and left-angled, for an easier treatment of hard-to-reach regions (palatal canals of upper premolars and molars, lingual canals of lower molars). The NiTi needles are by design universal and can be indicated for most orthograde and retrograde cases of anterior and posterior teeth.

The intra-cannula plunger inside the needle is intentionally longer than the needle itself (12.19), so that it will not only deliver the MTA in the retropreparation, but will also act as a plugger and thus begins to compact the material in the deepest portion of the prepared cavity. The risk of air bubbles can therefore be avoided. As a result, the retrograde root canal filling will always be well compacted. The plungers are made of a Polyoxymethylene (POM) material, which can easily navigate even a triple-bent needle.

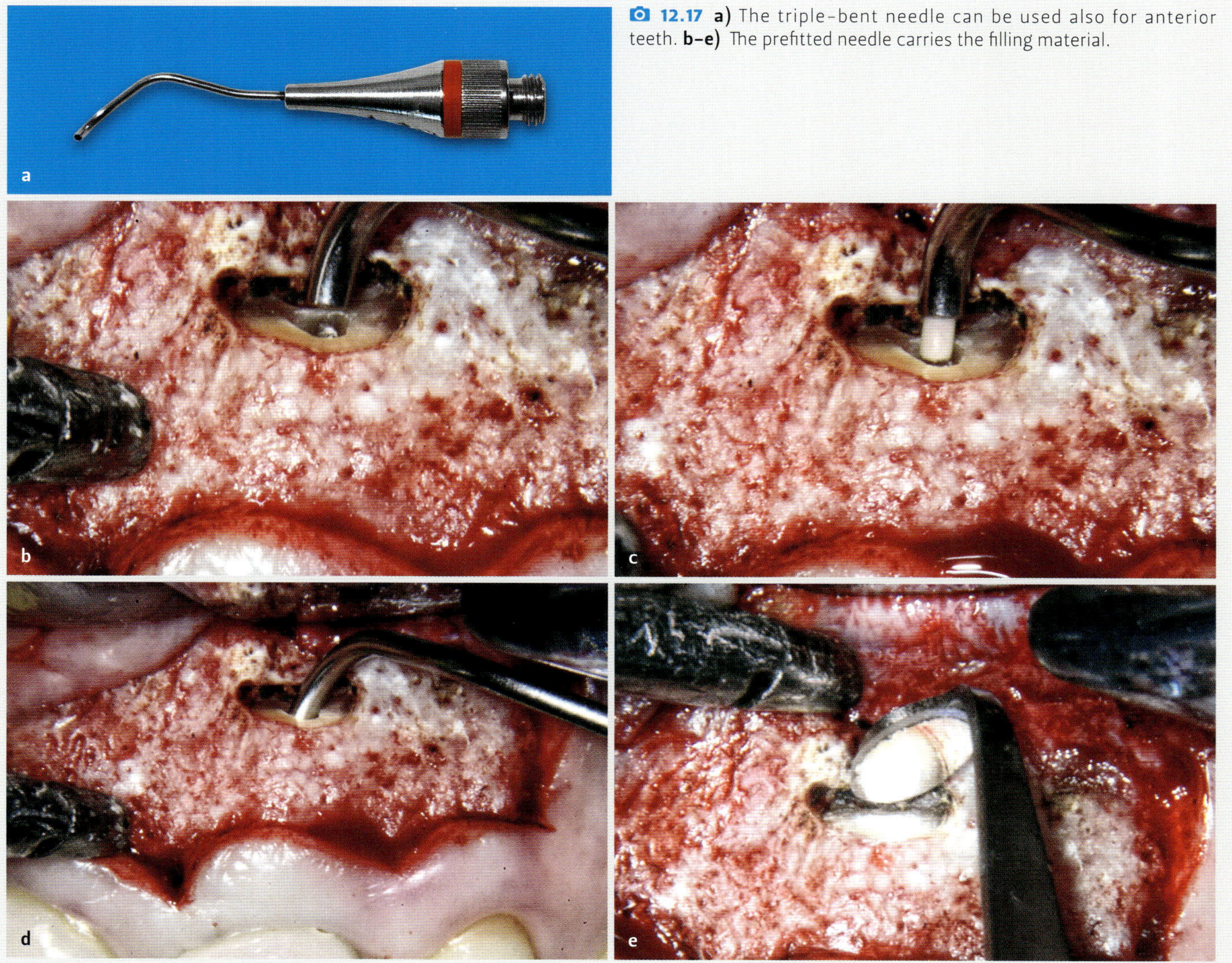

12.17 **a)** The triple-bent needle can be used also for anterior teeth. **b–e)** The prefitted needle carries the filling material.

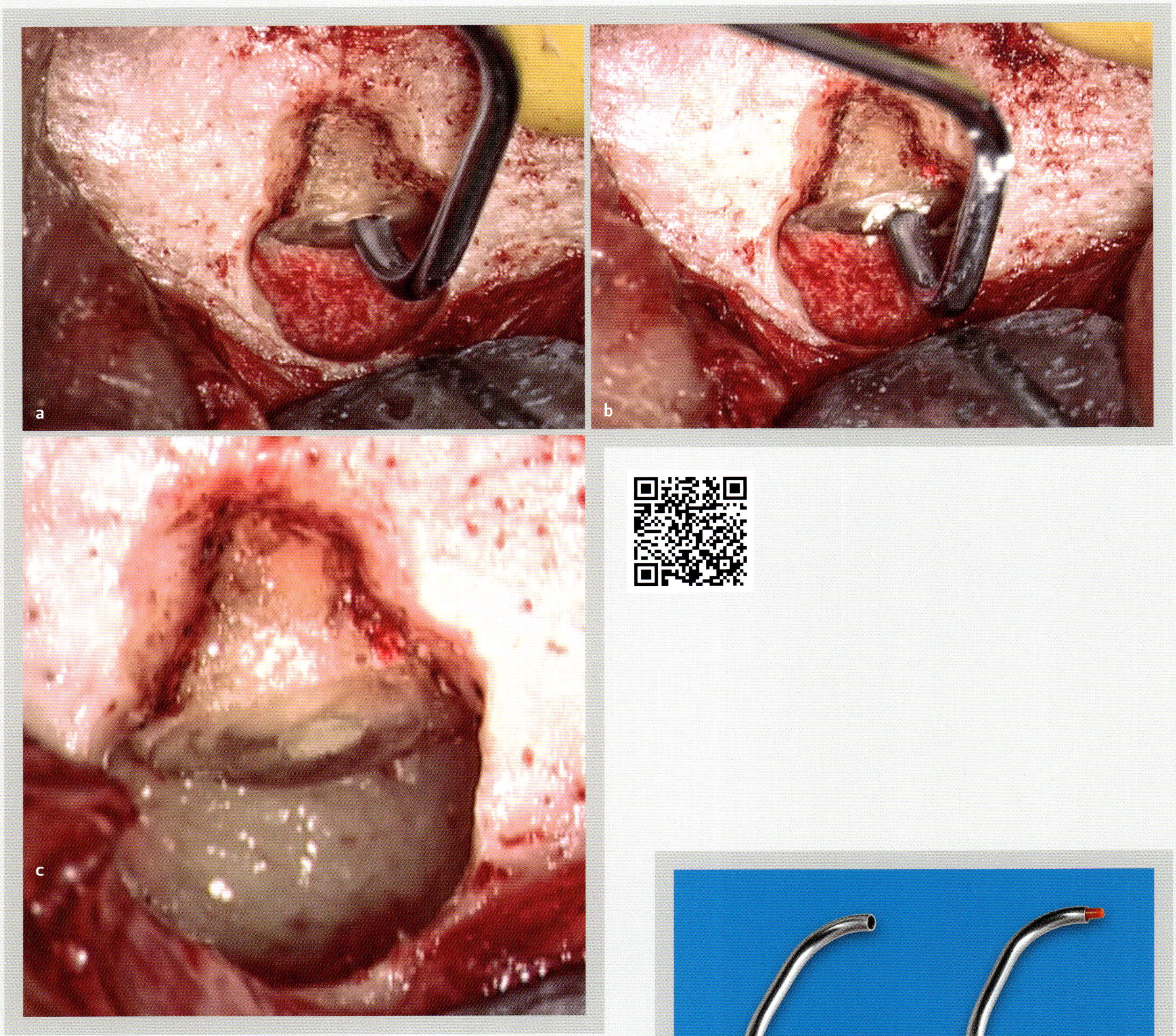

12.18 a–c) The triple-bent needle carries the root-end filling material in a lower second premolar.

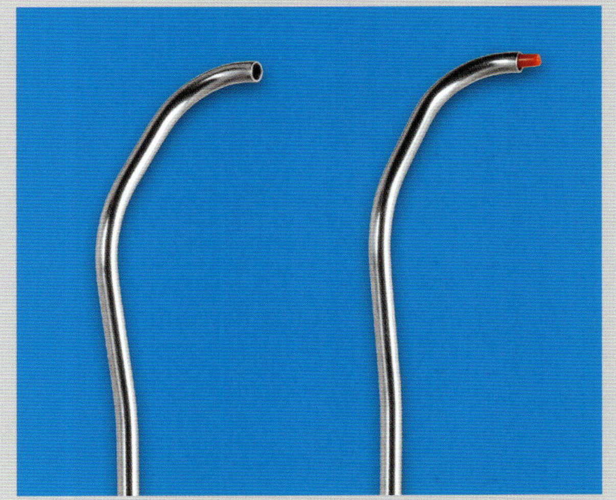

12.19 The intra-cannula plunger inside the needle is intentionally longer than the needle itself in order to act as a plugger, beginning to compact the filling material in the deepest portions of the prepared cavity.

Another advantage of using the MAP System during surgery is the perfect control of the obturating material, which will be laid in the retrocavity without any dispersion in the surrounding bone and soft tissue.

Once the retrocavity has been prepared using the ultrasonic retrotips, the bleeding of the bony crypt is under control, the root-end preparation is dried with the Stropko and checked with a microsurgical mirror at high magnification under the microscope, the operator asks the dental assistant to mix the MTA to the correct consistency and then to load the prefitted applicator syringe (see 12.17b-e). The consistency of MTA must be neither too wet nor too dry. If the mix is too wet, it will be difficult to compact the material properly into the cavity. In this situation a gentle blow of air from the Stropko irrigator will provide the right consistency (12.20). If it is too dry, it will be difficult to extrude the material from the needle and the syringe can remain blocked. Should the latter be the case, it is essential to avoid pushing too hard. The POM plunger is insufficiently rigid and will remain bent next to the bayonet catch, and therefore need replacing. For this reason, is always advisable to have two syringes ready for use and the needles should not be packed too tightly. It is also important that the dental assistant disassembles and cleans the carrier immediately after surgery because the material inside the needle may set and block it. If this happens, the set material can be easily removed using the MAP System cleaning curette or a thin ultrasonic tip to disintegrate it and make the needle clean again, without damaging the metal.

During the placement of MTA in the retrocavity, the dental assistant is asked to touch the metal plugger with an ultrasonic tip (12.21) in order to release the entrapped air, to improve the adaptation to the cavity walls and to improve the density of the obturating material. The material is always carried in excess, condensed with a big burnisher (12.22) and then is finished with a small spatula (12.23) and a microsurgical brush (12.24) to the level of the resected (12.25).

The MTA is hydrophilic and requires moisture to set. The necessary moisture will come from the blood which will fill the bony crypt immediately after surgery. If ferric sulfate has been used, it is important now to curette and irrigate in order to stimulate the bleeding which will provide the moisture for the MTA (12.26a-c). While doing this irrigation the operator has to be careful not to expose the freshly mixed MTA to excessive fluids because it could be washed out, with a consequent detrimental effect on its sealing ability.

The only disadvantages of ProRoot® MTA is the long setting time and the high cost. Recently, several modified types of MTA-like materials have been developed and marketed, like PD White MTA, which - accordingly to the manufacturer - has a much shorter setting time, of about 15 minutes. However, this as - well as other relatively new products - is in need of research-based conclusions.

Bioceramics

Bioceramic-based materials have been recently introduced in endodontic practice because of their advantageous physical and biological properties. Bioceramics are the result of the combination between calcium silicate and calcium phosphate that are applicable for biomedical and dental use.[44]

Bioceramics refers to a wide range of specially designed ceramics used for the repair, reconstruction, and replacement of diseased or damaged parts of the body.[20] The first generation bioceramic used in dentistry has been MTA, which belongs to the category of tricalcium silicate-base cements. Tricalcium silicate is the component responsible of sealability and biocompatibility of MTA.[20] Recently other bioactive tricalcium silicate and phosphate cements have been introduced, and EndoSequence Root Repair Material (RRM) (Brasseler USA, Savannah, GA, USA) is available to endodontists since 2010 and is one of the most popular. Its indications are similar to MTA. According to the manufacturer it is composed of calcium silicates, monophasic calcium phosphate, zirconium oxide, tantalum oxide, along with filler and thickening agents.[45] Many *in vitro* and *in vivo* studies have shown that RRM is biocompatible, nontoxic, nonshrinking, and chemically stable within the biological environment.[46–48] In addition, RRM has many desirable clinical properties; it is premixed, its handling characteristics are similar to an intermediate restorative material, has optimal radiopacity,[44] and does not cause tooth discoloration.[49] It has been proposed that bioceramic-based materials are able to form hydroxyapatite when in contact with moisture and ultimately form a bond between dentin and the filling material.[44] The reported setting time of RRM has been inconsistent and ranges from 4 hours to more than 48 hours.[50] All of these characteristics can explain the high level of success when used as a retrofilling material. RRM comes premixed with an intermediate restorative material-like consistency and therefore is easier to handle.[50] The retrospective study of Shinbori et al.[45] shows promising results of RRM used in endodontic microsurgery. The high success rate observed in their study is comparable to that reported when MTA is used as the retrofilling material,[51,52] suggesting RRM is a viable alternative to MTA as a root-end filling material.

Membranes and Bone Grafts

A frequently asked question is whether a bone graft should be placed in the bony crypt and a membrane over the surgical site as a matter of routine.[53] An ex-

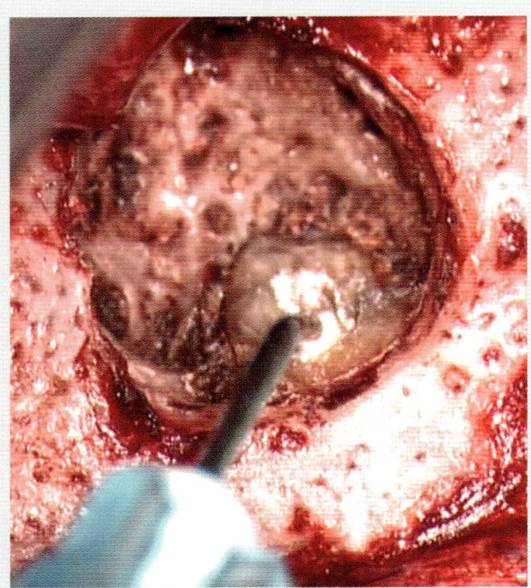

12.20 If the mix is too wet, a gentle blow of air from the Stropko irrigator will provide the right consistency, making the mix a little dryer.

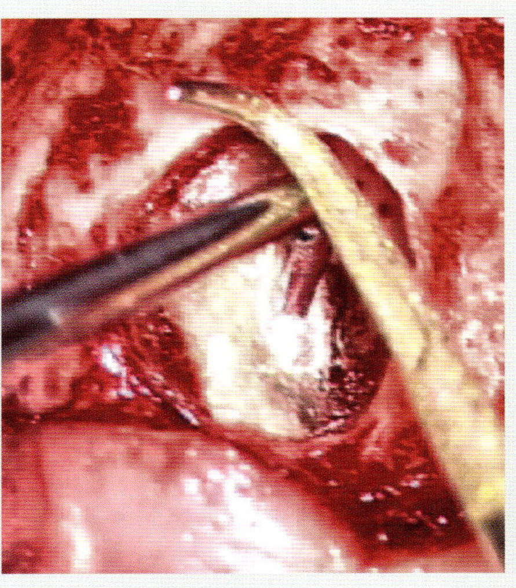

12.21 The ultrasonic tip is in contact with the metal plugger to improve the adaptation of MTA to the dentinal walls of the cavity.

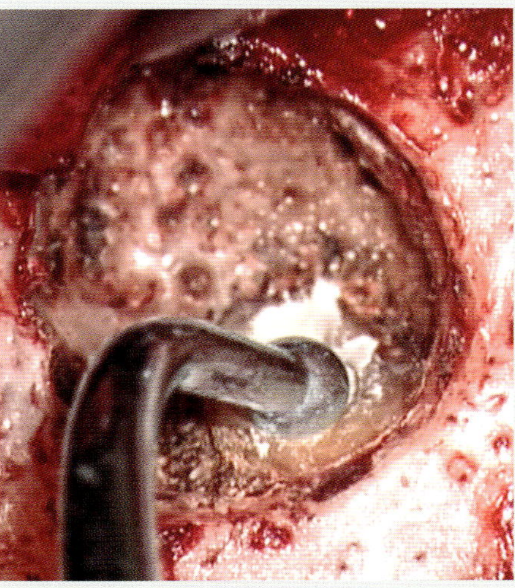

12.22 The excess material is condensed with a ball burnisher.

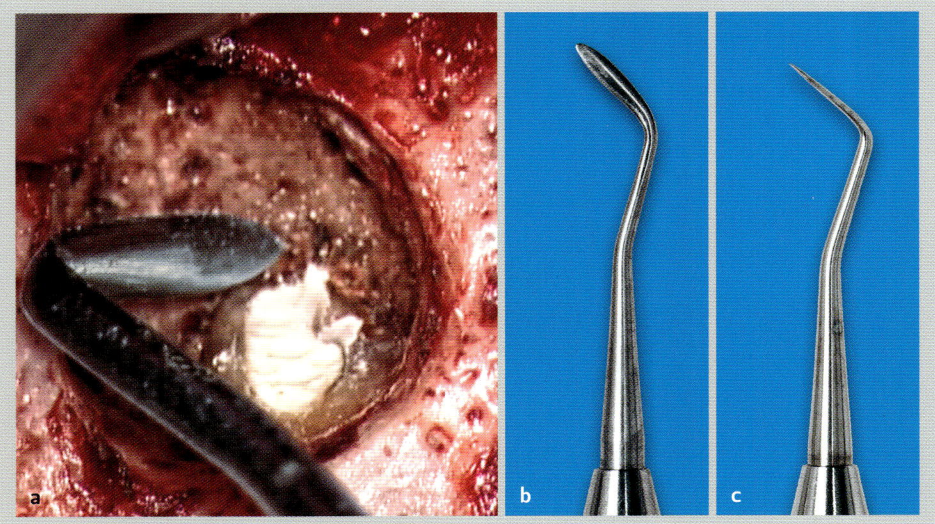

12.23 **a–c)** A small spatula with sharp edges removes the excess material and finishes the root-end filling.

haustive answer to this question has been given by Lin et al. in their article.[54]

Guided tissue regeneration is a technique for enhancing and directing cell growth to repopulate specific parts of the periodontium that have been damaged by periodontal diseases, tooth diseases, or trauma.[55] Guided tissue regeneration by using membrane barriers and/or bone grafting materials has also been used in periapical surgery to enhance new bone formation.[56–61] Those studies were mainly focused on new bone formation and did not address formation of periodontal ligament (PDL) and cementum, which are also components of the periapical tissues. Application of guided tissue regeneration concepts to periapical surgery is primarily based on extensive studies of periodontal regenerative therapy. However, there are significant differences in the application of guided tissue regeneration in periodontal regenerative therapy and in periapical surgery. Wound healing can result in either regeneration or repair, depending on several factors, like the nature of wound, availability of progenitor/stem cells, growth/differentiation factors.[54]

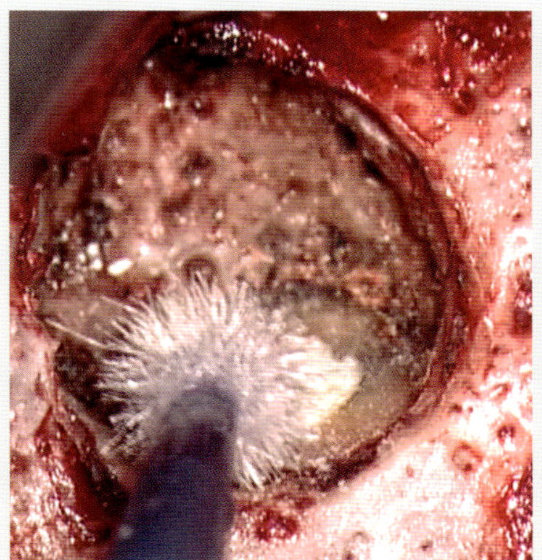

12.24 A microsurgical brush completes the finishing of the resected surface.

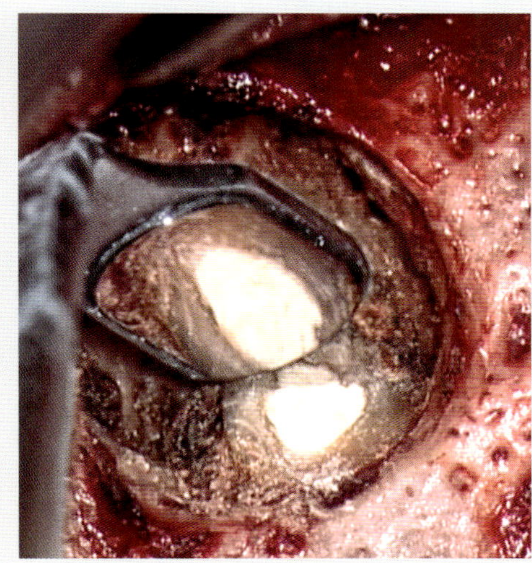

12.25 The microsurgical mirror shows the finished root-end filling.

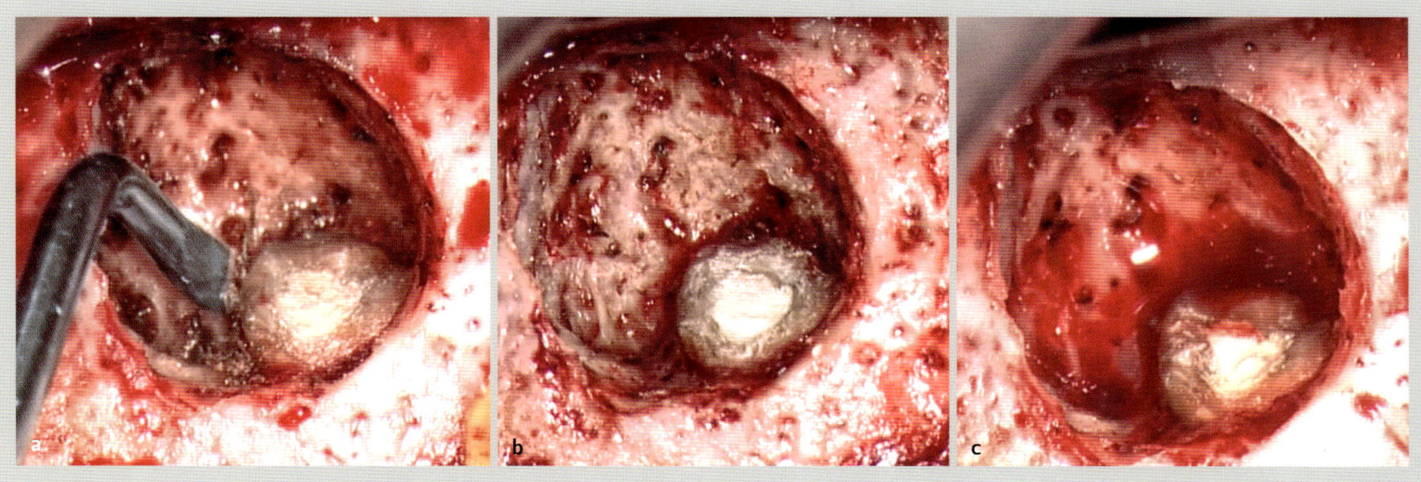

12.26 a–c) The bony crypt is curetted under irrigation to stimulate bleeding.

Regeneration represents the replacement of damaged tissue by the cells of the same tissue. *Repair* represents the restoration of the destroyed tissue by new tissue different from the original tissue. It does not reconstitute the architecture and functions of the original tissue, which means that in periapical surgery, the resected root-end cannot be regenerated. Regeneration of periapical tissues after periapical surgery requires [62] recruitment of progenitor/stem cells to differentiate into committed osteoblasts, PDL cells, and cementoblasts. Lack of any one of these elements would result in repair rather than regeneration.[63] It seems that if both buccal and palatal/lingual cortical plates are lost as a result of apical periodontitis lesions or periapical surgery, periapical wounds will most probably heal by scar tissue formation.[64–66] Studies have shown no difference in bone tissue healing if only the buccal cortical plate was destroyed, whether or not a membrane barrier was used in periapical surgery.[67,68] On the basis of limited controlled clinical trials, there is no conclusive evidence to demonstrate that the application of membrane barriers in large or through-and-through bony lesions/defects has a better long-term outcome than a control group in periapical surgery.[54] By definition,[55] application of membrane barriers in periapical surgery does not appear to meet the concept of guided tissue regeneration. In contrast, in periodontal regenerative therapy membrane barriers serve to guide progenitor/stem cells to repopulate their specific parts of the periodontium. Clinically, the best application of membrane barriers in periapical surgery appears to be in combined endodontic-periodontal or periodontal-endodontic lesions[69] or large periapical lesions communicating with the alveolar crest.[70,71] In this kind of apicomarginal bony defect, the PDL and cementum are destroyed. Accordingly, application of a membrane barrier is indicated during periapical surgery to prevent apical migration of junctional epithelium along the denuded root surface into the periapical wound and to induce selective repopulation with cells of the connective tissue attachment.[60–71] In combined endodontic-periodontal or periodontal-endodontic lesions, the use of a membrane to manage the lesions is directed at the periodontal tissue rather than periapical tissue regeneration.[54]

As far as bone grafts are concerned, bone grafting materials, except autogenous bone grafts, are foreign to the host's tissue and can interfere with the normal wound healing process, resulting in delayed healing or a foreign body reaction.[72,73]

Biologically, a blood clot is a better space filler than all bone grafting materials.[54] A blood clot is the host's own biologic product and is essential to tissue wound healing and provides an excellent natural scaffold for wound healing. Without a blood clot, tissue wound healing would be impaired,[72,73] as in a dry socket after tooth extraction. Bone grafts alone without a blood clot or angiogenic factors are unlikely to be capable of promoting periapical wound healing.[74]

In conclusion, except in apicomarginal bony defects caused by combined periodontal-endodontic or endodontic-periodontal lesions [69,71] or in large periapical lesions communicating with the alveolar crest,[70,71] the use of membrane barriers in periapical surgery has not been shown to have a clear benefit in regenerating periapical tissues. The ability of bone grafts to induce new bone formation has been well-documented.[56–61,75–80] However, new PDL and cementum regeneration in periapical surgery has not been shown to benefit from the use of bone grafts.

Simply applying a membrane barrier and/or bone graft during periapical surgery might not result in complete regeneration of the periapical tissues, because these biomaterials are not capable of recruiting progenitor/stem cells and inducing these undifferentiated mesenchymal cells to differentiate into PDL cells and cementoblasts after periapical surgery.[54]

Regardless of the size of periapical lesions, persistence of root canal infection is the primary cause of inflamed periapical tissues not to heal after endodontic therapy.[81] Therefore membrane barriers and/or bone grafts by themselves will never be able to prevent periapical surgery failures (📷 10.22).

Without using membrane barriers and/or bone grafts in periapical surgery for large apical periodontitis lesions, complete periapical tissue regeneration has been observed histologically in many animal and human studies.[66,82–87]

REFERENCES

1. **Farrar JN.** *Radical and heroic treatment of alveolar abscess by amputation of roots of teeth, with description and application of the cantilever crown.* Dent Cosmos. 1884;26:135-139.
2. **Omnell KA.** *Electrolytic precipitation of zinc carbonate in the jaw; An unusual complication after root resection.* Oral Surg Oral Med Oral Pathol. 1959;12:846-952.
3. **Agrabawi J.** *Sealing ability of amalgam, SuperEBA cement, and MTA when used as retrograde filling materials.* Br Dent J. 2000;11:188(5):266-268.
4. **Frank AL et al.** *Long-term evaluation of surgically placed amalgam fillings.* J Endod. 1992;18:391-398.
5. **Saatchi M, Shadmehr E, Talebi SM, Nazeri M.** *A prospective clinical study on blood mercury levels following endodontic root-end surgery with amalgam.* Iran Endod J. 2013;8(3):85-88.
6. **Dorn SO, Gartner AH.** *Retrograde filling materials: a retrospective success-failure study of amalgam, EBA, and IRM.* J Endod. 1990;16:391-393.
7. **Rahbaran S, Gilthorpe MS, Harrison SD, Gulabivala K.** *Comparison of clinical outcome of periapical surgery in endodontic and oral surgery units of a teaching dental hospital: a retrospective study.* Oral Surg Oral Med Oral Pathol Oral Radiol Endod. 2001;91:700-709.
8. **Wesson CM, Gale TM.** *Molar apicectomy with amalgam root-end filling: results of a prospective study in two district general hospitals.* Br Dent J. 195:707-14, 2003.
9. **Cook D, Taylor P.** *Tissue reactions to improved zinc oxide-eugenol cements.* J Dent Child. 1973;40:199-207.
10. **Blackman R, Gross M, Seltzer S.** *An evaluation of the biocompatibility of a glass ionomer-silver cement in rat connective tissue.* J Endod. 1989;15:76-79.
11. **Abdal AK, Retief DH.** *The apical seal via the retrosurgical approach. I. A preliminary study.* Oral Surg. 1982;53:614-621.
12. **Bondra DL, Hartwell GR, MacPherson MG, Portell FR.** *Leakage in vitro with IRM, high copper amalgam, and EBA cement as retrofilling materials.* J Endod. 1989;15:157-160.
13. **Sullivan JE Jr, Da Fiore PM, Heuer MA, Lautenschlager EP, Koerber A.** *Super-EBA as an endodontic apical plug.* J Endod. 1999;25:559-561.
14. **Pitt Ford TR, Andreasen JO, Dorn SO, Kariyawasam SP.** *Effect of Super-EBA as a root end filling on healing after replantation.* J Endod. 1995;21:13-15.
15. **Oynick J, Oynick T.** *A study of a new material for retrograde fillings.* J Endod. 1978;4:203-206.
16. **Rubinstein R, Kim S.** *Long-term follow-up of cases considered healed one year after apical microsurgery.* J Endod. 2002;25:378-83.
17. **Song M, Shin SJ, Kim E.** *Outcomes of endodontic micro-surgery: A prospective clinical study.* J Endod. 2011;37:316-320.
18. **Biggs JT, Benenati FW, Powell SE.** *Ten-year in vitro assessment of the surface status of three retrofilling materials.* J Endod. 1995;21:521-525.
19. **Stropko J.** *Micro-Surgical Endodontics.* In: Castellucci A, ed. *EndodonticS*, vol. III. Florence, Italy: Il Tridente; 2005:342-411.
20. **Shin S, Chen I, Karabucak B, Baek S, Kim S.** *MTA and bioceramic root-end filling materials.* In: Kim S, Kratchman S, eds. *Microsurgery in Endodontics.* New Jersey: Wiley Blackwell; 2018:91-99.
21. **Torabinejad M, Watson TF, Pitt Ford TR.** *Sealing ability of a mineral trioxide aggregate when used as a root end filling material.* J Endod. 1993; 19:591-595.
22. **Torabinejad M, Hong C-U, Lee S-J, Monsef M, Pitt-Ford TR.** *Investigation of mineral trioxide aggregate for root-end filling in dogs.* J Endod. 1995;21:603-607.
23. **Torabinejad M, Chivian N.** *Clinical applications of mineral trioxide aggregate.* J Endod. 1999;25:197-203.
24. **Agrabawi J.** *Sealing ability of amalgam, SuperEBA cement, and MTA when used as retrograde filling materials.* Br Dent J. 2000;11:188(5):266-268.
25. **Holland R, Souza V, Nerj MJ, et al.** *Reaction of rat connective tissue to implanted dentin tubes filled with a white mineral trioxide aggregate.* Braz Dent J. 2002;13(1): 23-26.
26. **Ferris D, Baumgartner JC.** *Perforation repair comparing two types of mineral trioxide aggregate.* J Endod. 2004;30:422- 424.
27. **Al-Hezaimi K, Naghshbandi J, Oglesby S, Simon J, Rotstein I.** *Human saliva penetration of root canals obturated with two types of mineral trioxide aggregate cements.* J Endod. 2005;31:453- 456.
28. **Faraco Junior IM, Holland R.** *Response of the pulp of dogs to capping with mineral trioxide aggregate or calcium hydroxide cement.* Dent Traumatol. 2001;17:163- 166.
29. **Faraco Junior IM, Holland R.** *Histomorphological response of dogs' dental pulp capped with white mineral trioxide aggregate.* Braz Dent J. 2004;15:104 - 108.
30. **Torabinejad M, Hong CU, McDonald F, Pitt Ford TR.** *Physical and chemical properties of a new root-end filling material.* J Endod. 1995;21:349.
31. **Koh ET, McDonald F, Pitt Ford TR, Torabinejad M.** *Cellular response to mineral trioxide aggregate.* J Endod. 1998;24:53.
32. **Koh ET, Torabinejad M, Pitt Ford TR, Brady K.** *Mineral trioxide aggregate stimulates a biological response in human osteoblasts.* J Biomed Mater Res. 1997;37:432.
33. **Pitt Ford TR, Torabinejad M, Abedi HR, Bakland LK, Kariyawasam SP.** *Mineral trioxide aggregate as a pulp capping material.* J Am Dent Assoc. 1996;127:1491.
34. **Bates CF, Carnes DL, Del Rio CE.** *Longitudinal sealing ability of mineral trioxide aggregate as a root end filling material.* J Endod. 1996;22:575-578.
35. **Nakata TT, Bae KS, Baumgartner JC.** *Perforation repair comparing mineral trioxide aggregate and amalgam.* Abs. no. 40. J Endod. 1997;23:259.

36. Torabinejad M, Higa RK, McKendry DJ, Pitt Ford TR. *Dye leakage of four root-end filling materials: effects of blood contamination.* J Endod. 1994;20:159-163.

37. Torabinejad M, Hong CU, Pitt Ford TR, Kettering JD. *Cytotoxicity of four root end filling materials.* J Endod. 1995;21:489-492.

38. Torabinejad M, Rastegar AF, Kettering JD, Pitt Ford TR. *Bacterial leakage of mineral trioxide aggregate as a root end filling material.* J Endod. 1995;21:109-112.

39. Torabinejad M, Watson TF, Pitt Ford TR. *The sealing ability of a mineral trioxide aggregate as a retrograde root filling material.* J Endod. 1993;19:591-595.

40. Chen I, Karabucak B, Wang C, Wang H-G, Koyama E, Kohli MR, Nah H-D, Kim S. *Healing after root-end microsurgery by using mineral trioxide aggregate and a new calcium silicate-based bioceramic material as root-end filling materials in dogs.* J Endod. 2015;41(3):389-399.

41. Lee E. *A new mineral trioxide aggregate root-end filling technique.* J Endod. 2000;26:764-766.

42. Lee ES. *Think outside the syringe.* Endodontic Practice. 2000;3:26-28.

43. Castellucci A, Papaleoni M. *The MAP System: a perfect carrier for MTA in clinical and surgical endodontics.* Roots. 2009;3:18-22.

44. Candeiro GT, Correia FC, Duarte MA, et al. *Evaluation of radiopacity, pH, release of calcium ions, and flow of a bioceramic root canal sealer.* J Endod. 2012;38: 842-5.

45. Shinbori N, Grama AM, Patel Y, Woodmansey K, He J. *Clinical outcome of endodontic microsurgery that uses EndoSequence BC Root Reapair Material as the root-end filling material.* J Endod. 2015;41(5): 607-612.

46. Ma J, Shen Y, Stojicic S, Haapasalo M. *Biocompatibility of two novel root repair materials.* J Endod. 2011;37:793-798.

47. Damas BA, Wheater MA, Bringas JS, Hoen MM. *Cytotoxicity comparison of mineral trioxide aggregates and EndoSequence Bioceramic root repair materials.* J Endod. 2011;37:372-375.

48. Bosio CC, Felippe GS, Bortoluzzi EA, et al. *Subcutaneous connective tissue reactions to iRoot SP, mineral trioxide aggregate (MTA) Fillapex, DiaRoot BioAggregate and MTA.* Int Endod J. 2014;47:667-674.

49. Walsh RM, Woodmansey KF, Glickman GN, He J. *Evaluation of compressive strength of hydraulic silicate-based root-end filling materials.* J Endod. 2014;40:969-972.

50. Charland T, Hartwell GR, Hirschberg C, Patel R. *An evaluation of setting time of mineral trioxide aggregate and EndoSequence root repair material in the presence of human blood and minimal essential media.* J Endod. 2013;39:1071-1072.

51. Song M, Kim E. *A prospective randomized controlled study of mineral trioxide aggregate and super ethoxy-benzoic acid as root-end filling materials in endodontic microsurgery.* J Endod. 2012;38:875-879.

52. Song M, Nam T, Shin S, Kim E. *Comparison of clinical outcomes of endodontic microsurgery: 1 year versus long-term follow-up.* J Endod. 2014;40:490-494.

53. Rubinstein R, Fayad MI. *Apical microsurgery: application of armamentaria, materials, and methods.* In: Torabinejad M, Rubinstein R, eds. *The art and science of contemporary surgical endodontics.* Surrey: Quintessence Publishing Co Inc; 2017:155-178.

54. Lin L, Chen MY-H, Ricucci D, Rosenberg PA. *Guided tissue regeneration in periapical surgery.* J Endod. 2010;36(4):618-625.

55. Guided tissue regeneration, periodontal. *Available at: http://www.symptomstoday. com/medical/guided_tissue_regeneration_periodontal.htm. Accessed March 2010.*

56. Saad AY, Abdellatief EM. *Healing assessment of osseous defects of periapical lesions associated with failed endodontically treated teeth with use of freezedried bone allograft.* Oral Surg Oral Med Oral Pathol. 1991;71:612-617.

57. Pinto VS, Zuolo ML, Mellonig JT. *Guided bone regeneration in the treatment of a large periapical lesion: a case report.* Pract Periodontic Aesthe Dent. 1995;7: 76-82.

58. Taschieri S, Del Fabbro M, Testori T, Saita M, Weinstein R. *Efficacy of guided tissue regeneration in the management of through-and through lesions following surgical endodontics: a preliminary study.* Int J Periodontics Restorative Dentistry. 2008;28: 265-271.

59. Apaydin ES, Torabinejad M. *The effect of calcium sulfate on hard-tissue healing after periapical surgery.* J Endod. 2004;30:17-20.

60. Beck-Coon RJ, Newton CW, Kafrawy AH. *An in vivo study of the use of a nonresorbable ceramic hydroxyapatite as an alloplastic graft material in periapical surgery.* Oral Surg Oral Med Oral Pathol. 1991;71:483-488.

61. Yoshikawa G, Murashima Y, Wadachi R, Sawada N, Suda H. *Guided bone regeneration (GBR) using membrane and calcium sulfate after apicectomy: a comparative histomorphometrical study.* Int Endod J. 2002;35:255-263.

62. Langer R, Vacanti JP. *Tissue engineering.* Science 1993;260:920-6.

63. Ivanovski S, Gronthos S, Shi S, Bartold PM. *Stem cells in the periodontal ligament.* Oral Disease. 2006;12:358-63.

64. Dahlin C, Linde A, Gottlow J, Nyman S. *Healing of bone defects by guided tissue regeneration.* Plast Reconstr Surg. 1988;81:672-676.

65. Dahlin C, Gottlow J, Linde A, Nyman S. *Healing of maxillary and mandibular bone defects using a membrane technique: an experimental study in monkeys.* Scand J Plast Reconstr Hand Surg. 1990;24:13-19.

66. Andreasen JO, Rud J. *Modes of healing histologically after endodontic surgery in 70 cases.* Int Oral Surg. 1972;1:148-160.

67. Bohning BP, Davenport WD, Jeansonne BJ. *The effect of guided tissue regeneration on the healing of osseous defects in rat calvaria.* J Endod. 1999;25:81-84.

68. Garrett K, Kerr M, Hartwell G, O'Sullivan S, Mayer P. *The effect of a bioresorbable matrix barrier in endodontic surgery on the rate of periapical healing: an in vivo study.* J Endod. 2002;28:503-506.

69. **Britain SK, von Arx T, Schenk RK, et al.** *The use of guided tissue regeneration principles in endodontic surgery for induced chronic periodontic-endodontic lesions: a clinical, radiographic and histological evaluation.* J Periodontol. 2005;76: 450-460.

70. **Rankow HJ, Krasner PR.** *Endodontic applications of guided tissue regeneration in endodontic surgery.* J Endod. 1996;22:34-43.

71. **Pompa DG.** *Guided tissue repair of complete buccal dehiscences associated with periapical defects: a clinical retrospective study.* J Am Dent Assoc. 1997;128: 989-997.

72. **Cotran RS, Kumar V, Collins T.** *Robbin's pathologic basis of disease.* 6th ed. Philadelphia: WB Saunders; 1999.

73. **Majno G, Joris I.** *Cell, tissue, and disease.* 2nd ed. Oxford: Oxford University Press; 2004.

74. **Laurell L, Gottlow J.** *Guided tissue regeneration update.* Int Dent J. 1998;48: 386-398.

75. **Pecora G, Andreana S, Margarone JE, Covani U, Sottosanti JS.** *Bone regeneration with a calcium sulfate barrier.* Oral Surg Oral Med Oral Pathol Oral Radiol Endod. 1997;84:424-429.

76. **Pecora G, Leonardis De, Ibrahim N, Bovi M, Cormelini R.** *The use of calcium sulfate in the surgical treatment of a "through and through" periradicular lesion.* Int Endod J. 2001;34:189-197.

77. **Taschieri S, Del Fabbro M, Testori T, Weinstein R.** *Efficacy of xenogenic bone grafting with guided tissue regeneration in the management of bone defects after surgical endodontics.* J Oral Maxillofac Surg. 2007;65:1121-1127.

78. **Tobon SI, Arismendi JA, Marin ML, Mesa AL, Valencia JA.** *Comparison between a conventional technique and two bone regeneration techniques in periradicular surgery.* Int Endod J. 2002;35:635-641.

79. **Demiralp B, Kecali HG, Muhtarogullari M, Serperr A, Demiralp B, Eratalay K.** *Treatment of periapical inflammatory lesion with the combination of platelet-rich plasma and tricalcium phosphate: a case report.* J Endod. 2004;30: 796-800.

80. **Stassen LFA, Hislop WS, Still DM, Moos KF.** *Use of anorganic bone in periapical defcts following apical surgery: a prospective trial.* Br J Oral Maxillofacial Surg. 1994;32:83-85.

81. **Nair PNR.** *Pathogenesis of apical periodontitis and the causes of endodontic failures.* Crit Rev Oral Biol Med. 2004;15:348-381.

82. **Andreasen JO, Rud J, Munksgaard EC.** *Retrograde filling with resin and a dentin bonding agent: preliminary histologic study of tissue reactions in monkeys.* Danish Dent J. 1989;93:195-197.

83. **Andreasen JO, Munksgaard EC, Fredebo L, Rud J.** *Periodontal tissue regeneration including cemtogenesis adjacent to dentin-bonded retrograde composit fillings in humans.* J Endod. 1993;19:151-153.

84. **Apaydin ES, Shabahang S, Torabinejad M.** *Hard-tissue healing after application of fresh or set MTA as root-end-filling material.* J Endod. 2004;30:21-24.

85. **Baek S-H, Plenk H, Kim S.** *Periapical tissue responses and cementum regeneration with amalgam, Super EBA, and MTA as root-end filling materials.* J Endod. 2005;31: 444-449.

86. **Tanomaru-Filho M, Luis MR, Leonardo MR, Tanomaru JMG, Silva LAB.** *Evaluation of periapical repair following retrograde filling with different root-end filling materials in dog teeth with periapical lesions.* Oral Surg Oral Med Oral Pathol Oral Radiol Endod. 2006;102:127-132.

87. **Tsesis I, Faivishevsky V, Kfir A, Rosen E.** *Outcome of surgical endodontic treatment performed by a modern technique: a mets-analysis of literature.* J Endod. 2009;35: 1505-1511.

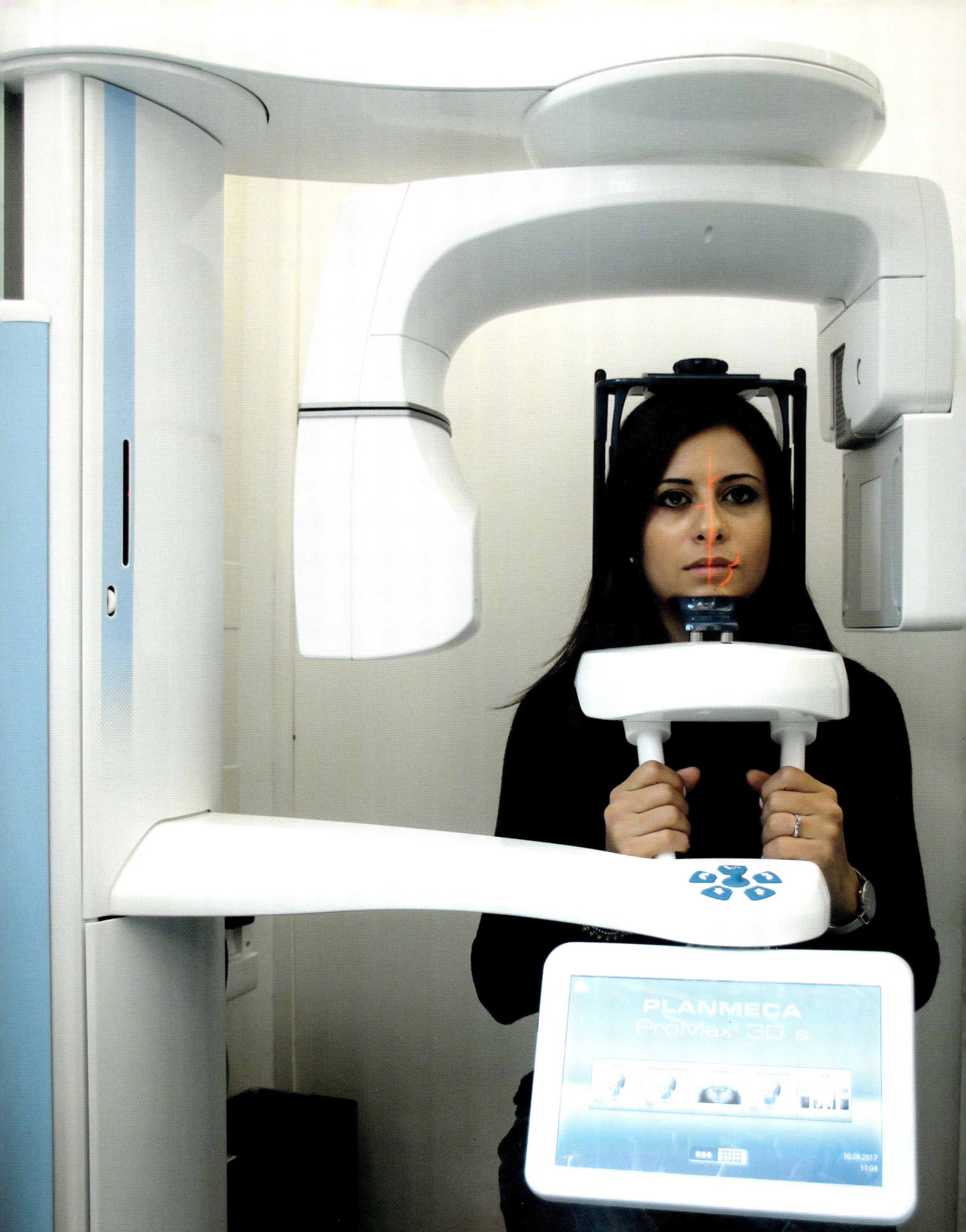
PLANMECA
ProMax® 3D s
30.09.2017
11:04

The Use of Cone Beam Computed Tomography (CBCT) in Microsurgical Endodontics

Arnaldo Castellucci, MD, DDS,
Massimo Gagliani, MD, DDS, *Fabio Gorni*, MD, DDS

In no other branch of dentistry does radiology play such an important role as in endodontics.

The discovery of X-rays by Wilhelm Conrad Roentgen in 1895 had such a profound impact on the entire medical world that it has come to be considered one of the most revolutionary achievements in the history of medical science.

In the field of dentistry, endodontics is surely the branch that has benefited most from this discovery, not only because of continual technical and technological improvements,[1] but mainly because the use of X-rays has brought dentists "out of the dark", allowing them to visualize areas not accessible by other diagnostic means.

Before this development dentists could only attempt, with greater or lesser success, to reach a diagnosis and implement a therapeutic approach to endodontic problems.

The advent of the first oral radiography equipment permitted visualization for the first time of the changes that occur in the bone surrounding the apices of nonvital teeth, as well as the results of endodontic therapy.

In this way, endodontics ceased to be simply an empirical pursuit; from that moment on, it became a scientific discipline.[2]

Today, the X-ray machine must be considered as an integral part of the dental equipment, especially in endodontic practice. Having to work on the root canals of a patient without the help of this essential diagnostic apparatus is inconceivable.

However, the radiograph is a two-dimensional representation of three-dimensional structures and objects. To extract three-dimensional information, it is necessary to take several off-angle X-rays along the horizontal plane, applying the "buccal object rule"

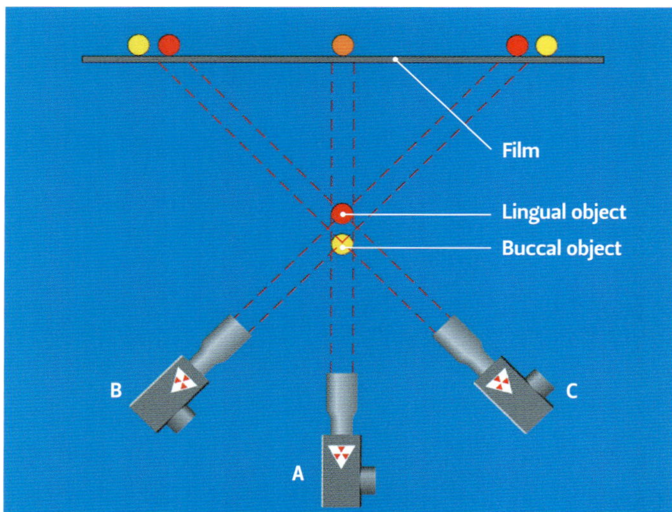

13.1 The Buccal Object Rule. The only method that allows one to visualize the third dimension in a bi-dimensional radiograph. With an orthoradial projection **(a)**, the two objects appear superimposed. With an oblique projection **(b, c)**, the two objects cease to be superimposed and become easily recognizable when the angulation of the X-ray machine is known: the buccal object (the one closest to the radiographic source) is displaced in the same direction as the X-rays.

(13.1),[3] but this is not enough. The traditional bi-dimensional radiographs have several limitations.

First of all, they are interpreted and not read, as was demonstrated by Goldman et al.[4,5] in 1972 and 1974. They found that when evaluating healing in periapical lesions using periapical radiographs, there was a low level of agreement between six examiners (47%) even when the same examiners evaluated the same films at two different moments in time (19-80% respectively).

Another limitation is represented by the size of the lesion. The detection rate depends on the percentage of mineralized tissue loss in comparison with the total amount of surrounding bone, which in turn depends on its density and thickness.[6,7] The visibility of the lesion also depends on the location of the defect.[8-10] Bender & Seltzer[6,11] and more recently Patel and Durak[12] demonstrated that periapical lesions confined to the cancellous bone without any considerable demineralization of the cortical plate are not easily visualized in radiographs (13.2). They concluded that better visualization occurred when the cortical bone plate became eroded.

Another concern that has been listed by Patel et. al.[13] is anatomic noise. The superimposition of overlying anatomy or the density of the cortical bone may also blur the area of interest, consequently reducing it in contrast, simulating radiolucencies or hiding existing radiolucencies (13.3), with the result that the radiographic image becomes more difficult to interpret.[13] These anatomical interferences can vary in radiodensity and are referred to as anatomical noise.[14]

Finally, geometric distortion and image reproducibility are other drawbacks of traditional radiology. In clinical practice, the so-called "long cone and paralleling technique" should be performed with the film or sensor placed as parallel as possible to the tooth and perpendicular to the radiographic beam to produce geometrically accurate images.[14-16] Factors such as the inclination of the alveolar process, the patient's compliance, a particularly unfavorable shape of the oral cavity, etc. may impair its impeccable execution with consequent elongation or image foreshortening.[17,18] Furthermore, pretreatment, post-treatment and follow-up radiographs should be standardized representing a snapshot in time of the area of interest.[19] Although customized stents have been largely used to reduce the risk of under- or over-estimation of the degree of healing, serial radiographs might still show several inconsistencies. In studies that investigated the implementation of quality assurance requirements, 8.5% of the images were classified as distorted, elongated or foreshortened.[13,20] Cone beam computed tomography has demonstrated an ability to overcome all of the above-mentioned limitations of traditional X-rays.

Basic Principles of CBCT

The method of obtaining the patient's data volume in CBCT differs significantly from that of conventional medical computed tomography (CT). In medical CT scanning (previously termed CAT: Computed Axial Tomography), the patient's region of interest, such as the head or other body part, is selected. As the X-ray source rotates around the region of interest 60 times per minute, multiple sensors detect the X-ray beam. This type of image acquisition is very precise, but the data acquired is voluminous, and the patient absorbs a very

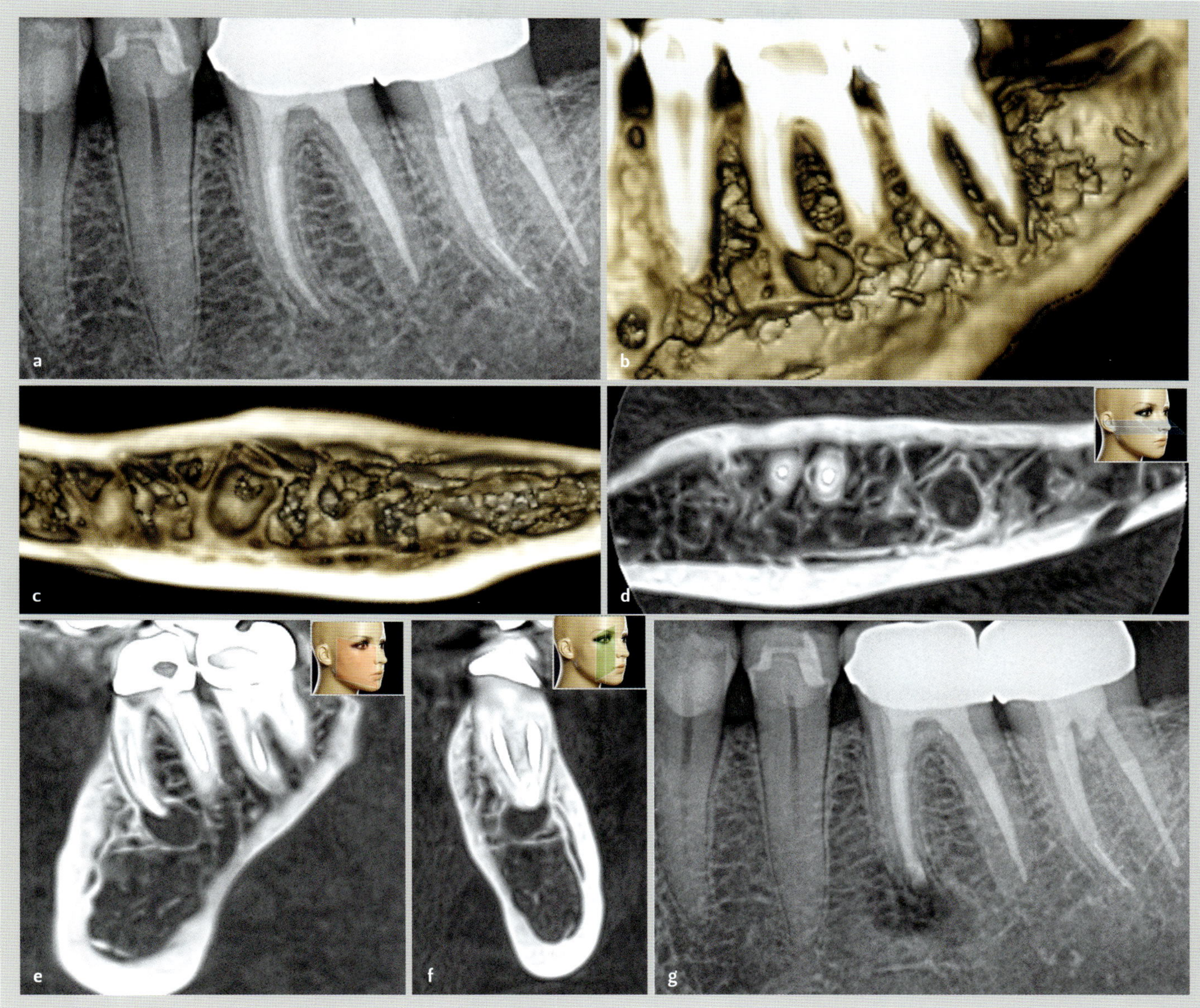

13.2 **a)** Preoperative radiograph of the lower left first molar. A small radiolucency seems to be present at the apex of the mesial root. **b)** 3D CBCT rendering demonstrating a round lesion at the apex of the mesial root. **c, d)** 3D CBCT rendering and CBCT axial view showing that the lesion did not involve the cortical bone, and this is the reason why the lesion was not easily recognizable in the periapical radiograph. **e)** CBCT sagittal view. **f)** CBCT coronal view. **g)** Postoperative radiograph.

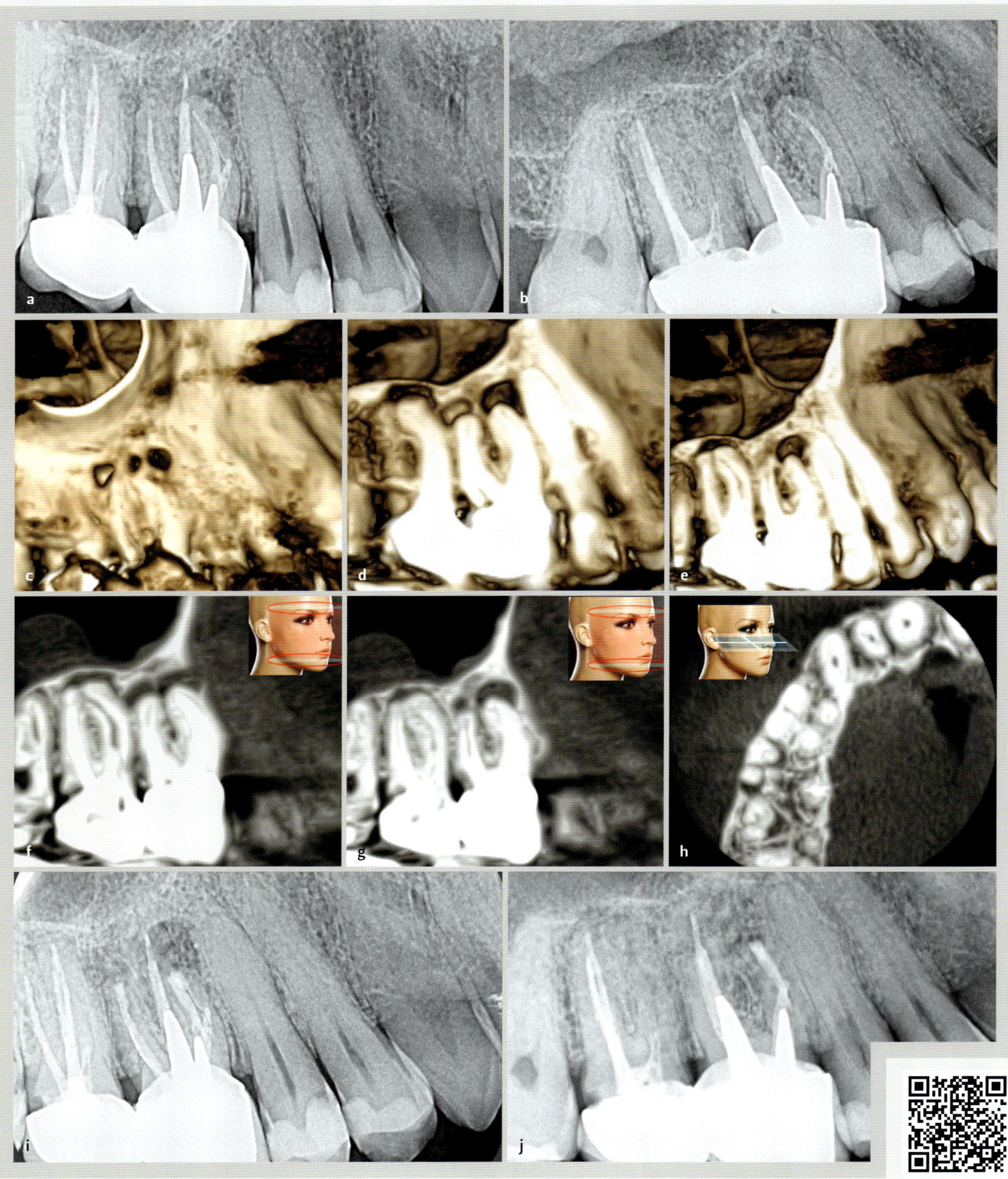
a
b
c
d
e
f
g
h
i
j

large dose of radiation.[21] A typical CT scan for a maxillary implant site assessment may have a radiation dose as high as 2100 mSV, equivalent to the dose from about 375 panoramic film or digital images.[22] Compared with medical CT, CBCT doses are between 76.2% and 98.5% lower, at around 40 to 500 mSV.[22]

Unlike conventional CT, CBCT uses a narrow cone-shaped beam which rotates 360° around the patient (13.4).

CBCT is accomplished by using a rotating platform to which an X-ray source and detector are fixed. A cone-shaped source of ionizing radiation is directed through the middle of the region of interest, and the transmitted, attenuated radiation is projected onto an area of an X-ray detector on the opposite side. The X-ray source and detector rotate around a fixed fulcrum within the region of interest. During the exposure sequence, hundreds of planar projection images are acquired of the field of view (FOV) in an arc of at least 180°. The projection images are then integrated by software to construct an image volume. In this single rotation, the CBCT provides precise, essentially immediate and accurate three-dimensional radiographic images.[23] The resulting information is digitally reconstructed and interpreted to create an interface whereby the clinician can three-dimensionally interpret "slices" of the patient's tissues in a multitude of planes: axial, sagittal and coronal (13.5).

The **axial** plane allows the clinician to evaluate the volume in a coronal to apical direction. This plane allows for visualization of perforations, expansion of cortical plates, the number of root canals present inside a root, etc.

The **coronal** plane runs from mesial to distal or from anterior to posterior. This plane illustrates the relationships between roots and the maxillary sinus, as well as the thickness of palatal/lingual buccal cortical plates.

The **sagittal** plane runs from lateral to medial or from buccal to palatal/lingual planes. This plane is useful to examine anterior teeth.

← **13.3** **a)** Preoperative radiograph of the upper right first molar. The patient was referred for surgical therapy of the mesiobuccal root of the upper right first molar. **b)** An off-angle radiograph appears to confirm that the only root involved with the periapical lesion is the mesiobuccal root. **c)** The CBCT is showing that the cortical bone adjacent to the distobuccal root has been resorbed. **d, e)** Another periapical lesion involves the second molar. **f, g)** The sagittal view better shows the upper first molar lesions on both buccal roots, and the lesions at the apices of both roots of the second molar, whose MB1 appears completely empty. **h)** The axial view shows the lesions of the first and second molars, involving the palatal aspect of the two roots. It is now obvious why these lesions were not visible in the periapical radiograph. **i)** Postoperative radiograph. **j)** Two-year recall.

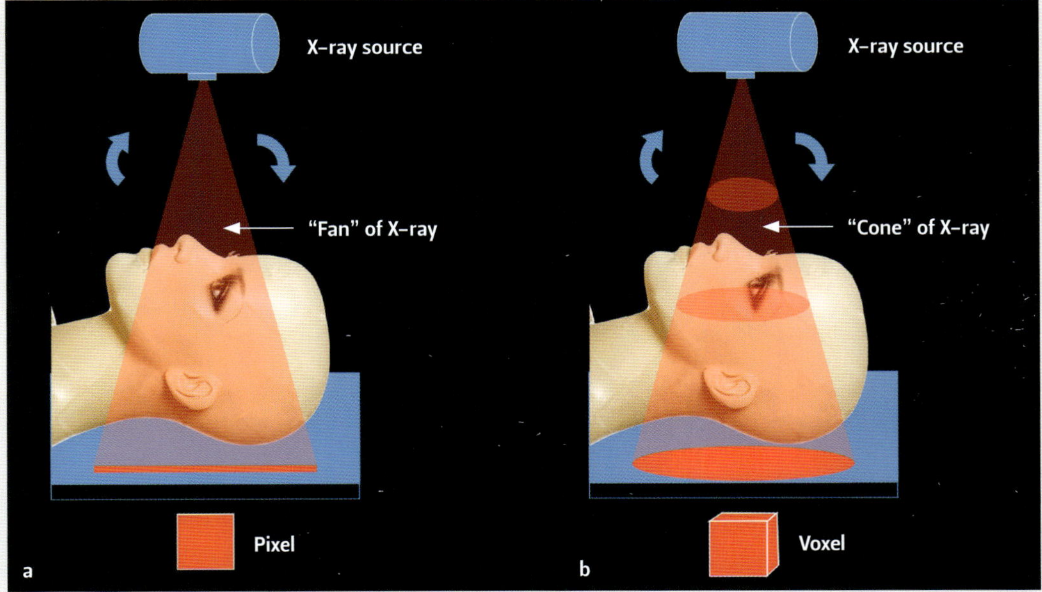

13.4 **a)** Traditional medical CT detector equipment with the X-ray source that rotates 360° around the patient about 60 times per minute. The thickness of each image slice is determined by the distance (usually between 1 and 100 mm) that the patient is moved through the gantry. This exposes the patient to a large dose of X-rays. The digital image is displayed on the computer in "pixels" to represent a 2D image. **b)** A cone beam device, using the cone-shaped beam, rotates around the patient. The exposure factors are similar to those used for exposing traditional dental radiographs, so the X-ray dose to which the patient is exposed is substantially reduced. The digital image is displayed on the computer in "voxels" to represent a 3D image.

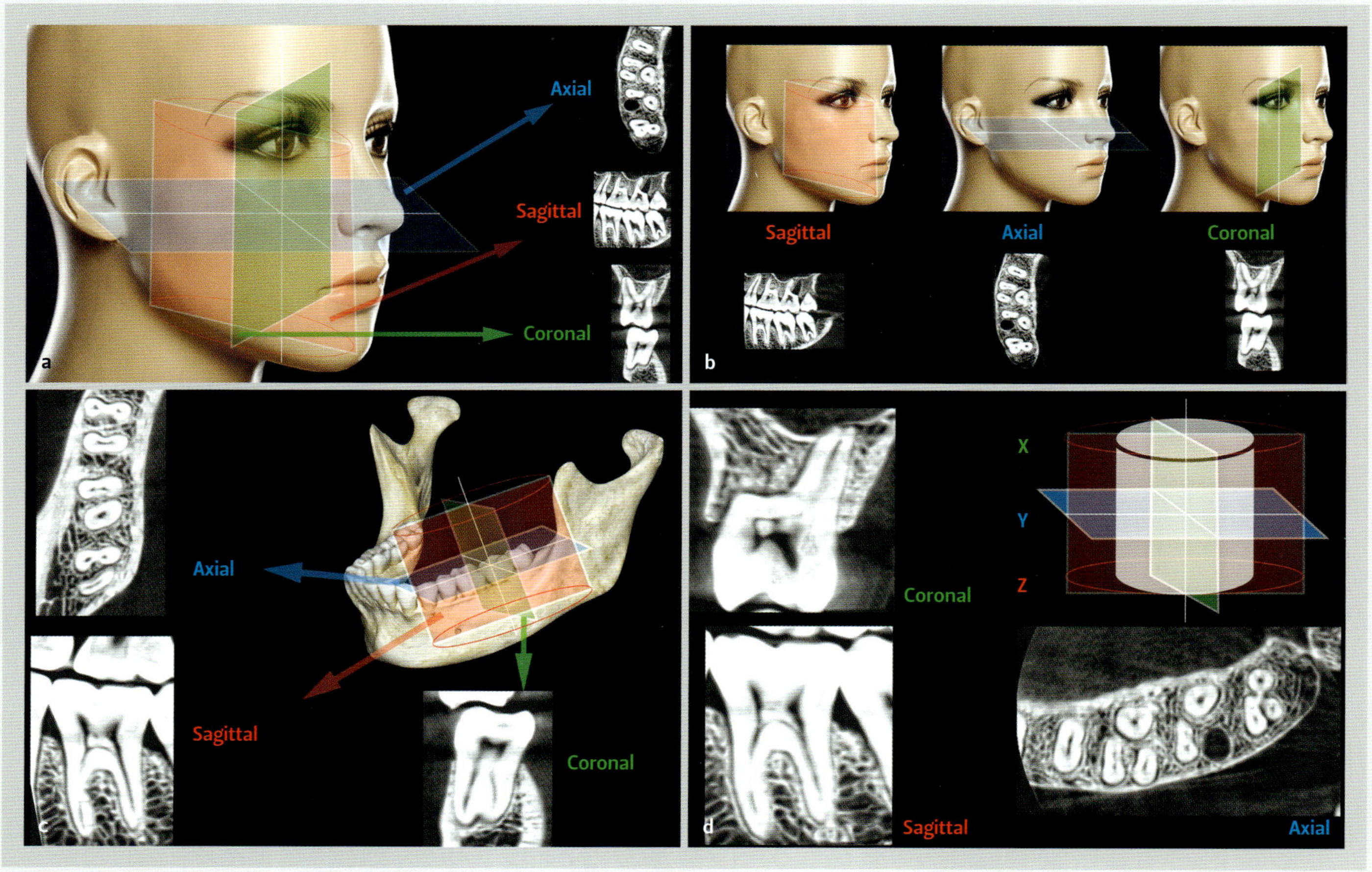

13.5 a–d) The CBCT allows the capture, storage and presentation of radiographic images in various horizontal and vertical planes: axial, sagittal, coronal.

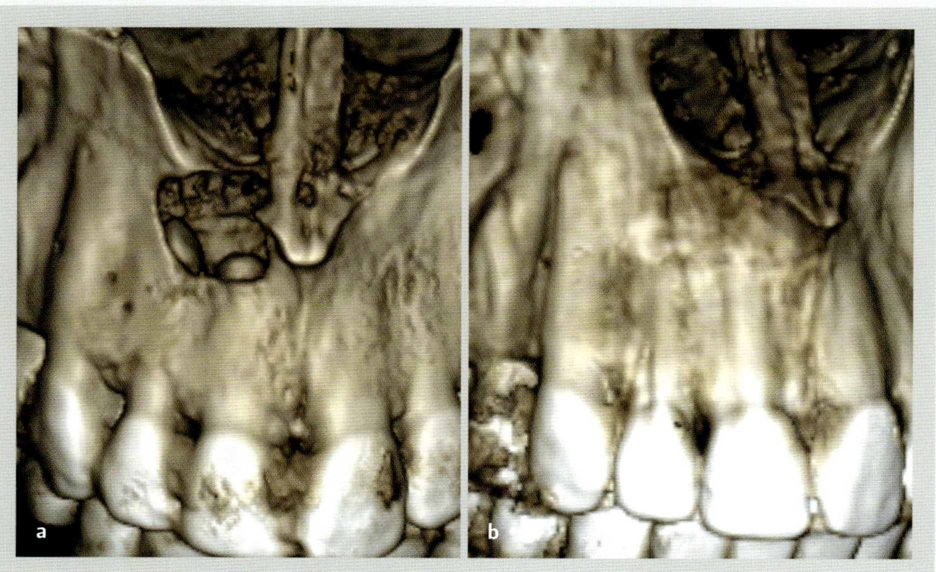

13.6 a) 3D CBCT rendering demonstrating a large lesion involving the upper right central and lateral incisors. **b)** One-year recall.

Volume-rendering reconstructions are also possible, and they are important in order to visualize anatomical structures more effectively (13.6).[24] CBCT is a simple, valuable, reproducible, reliable, relatively economical and task-specific imaging modality exposing the patient to a relatively low radiation dose and providing the maximum amount of information to the clinician, when performed with the right equipment and acquisition protocols. Dentists and dental specialists continue to be amazed at the incredibly precise and profound information produced by CBCT scans, and they realize that the data they receive will influence their treatment decisions like no other imaging modality used in the profession in the past 100 years. CBCT makes clinical decision making easier and more precise, patient treatment decisions more accurate, and visualization of the X-ray data more meaningful. Dentistry is moving away from "radiographic interpretation" and into "disease visualization".[21]

Indications

The use of CBCT finds its best indications in both non-surgical and surgical retreatments.

In 2003, Rigolone et al.[25] proposed the use of low-dose cone beam tomography to verify the surgical access to the palatal root before microsurgical endodontics. Since then, preoperative CBCT has been used widely. It provides an enormous amount of information, even when compared to more innovative digital periapical radiographies[26,27] and it is a fundamental guide in the decision-making process,[28-30] preparation and execution of the surgical procedure.

Rodriguez et al.[31] reported that CBCT imaging had a substantial impact on endodontic decision making even among specialists, particularly in high difficulty cases, leading to a less conservative approach to these cases. These were particularly stressed when general practitioners were involved in the study.[32]

It is possible to detect small lesions not visible on the traditional X-ray, to know in advance if there is a bony fenestration (2.46, 2.47), and the thickness of the cortical bone.[33-35] In situations where patients have poorly localized symptoms associated with an untreated or previously root-filled tooth, and clinical and periapical X-rays show no evidence of disease, CBCT may be indicated to detect the presence of previously undiagnosed periapical disease (13.7).[36]

In addition, CBCT seems a more reproducible examination, not influenced by evaluator's experience and knowledge.[37,38] All these features will be further improved by new software recently included in viewing programs.[39]

In conclusion, it is recognized that CBCT analysis provides a huge amount of information about the identification of important landmarks to be evaluated before the surgical procedure (13.1).

As reported in 13.1, it is quite easy to separate anatomical features related to tooth position in the upper and lower jaw and tooth characteristics such as abnormal root anatomies, infrequent root canal composition, iatrogenic root perforations, root fractures, and root internal and external resorptions.

All these last pathologies might lead to a surgical intervention but are out of the remit of this book; however, we can say that CBCT analysis may clearly disclose internal and external root resorptions with a higher level of accuracy when compared with traditional X-ray analyses.[40-42]

Some concern about the reliability of CBCT analysis in identifying vertical root fractures has been raised

13.1 Anatomical features to be evaluated before endodontic surgery intervention

· Mandibular canal	(13.8)
· Mental nerve	(13.9, 13.10)
· Maxillary sinus	(13.11)
· Adjacent vital teeth	(6.12)
· Tooth anatomy	(13.12)
· Tooth (root canal) perforations	(13.13)
· Tooth fractures	(13.14)
· Tooth internal or external resorption	(13.15, 13.16)

Cont'd on page 250

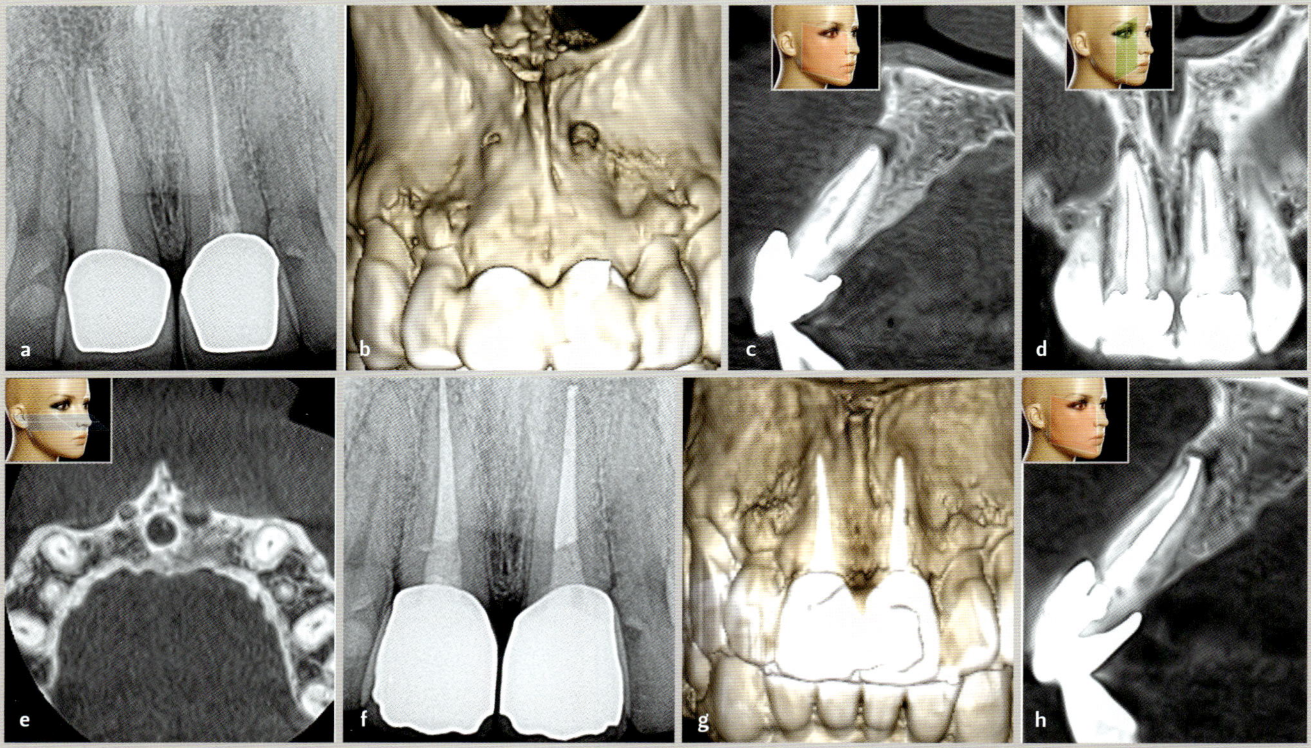

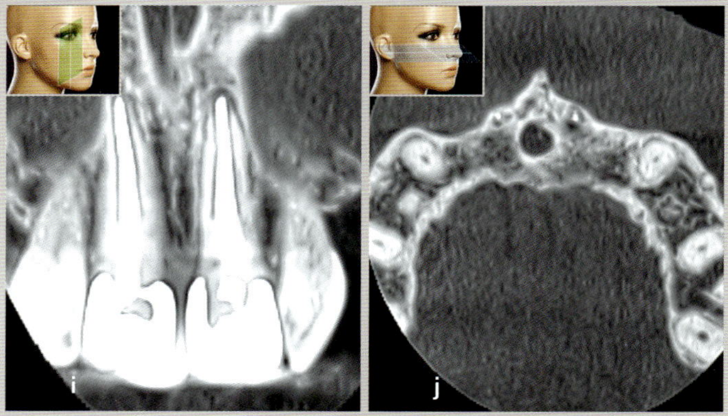

13.7 **a)** Preoperative radiograph of the two central incisors. Two small periapical lesions are quite difficult to recognize. **b)** 3D CBCT rendering demonstrating both lesions. **c)** CBCT sagittal view confirming the lesion of the upper left central incisor, involving the cortical bone. **d)** CBCT coronal view. **e)** CBCT axial view. **f)** Eight-month recall after nonsurgical retreatment. **g)** 3D CBCT rendering demonstrating the healing of the cortical bone. **h)** CBCT sagittal view. **i)** CBCT coronal view. **j)** CBCT axial view.

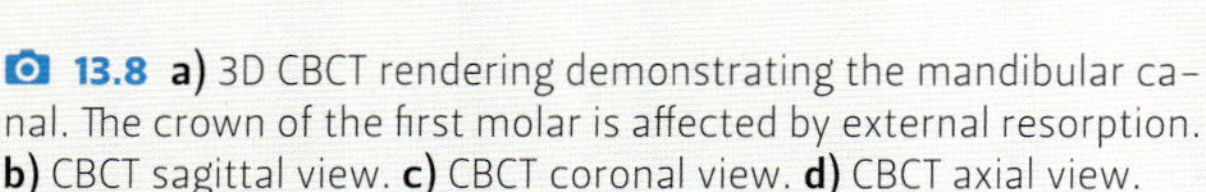

13.8 **a)** 3D CBCT rendering demonstrating the mandibular canal. The crown of the first molar is affected by external resorption. **b)** CBCT sagittal view. **c)** CBCT coronal view. **d)** CBCT axial view.

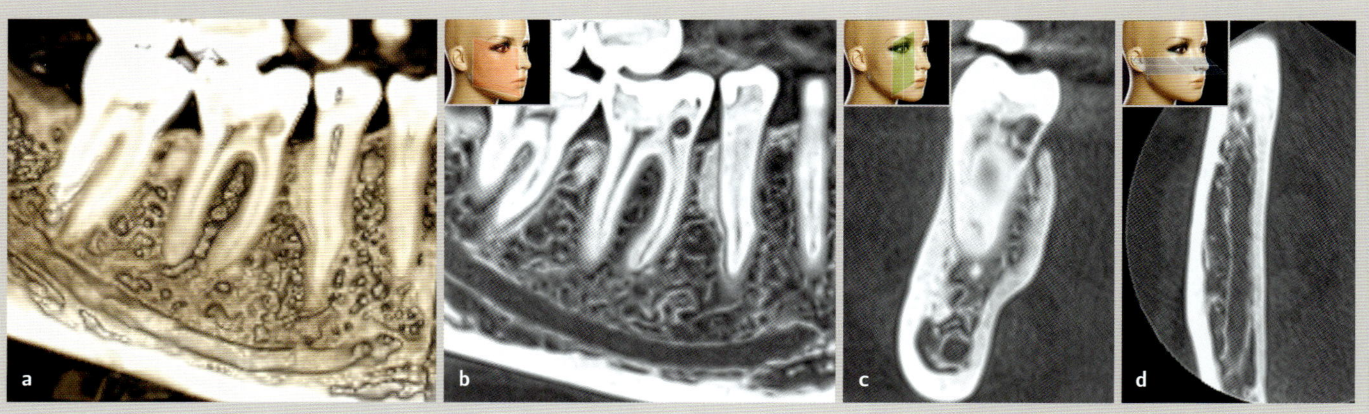

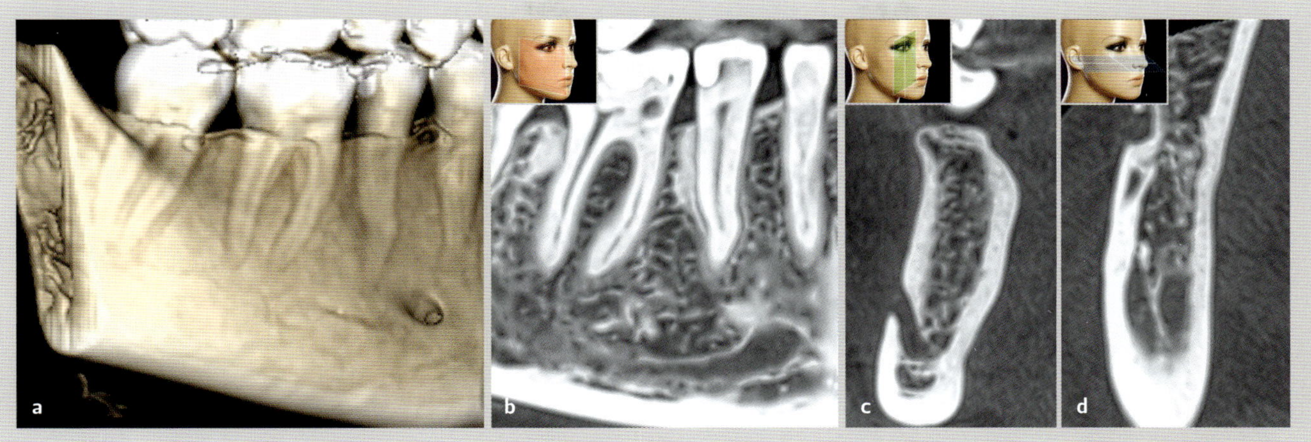

13.9 **a)** 3D CBCT rendering demonstrating the mental foramen. **b)** CBCT sagittal view. **c)** CBCT coronal view. **d)** CBCT axial view.

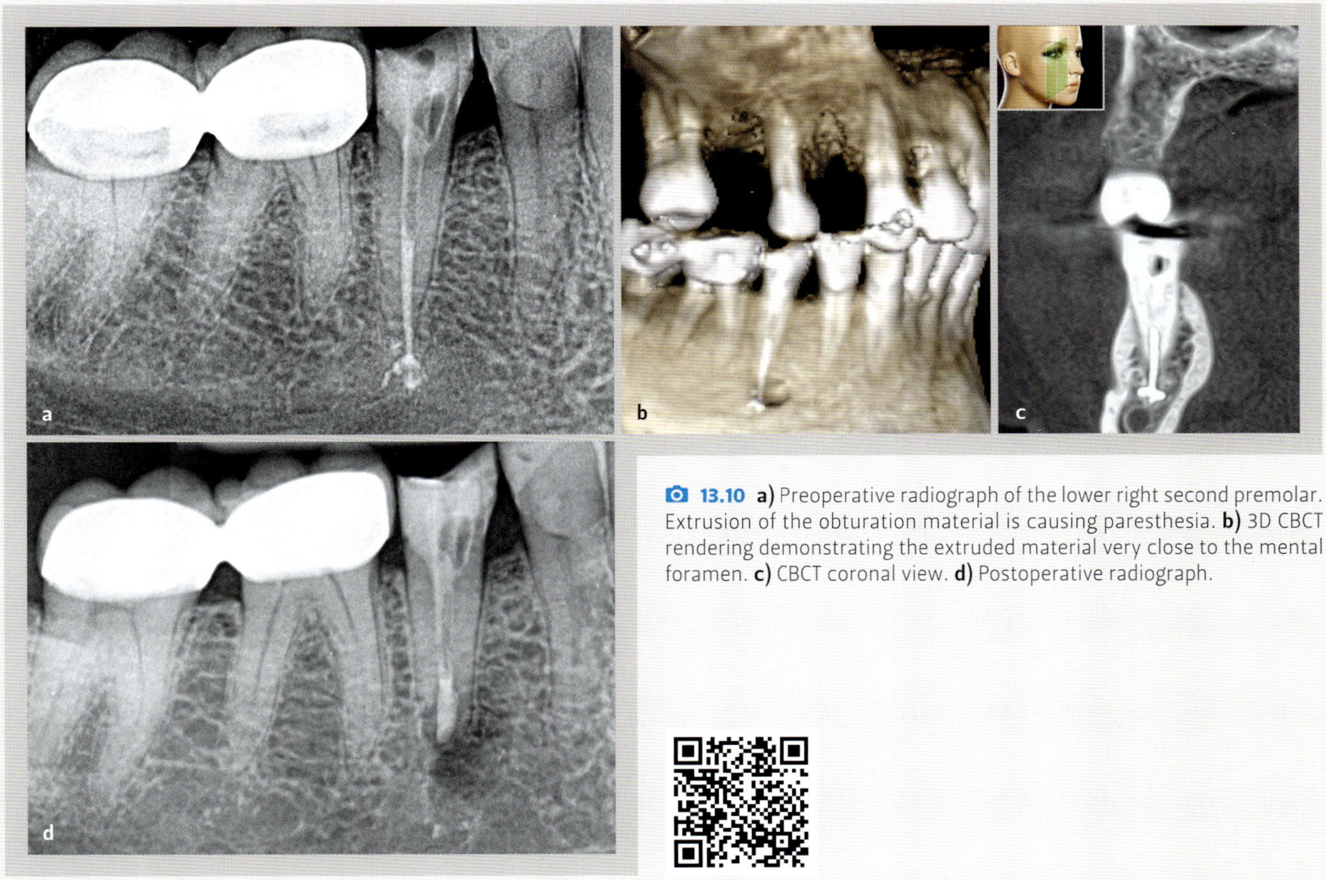

13.10 **a)** Preoperative radiograph of the lower right second premolar. Extrusion of the obturation material is causing paresthesia. **b)** 3D CBCT rendering demonstrating the extruded material very close to the mental foramen. **c)** CBCT coronal view. **d)** Postoperative radiograph.

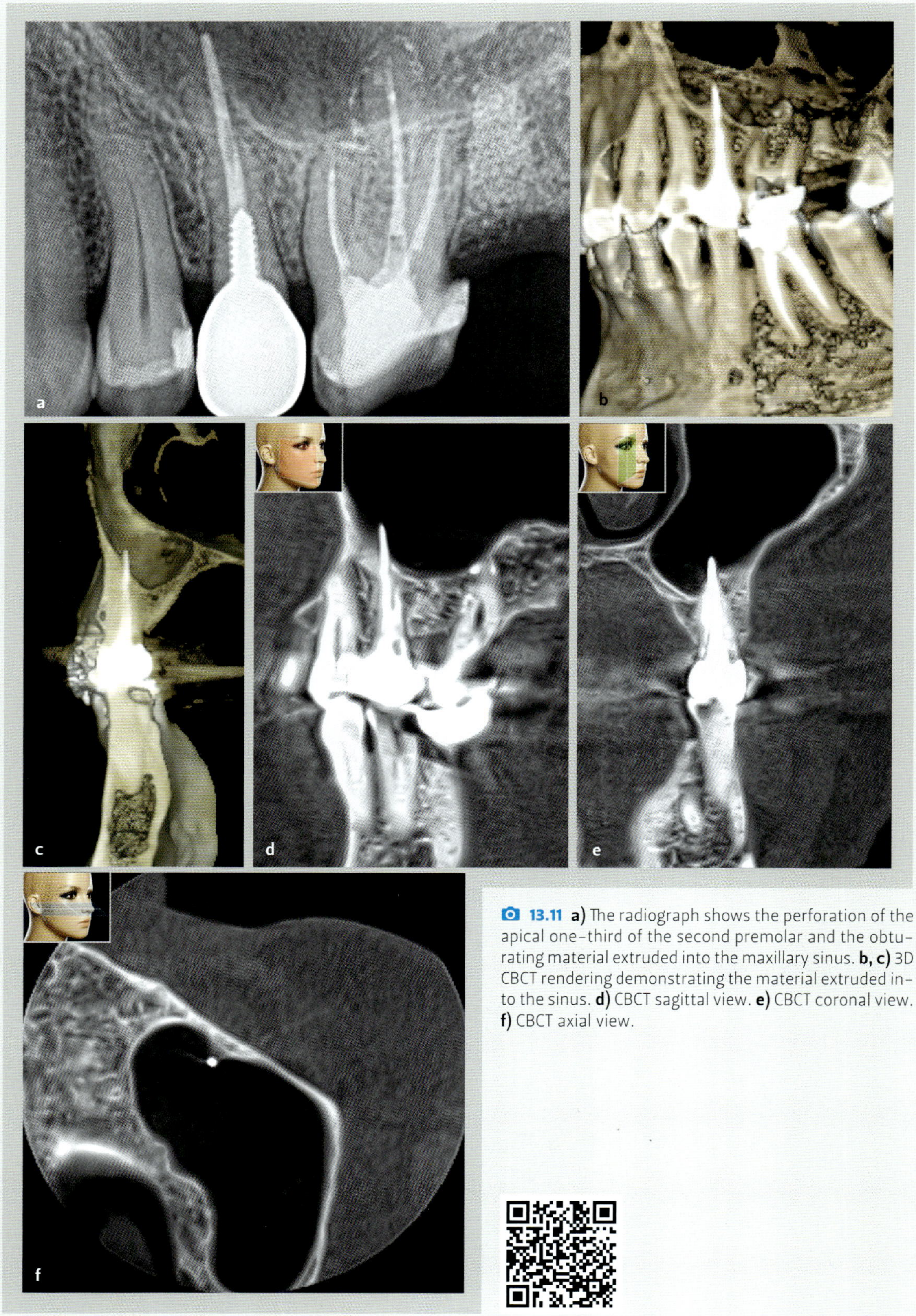

13.11 **a)** The radiograph shows the perforation of the apical one-third of the second premolar and the obturating material extruded into the maxillary sinus. **b, c)** 3D CBCT rendering demonstrating the material extruded into the sinus. **d)** CBCT sagittal view. **e)** CBCT coronal view. **f)** CBCT axial view.

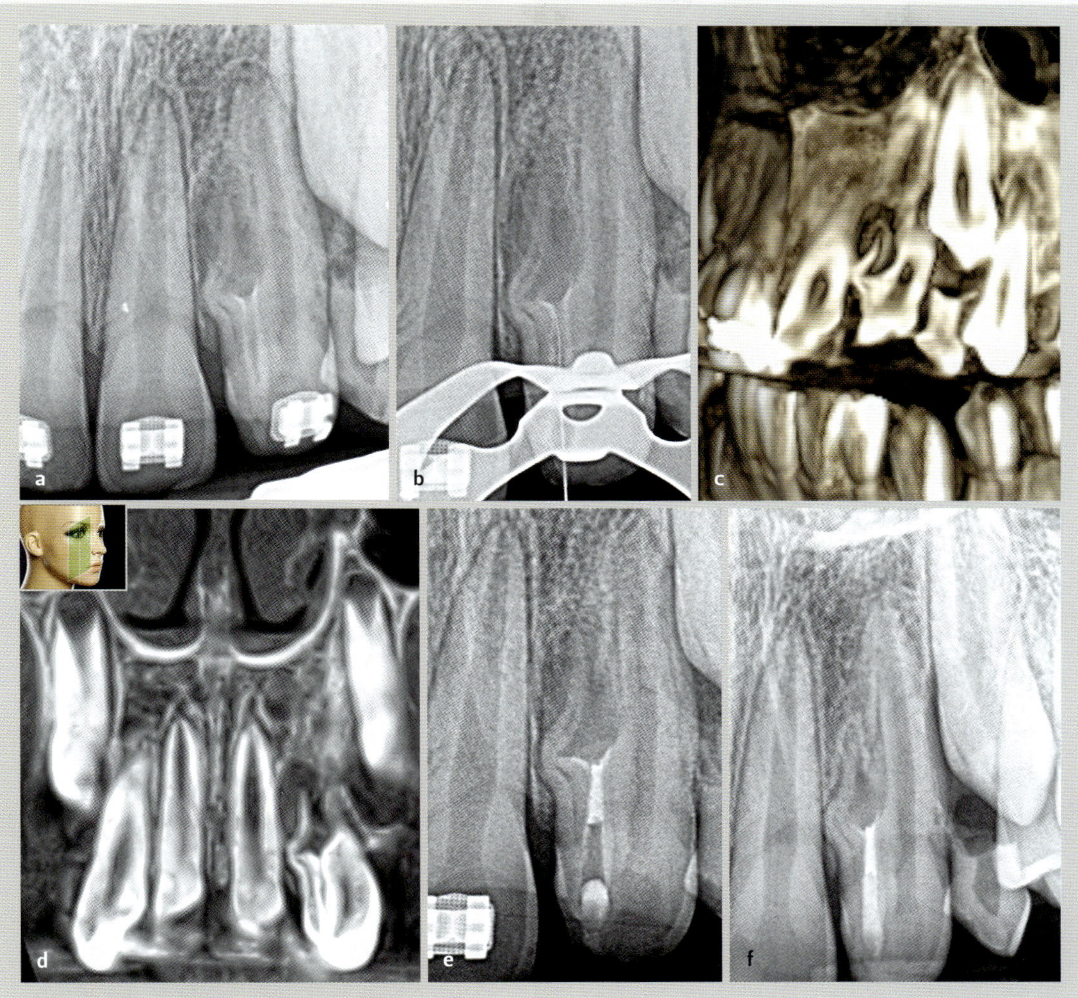

13.12 **a)** The upper left lateral incisor is a dens invaginatus. **b)** Intraoperative radiograph. **c)** 3D CBCT rendering demonstrating the unusual anatomy and the lesion. **d)** CBCT coronal view. **e)** Postoperative radiograph. **f)** One-year recall.

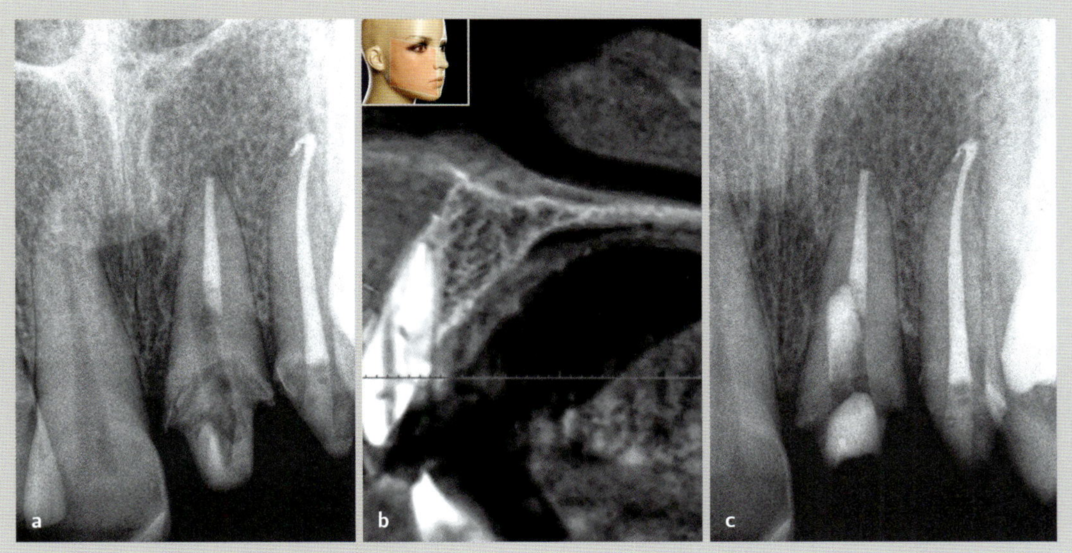

13.13 **a)** Preoperative radiograph of the upper left central incisor. A carbon fiber post has been cemented in the wrong position. **b)** CBCT sagittal view demonstrating the buccal perforation. **c)** The perforation was sealed with white MTA.

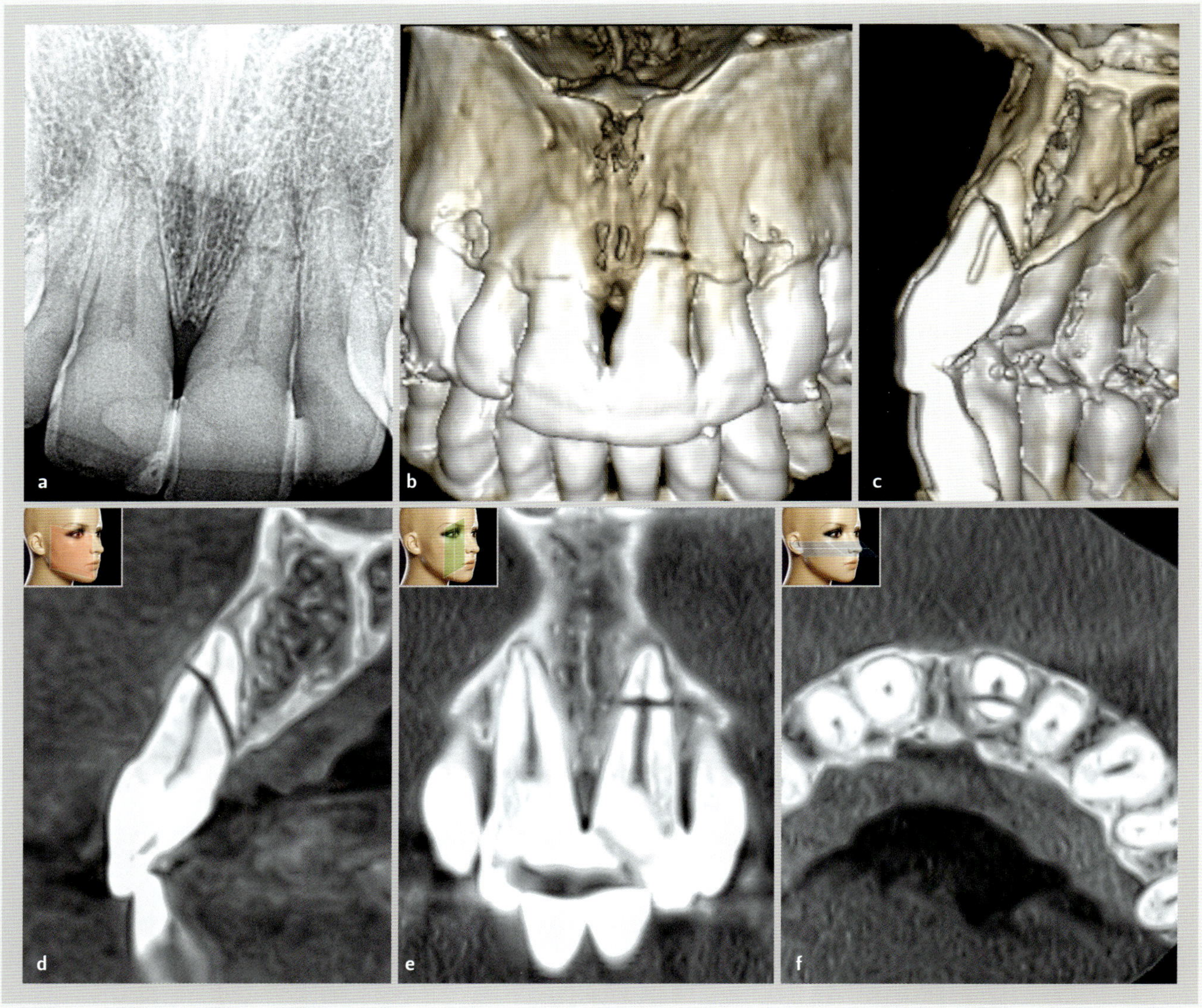

13.14 **a)** Preoperative radiograph of the upper left central incisor. The patient has a horizontal root fracture due to a car accident. **b, c)** 3D CBCT rendering demonstrating the horizontal root fracture. **d)** CBCT sagittal view. **e)** CBCT coronal view. **f)** CBCT axial view.

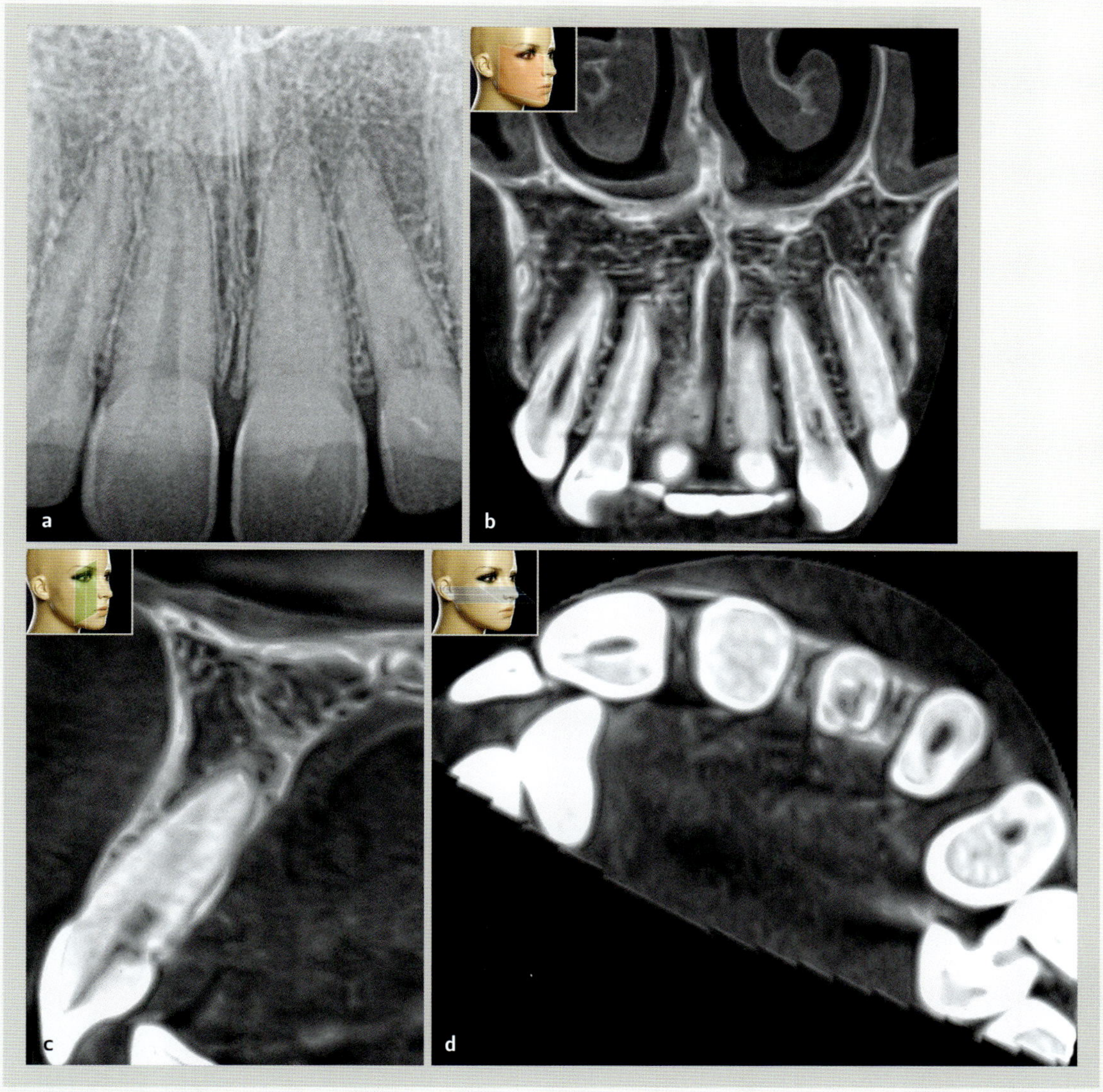

13.15 **a)** The upper left lateral incisor has external resorption. **b)** CBCT coronal view. **c)**. CBCT sagittal view demonstrating the defect starting from the palatal cervical area. **d)** CBCT axial view.

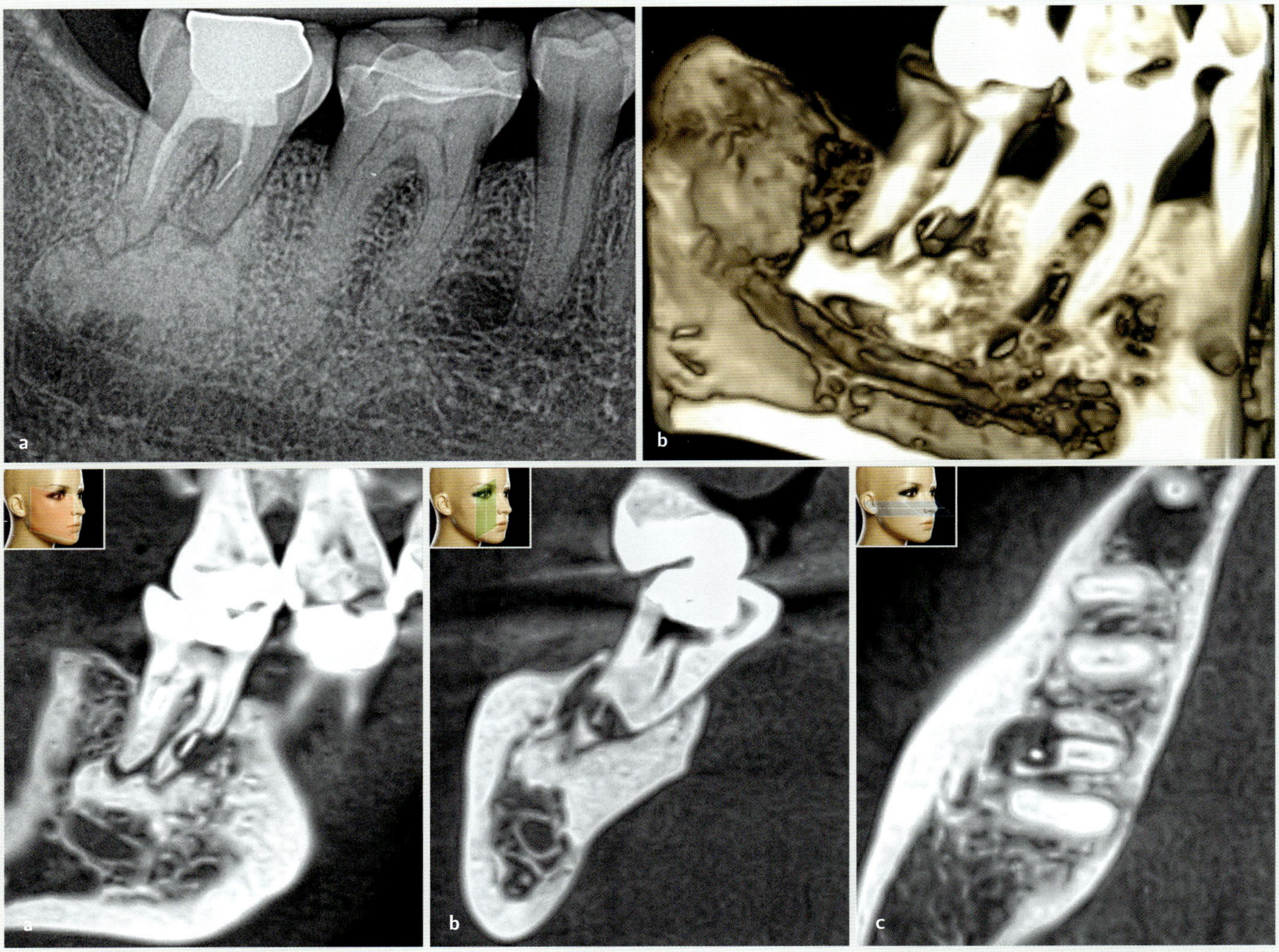

13.16 **a)** Preoperative radiograph of the lower right second molar. A broken instrument is present in the mesial root. **b)** 3D CBCT rendering demonstrating the broken instrument inside an area of root resorption. **c)** CBCT sagittal view. **d)** CBCT coronal view. **e)** CBCT axial view.

Cont'd from page 243

by Costa et al.[43,44] when intracanal posts were inserted. It might be due to the type of CBCT used and the large field of view (FOV) utilized. In other studies,[45–48] the accuracy of the 3D X-ray examination has been assessed, and a substantial agreement over its efficacy in detecting not only vertical root fracture, but also horizontal ones, has been achieved. Similar results were reported when diagnosing a perforation before performing any type of root canal treatment or microsurgical endodontics.[49]

Root anatomies and canal abnormalities

CBCT may detect root canal anatomies that are peculiar for some teeth; for instance, a typical example is the undisclosed second root canal in the mesial root of maxillary molar (MB2), which is frequently detected by CBCT.[50,51]

Peculiar root anatomies are also related to upper premolars with three roots, the first being more frequent than the second.[52] In the case presented (13.17), a huge periapical lesion has been assessed both on 2D and

13.17 **a)** 2D X-ray compared to 3D CBCT image; in both cases, the periapical involvement of the premolar is quite clear. The CBCT analysis clearly shows the buccal lesion related to unusual tooth anatomy. **b)** CBCT sagittal view demonstrating the large dimension of the lesion. **c)** CBCT axial views better define the area of periapical resorption. **d)** The operative surgical field shows a large bone cavity distal to the distobuccal root of this premolar with peculiar anatomy. **e, f)** A higher magnification view of the apical area with the two root-ends exposed. **g, h)**. The two root-end cavities filled. **i)** The addition of heterologous bone is provided to obtain a more precise bone formation. **j)** The placement of a membrane completed the surgical procedure. **k)** The entire procedure was completed with a tight suture. **l)** The 2D X-rays before and after the treatment, at the follow-up. **m, n)** CBCT axial view confirming satisfactory healing. **o, p)** CBCT sagittal and coronal views (*Courtesy of Dr. Fabio Gorni*).

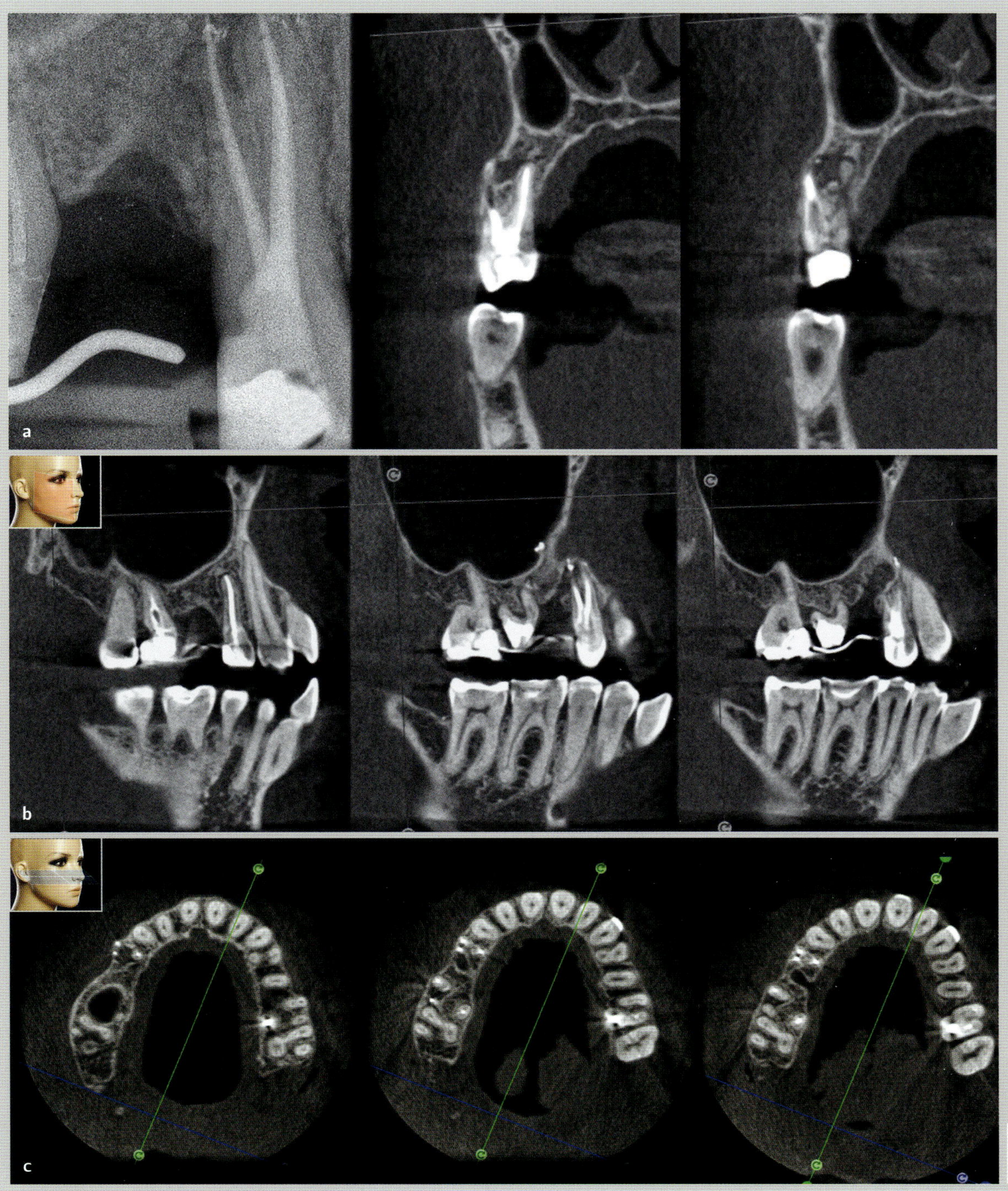

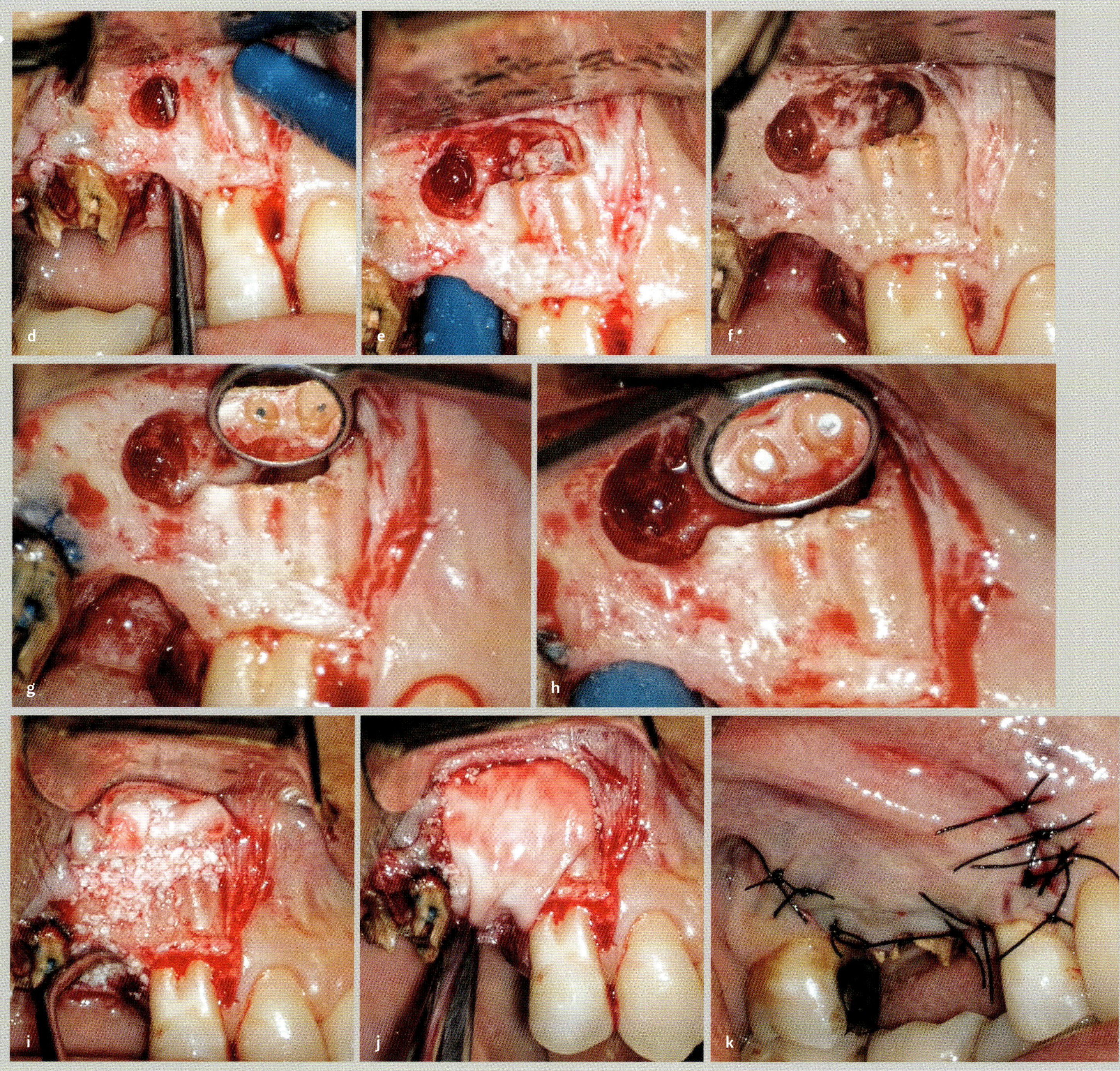
d
e
f
g
h
i
j
k

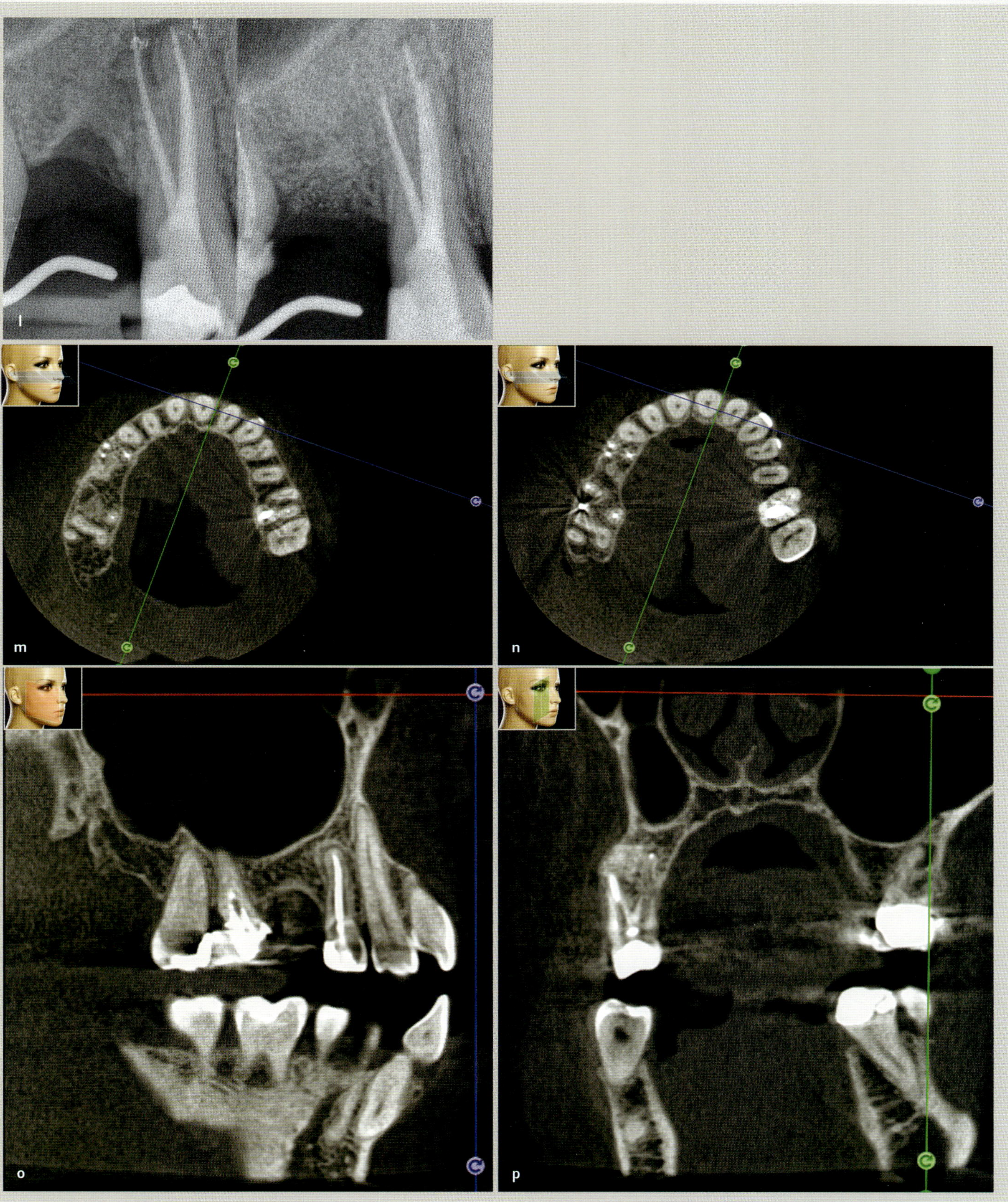
l
m
n
o
p

13.18 **a)** The 2D X-ray of this lower right first premolar shows a lesion of endodontic origin. The 3D CBCT sagittal and coronal views show the presence of a bifurcation in the apical one third. **b)** CBCT axial view clearly demonstrates the dimension of the lesion toward the lingual area and the second uninstrumented root canal. **c)** CBCT axial view demonstrating the extension of the periapical radiolucency. **d)** Preoperative radiograph and postoperative radiograph after root end obturation. **e)** The microsurgical field shows the buccal canal sealed and the orifice of the unsealed lingual canal. **f)** The ultrasonic retrotip inserted in the bony crypt to carry out the root-end preparation. **g, h)** The two root-end cavities and the isthmus have been prepared and sealed (*Courtesy of Dr. Fabio Gorni*).

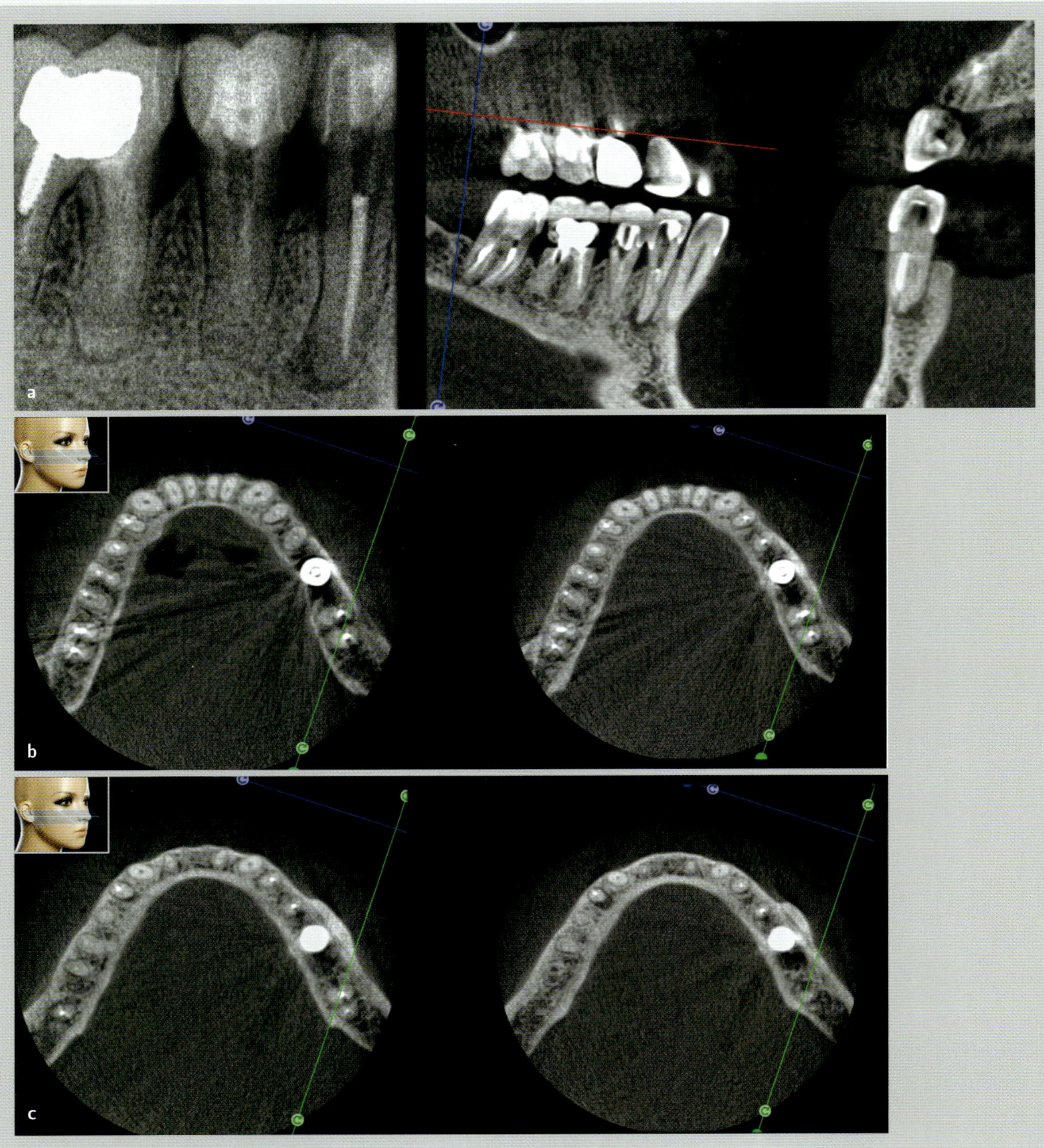

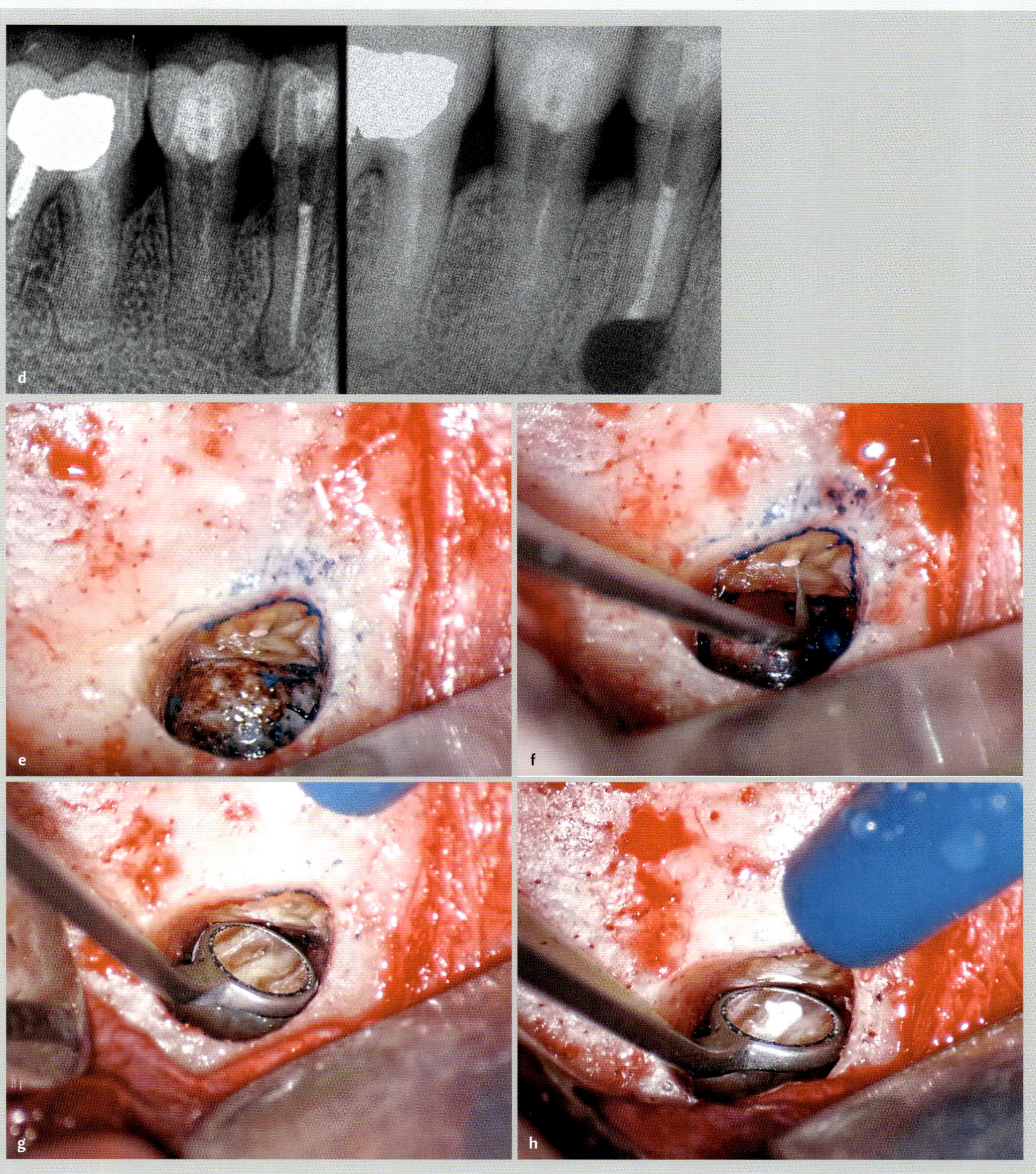
d
e
f
g
h

13.19 a) The orthopanoramic view shows a large lesion related to the upper right lateral incisor. **b)** The 2D radiograph shows a suspect area. **c)** CBCT axial view demonstrating unusual anatomy of the upper right central incisor. **d)** A second CBCT axial view confirms that the periapical lesion involves both the lateral and the central incisors. **e)** The third CBCT axial view demonstrates major destruction of the buccal cortical bone. **f, g)**. CBCT coronal views confirming the involvement of the two incisors. **h)** The unusual anatomy of the central incisor is discovered with a wide mucogingival flap. **i)** The two root apices prepared for the retrofilling. **j)** Another phase of the surgical procedure. **k, l)** The two apices isolated after microsurgical toilette of the bone cavities (*Courtesy of Dr. Fabio Gorni*).

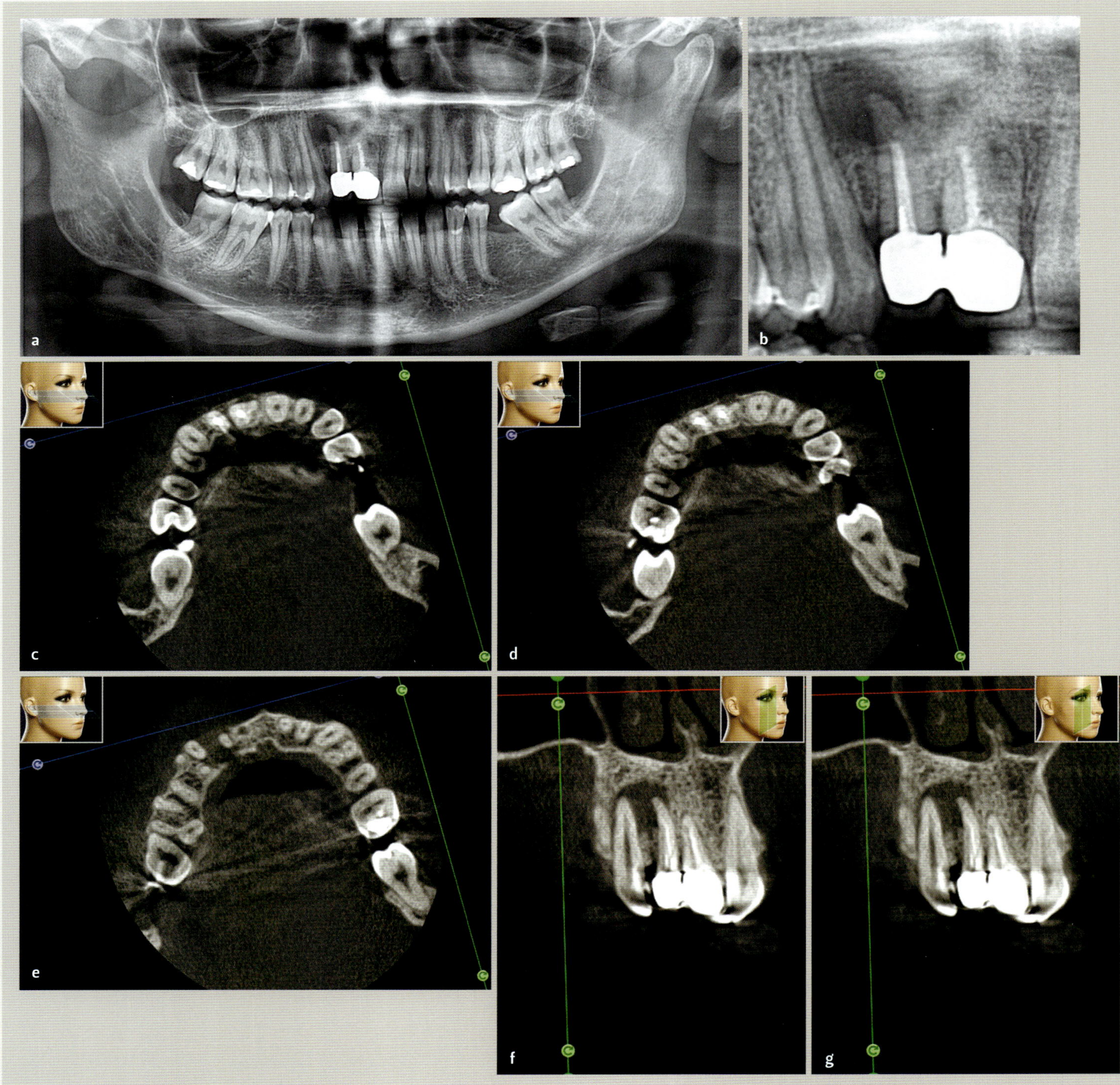

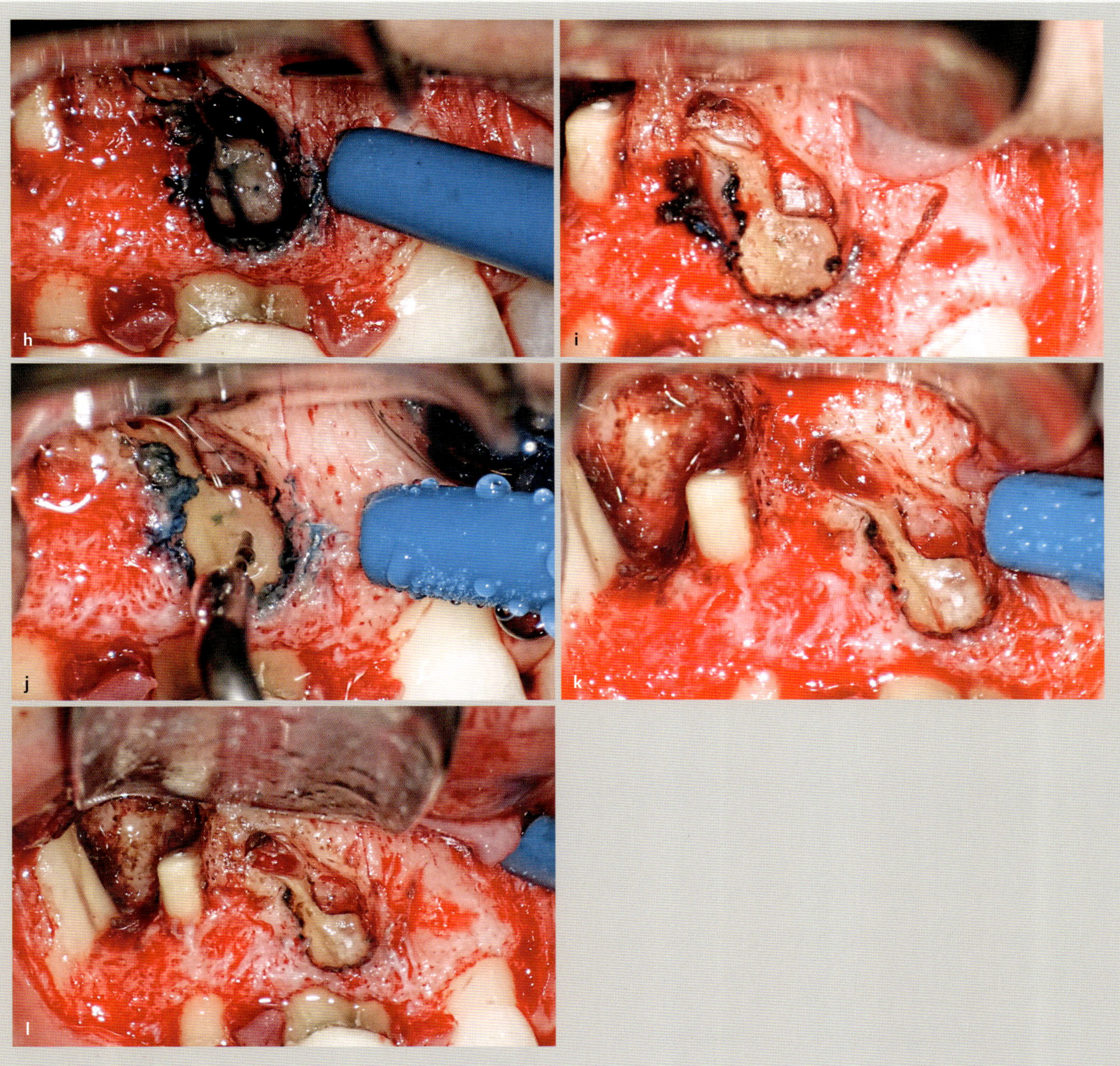
h
i
j
k
l

3D radiographs, revealing a typical three root morphology of the first upper premolar. During surgical access, owing to the osseous lesion, a graft with bovine bone and a membrane was performed in order to have better and faster healing. A one-year-recall resulted in a positive outcome.

In lower premolars, bifurcations in the apical third are quite common and frequently lead to periapical pathosis in teeth that have been previously sealed. In the case reported in 3.18 the canal bifurcation might have been suspected, but only with an accurate CBCT analysis could be evaluated properly for microsurgical endodontics.

Sometimes CBCT examination brings to light different evidence, not suspected by the periapical radiograph. In the case described in 3.19, a wide periapical lesion was clearly evident in a two-dimensional X-Ray but, in order to investigate the involvement of the canine, a CBCT was requested. In the subsequent analysis, an abnormal root canal configuration of the upper central incisor was observed, and a periapical lesion of endodontic origin was localized around the root not detected by the first periapical radiograph.

Other suitable indications proposed were for the locations of separated instrument localizations.[53,54] In these studies, the Authors outlined a lower accuracy for CBCT when intracanal obturation was present but suggested its use for the detection of the root canal in which the instrument was broken when multi-rooted teeth were involved.

Maxillary and Mandibular Anatomy: A Radiographic Analysis

CBCT has particular features useful for microsurgery treatment planning; its use has strategic value, either for the diagnostic part or even for the surgical procedure, the last being quite dangerous in some areas of the upper and lower jaw.

In the upper jaw it is quite common in posterior teeth to have a communication with the sinus, frequently demonstrating a pathological thickening of the inner mucosa;[55] sometimes, the roots are localized inside the sinus, and this should be taken into consideration for the management of the surgical procedure (13.20).[56]

In the lower jaw, the mental foramen[57,58] and the mandibular canal[59,60] are the two anatomical structures that should be taken into account when planning microsurgical procedures.

Sometimes the apex and inferior alveolar nerve are so close that apical extrusion of sealing material might lead to mental nerve paresthesia (6.10).[61] In the case illustrated in 13.21, the two-dimensional radiograph didn't show any pathologic sign around the apex of the lower premolar, but the CBCT clearly depicted a compression of the extruded periapical material onto the inferior alveolar nerve. This led the operator to widen the surgical access[62] to expose the mental foramen and to have better visibility of the operative field (6.8b).

Concluding Remarks

The use of the CBCT is important for both diagnostic and surgical phases; the limited field of view (FOV) prevents excessive radiation doses to the patient, and also provides an improved resolution of the images obtained, facilitating a more precise analysis.

From this perspective, follow-up examinations can be more safely performed and may furnish more precise information about the treatment outcome.

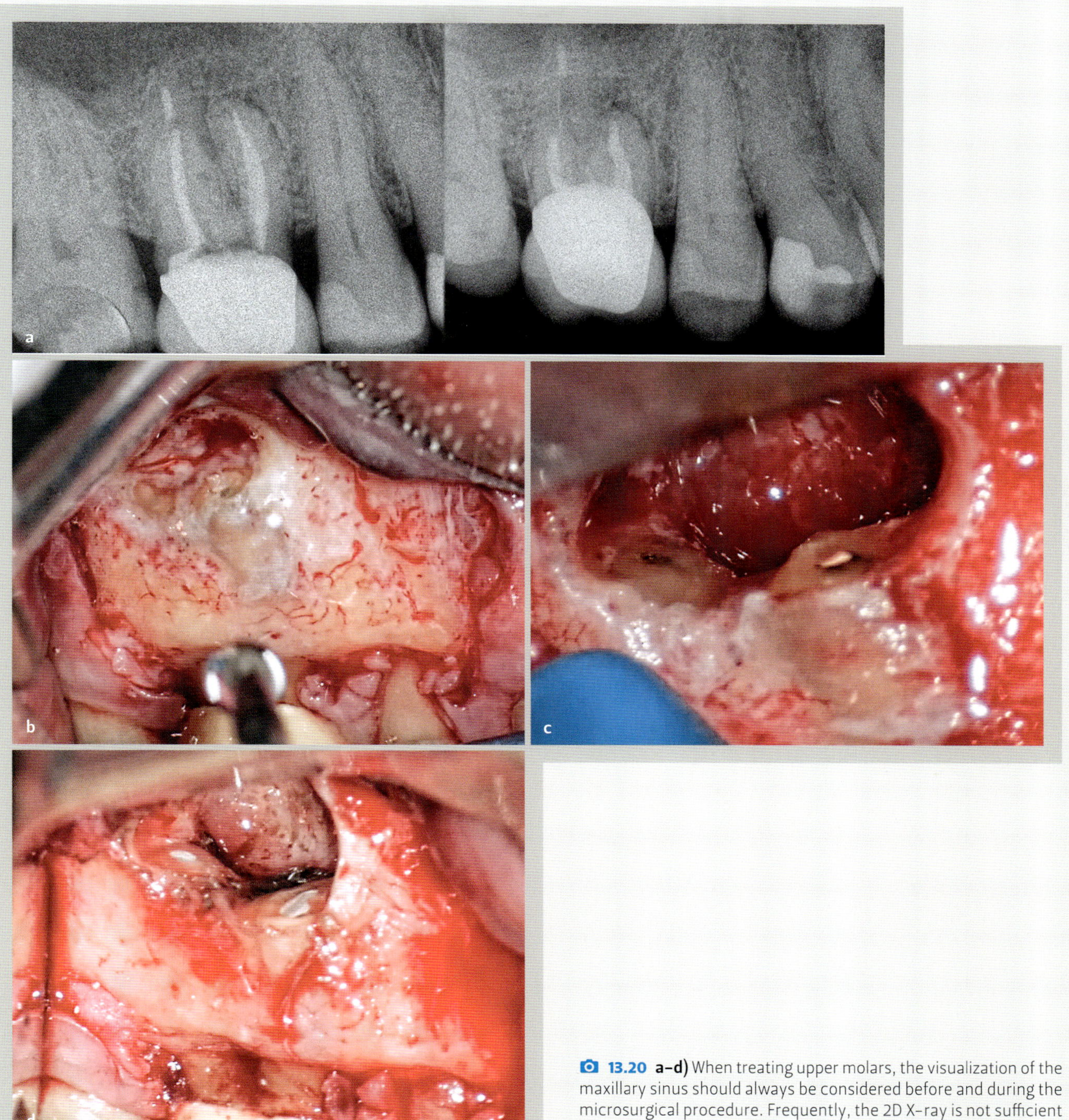

13.20 **a–d)** When treating upper molars, the visualization of the maxillary sinus should always be considered before and during the microsurgical procedure. Frequently, the 2D X-ray is not sufficient to show the relationship between roots and maxillary sinus (*Courtesy of Dr. Fabio Gorni*).

13.21 a) The 2D X-ray does not demonstrate any sign of apical periodontitis, but the symptoms referred by the patient are clearly related to the mental nerve compression. **b)** CBCT sagittal view confirming the close relationship between the extruded obturation material and the mental nerve. **c)** CBCT coronal view. **d)** Another CBCT coronal view demonstrating a large amount of extruded material in contact with the mandibular canal. **e)** The wide flap verifies the position of the mental foramen. **f–h)** A cautious apical resection permits complete removal of the extruded material. **i)** The apical resection after completion. **j)** The root-end filling material in place. **k)** CBCT sagittal view. Sufficient distance from the mental nerve is now available for the connective tissue to heal. **l)** CBCT coronal view (*Courtesy of Dr. Fabio Gorni*).

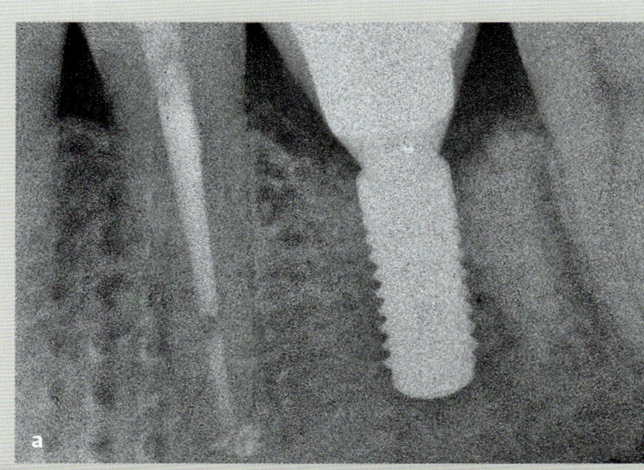

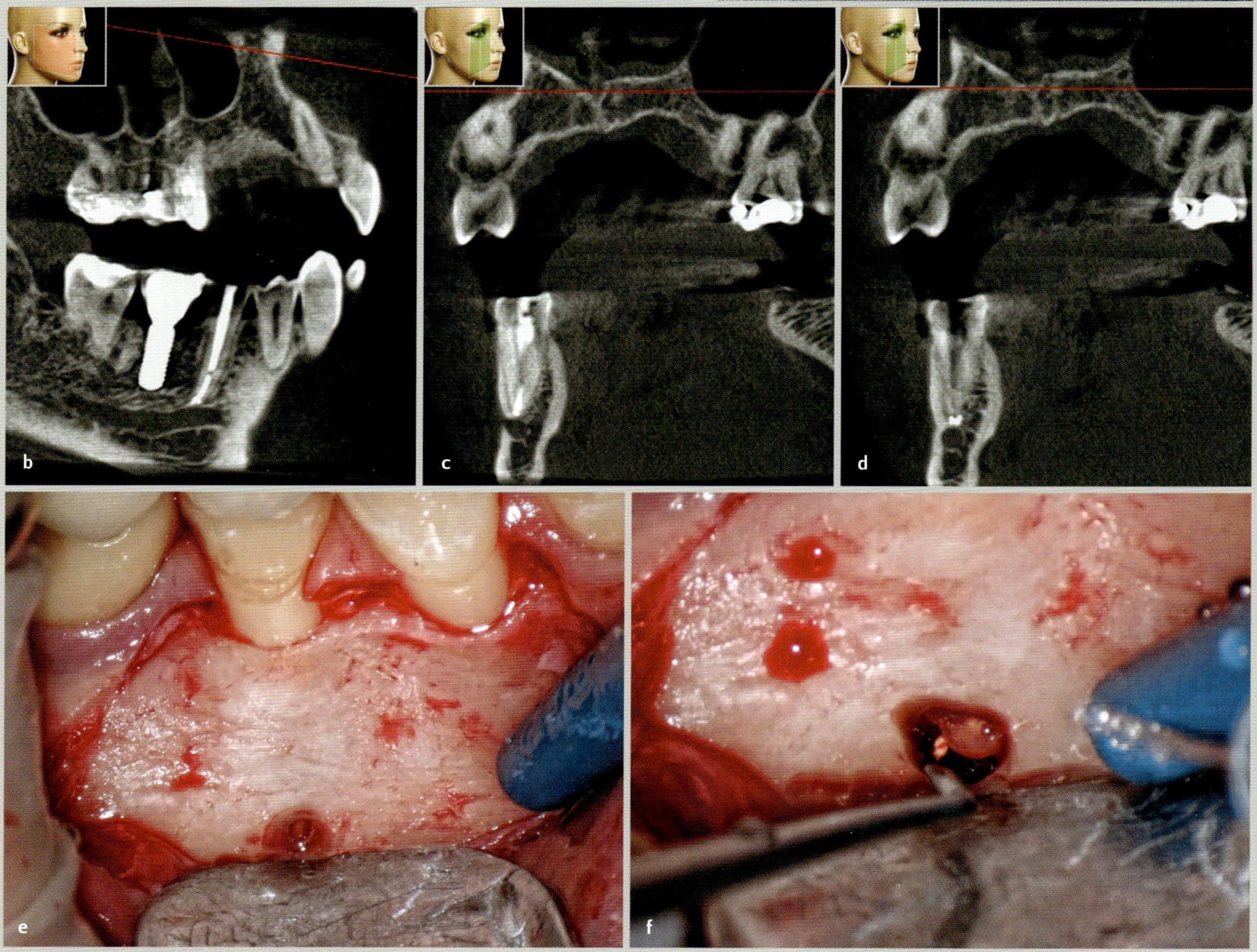

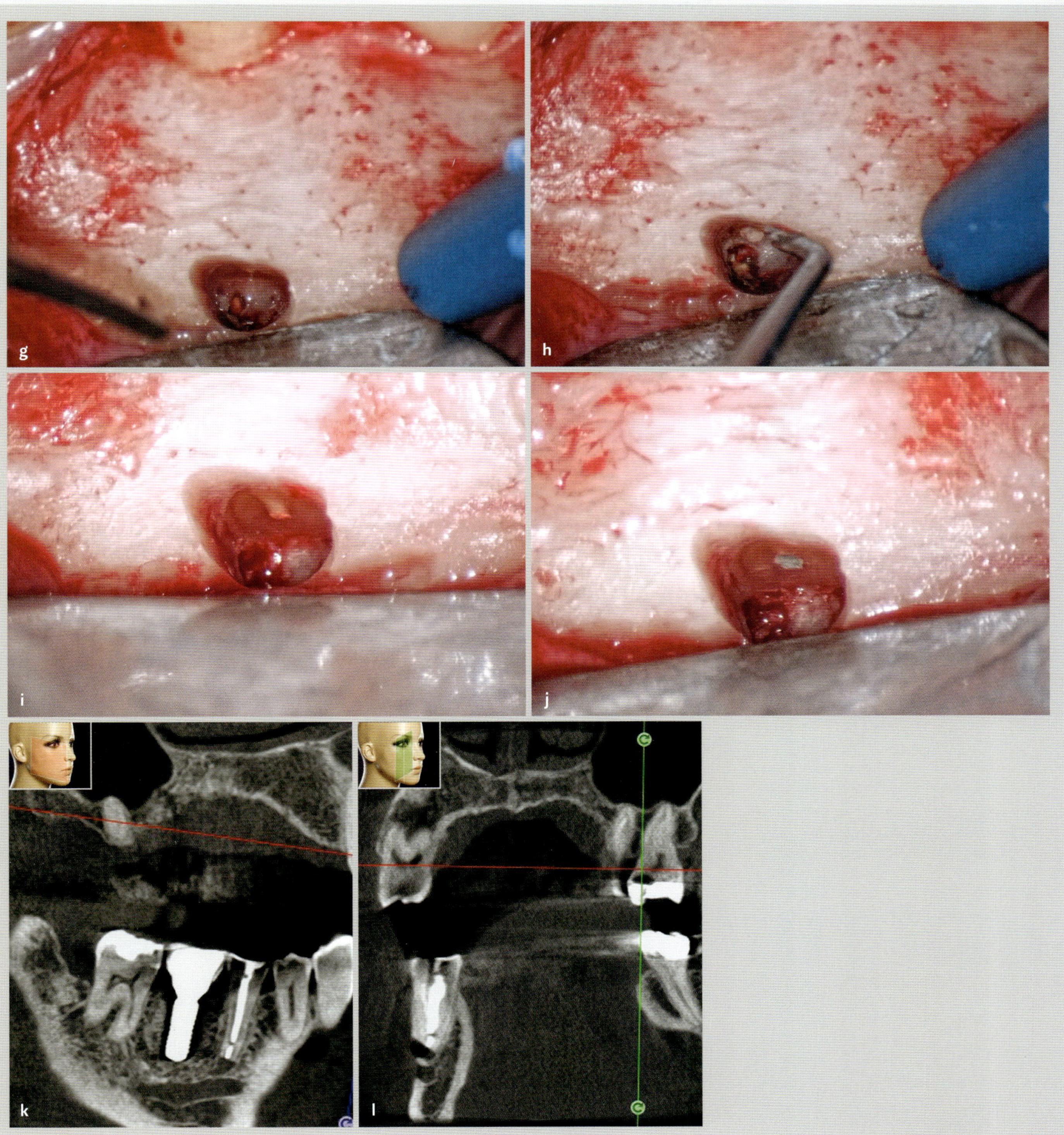
g
h
i
j
k
l

REFERENCES

1. Richards AG, Colquitt WN. *Reduction in dental X-ray exposures during the past 60 years.* J Am Dent Assoc. 1981;103:713.
2. Grossman LI. *A brief history of endodontics.* J Endod. Special Issue. 1982;8:536.
3. Richards AG. *The buccal object rule.* Tenn State Dent Assoc. 1953;33:263.
4. Goldman M, Pearson AH, Darzenta N. *Endodontic success - Who's reading the radiograph?* Oral Surg Oral Med Oral Pathol. 1972;33(3):432-7.
5. Goldman M, Pearson AH, Darzenta N. *Reliability of radiographic interpretations.* Oral Surg Oral Med Oral Pathol. 1974;38(2):287-93.
6. Bender IB, Seltzer S. *Roentgenographic and direct observation of experimental lesions in bone:* I. 1961. J Endod. 2003;29(11):702-6.
7. Brynolf I. *Roentgenologic periapical diagnosis. I. Reproducibility of interpretation.* Sven Tandlak Tidskr. 1970;63(5):339-44.
8. Cheung GS, Wei WL, McGrath C. *Agreement between periapical radiographs and cone-beam computed tomography for assessment of periapical status of root filled molar teeth.* Int Endod J. 2013;46(10):889-95.
9. Patel S, Wilson R, Dawood A, Mannocci F. *The detection of periapical pathosis using periapical radiography and cone beam computed tomography - part 1: pre-operative status.* Int Endod J. 2012;45(8):702-10.
10. Stavropoulos A, Wenzel A. *Accuracy of cone beam dental CT, intraoral digital and conventional film radiography for the detection of periapical lesions. An ex vivo study in pig jaws.* Clin Oral Investig. 2007;11(1):101-6.
11. Bender IB, Seltzer S. *Roentgenographic and direct observation of experimental lesions in bone: II. 1961.* J Endod. 2003;29(11):707-12.
12. Patel S, Durack C. *Apical Periodontitis.* In: Patel S, Harvey S, Shemesh H. Durak C. *Cone Beam Computed Tomography in Endodontics.* New Malden: Quintessence Publishing Co. Ltd.; 2016:81.
13. Patel S, Dawood A, Whaites E, Pitt Ford T. *New dimensions in endodontic imaging: part 1. Conventional and alternative radiographic systems.* Int Endod J. 2009;42(6):447.
14. Durack C, Patel S. *Cone beam computed tomography in endodontics.* Braz Dent J. 2012;23(3):179-91.
15. Peters C, Peters OA. *Cone beam computed tomography and other imaging techniques in the determination of periapical healing.* Endod Topics. 2012;26(1):57.
16. Todd R. *Dental Imaging-2D to 3D: a historic, current, and future view of projection radiography.* Endod Topics. 2014;31:36.
17. Lofthag-Hansen S, Huumonen S, Gröndahl K, Gröndahl HG. *Limited cone-beam CT and intraoral radiography for the diagnosis of periapical pathology.* Oral Surg Oral Med Oral Pathol Oral Radiol Endod. 2007;103(1):114-9.
18. Estrela C, Bueno MR, Leles CR, Azevedo B, Azevedo JR. *Accuracy of cone beam computed tomography and panoramic and periapical radiography for detection of apical periodontitis.* J Endod. 2008;34(3):273-9.
19. Ørstavik D, Pitt Ford TR. *Essential Endodontology– Prevention and Treatment of Apical Periodontitis.* 2nd ed. Oxford: Blackwell Munksgaard, 2008.
20. Scarfe WC, Levin MD, Gane D, Farman AG. *Use of cone beam computed tomography in endodontics.* Int J Dent. 2009;63:45.
21. Miles DA. *Atlas of Cone Beam Imaging for Dental Applications.* 2nd ed. New Malden: Quintessence Publishing Co. Ltd.; 2013:2-14.
22. Ludlow JB, Davies-Ludlow LE, Brooks SL. *Dosimetry of two extraoral direct digital imaging devices: NewTom cone beam CT and Orthophos Plus DS panoramic unit.* Dentomaxillofac Radiol. 2003;32:229.
23. American Association of Endodontists, Colleagues for excellence. *Cone beam computed tomography in endodontics.* 2011.
24. Tanimoto H, Arai Y. *The effect of voxel size on image reconstruction in cone-beam computed tomography.* Oral Radiol. 2009;25:149-153.
25. Rigolone M, Pasqualini D, Bianchi L, Berutti E, Bianchi SD. *Vestibular surgical access to the palatine root of the superior first molar: "low-dose cone-beam" CT analysis of the pathway and its anatomic variations.* J Endod. 2003;29(11):773-775.
26. Patel S, Durack C, Abella F, Shemesh H, Roig M, Lemberg K. *Cone beam computed tomography in Endodontics - a review.* Int Endod J. 2015;48(1):3-15.
27. Parker J, Mol A, Rivera EM, Tawil P. *CBCT uses in clinical endodontics: the effect of CBCT on the ability to locate MB2 canals in maxillary molars.* Int Endod J. 2016.
28. Davies A, Mannocci F, Mitchell P, Andiappan M, Patel S. *The detection of periapical pathoses in root filled teeth using single and parallax periapical radiographs versus cone beam computed tomography - a clinical study.* Int Endod J. 2015;48(6):582-592.
29. Venskutonis T, Plotino G, Tocci L, Gambarini G, Maminskas J, Juodzbalys G. *Periapical and endodontic status scale based on periapical bone lesions and endodontic treatment quality evaluation using cone-beam computed tomography.* J Endod. 2015;41(2):190-196.
30. Gambarini G, Piasecki L, Miccoli G, Gaimari G, Nardo DD, Testarelli L. *Cone-beam computed tomography in the assessment of periapical lesions in endodontically treated teeth.* Eur J Dent. 2018;12(1):136-143.
31. Rodriguez G, Abella F, Duran-Sindreu F, Patel S, Roig M. *Influence of Cone-beam Computed Tomography in Clinical Decision Making among Specialists.* J Endod. 2017;43(2):194-199.
32. Rodriguez G, Patel S, Duran-Sindreu F, Roig M, Abella F. *Influence of Cone-beam Computed Tomography on Endodontic Retreatment Strategies among General Dental Practitioners and Endodontists.* J Endod. 2017;43(9):1433-1437.
33. Lopez FU, Kopper PM, Cucco C, Della Bona A, de Figueiredo JA, Vier-Pelisser FV. *Accuracy of cone-beam computed tomography and periapical radiography in apical periodontitis diagnosis.* J Endod. 2014;40(12):2057-2060.
34. Kanagasingam S, Lim CX, Yong CP, Mannocci F, Patel S. *Diagnostic accuracy of periapical radiography and cone beam computed tomography in detecting apical periodontitis using histopathological findings as a reference standard.* Int Endod J. 2017;50(5):417-426.
35. Lo Giudice R, Nicita F, Puleio F, Alibrandi A, Cervino G, Lizio AS, et al. *Accuracy of Periapical Radiogra-*

phy and CBCT in Endodontic Evaluation. Int J Dent. 2018;2018:2514243.

36. Cotton TP, Geisler TM, Holden DT, Schwartz SA, Schindler WG. *Endodontic applications of cone-beam volumetric tomography.* J Endod. 2007;33:1121-1132.
37. Barnett CW, Glickman GN, Umorin M, Jalali P. *Interobserver and Intraobserver Reliability of Cone-beam Computed Tomography in Identification of Apical Periodontitis.* J Endod. 2018;44(6):938-940.
38. Beacham JT, Geist JR, Yu Q, Himel VT, Sabey KA. *Accuracy of Cone-beam Computed Tomographic Image Interpretation by Endodontists and Endodontic Residents.* J. Endod. 2018;44(4):571-575.
39. Bueno MR, Estrela C, Azevedo BC, Diogenes A. *Development of a New Cone-Beam Computed Tomography Software for Endodontic Diagnosis.* Braz Dent J. 2018;29(6):517-529.
40. Mavridou AM, Pyka G, Kerckhofs G, Wevers M, Bergmans L, Gunst V, et al. *A novel multimodular methodology to investigate external cervical tooth resorption.* Int Endod J. 2016;49(3):287-300.
41. Vaz de Souza D, Schirru E, Mannocci F, Foschi F, Patel S. *External cervical resorption: a comparison of the diagnostic efficacy using 2 different cone-beam computed tomographic units and periapical radiographs.* J Endod. 2017;43(1):121-125.
42. Deliga Schroder AG, Westphalen FH, Schroder JC, Fernandes A, Westphalen VPD. *Accuracy of digital periapical radiography and cone-beam computed tomography for diagnosis of natural and simulated external root resorption.* J Endod. 2018;44(7):1151-1158.
43. Costa FF, Gaia BF, Umetsubo OS, Pinheiro LR, Tortamano IP, Cavalcanti MG. *Use of large-volume cone-beam computed tomography in identification and localization of horizontal root fracture in the presence and absence of intracanal metallic post.* J Endod. 2012;38(6):856-859.
44. Costa FF, Pinheiro LR, Umetsubo OS, dos Santos O, Jr, Gaia BF, Cavalcanti MG. *Influence of cone-beam computed tomographic scan mode for detection of horizontal root fracture.* J Endod. 2014;40(9):1472-1476.
45. Brady E, Mannocci F, Brown J, Wilson R, Patel S. *A comparison of cone beam computed tomography and periapical radiography for the detection of vertical root fractures in non-endodontically treated teeth.* Int Endod J. 2014;47(8):735-746.
46. Ma RH, Ge ZP, Li G. *Detection accuracy of root fractures in cone-beam computed tomography images: a systematic review and meta-analysis.* Int Endod J. 2016;49(7):646-654.
47. Talwar S, Utneja S, Nawal RR, Kaushik A, Srivastava D, Oberoy SS. *Role of cone-beam computed tomography in diagnosis of vertical root fractures: a systematic review and meta-analysis.* J Endod. 2016;42(1):12-24.
48. Dutra KL, Pacheco-Pereira C, Bortoluzzi EA, Flores-Mir C, Lagravere MO, Correa M. *Influence of intracanal materials in vertical root fracture pathway detection with cone-beam computed tomography.* J Endod. 2017;43(7):1170-1175.
49. Khojastepour L, Moazami F, Babaei M, Forghani M. *Assessment of root perforation within simulated internal resorption cavities using cone-beam computed tomography.* J Endod. 2015;41(9):1520-1523.
50. Vizzotto MB, Silveira PF, Arus NA, Montagner F, Gomes BP, da Silveira HE. *CBCT for the assessment of second mesiobuccal (MB2) canals in maxillary molar teeth: effect of voxel size and presence of root filling.* Inter Endod J. 2013;46(9):870-876.
51. Studebaker B, Hollender L, Mancl L, Johnson JD, Paranjpe A. *The incidence of second mesiobuccal canals located in maxillary molars with the aid of cone-beam computed tomography.* J Endod. 2018;44(4):565-570.
52. Sousa TO, Haiter-Neto F, Nascimento EHL, Peroni LV, Freitas DQ, Hassan B. *Diagnostic accuracy of periapical radiography and cone-beam computed tomography in identifying root canal configuration of human premolars.* J Endod. 2017;43(7):1176-1179.
53. Rosen E, Venezia NB, Azizi H, Kamburoglu K, Meirowitz A, Ziv-Baran T, et al. *A comparison of cone-beam computed tomography with periapical radiography in the detection of separated instruments retained in the apical third of root canal-filled teeth.* J Endod. 2016;42(7):1035-1039.
54. Ramos Brito AC, Verner FS, Junqueira RB, Yamasaki MC, Queiroz PM, Freitas DQ, et al. *Detection of fractured endodontic instruments in root canals: comparison between different digital radiography systems and cone-beam computed tomography.* J Endod. 2017;43(4):544-549.
55. Lu Y, Liu Z, Zhang L, Zhou X, Zheng Q, Duan X, et al. *Associations between maxillary sinus mucosal thickening and apical periodontitis using cone-beam computed tomography scanning: a retrospective study.* J Endod. 2012;38(8):1069-1074.
56. Nunes CA, Guedes OA, Alencar AH, Peters OA, Estrela CR, Estrela C. *Evaluation of periapical lesions and their association with maxillary sinus abnormalities on cone-beam computed tomographic images.* J Endod. 2016;42(1):42-46.
57. Carruth P, He J, Benson BW, Schneiderman ED. *Analysis of the size and position of the mental foramen using the CS 9000 cone-beam computed tomographic unit.* J Endod. 2015;41(7):1032-1036.
58. Chong BS, Gohil K, Pawar R, Makdissi J. *Anatomical relationship between mental foramen, mandibular teeth and risk of nerve injury with endodontic treatment.* Clin Oral Investig. 2017;21(1):381-387.
59. Wang X, Chen K, Wang S, Tiwari SK, Ye L, Peng L. *Relationship between the mental foramen, mandibular canal, and the surgical access line of the mandibular posterior teeth: a cone-beam computed tomographic analysis.* J Endod. 2017;43(8):1262-1266.
60. Ugur Aydin Z, Goller Bulut D. *Relationship between the anatomic structures and mandibular posterior teeth for endodontic surgery in a Turkish population: a cone-beam computed tomographic analysis.* Clin Oral Investig 2019 Feb 2.
61. Gambarini G, Plotino G, Grande NM, Testarelli L, Prencipe M, Messineo D, et al. *Differential diagnosis of endodontic-related inferior alveolar nerve paraesthesia with cone beam computed tomography: a case report.* Int Endod J. 2011;44(2):176-181.
62. von Arx T, Friedli M, Sendi P, Lozanoff S, Bornstein MM. *Location and dimensions of the mental foramen: a radiographic analysis by using cone-beam computed tomography.* J Endod. 2013;39(12):1522-1528.

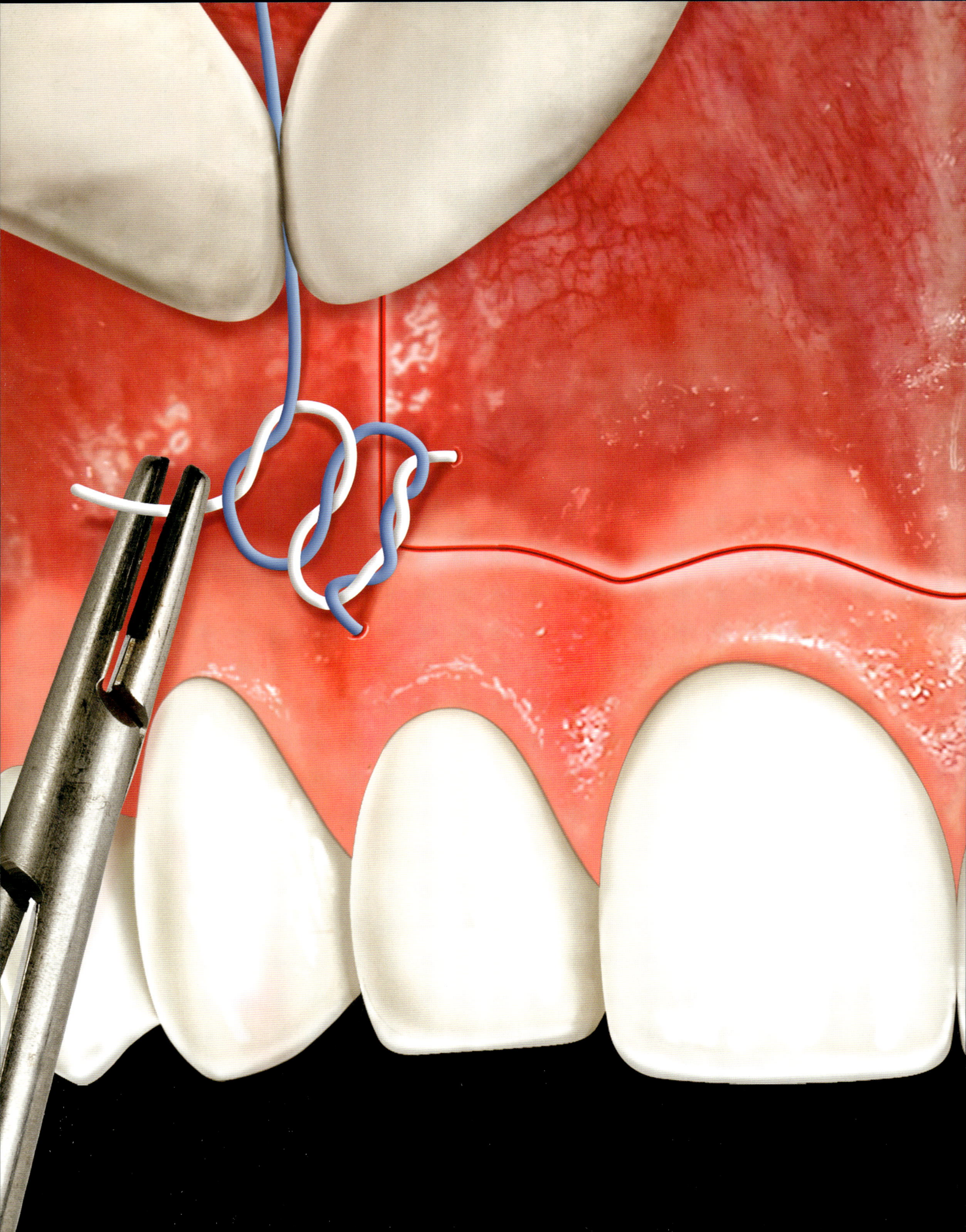

Sutures

Once the root-end filling material has been positioned and the marginal adaptation has been checked at high magnification under the operating microscope, before suturing it is advisable to take a postoperative radiograph to make sure that the procedure has been done correctly. The flap elevator is removed, the flap is temporarily repositioned and a moist sterile gauze is positioned between the flap and the lip, firm finger pressure is applied to restore elasticity to the tissue and to rehydrate the flap. Then the film holder is introduced in the mouth and the radiograph is taken.

After checking the postoperative radiograph, the elevated soft tissue can be sutured.

As already mentioned before, the suture can and should be done using the operating microscope. Suturing under the microscope has the advantage of being more accurate in repositioning the flap, allowing perfect healing by primary intention, without any scar tissue. The author disagrees with people who recommend the use of the microscope for osteotomy, curettage, apicoectomy, apical preparation, retrofilling and documentation but not for the incision as well as for suturing.[1] Suturing under the microscope can be difficult sometimes, especially in posterior regions, but the accuracy in reapproximation provided by the microscope cannot be compared with that provided by the use of loops or, even worst, by the naked eye.

Reapproximation and Compression

After irrigation with saline solution to remove debris, the wound edges are carefully reapproximated in the same position as before surgery to allow healing by primary intention.[2] After the flap is back in place, compression of the wound is essential to enhance intravascular clotting and for the creation of a thin fibrin clot between the flap and the bone and a thin hiatus between the wound edges.[3–6] The compression is maintained for 3 to 5 minutes with firm finger pressure using a moist sterile gauze (14.1). The goal of the compression is to avoid the formation of a coagulum in the dissectional wound between the flap and the bone. If a coagulum forms, healing is delayed, because the coagulum needs to be reorganized before epithelial attachment can be accomplished.[3,7]

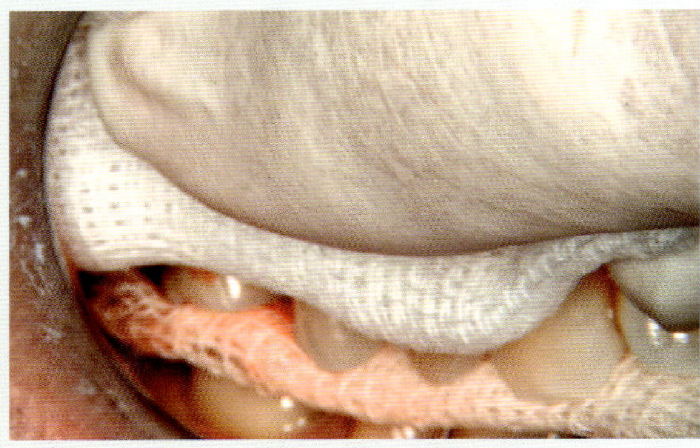

14.1 The flap is compressed for a few minutes before suturing.

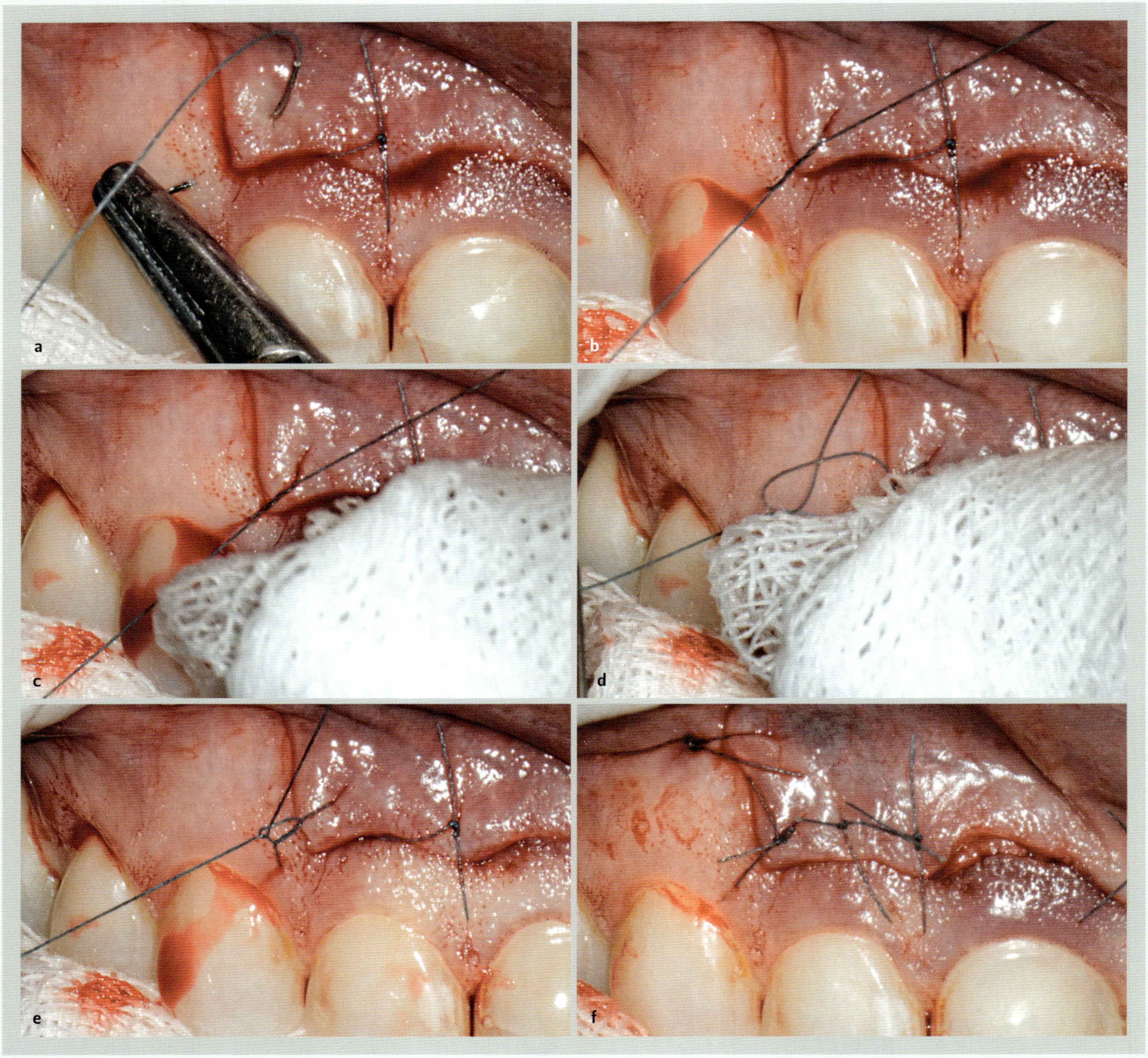

14.2 a–f) During suturing, the dental assistant keeps compressing the flap so that the knot doesn't become loose.

While suturing, the repositioned flap should be gently compressed with a saline-moistened piece of gauze by the dental assistant to keep the knot in place while it is being tightened (14.2) and to create a thin fibrin layer between flapped tissue and cortical bone.[6,8] Replacement of a thin blood cloth with parallel fibrin fibers by new fibrous tissue results in collagen adhesion.[2]

Selection of the Suture

Historically, silk has been the suture of choice for many clinicians and still is for many oral surgeons and maxillofacial surgeons. Accordingly, non-absorbable silk sutures are easy to tie and handle but are no longer recommended as they exhibit a wicking effect by which they conduct fluid and bacteria into the surgical site.[9,10] They allow rapid bacterial colonization (14.3) within 24 hours which causes high inflammation of the wound site[3,11,12] and are uncomfortable to remove because of ingrowth of tissue.[13] Parikoh et al.[14] showed after 3, 5 and 7 days that the whole surface of silk sutures was covered with a thick layer of bacterial plaque and debris, while the polyvinylidene fluoride suture (PVDF) had less debris and a smaller area of contamination. On the other hand, PVDF is difficult to handle and patients often complain that the tag ends of the suture are stiff and irritating the oral mucosa. The same is true for other monofilament suture materials like Supramid®, a polyglycolic acid suture (Supramid®, S. Jackson Inc.) which seems to inhibit bacterial transmission (14.4).[15] Nylon (like any other monofilament synthetic sutures) is colonized more slowly, allows less bacterial migration but is too rigid and often patients complain because the suture is irritating to the lip or the cheek.

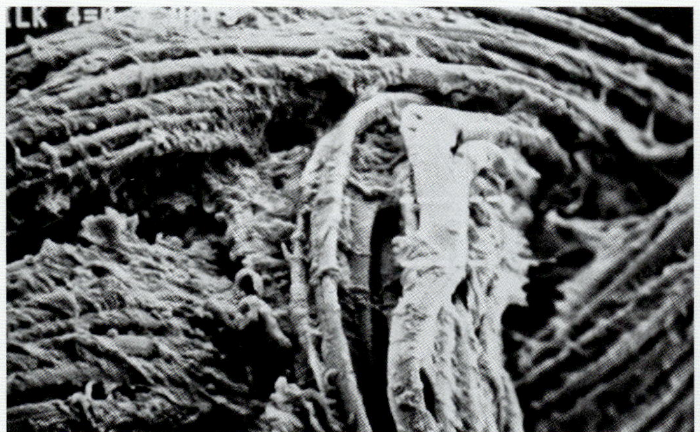

14.3 Black silk sutures accumulate bacterial plaque very quickly (*Courtesy of Dr. Gary Carr*).

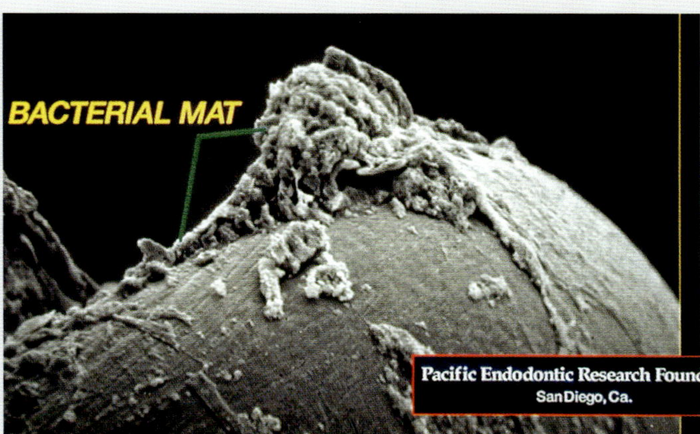

14.4 Supramid accumulates less bacterial plaque compared to silk (*Courtesy of Dr. Gary Carr*).

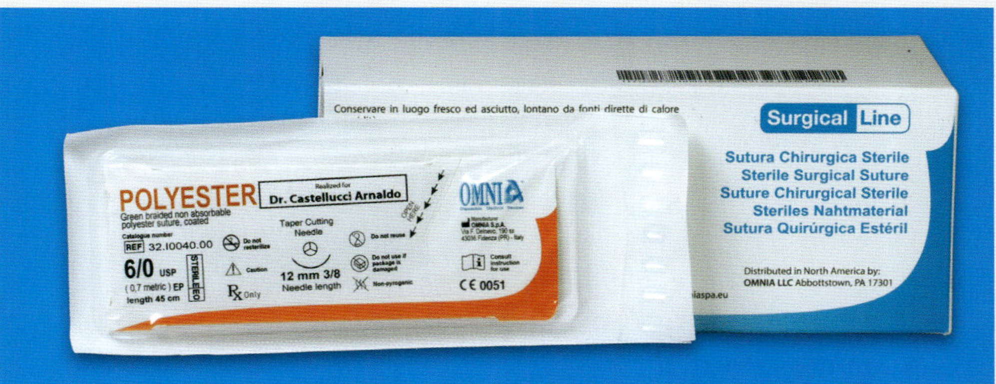

14.5 The 6-0 polyester suture coated with a thin layer of wax (Omnia S.p.A., Italy) doesn't accumulate bacterial plaque.

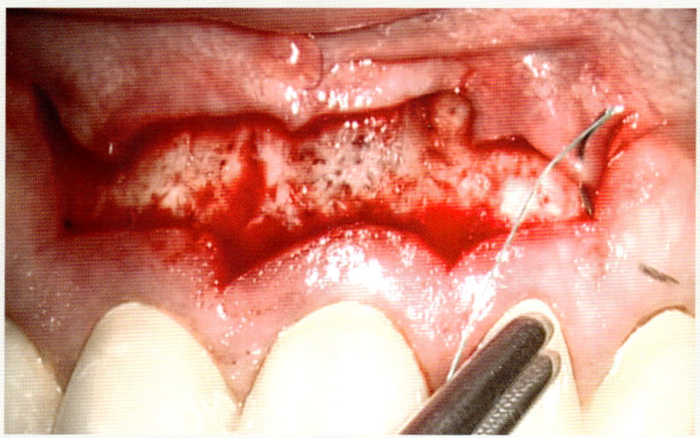

14.6 The needle always goes from unattached to attached tissue, and the entrance and the exit should be equidistant from the incision.

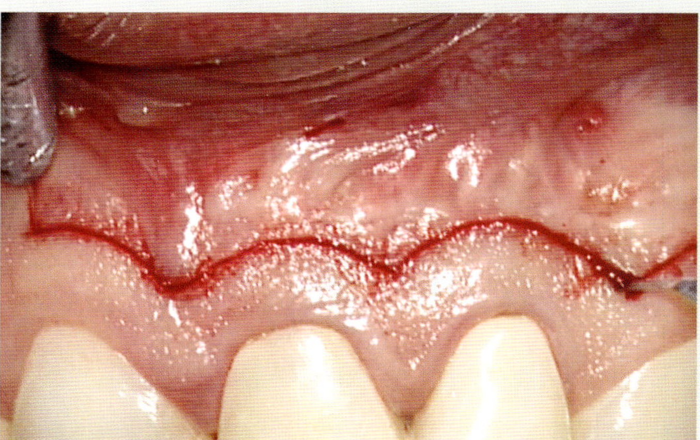

14.7 The scalloped incision facilitates the re-approximation and the suturing.

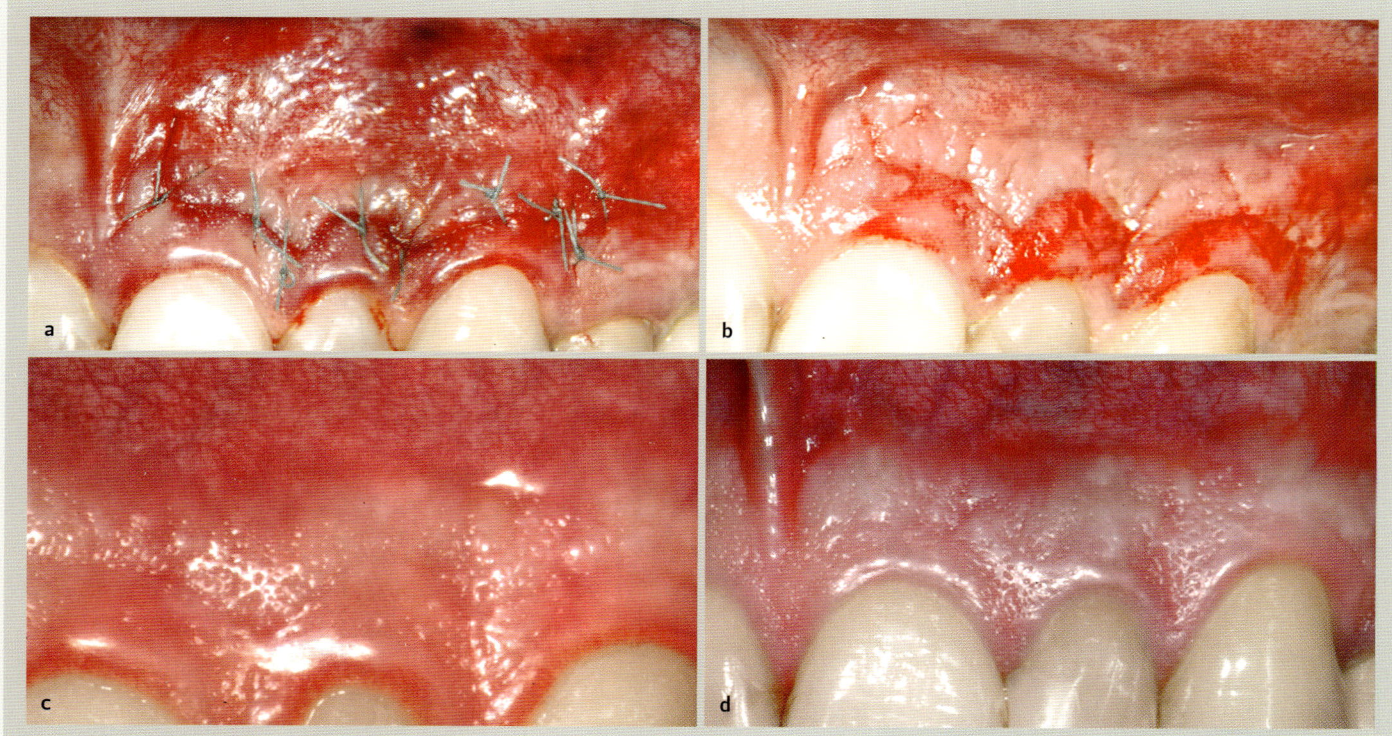

14.8 **a)** The submarginal flap has been sutured with 6-0 Tevdek. **b)** The sutures were removed after 24 hours. **c)** Nice healing after 15 days. **d)** 17-year recall: the complete absence of scarring.

As already described in Chapter 3, the most recommended suturing material today is the 6-0 braided polyester suture like Tevdek® (Genzyme Biosurgery, MA, USA), composed of poly(ethylene terephthalate), prepared from fibers of linear polyesters coated with Polytetrafluoroethylene (PTFE or Teflon®) (Genzyme Corp. MA, USA), or the 6-0 polyester coated with a thin layer of wax (Omnia S.p.A., Italy) (14.5). The polyester sutures have the characteristic of not accumulating plaque, even when they remain in place longer than intended (3.32).

It is very easy to handle, very resistant to bacterial colonization and is nonirritating. For the submarginal flap, the needle should be a tapered point needle 3/8 circle, which is preferable to the reverse cutting type needle because it does not tend to cut or tear the tissue. For the marginal flap, the reverse cutting needle is better indicated because its larger size will facilitate passing through the contacts when doing a continuous sling suture.

For the submarginal flap, the needle should enter about 2 mm apical to the incision and exit about 2 mm coronal to the incision, always going from unattached to attached tissue. This means that the entrance and the exit should be equidistant from the incision so that later it will be easy to cut the suture with appropriate scissors (14.6). Thanks to the scallops (14.7), reapproximation and suturing will be easy, the tissue will return to its original place and after 24/48 hours will be possible to appreciate the nice healing without inflammation and later without any scar tissue (14.8).

For the marginal flap, the sling or the mattress suture can be used.

Needle Holders

As far as the needle holders are concerned, traditionally they were designed to be held like a pair of scissors, and they were quite uncomfortable and not so easy to handle. Much more comfortable is the Castroviejo (14.9) that can be held in the hand of the operator and having a round cross-section makes the introduction of the needle into the soft tissues a lot easier.

Suturing Technique

While suturing, as already stated, the repositioned flap should be gently compressed with a saline-moistened piece of gauze by the dental assistant to maintain the tissue in the right position while the doctor is suturing, to keep the knot in place while it is being tightened, to avoid the knot from becoming loose and to create a thin fibrin layer between flapped tissue and cortical bone.[6,8] Replacement of a thin blood clot with parallel fibrin fibers by new fibrous tissue results in collagen adhesion.[2]

The suture is performed using the microscope at low magnification (2.5×–4.5×). The Castroviejo needle holder grasps the needle close to the filament, to avoid grasping and deform the sharp end. The needle is perpendicular to the holder (14.10) so that the doctor has good visibility and can easily control the direction of the needle itself. While the second dental assistant helps by gently retracting the cheek or the lips, the first one will help with the suction and compressing the flap against the bone while the doctor is tying the knots. The suture is always performed passing from the unat-

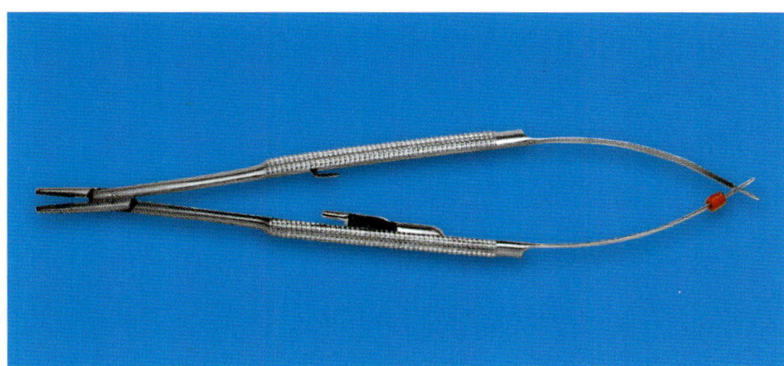

14.9 The Castroviejo needle holder.

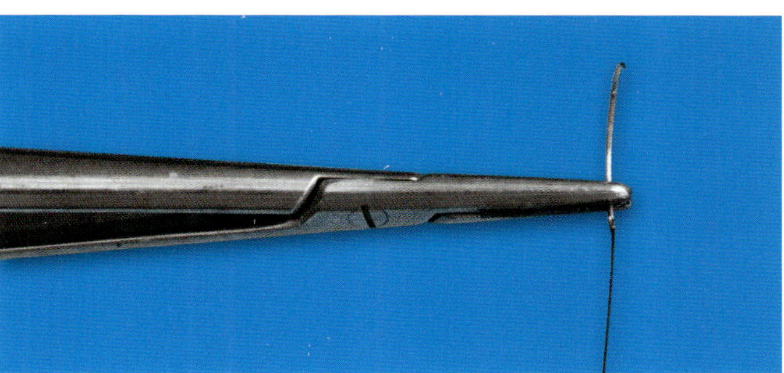

14.10 The Castroviejo needle holder grasps the needle close to the filament.

tached tissue (the flap side) to the attached tissue. Once the needle exits from the attached tissue, the doctor will pull the suture with the other hand until 2–3 cm will remain apical to the incision. Doing this, the needle holder maintains the suture parallel to the tissue, in order not to tear it, and the doctor folds the suture in his/her hand (📷 14.11). Now the doctor makes two loops around the beaks of the holder and starts to pull the knot tighter (📷 14.12). To keep the tissue in position and the knot gently tight, the dental assistant continues compressing the flap and maintaining pressure until the doctor is ready with the second loop and then the third one. This is performed each time by going in a different direction, from clockwise to counterclockwise and back to clockwise (📷 14.13). After checking the ideal reapproximation, the doctor cuts the suture and pushes the knot apical to the incision, exactly at the puncture site of the needle, in order to move the knot away from the incision line as much as possible, to prevent plaque accumulation over the incision itself. This is done because the suture knot collects food, debris, bacteria, and plaque. If left over the incision line, the knot may cause delayed healing responses.[2]

The suture is continued until there are no more gaps between the flap and the attached gingiva and an adequate reapproximation is achieved (📷 14.14). The last knots are positioned in the releasing incisions in case there is a need, which doesn't happen all the times. The suture of the releasing incision doesn't have to be tight but rather quite loose. If made too tight, its removal will be more difficult for the surgeon and will cause more discomfort for the patient.

In the case of nonresorbable, monofilament sutures, the remaining free ends of the suture can be seared to eliminate suture irritation of the patient's lips or cheeks (📷 7.20l).

When the suturing is completed, the doctor will gently compress the flap again with a moistened sterile gauze to improve the approximation and to permit a very thin fibrin clot under the flap, that will accelerate the healing.[16]

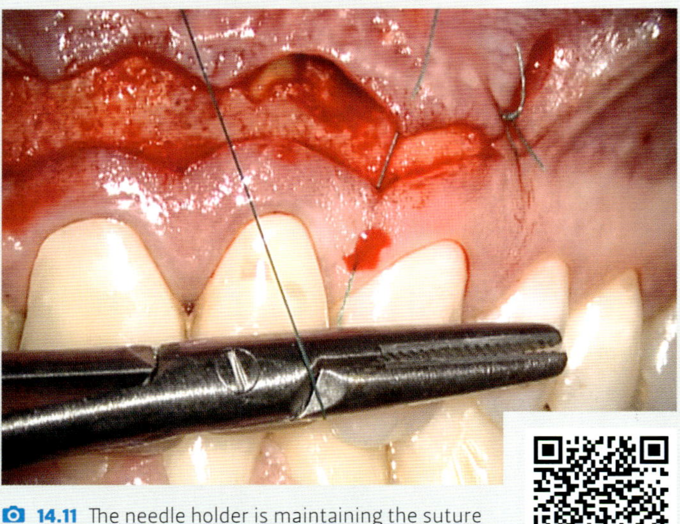

📷 **14.11** The needle holder is maintaining the suture parallel to the tissue, in order not to tear it, while the doctor folds the suture in his/her hand.

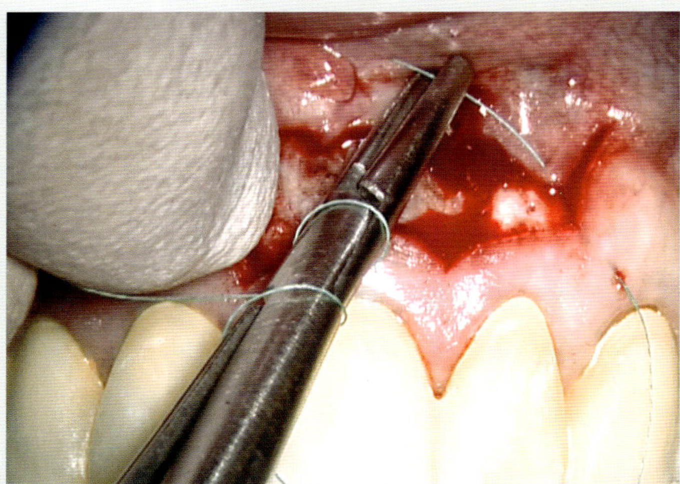

📷 **14.12** The doctor is winding the suture twice around the beaks of the needle holder in a clockwise direction.

→ 📷 **14.13** **a)** The suture has been inserted through the flap edges leaving about 3–4 cm out of the unattached tissue. **b)** The long portion of the suture has been wound twice around the needle holder in a clockwise direction. **c)** The needle holder is grasping the short portion to make the knot tight. **d)** The needle holder and the fingers of the doctor apply tension to the suture to make the knot tighter. **e)** The long portion of the suture has been wound once in a counter-clockwise direction around the beaks of the needle holder, which is now grasping the short portion of the suture. **f)** The knot is made tighter with tension. **g)** The long portion of the suture has been wound once more in a clockwise direction around the beaks of the needle holder, which is now grasping the short portion of the suture. **h)** More tension will now make the knot a bit tighter.

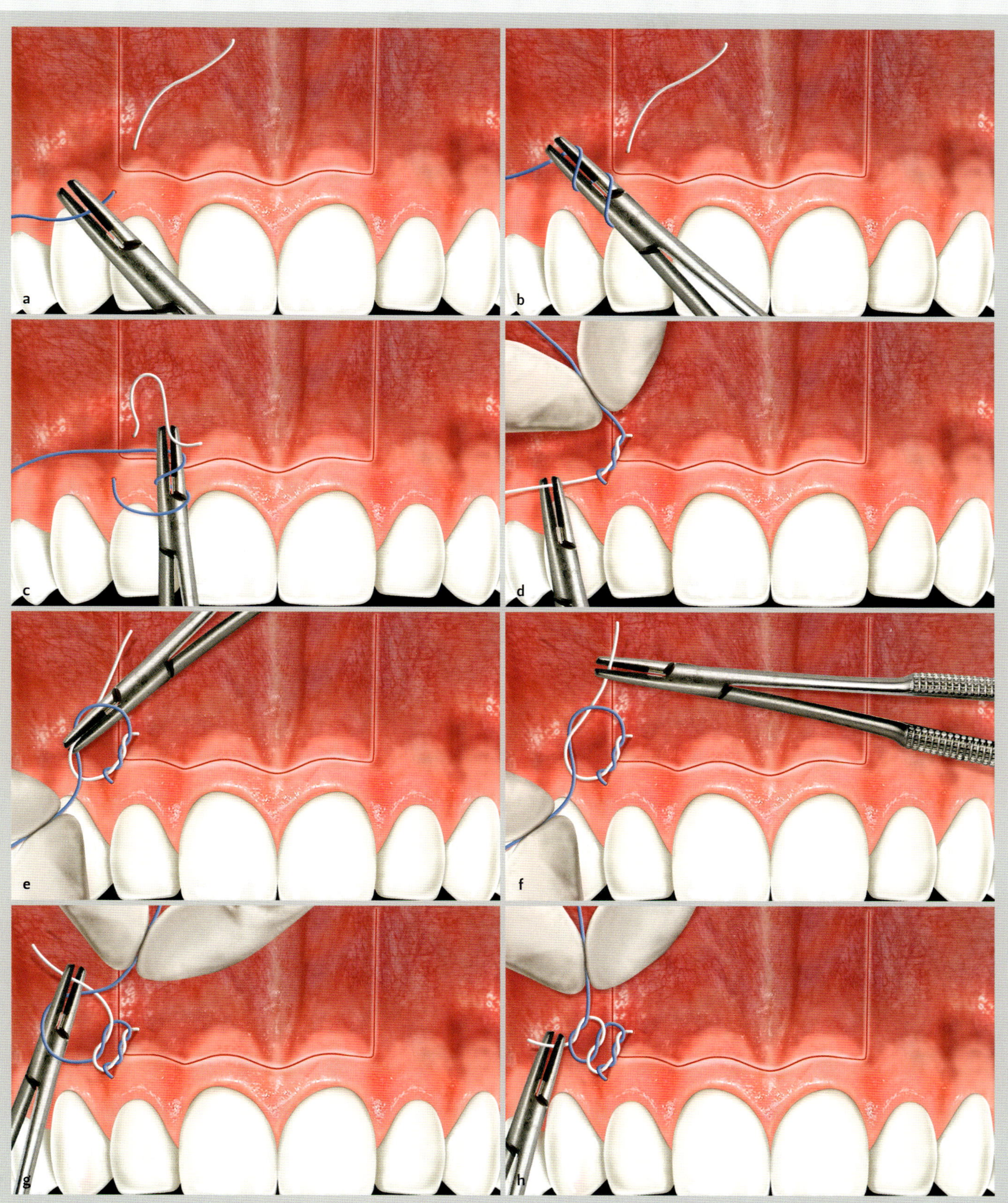
a
b
c
d
e
f
g
h

Postoperative Instructions

After suturing the patient can leave the office, having the ice packs already applied to the face over the involved area and therefore ice packs should be available in the office (14.15). Pressure to the surgical area with the ice pack is probably more important than the application of cold. The latter may give a reduction in blood flow and has an analgesic function.[3]

The patient should be informed that postoperatively he/she will experience very little or quite often no pain. It is unusual for a patient to experience pain that cannot be managed by mild to moderate analgesics.[17]

The second or third day after surgery he/she will also experience some little swelling. If patients already had this kind of surgery years before, performed with old protocols, they should know that they must forget their previous experience (14.16) because now their discomfort will be absolutely minimum and of short duration.

The postoperative recommendations are the following:

- continue to apply ice packs for a minimum of 15 minutes per hour for the first 5/6 hours.
- observe a soft and not too warm diet for the same day
- brush their teeth being very gentle in the operated area in order not to dislodge the flap, only on the occlusal or incisal surfaces of the teeth and rinse with chlorhexidine 0.2% twice a day for the next two or three days
- assume the prescribed medications as indicated
- come back for the suture removal after one or two days.

Usually, there is no need to prescribe antibiotics unless it is indicated by the medical history of the patient. In such a case, routine antibiotics are commonly used.

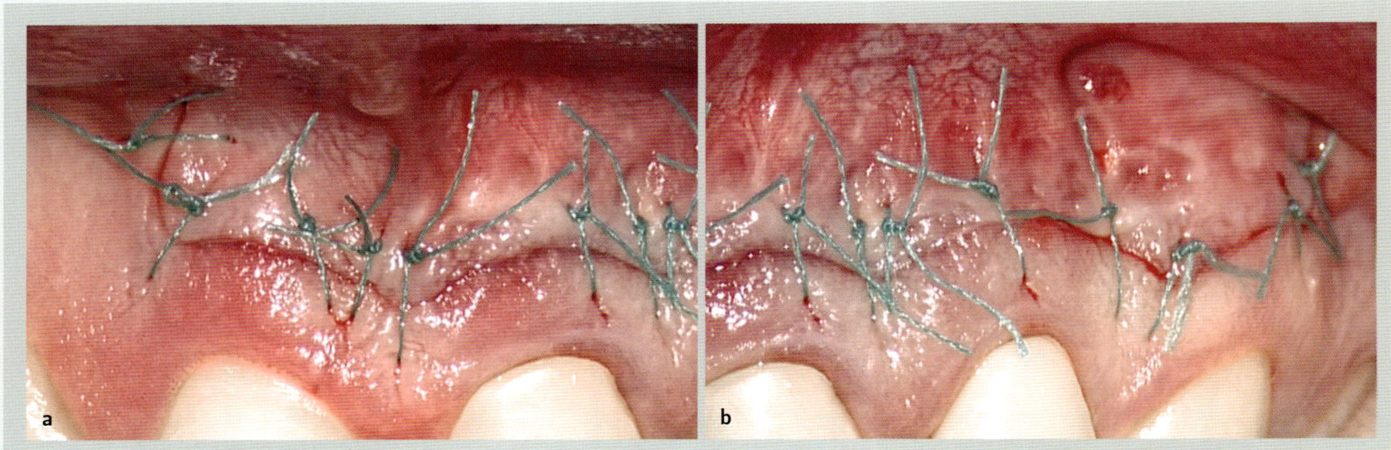

14.14 The suture is continued until there are no more gaps between the flap and the attached gingiva and an adequate re-approximation is achieved. **a)** Right quadrant. **b)** Left quadrant.

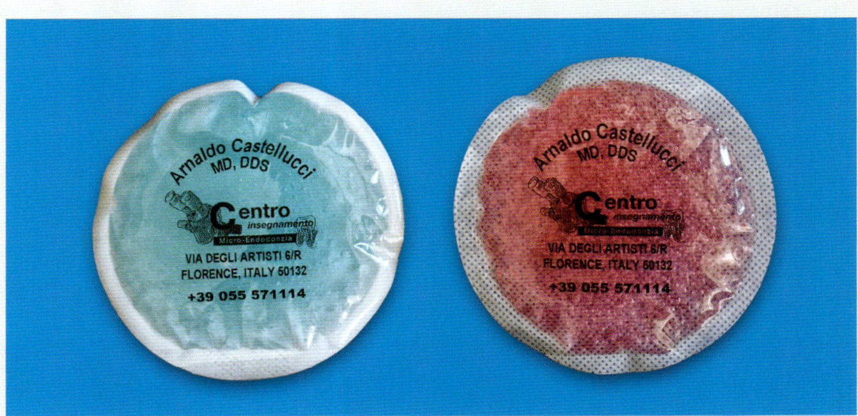

14.15 Ice packs made by Accurate Manufacturing (Swansea, SC, USA) can be customized with the logo of the doctor's office.

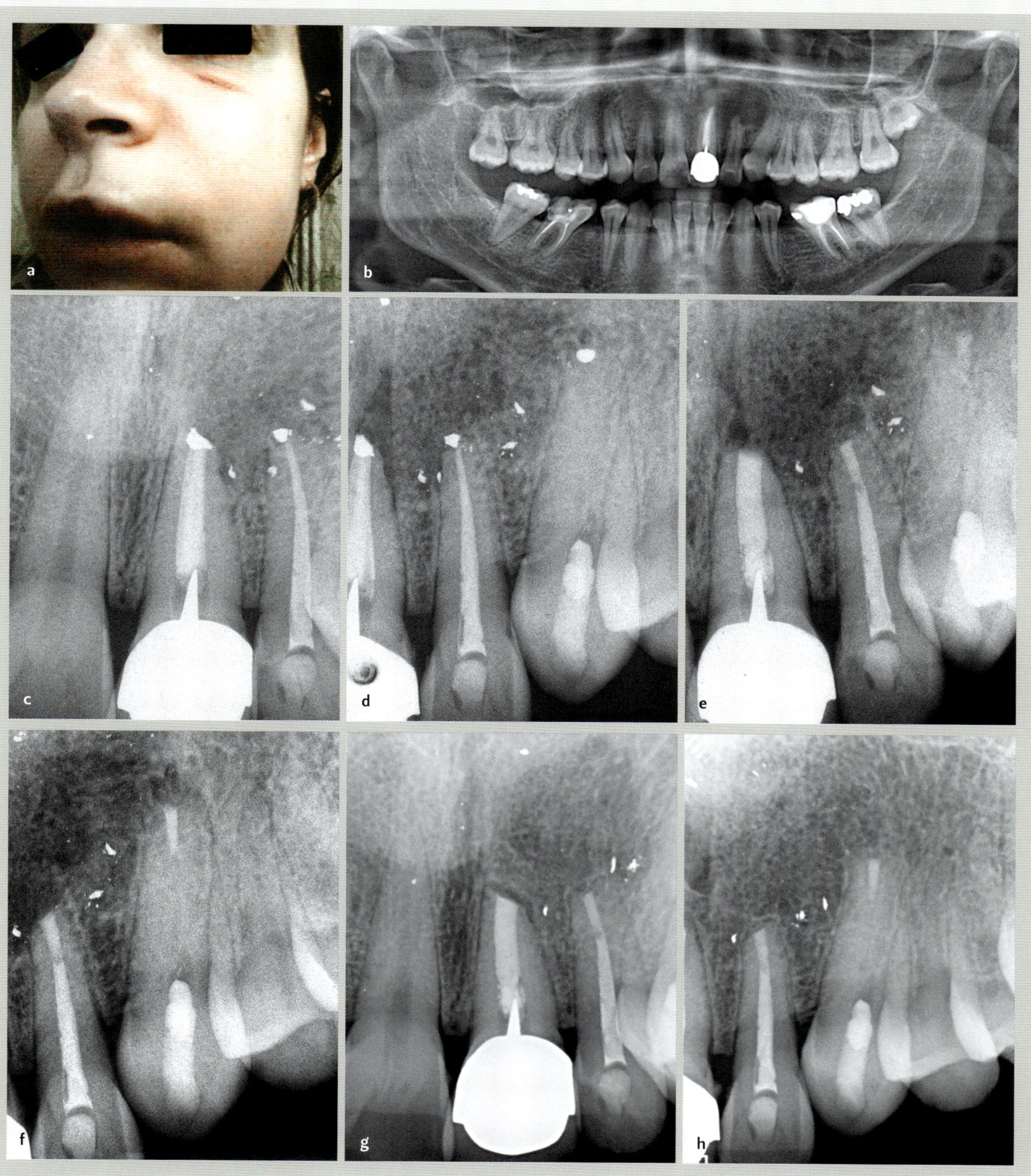

14.16 **a)** The young female patient had surgery in the upper left central and lateral incisors and cuspid, made by an oral surgeon who used the old protocol, without magnification, traumatizing the soft tissues during the surgical procedure, using burs and amalgam. **b)** Preoperative radiograph. The upper cuspid was vital and had nothing to do with the lesion. **c, d)** Postoperative radiographs after the surgical procedure in general anesthesia. One month later the sinus tract has not healed, and the diagnosis and treatment plan made by the oral surgeon was "vertical root fracture of three teeth, extractions and implants". **e, f)** Postoperative radiographs after the microsurgical endodontics procedure. **g, h)** Five-year recall.

As an anti-inflammatory and postsurgical analgesia, a non steroidal anti-inflammatory is usually prescribed (ibuprofen 600 mg) twice a day until the discomfort disappears, usually for the first two or three days. The patient should be warned not to take aspirin for pain prior to surgery or after.

The patient is then scheduled 15 days after surgery for a follow-up visit, to check the healing and now one can expect to find that the incision is almost not visible anymore.

Suture Removal

Just as the suturing was done under the operating microscope, so should the suture removal also be done under low range magnification. Especially if the suture used was 6-0 or 7-0, then the use of magnification is highly suggested.

Ideally, the suture must keep the soft tissue in place during the time of healing and should not encourage colonization of bacteria.

According to Gutmann and Harrison,[3] the key to preventing sutures from having a negative effect on wound healing following surgery is their early removal. The primary purpose for placing sutures following surgical endodontics is to approximate the edges of the incisional wound and provide stabilization until the epithelium and the myofibroblast-fibronectin network provides a sufficient barrier to dislodgment of the flapped tissues. This usually occurs within 48 hours following surgery.[18]

If repositioning has been accurate as it should be, healing occurs by primary intention in 24-48 hours and this is the reason why suture removal is indicated after 24-48 hours.[13,19] In earlier days, the suturing process was solely regarded as bringing the wound edges together and keeping them in this position until the body has healed the defect. It was customary to leave the sutures in place

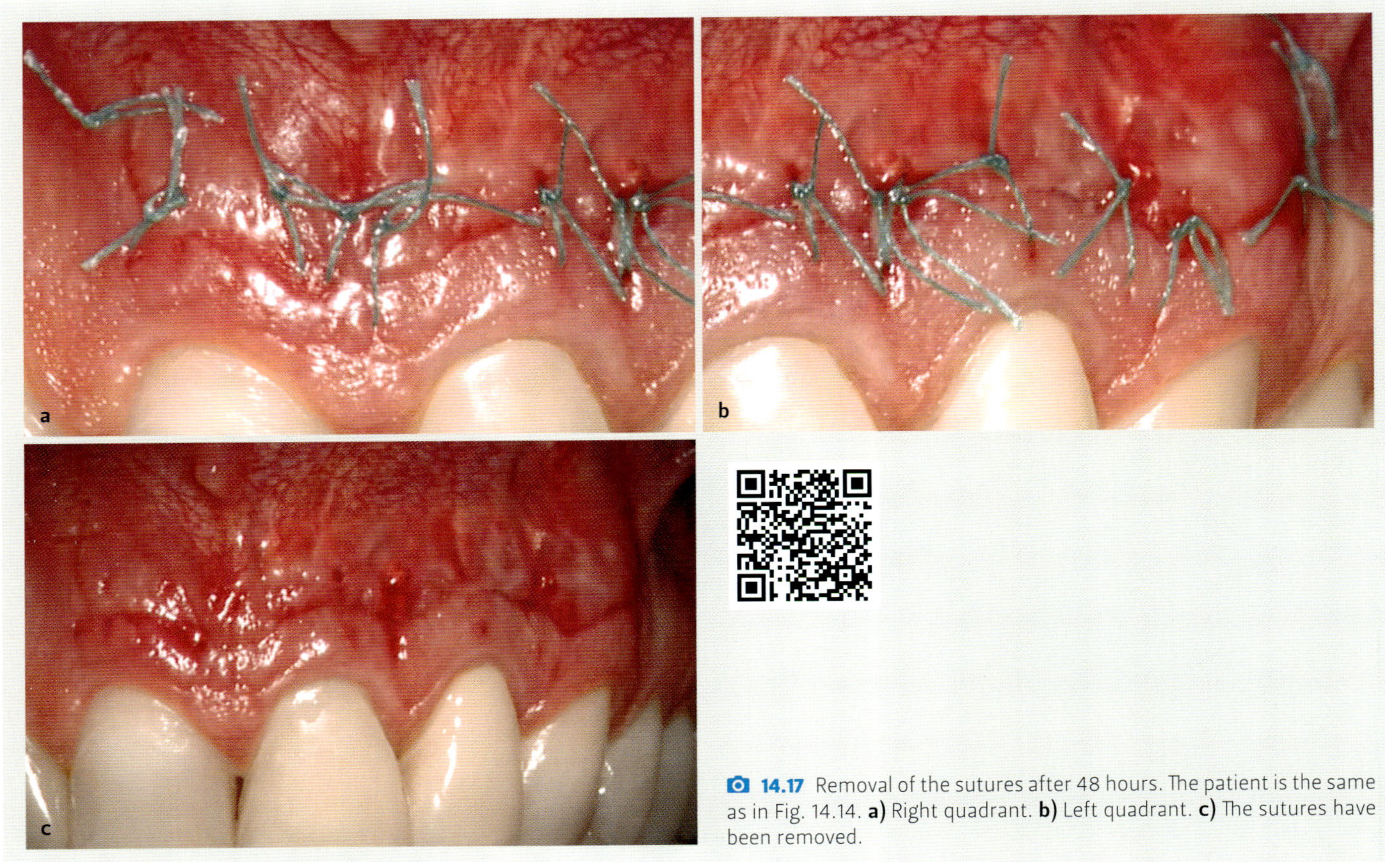

14.17 Removal of the sutures after 48 hours. The patient is the same as in Fig. 14.14. **a)** Right quadrant. **b)** Left quadrant. **c)** The sutures have been removed.

for 7 to 10 days and the clinical findings seemed to confirm the protocol.[20] When left in place for such a long period of time, the suture has no function and is simply an irritant: soon it will be completely covered by bacteria and will cause inflammation and delayed healing by secondary intention. This phenomenon is most predominant with multifilament materials which have a wicking action, and this is the reason why some materials like silk are no longer recommended today.[13]

While the periodontists are dealing with diseased tissue, and quite often reposition the flap laterally, apically, coronally so that healing comes by secondary intention, our flaps are passively elevated and passively repositioned exactly in their original place, so that healing will progress by primary intention. This is true especially if the tissue has not been traumatized during the surgical procedure and everything has been performed gently under the microscope.

According to Ruben et al.[21], the epithelial creep occurs at a rate of about 1 mm per side per 24 hours. The formation of the epithelial seal in humans takes about 28 hours to form. The subsequent epithelial barrier is evident after 36 to 42 hours.[22]

That means that if the reapproximation performed under the microscope has been precise, the gap left by the incision is completely closed after 24 hours and the

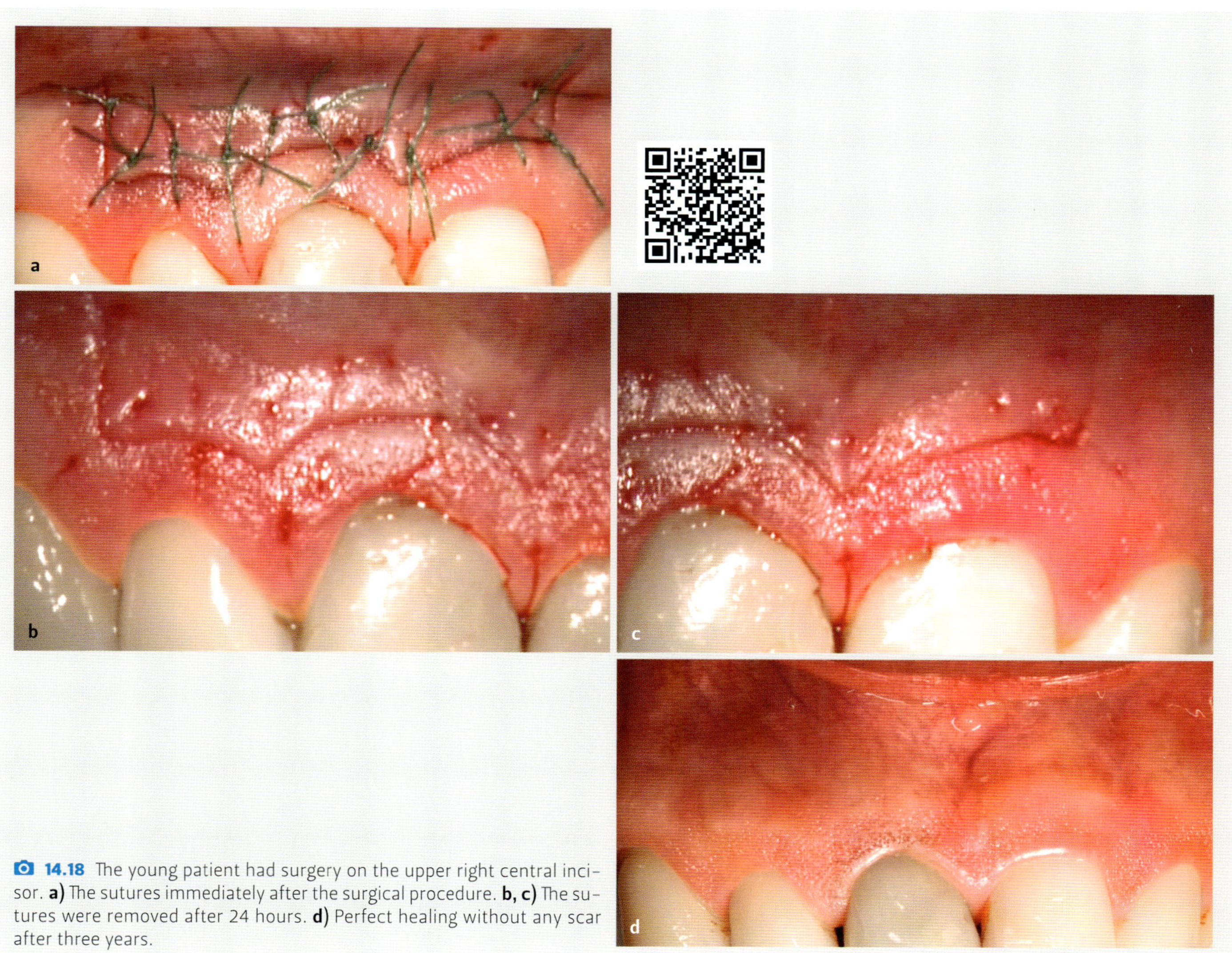

14.18 The young patient had surgery on the upper right central incisor. **a)** The sutures immediately after the surgical procedure. **b, c)** The sutures were removed after 24 hours. **d)** Perfect healing without any scar after three years.

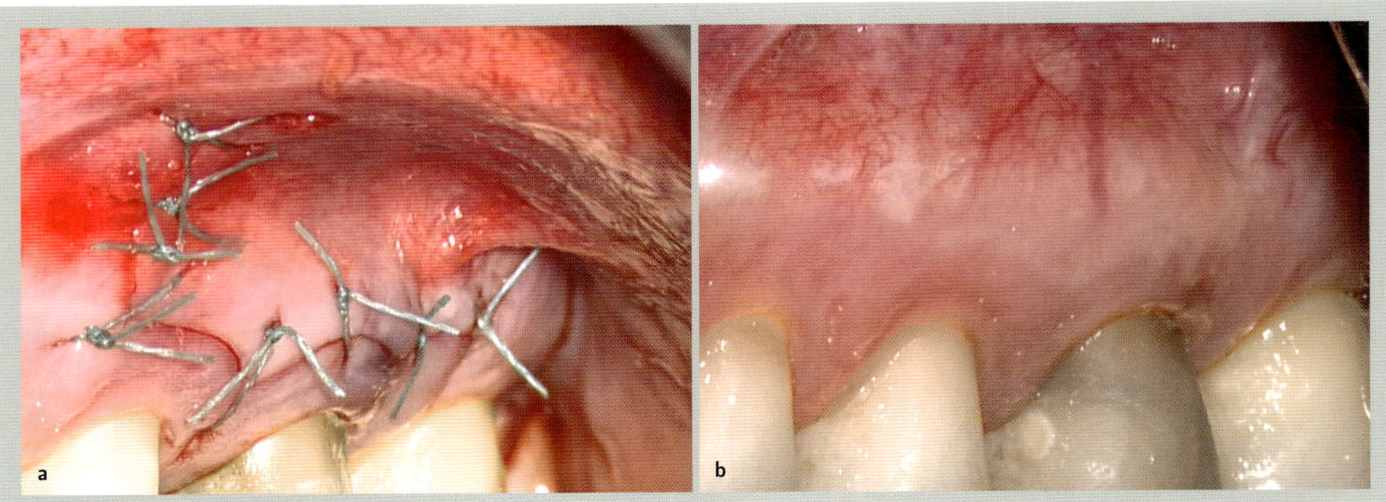

14.19 **a)** The female patient had surgery on the upper left first molar and the sutures have just been placed. **b)** The sutures were removed after 24 hours and the three-year recall shows the absence of any scar.

suture has completed its task (14.17, 14.18). In other words, there is no need to keep the suture any longer. Now it is just a foreign body that can only attract bacterial plaque, cause inflammation, delay healing and later will be responsible for a scar. On the other hand, once the procedure has been performed under the microscope with a nice scalloped incision, passive flap elevation and retraction, passive and precise repositioning, careful suturing with a 6-0 filament, then the suture can be removed after 24/48 hours, resulting in very little or no scarring at all (14.19). Of course, if the patient for some reason cannot come for the removal of the sutures before of two or three days, there is no problem (3.32) but for sure the sutures should not remain in place for more than one week and this should be avoided.[3,23]

Before the removal, the sutures and surrounding mucosa should be cleaned with a moist gauze containing a mild disinfectant. This helps to destroy bacteria and remove plaque and debris that have accumulated on the sutures, thus reducing the inoculation of bacteria into the underlying tissues as the suture is pulled through.[18] The suggested scissors are the safety-ended suture scissors (Laschal Surgical) having blunt blades (14.20). While the dental assistant is gently retracting the lips or the cheek, the operator holds in his/her left hand the Castroviejo needle older to grasp the apical tag of the suture. Holding the safety-ended scissors with the right hand he/she cuts the most coronal loop of the suture and then pulls it out. This way the portion of the filament that was exposed to the oral cavity will not be pulled through the flap and will not carry bacteria inside the tissue (14.21).

Healing Mechanism of Surgical Wounds

The principle of healing after microsurgical endodontics is almost the same as nonsurgical root canal therapy. The main difference is that healing after surgery requires a blood clot formation.

Surgical wounding causes disruption of the microvasculature supplying the mucoperiosteal tissues and

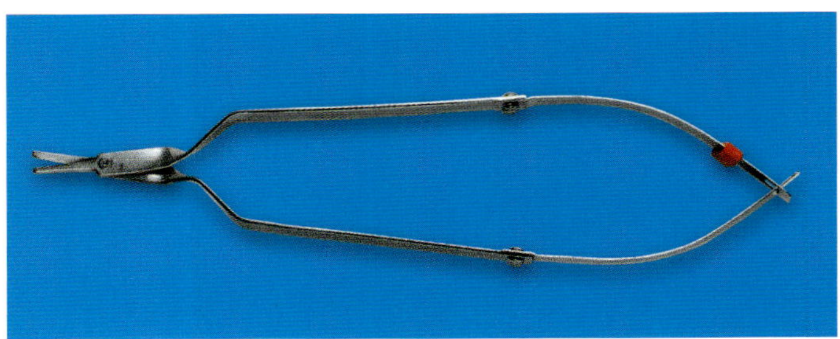

14.20 Scissors made by Laschal Surgical (Kisco, NY, USA) have blunt blades and are very safe and easy to use.

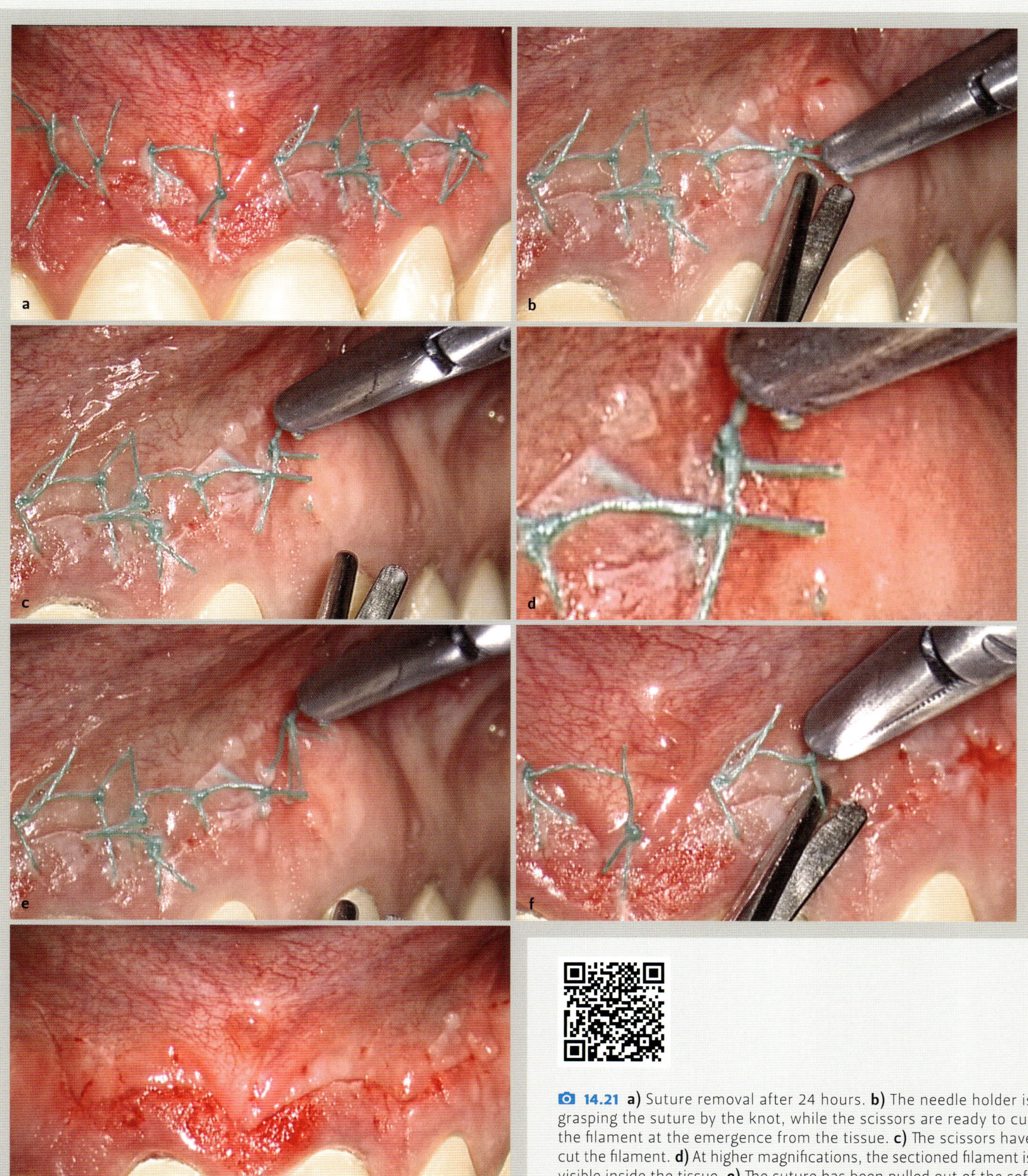

14.21 **a)** Suture removal after 24 hours. **b)** The needle holder is grasping the suture by the knot, while the scissors are ready to cut the filament at the emergence from the tissue. **c)** The scissors have cut the filament. **d)** At higher magnifications, the sectioned filament is visible inside the tissue. **e)** The suture has been pulled out of the soft tissue without carrying bacteria through the flap. **f)** Another suture is going to be removed, following the same approach. **g)** The suture removal has been completed.

the first requirement is to effect hemostasis and arrest the flow of blood.[24] Vascular injury releases plasma fractions, like fibrinogen, and formed elements, like platelets, into the surrounding tissues. Extrinsic and intrinsic clotting mechanisms are triggered, each giving rise to a cascading sequence of events leading to clot formation.[25] The crucial step in both clotting mechanisms is the conversion of fibrinogen to fibrin so that a *fibrin clot* is formed.[5,26] The properly formed, thin fibrin clot is essential for rapid, primary intention healing and forms the initial seal between the oral environment and the wound edges of the injured mucoperiosteal tissues.[24] The importance of the thin fibrin clot in wound healing is made pointedly obvious when early hemostasis is not accomplished and blood continues to leak into the wound site. Healing is delayed by the formation of a coagulum, which occupies excessive space and is associated with inadequate reapproximation of wound edges, leading to second intention healing and scar formation.[16,21,26] A large coagulum is clinically observable as a mucoid mass between gaping wound edges. If it forms between the flap and cortical bone, it is commonly referred to as a hematoma.[27] Coagulum formation greatly inhibits wound healing because it acts as a barrier, as opposed to a pathway for inflammatory and reparative cells and must first be resorbed before connective tissue healing can be initiated.[16,28]

Epithelial cells in the wound edges undergo specific changes within hours after surgical wounding.[24] The migrating cells move as a monolayer or sheet of cells, which may be several cells in thickness, toward the center of the surface of the wound until cellular contact is made with epithelial cells migrating from the opposing wound edge.[28,29] Contact of the opposing epithelial cells from the wound edges establishes the *epithelial seal* (or epithelial bridge).[30,31] Once the seat is established, the epithelial cells differentiate, undergo mitosis at an accelerated rate, and soon reform the definitive layers of stratified squamous epithelium through the process of maturation.[26,28,32] With stratification or layering, an effective *epithelial barrier* now exists and underlying connective tissue healing can progress without interference from the irritants of the oral cavity.[21,31] In addition to preventing the ingress of oral irritants, the epithelial barrier is of clinical significance for two other reasons.[24] The barrier inhibits the loss of tissue fluids, which are the source of nutrients for the connective tissue cells which will effect a repair. It thus greatly enhances healing by maintaining tissue hydration.[21] And, it is the epithelial barrier that provides a tremendous increase in wound strength (i.e., resistance to dislodgement or separation of the wound edges).[16,27]

The thin *epithelial seal* is established at 24 hours, a multilayered seal between 48 and 72 hours, and *epithelial barrier* formation occurs between 72 and 96 hours. Collagen fibers are formed in the wound site between 24 and 48 hours.

Knowing all this, it is obvious that sutures can be safely removed after 24/48 hours.

REFERENCES

1. **Lui JN, Khin MM, Krishnaswamy G, Chen NN.** *Prognostic factors relating to the outcome of endodontic microsurgery.* J Endod. 2014;40(8):1071-1076.
2. **Peters LB, Wesselink PR.** *Soft tissue management in endodontic surgery.* Dent Clin North Am. 1997;41:513-28.
3. **Gutmann JL, Harrison JW.** *Surgical Endodontics.* St Louis, Missouri: Ishiyaku EuroAmerica; 1994.
4. **Levine HL.** *Periodontal flap surgery with gingival fiber retention.* J Periodontol. 1972;43:91-98.
5. **Levine HL, Stahl SS.** *Repair following periodontal flap surgery with the retention of gingival fibers.* J Periodontol. 1972;43:99-103.
6. **Selvig KA, Torabinejad M.** *Wound healing after mucoperiosteal surgery in the cat.* J Endod. 1996;22:507-515.
7. **Hiatt WH, Stallard RE, Butler ED, et al.** *Repair following mucoperiosteal flap surgery with full gingival retention.* J Periodontol. 1968;39:11-16.
8. **Harrison J, Jurosky K.** *Wound healing in the tissues of the periodontium following periradicular surgery. 2. The dissectional wound.* J Endod. 1991;17:544-552.
9. **Lilly GE.** *Reaction of oral tissues to sutures materials.* Oral Surg. 1968;26:128-133.
10. **Lilly GE, Armstrong JH, Salema JE, et al.** *Reaction of oral tissues to sutures materials. Part II.* Oral Surg. 1968;26:592-599.
11. **Lilly GE, Armstrong JH, Cutcher JL.** *Reaction of oral tissues to sutures materials. Part III.* Oral Surg. 1969;28:432-438.
12. **Lilly GE, Cutcher JL, Jones TC, et al.** *Reaction of oral tissues to sutures materials. Part IV.* Oral Surg. 1972;33:152-157.
13. **Selvig KA, Biagiotti GR, Leknes KN, Wikesjo UM.** *Oral tissue reactions to suture materials.* Int J Periodontics Restorative Dent. 1998;18:474-487.
14. **Parikoh M, Asgary S, Eghbal MJ, Stowe S, Kakoel S.** *A scanning electron microscope study of plaque accumulation on silk and PVDF suture materials in oral mucosa.* Int Endod J. 2004;37:776-781.
15. **Lilly GE, Osbon DB, Hutchinson RA, Heflich RH.** *Clinical and bacteriologic aspects of polyglycolic acid sutures.* J Oral Surg. 1973;31:103-105.
16. **Hiatt WH, Stallard RE, Butler ED, Badget B.** *Repair following mucoperiosteal flap surgery with full gingival retention.* J Periodontol. 1968;39:11-16.
17. **Seymour RA, Meedhan JG, Blair GS.** *Postoperative pain after apicoectomy. A clinical investigation.* Int Endod J. 1986;19:242-7.
18. **Glickman GN, Hartwell GR.** *Endodontic Surgery.* In: Ingle JI, Bakland LK, Baumgartner JC, eds. *Endodontics. 6th ed.* PMPH-USA. 2008:1233-1294.
19. **Harrison J, Jurosky K.** *Wound healing in the tissues of the periodontium following periradicular surgery. I. The incisional wound.* J Endod. 1991;17:425-35.
20. **Velvart P, Peters CI.** *Soft tissue management in endodontic surgery.* J Endod. 2005;31(1):4-16.
21. **Ruben MP, Smuckler H, Schulman SM, Kon S, Bloom AA.** *Healing of periodontal surgical wounds.* In: Goldman HM, Cohen DW, eds. *Periodontal therapy.* 6th ed. St. Louis: The CV Mosby Co; 1980:640-754.
22. **Mittleman HR, Toto PD, Sicher H, et al.** *Healing in the human attached gingiva.* Periodontics. 1964;2:106-114.
23. **Carr GB.** *Surgical Endodontics.* In: Cohen S, Burns RC, eds. *Pathways of the pulp.* 6th ed. St. Louis: Mosby-Year book;1994:535-538.
24. **Harrison JW.** *Healing of surgical wounds in oral mucoperiosteal tissues.* J Endod. 1991;17(8):401-408.
25. **Boucek RJ.** *Factors affecting wound healing.* Otolaryngol Clin North Am. 1984;17:243-264.
26. **Krawczyk WS.** *Wound healing in the oral cavity.* In: Shaw JH, Sweeney EA, Cappuccino CC, et al. eds. *Textbook of oral biology.* Philadelphia: WB Saunders; 1978:937-54.
27. **Harrison JW, Gutmann AL (eds.).** *Surgical wound healing. Surgical endodontics.* Boston: Blackwell Scientific Publications; 1991:300-37.
28. **Melcher AH.** *Healing of wounds in the periodontium.* In: Melcher AH, Bowen WH, eds. *Biology of the periodontium.* London: Academic Press; 1969:499-529.
29. **Ordman LN, Gillman T.** *Studies of the healing of cutaneous wounds. Part II. The healing of epidermal, appendageal, and dermal injuries inflicted by suture material in the skin of pigs.* Arch Surg. 1966;93:883-910.
30. **Ordman LN, Gillman T.** *Studies in the healing of cutaneous wounds. Part III. A critical comparison in the pig of the healing of surgical incisions closed with sutures or adhesive tape based on tensile strength and clinical and histologic criteria.* Arch Surg. 1966;93:911-928.
31. **Ordman LN, Gillman T.** *Studies in the healing of cutaneous wounds. Part I. The healing of incisions through the skin of pigs.* Arch Surg. 1966;93:857-882.
32. **Sciubba J J, Waterhouse JP, Meyer J.** *A fine structural comparison of the healing of incisional wounds of mucosa and skin.* J Oral Pathol. 1978;7:214-227.

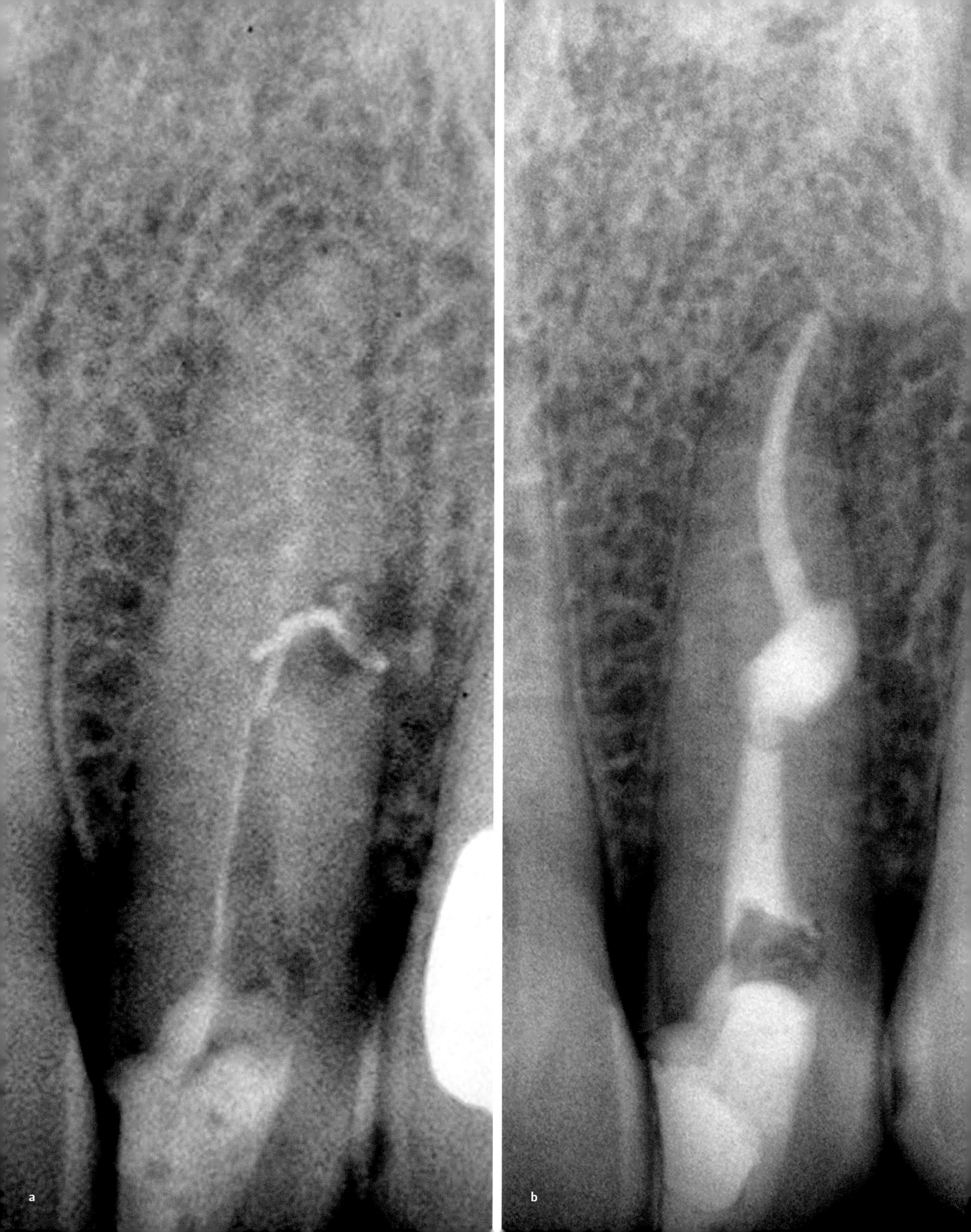
a
b

Prognosis of Microsurgical Endodontics

Arnaldo Castellucci, MD, DDS,
Massimo Gagliani, MD, DDS

Microsurgical endodontics has radically changed the prognosis of surgical root canal treatments in the last few decades; several instruments and techniques have been developed to enhance the operator's possibilities of treating resected root apices properly.

Diagnostic devices such as the CBCT modified the preoperative investigations,[1,2] and magnifications[3,4] while ultrasonic retrotips[5] have simplified clinical procedures and biocompatible retrofilling materials[6] have improved the healing rate in periapical surgery.[7]

All of these variables should be taken into account when a periapical radiolucency is examined by expert endodontists; the decision-making process is quite complicated and going straight to the surgical approach rather than to the orthograde one is still concerning.[8-10]

← 2.12 a) Preoperative radiograph of the upper left lateral incisor. b) Seventeen-year follow-up.

There is no clear consensus on this. Furthermore, the right decision is often the final solution after several attempts have been made, most of them time-consuming for both the patient and the dentist.[11,12]

There is still an area, of the diagnostic process, related to root apical microfractures that can, sometimes, lead to the decision for periapical surgery even if the right choice would be extraction.[13-15] In these cases, a prognosis of apicoectomy is worsened by the inclusion of the teeth that have been misdiagnosed for apical surgery.

Overview of Longitudinal Studies in Microsurgical Endodontics

As reported above, the changes in operative conditions have been developed over the last thirty years;[7] outcomes are strongly related to the number of variables involved in the studies examined and should be considered during everyday practice.

The absence of either the instruments or the devices might lead to a poorer outcome.[16]

Among all the variables, magnification, ultrasonic retrotips and obturating materials might play a significant role in the outcome,[7,17,18] the preoperative conditions being similar. On the other hand, the size of periapical lesion,[19] presence or absence of a sinus tract as well as periodontal status[20] could be clinical variables to consider in the decision-making process and may lead to a successful outcome in microsurgical endodontics.

Although dated, longitudinal clinical comparisons of nonsurgical retreatment and surgical endodontics never succeeded in demonstrating a significant difference in the outcomes for both procedures.[21–23] Riis et al.[24] suggested a faster healing process in surgical endodontics but no conclusive answers were achieved in the study.

Recently, microsurgical endodontics – as also reported in Chapter 1 and 2 of this book – might guarantee a successful outcome in a high percentage of case: more than 90% in a period of 3 to 5 years.[25]

In a recent systematic review on apicoectomy,[26] i.e. root end resection and retrofill using biocompatible materials such as Mineral Trioxide Aggregate (MTA), the Authors reported satisfactory results but not superior to cases where zinc-oxide reinforced cements (e.g. Super-EBA, Bosworth, USA, or IRM, Dentsply-Sirona, USA) were used.

The surgical solution is also suitable in secondary interventions: Gagliani, Gorni et al.[27] reported a success rate in re-intervention slightly inferior to the one obtained in primary endodontic surgery, confirming the previous review of Peterson and Gutmann.[28]

Long-term Clinical and Radiographic Evaluations

Recall Time

Patients treated for root apical resection and retrograde sealing should be scheduled for recall evaluation every year for a total of three/four years at the minimum.

Clinical and Radiological Recall Evaluations

Routine clinical and radiographic examination procedures should be used to evaluate any evidence of signs and/or symptoms, such as the following: loss of function, tenderness to percussion or palpation, subjective discomfort, mobility, sinus tract formation, infection or swelling, and periodontal pocket formation.[29] Patients should demonstrate the absence of any clinical signs/symptoms and radiographically the previous radiolucency (if present preoperatively) must be completely healed, with the formation of healthy bone and periodontal ligament (📷 15.1).

When evaluating the radiographic healing, particular attention should be paid to evaluate the presence of scar tissue. Everett[30] and Penick[31] described the presence of scar tissue in cases that were perfectly healed after periapical surgery as well as after conservative endodontic therapy. In both cases, particularly frequent after treating large lesions, the periapical repair happens due to dense fibrous connective tissue formation. This tissue is radiotransparent and could be misinterpreted as a failure. Of course, the radiolucency must be separated from the root apex, which should be surrounded by healthy bone (📷 15.2). If the radiolucency, on the other hand, is in contact with the treated tooth apex, it must be considered as a failure and not just a scar.

Recently the use of Cone Beam Computed Tomography (CBCT) changed the perspective of the evaluation processes during healing time. Torabinejad et al.[32] proposed a new scale for this procedure, but these strict criteria may influence one to make a misleading judgment, more oriented towards radiographic appearance rather than the tooth's clinical behavior.

Concluding Remarks

The introduction of microsurgery for surgical endodontics minimizes trauma and enhances the outcome of results. When using magnification and illumination resected roots reveal intricate anatomical details. In conjunction with ultrasonic root-end preparation and tight sealing of the root-end cavity with biocompatible materials, the requirements for mechanical and biological success are more adequately fulfilled.

15.1 a) Preoperative radiograph of the upper left central and lateral incisors. Periapical surgery was performed by an oral surgeon on both teeth a few months before. Only the central incisor has a root-end filling. No radiolucency is evident at the apex of both teeth but the patient has complained about pain. **b)** A scar shows that the patient has already had surgery on these teeth. **c)** After raising the flap, the root apexes appear surrounded by some bone graft material. **d)** The apex of the central incisor has been resected. **e)** The root-end preparation of the central incisor. **f, g)** The root apex of the lateral incisor had not even been resected by the previous operator. **h)** Root-end filling with White MTA of the central incisor. **i)** Root-end filling with White MTA of the lateral incisor. **j)** The ultrasonic tip Start-X® #3 (Maillefer) is used to remove all the previous bone graft material, that is still filling the bony crypt; it was simulating a perfect healing of the endodontic lesion and is responsible for the absence of any radiolucency visible at the apex of both teeth. **k)** Postoperative radiograph. **l)** Three-year recall.

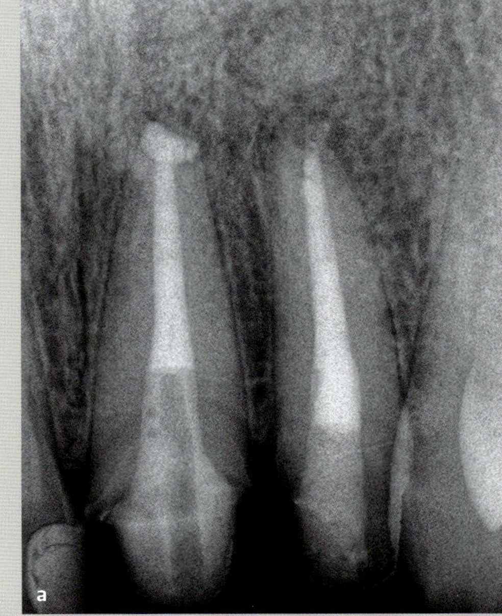

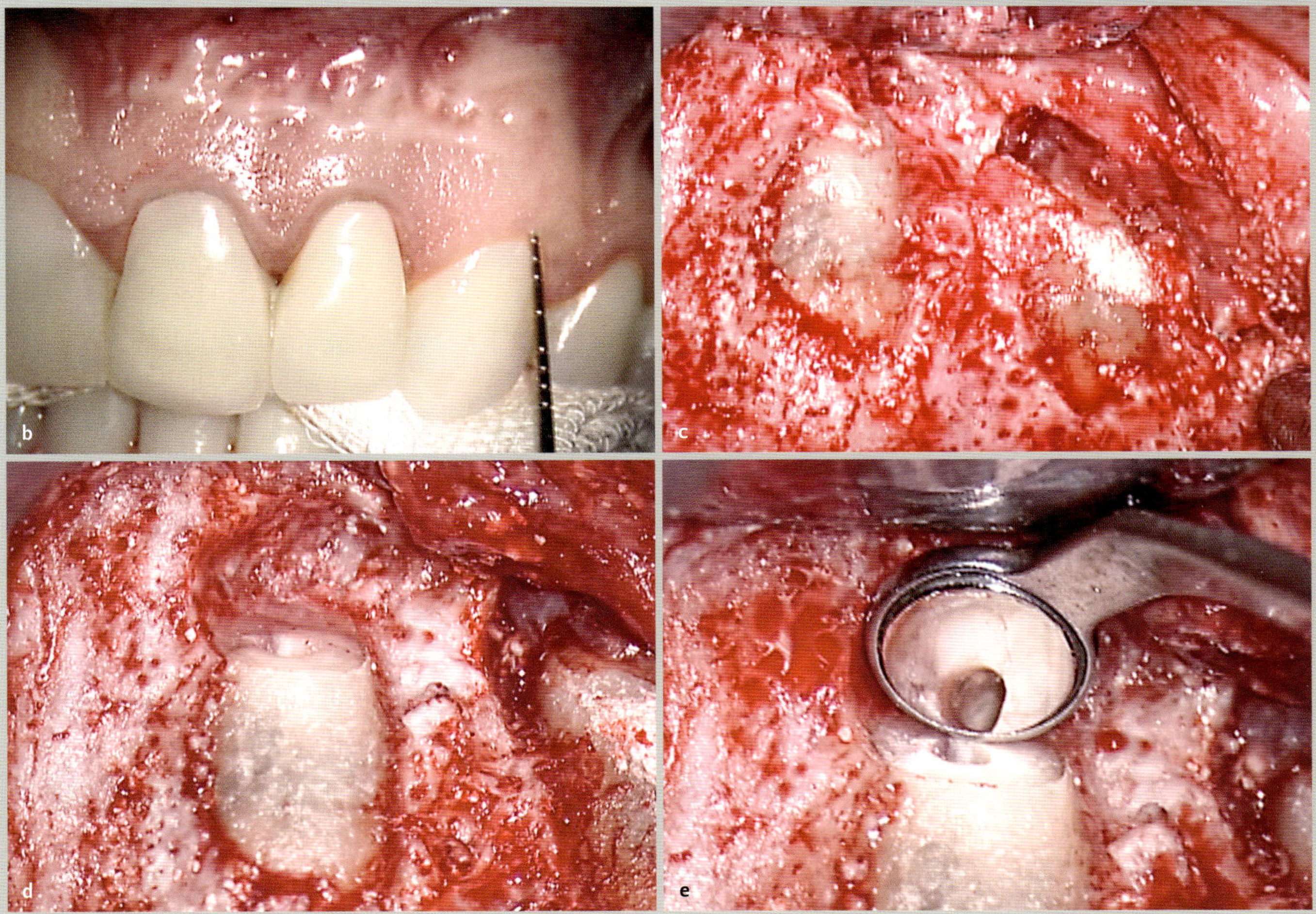

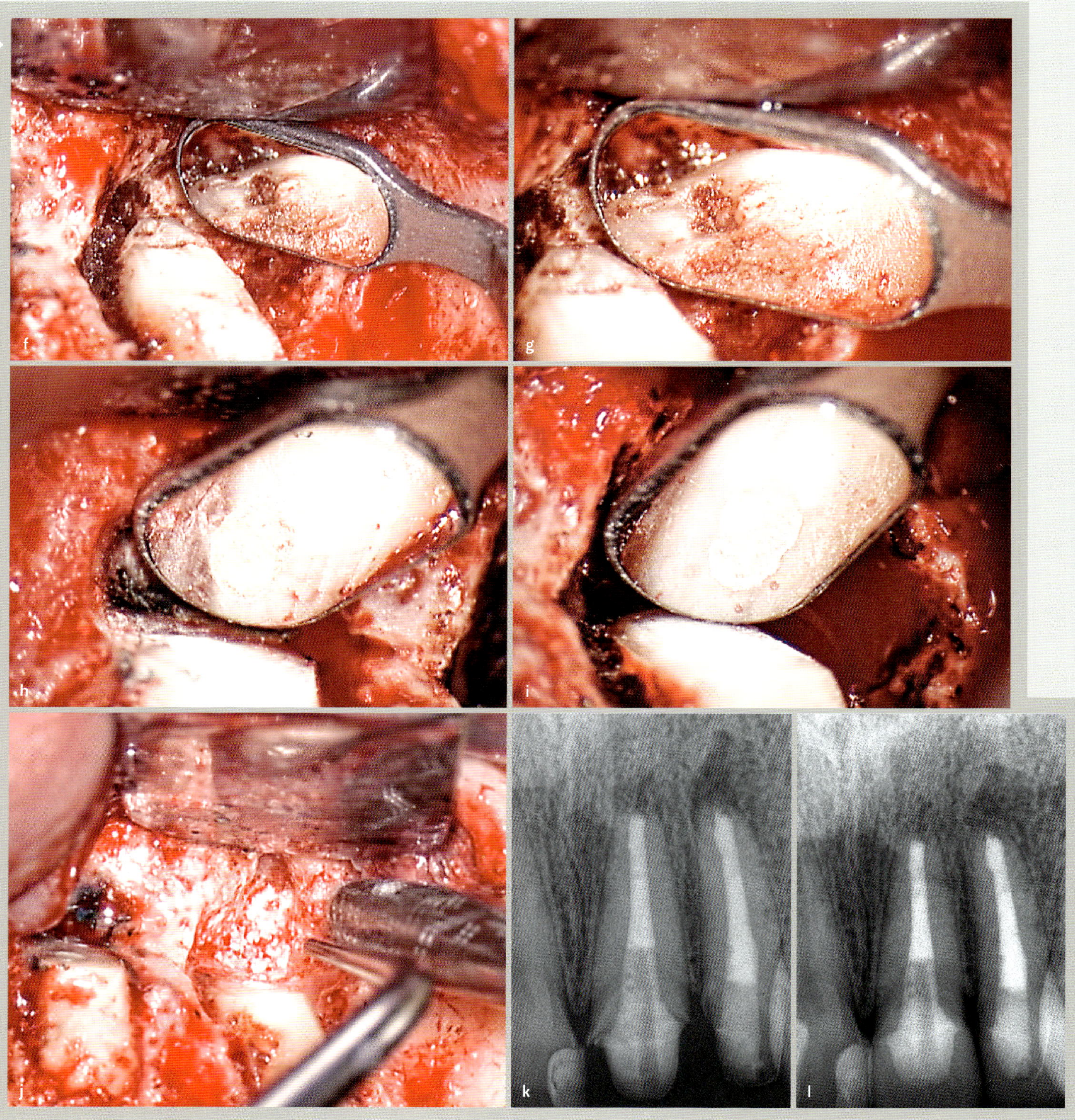
f
g
h
i
j
k
l

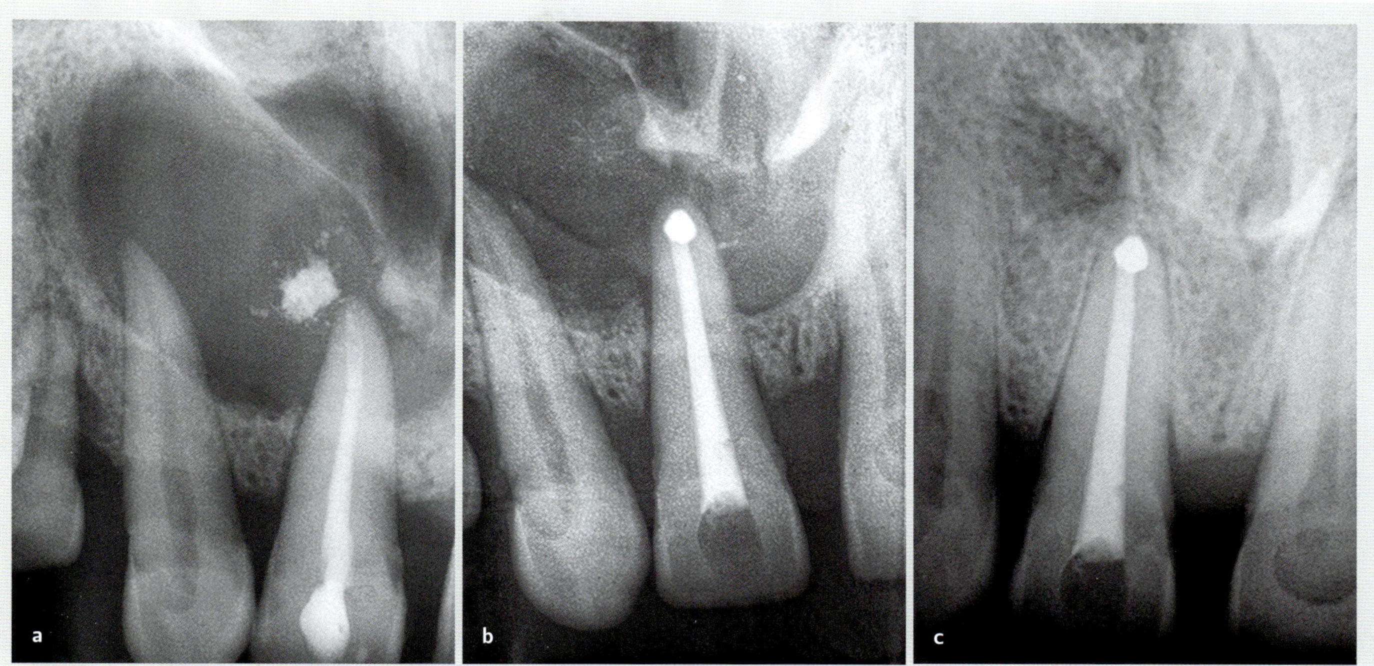

15.2 **a)** Preoperative radiograph of the upper right lateral incisor. The large lesion is involving the adjacent central incisor on one side and the cuspid on the other side, being both vital. **b)** Postoperative radiograph. **c)** Four-year recall. A radiolucency is evident apical to the lateral incisor, between the lateral and the cuspid, not in contact with any apex. The apex of the lateral incisor is surrounded by healthy bone; therefore, the radiolucency can be attributed to the presence of scar tissue, as a result of the healing of the previous large lesion.

Microsurgery alone will not accelerate epithelial healing rates, but through perfect tissue adaptation of wound edges, it can create smaller distances for epithelial migration during the healing process. More rapid soft tissue healing is a result of reduced tissue trauma and enhanced wound closure after microsurgical procedures.

To achieve these goals, several measures are necessary, including accurate preoperative treatment planning for the condition and quality of the tissue to be manipulated. Minimal trauma should be inflicted during incision and raising of the flap. Both the flap and unreflected tissue that remain on the tooth surface should be kept moist during the entire procedure, especially in situations where excellent hemostasis can be achieved. Finally, delicate handling of the soft tissues during suturing is mandatory, with wound edges being reapproximated without tension and held in place with nonabsorbable atraumatic sutures.[33]

Microsurgical endodontics is effective in saving natural teeth and the long-term success rates have currently reached a peak and should be brought into comparison with orthograde retreatment and implantology.[34]

As mentioned above, the success rate in microsurgical endodontics was reported to be significantly greater than the one achieved by traditional root-end surgery.

It's questionable whether microsurgical techniques are always needed in endodontic retrograde treatment; recent meta-analysis concluded that the use of traditional root-end surgery techniques should no longer be considered a state of the art.[35,36]

The influence of the equipment used during microsurgical endodontics is well known and universally accepted as a legitimate standard of care.

REFERENCES

1. Rosen E, Taschieri S, Del Fabbro M, Beitlitum I, Tsesis I. *The diagnostic efficacy of cone-beam computed tomography in endodontics: a systematic review and analysis by a hierarchical model of efficacy.* J Endod. 2015;41(7):1008-1014.
2. Kruse C, Spin-Neto R, Wenzel A, Vaeth M, Kirkevang LL. *Impact of cone beam computed tomography on periapical assessment and treatment planning five to eleven years after surgical endodontic retreatment.* Int Endod J. 2018;51(7):729-737.
3. Taschieri S, Del Fabbro M, Testori T, Weinstein R. *Microscope versus endoscope in root-end management: a randomized controlled study.* Int J Oral Maxillofacial Surg. 2008;37(11):1022-1026.
4. Del Fabbro M, Taschieri S. *Endodontic therapy using magnification devices: a systematic review.* J Dent. 2010;38(4):269-275.
5. Tsesis I, Rosen E, Schwartz-Arad D, Fuss Z. *Retrospective evaluation of surgical endodontic treatment: traditional versus modern technique.* J Endod. 2006;32(5):412-416.
6. Kohli MR, Berenji H, Setzer FC, Lee SM, Karabucak B. *Outcome of Endodontic Surgery: A Meta-analysis of the Literature-Part 3: Comparison of Endodontic Microsurgical Techniques with 2 Different Root-end Filling Materials.* J Endod. 2018;44(6):923-931.
7. Tsesis I, Rosen E, Taschieri S, Telishevsky Strauss Y, Ceresoli V, Del Fabbro M. *Outcomes of surgical endodontic treatment performed by a modern technique: an updated meta-analysis of the literature.* J Endod. 2013;39(3):332-339.
8. Alani A, Bishop K, Djemal S. *The influence of specialty training, experience, discussion and reflection on decision making in modern restorative treatment planning.* Br Dent J. 2011;210(4):e4.
9. Brignardello-Petersen R. *Evidence about success of endodontic treatment or retreatment versus tooth extraction and implant placement is not sufficient for making clinical decisions.* J Amer Dent Assoc. 2017;148(8):e110.
10. Burns LE, Visbal LD, Kohli MR, Karabucak B, Setzer FC. *Long-term evaluation of treatment planning decisions for nonhealing endodontic cases by different groups of practitioners.* J Endod. 2018;44(2):226-232.
11. Derhalli M, Mounce RE. *Clinical decision making regarding endodontics versus implants.* Comp Contin Educ Dent. 2011;32(4):24-26, 28-30, 32-25; quiz 36.
12. Stockhausen R, Aseltine R, Jr, Matthews JG, Kaufman B. *The perceived prognosis of endodontic treatment and implant therapy among dental practitioners.* Oral Surg Oral Med Oral Pathol Oral Radiol Endod. 2011;111(2):e42-47.
13. Song M, Jung IY, Lee SJ, Lee CY, Kim E. *Prognostic factors for clinical outcomes in endodontic microsurgery: a retrospective study.* J Endod. 2011;37(7):927-933.
14. Tawil PZ, Saraiya VM, Galicia JC, Duggan DJ. *Periapical microsurgery: the effect of root dentinal defects on short- and long-term outcome.* J Endod. 2015;41(1):22-27.
15. Maddalone M, Gagliani M, Citterio CL, Karanxha L, Pellegatta A, Del Fabbro M. *Prevalence of vertical root fractures in teeth planned for apical surgery. A retrospective cohort study.* Int Endod J.2018;51(9):969-974.
16. [No authors listed] *Evidence-based review of clinical studies on surgery.* J Endod. 2009;35(8):1094-1110.
17. Song M, Shin SJ, Kim E. *Outcomes of endodontic micro-resurgery: a prospective clinical study.* J Endod. 2011;37(3):316-320.
18. von Arx T. *Apical surgery: A review of current techniques and outcome.* Saudi Dent J. 2011;23(1):9-15.
19. Barone C, Dao TT, Basrani BB, Wang N, Friedman S. *Treatment outcome in endodontics: the Toronto study-phases 3, 4, and 5: apical surgery.* J Endod. 2010;36(1):28-35.
20. Kim D, Ku H, Nam T, Yoon TC, Lee CY, Kim E. *Influence of Size and Volume of Periapical Lesions on the Outcome of Endodontic Microsurgery: 3-Dimensional Analysis Using Cone-beam Computed Tomography.* J Endod. 2016;42(8):1196-1201.
21. Danin J, Stromberg T, Forsgren H, Linder LE, Ramskold LO. *Clinical management of nonhealing periradicular pathosis. Surgery versus endodontic retreatment.* Oral Surg Oral Med Oral Pathol Oral Radiol Endod. 1996;82(2):213-217.
22. Kvist T, Reit C. *Results of endodontic retreatment: a randomized clinical study comparing surgical and nonsurgical procedures.* J Endod. 1999;25(12):814-817.
23. Del Fabbro M, Taschieri S, Testori T, Francetti L, Weinstein RL. *Surgical versus non-surgical endodontic re-treatment for periradicular lesions.* Cochrane Database Syst Rev. 2007(3):CD005511.
24. Riis A, Taschieri S, Del Fabbro M, Kvist T. *Tooth Survival after Surgical or Nonsurgical Endodontic Retreatment: Long-term Follow-up of a Randomized Clinical Trial.* J Endod. 2018;44(10):1480-1486.
25. Torabinejad M, Corr R, Handysides R, Shabahang S. *Outcomes of nonsurgical retreatment and endodontic surgery: a systematic review.* J Endod. 2009;35(7):930-937.
26. Tang Y, Li X, Yin S. *Outcomes of MTA as root-end filling in endodontic surgery: a systematic review.* New Malden: Quintessence Publishing Co. Ltd.; 2010;41(7):557-566.
27. Gagliani MM, Gorni FG, Strohmenger L. *Periapical resurgery versus periapical surgery: a 5-year longitudinal comparison.* Int Endod J. 2005;38(5):320-327.
28. Peterson J, Gutmann JL. *The outcome of endodontic resurgery: a systematic review.* Int Endod J. 2001;34(3):169-175.

29. **Zuolo ML, Ferreira MO, Gutmann JL.** *Prognosis in periradicular surgery: a clinical prospective study.* Int Endod J. 2000;33:91-98.
30. **Everett FG.** *Apicoectomy followed by unusual radiographic finding.* Oral Surg. 1951;4:1531-1533.
31. **Penick EG.** *Periapical repair by dense fibrous connective tissue following conservative endodontic therapy.* Oral Surg. 1961;14:239-242.
32. **Torabinejad M, Rice DD, Maktabi O, Oyoyo U, Abramovitch K.** *Prevalence and Size of Periapical Radiolucencies Using Cone-beam Computed Tomography in Teeth without Apparent Intraoral Radiographic Lesions: A New Periapical Index with a Clinical Recommendation.* J Endod. 2018;44(3):389-394.
33. **Velvart P, Peters CI.** *Soft tissue management in endodontic surgery.* J Endod. 2005;31(1):4-16.
34. **Chercoles-Ruiz A, Sanchez-Torres A, Gay-Escoda C.** *Endodontics, Endodontic Retreatment, and Apical Surgery Versus Tooth Extraction and Implant Placement: A Systematic Review.* J Endod. 2017;43(5):679-686.
35. **Setzer FC, Shah SB, Kohli MR, Karabucak B, Kim S.** *Outcome of endodontic surgery: a meta-analysis of the literature-Part 1: Comparison of traditional root-end surgery and endodontic microsurgery.* J Endod. 2010;36(11):1757-65.
36. **Setzer FC, Kohli MR, Shah SB, Karabucak B, Kim S.** *Outcome of endodontic surgery: a meta-analysis of the literature-Part 2: Comparison of endodontic microsurgical techniques with and without the use of higher magnification.* J Endod. 2012;38(1):1-10.

Index

Page numbers in *italics* refer to figure and tables